Orthopedics: A Clinical Approach

Orthopedics: A Clinical Approach

Editor: Elvis Green

FOSTER ACADEMICS
www.fosteracademics.com

www.fosteracademics.com

Cataloging-in-Publication Data

Orthopedics : a clinical approach / edited by Elvis Green.
p. cm.
Includes bibliographical references and index.
ISBN 978-1-63242-756-4
1. Orthopedics. 2. Orthopedics--Diagnosis. 3. Orthopedics--Treatment. I. Green, Elvis.
RD731 .O78 2019
616.7--dc23

Foster Academics,
118-35 Queens Blvd., Suite 400,
Forest Hills, NY 11375, USA

ISBN 978-1-63242-756-4 (Hardback)

Printed and bound in China.

Contents

Preface

Every book is initially just a concept; it takes months of research and hard work to give it the final shape in which the readers receive it. In its early stages, this book also went through rigorous reviewing. The notable contributions made by experts from across the globe were first molded into patterned chapters and then arranged in a sensibly sequential manner to bring out the best results.

The branch of surgery which deals with the conditions associated with the musculoskeletal system is known as orthopedics. Doctors who have specialized in this field are called orthopedic surgeons. In order to treat disorders like musculoskeletal trauma, sports injuries, congenital disorders, spine disorders and infections related to the musculoskeletal system, orthopedic surgeons use both surgical as well as nonsurgical methods. Pediatric orthopedics, total joint reconstruction, spine surgery, orthopedic trauma, foot and ankle surgery, and musculoskeletal oncology are some of the sub-fields which fall under the scope of orthopedics. Two of the most common procedures performed by orthopedic surgeons are arthroscopy and arthroplasty. This book is a compilation of chapters that discuss the most vital concepts and emerging trends in the field of orthopedics. Different approaches, evaluations, methodologies and advanced studies on orthopedics have been included herein. This book, with its detailed analyses and data, will prove immensely beneficial to professionals and students involved in this area at various levels.

It has been my immense pleasure to be a part of this project and to contribute my years of learning in such a meaningful form. I would like to take this opportunity to thank all the people who have been associated with the completion of this book at any step.

Editor

1

Comparison of Atypical and Osteoporotic Femoral Shaft Fractures in the Elderly: A Multicenter Study

Takanori Miura,[1] Hiroaki Kijima,[2] Noriyuki Ishikawa,[3] Toshihito Ebina,[1] Takayuki Tani,[1] Shuichi Chida,[1] Tetsuya Suzuki,[3] Satoshi Yumto,[3] Hiroshi Tazawa,[3] Naohisa Miyakoshi,[2] and Yoichi Shimada[2]

[1]*Department of Orthopedic Surgery, Kakunodate General Hospital, 3-Iwase Kakunodatemachi, Semboku, Akita 014-0394, Japan*
[2]*Department of Orthopedic Surgery, Akita University Graduate School of Medicine, 1-1-1 Hondo, Akita 010-8543, Japan*
[3]*Department of Orthopedic Surgery, Akita Red Cross Hospital, Kamikitate Saruta, Aza-Naeshirosawa 222-1, Akita 010-1406, Japan*

Correspondence should be addressed to Takanori Miura; m08096tm@jichi.ac.jp

Academic Editor: Hiroshi Hashizume

Background. In atypical femoral fractures, owing to the high rates of complications and delayed healing that accompany the plate fixation, the most favorable treatment is intramedullary nailing. Although there is insufficient evidence, plate fixation is chosen due to anterolateral bowing of the femur. This study compared the bone healing time and rates of complications in atypical femoral shaft fractures and osteoporotic femoral shaft fractures. *Methods*. We searched the medical records of 3 institutions in Japan for patients with femoral shaft fractures who visited between 1 January 2010 and 31 December 2015. We identified 65 patients and excluded 37 among these due to high-energy injuries or being younger than 65 years. Among the remaining patients, we identified 17 and 11 women with atypical (AFF group) and osteoporotic femoral shaft fractures (OP group), respectively. *Results*. In surgical method, there were differences in intramedullary nailing (94.1% versus 27.2%) ($p < 0.01$). The mean bone healing time was 11.1 months versus 6.7 months in 2 groups ($p < 0.01$). Iatrogenic femoral fractures during intramedullary nail insertion were observed in both groups, and reoperation was only seen in atypical femoral fractures treated with a plate fixation, but there was no difference in the rate of complications (23.5% versus 9.1%). *Conclusions*. In the atypical femoral fracture group, intramedullary nailing was more chosen, but the bone healing time was delayed and plate fixation cases needed reoperation. There was no significant difference in the rate of complications between the 2 groups.

1. Introduction

Atypical femoral fracture (AFF) is a fracture that occurs at the femoral subtrochanteric or shaft region. The occurrence of this type of fracture is associated with the long-term use of bisphosphonates (BPs) and bowed femoral shaft stress fractures [1–4]. It is a common conception that atypical femoral shaft fractures heal poorly [1, 5], but there have been few reports comparing patients with AFF and the control group with respect to bone healing times [5]. Among the treatment options, intramedullary nail fixation is most favorable. But in some cases with a high degree of lateral femoral bowing, it is difficult to insert the intramedullary nail, and there are consequently high rates of intraoperative fractures and implant failure during the procedure in patients with AFF [6, 7]. However, the sample size available for the examination of AFF in a single institution is limited. The present multicenter study aimed to compare the bone healing time and rates of complications in patients with atypical femoral shaft fractures and those with osteoporotic femoral shaft fractures.

2. Materials and Methods

2.1. Inclusion Criteria. To identify patients with AFF of the femoral shaft and osteoporotic femoral shaft fractures, we reviewed digitized radiographs of all patients, from 3 institutions, who had sustained fractures of the femoral shaft and received acute treatment for them between 1 January 2010

Table 1: Patient characteristics and treatments.

Parameter	AFF ($n = 17$)	OP ($n = 11$)	p	Test
Male : Female	0 : 17	0 : 11	—	—
Age (years)	80.7 (77–88)	81.0 (65–96)	0.67	Mann–Whitney U test
Antiresorptive therapy (%)	88.2	18.2	<0.01	Fisher's exact test
Surgery (%)	100	81.8	0.40	Fisher's exact test
Intramedullary nail (%)	94.1	27.2	<0.01	Fisher's exact test
Fixation with plate (%)	5.9	36.3	0.06	Fisher's exact test
Replacement arthroplasty (%)	0	18.2	0.15	Fisher's exact test
Conservative treatment (%)	0	18.2	0.15	Fisher's exact test
Teriparatide treatment (%)	41.2	18.2	0.25	Fisher's exact test
Postoperative LIPUS treatment (%)	23.5	9.1	0.30	Fisher's exact test

and 31 December 2015. Patient medical and drug treatment histories were obtained from medical records. Patients with primary or secondary metabolic disorders of the skeleton apart from osteoporosis were excluded. Patients with AFF were identified by the radiographic pattern consisting of a transverse fracture line on the lateral side of the femoral shaft with focal thickening (callus reaction) around the fracture and no or minimal comminution, in accordance with the American Society for Bone and Mineral Research Task Force's major criteria, 2nd version [1]. Osteoporotic fractures were defined as spiral, oblique, or comminuted shaft fractures below the lesser trochanter and above the supracondylar flare, and this definition included periprosthetic fractures.

2.2. Study Patients. We identified 65 patients; however, we excluded 37 patients who had high-energy injuries or who were below 65 years of age. The remaining 28 patients were all above 65 years of age and sustained low-energy-mechanism injuries, such as a fall from standing height or lower. All patients with fractures were routinely asked by the admitting physician whether they were taking or had a history of taking BPs.

The mean follow-up time for patients with atypical fractures and osteoporotic femoral fractures was 17.26 months (range: 6–36 months) and 10.27 months (range: 3–28 months), respectively. No patients were lost to follow-up. No patients were recalled specifically for this study; all data were obtained from medical records or radiographs. Healing was judged by 2 observers using the following criteria: the ability to fully bear weight, lack of pain at the fracture site, and radiographic consolidation as observed on orthogonal plain radiographic views. All patients included in the current study had all clinical and radiographic data available for analysis. We determined differences in the continuous variables of interest (age and bone healing time) between the AFF (AFF group) and osteoporotic fractures group (OP group). The overall data were examined using descriptive statistics, with frequencies given for categorical variables and means and standard deviations for continuous variables. IBM SPSS Statistics Version V22.0 was used for all analyses.

3. Results

The demographic data are shown in Table 1. All patients were women; 17 patients had complete atypical femoral shaft fractures [average age: 80.7 years (range: 77–88 years)], and the remaining 11 had osteoporotic femoral shaft fractures [average age: 81.0 years (range: 65–96 years)]. There were no significant differences in age between the two groups (p = 0.67). The patients with AFF used BPs more often (15 patients, 88%) compared to those with osteoporotic femoral fractures (2 patients, 18%) ($p < 0.01$). For treatment, all patients with atypical fractures and 81.8% (9 of 11) with osteoporotic fractures underwent surgery ($p = 0.40$). In the group with AFF, intramedullary nail fixation was performed in 94.1% (16 of 17) and plate fixation in 5.9% (1 of 17). In the group with osteoporotic femoral fractures, intramedullary nail fixation was performed in 27.2% (3 of 11), plate fixation in 36.3% (4 of 11), replacement arthroplasty in 18.2% (2 of 11), and conservative treatment in 18.2% (2 of 11). Intramedullary nail fixation was used more frequently in the group with atypical femoral fractures (94.1% versus 27.2%; $p < 0.01$). Teriparatide was used in 41.2% (7 patients) with AFF and in 18.2% (2 patients) with osteoporotic femoral fractures ($p = 0.25$). Low-intensity pulsed ultrasound (LIPUS) therapy was performed postoperatively in 23.5% (4 patients) in the group with AFF and in 9.1% (1 patient) in the group with osteoporotic femoral fractures ($p = 0.30$).

The main results are shown in Table 2. We determined the mean bone healing time in the group with AFF to be 11.1 months (range: 5–28 months; SD: 6.1 months) and median bone healing time to be 10 months (6–14.5 months; interquartile range; 25–75); in the group with osteoporotic femoral fractures, we determined the mean bone healing time to be 6.7 months (range: 2.5–28 months; SD: 8.1 months) and median bone healing time to be 3.25 months (2.75–5.5 months; interquartile range: 25–75). This was a significant difference between the two groups ($p < 0.01$). There were no statistically significant differences in the rates of complications in the two groups (23.5% versus 9.1%; $p = 0.62$). In the group with AFF, intraoperative femoral fracture during

TABLE 2: Comparison of bone healing time and complication rates.

Parameter	AFF (n = 17)	OP (n = 11)	p	test
Bone healing time (months)	11.1 (5–28)	6.7 (2.5–28)	<0.01	Mann–Whitney U test
Complication (%)	23.5	9.1	0.62	Fisher's exact test
Intraoperative fracture (%)	11.8	9.1	0.66	Fisher's exact test
Implant failure (%)	5.9	0	0.61	Fisher's exact test
Reoperation (%)	5.9	0	0.61	Fisher's exact test

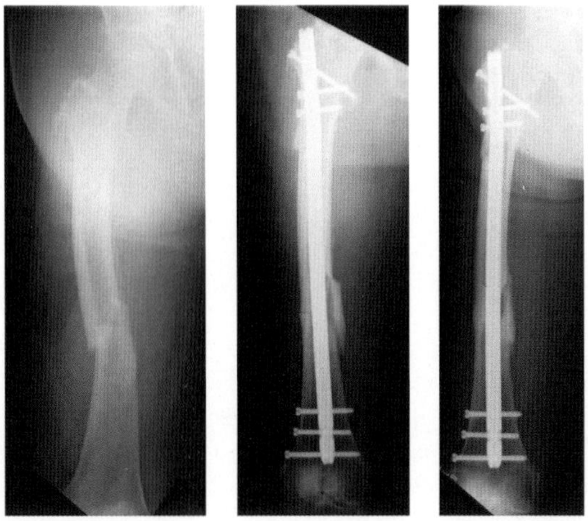

(a) (b) (c)

FIGURE 1: (a) AP radiographs of a patient with atypical femoral shaft fracture (b) treated with an intramedullary nail and intraoperative peri-implant fracture occurred. (c) Bone healed after 32 weeks from the index surgery.

intramedullary nail insertion occurred in 11.8% (2 cases) (Figure 1), and one plate failure occurred (5.9%); there were no nail failures. In the group with osteoporotic fractures, there was only 1 case of intraoperative fracture (9.1%) and no implant failures. There was 1 reoperation among the 17 patients with AFF, which was treated with BPs and fixation with a plate. There were no reoperations in the 11 patients with osteoporotic femoral shaft fractures. One patient had osteoarthritis of the hip, and the deformity was severe (Figure 2). We considered that antegrade intramedullary nail insertion would be difficult and performed plate fixation. But implant failure occurred, and retrograde nail fixation was performed 22 weeks after the index surgery. The time to union was 43 weeks after the first surgery (Figure 3). The patient reports having no pain and can walk with a cane.

4. Discussion

The present study demonstrated a statistically significant difference in the bone healing time between patients with atypical femoral shaft fractures and those with osteoporotic femoral shaft fractures (11.1 months versus 6.7 months, $p < 0.01$). However, the rate of complications was 23.5% (AFF) versus 9.1% (osteoporotic femoral shaft fractures) for the two groups, which was not significant, although we experienced 1 plate failure and required revision surgery with intramedullary nail fixation in the AFF group.

There have been reports showing that the long-term use of BPs, steroids, rheumatoid arthritis, femoral lateral bowing, and diabetes mellitus are associated with the risk of AFF [1, 4, 8–12]. A multifactorial etiology, including poor bone quality due to mutual interactions and mechanical stress, appears to be responsible for the occurrence of AFF [4, 6]. In particular, patients with severe lateral bowing of the femur are likely to sustain dynamic stress on the femoral shaft due to axial pressure [4]; as a result, femoral shat fractures are increased [2–4]. In surgical treatment, intramedullary nail fixation has been recommended [2], and plates were previously chosen as the fixation device owing to the technical impracticability of nailing due to bowing of the femur or cortex thickening [7]. However, in atypical femoral shaft fractures, fragility of the bone, lateral bowing of the femur, and varus moment arm are associated with high rates of complications [5, 7]. Lateral bowing of the femur was associated with difficulties in

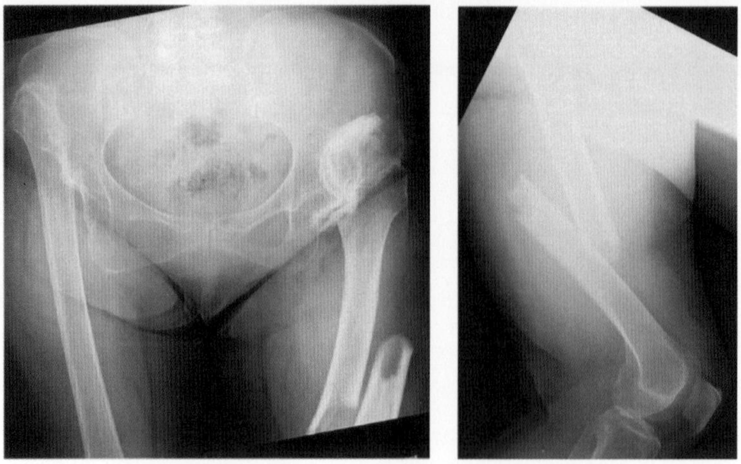

(a) (b)

FIGURE 2: (a) AP and (b) lateral radiographs show a characteristic atypical femoral fracture and severe osteoarthritis of the hip.

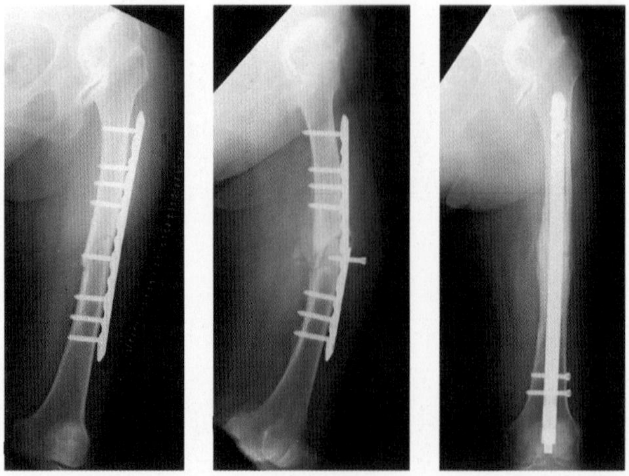

(a) (b) (c)

FIGURE 3: (a) AP image is shown, which was obtained after open reduction and internal fixation with an LCP plate. (b) AP radiographs obtained 22 weeks after fracture surgery show plate breakage. (c) AP image obtained 43 weeks after initial fracture surgery; reoperation was performed with retrograde intramedullary nailing.

nail insertion during the operation and iatrogenic fracturing during nail placement [5]. Delayed bone healing was associated with postoperative plate failure [7]. In the plate fixation procedure in particular, complications rates were high and outcomes poor [6, 7]. So, choosing the fixation material in atypical femoral shaft fractures is difficult.

First, this analysis revealed that atypical femoral shaft fractures delay bone healing. However, there were statistical differences in the rate of use of intramedullary nails; it took an average of 11.1 months until bone healing with AFF was considered to be a prominent feature of AFF. In the osteoporotic femoral shaft fractures group, due to existing implants, plate fixation was more chosen. Second, the rate of complications was 23.5% (AFF) versus 9.1% (osteoporotic femur fracture) between the two groups, which was not significant. Although we experienced 1 plate failure and required revision surgery with intramedullary nail fixation in the AFF patient, only 1 patient underwent plate fixation in the AFF group. But the 4 patients who underwent plate fixation in the osteoporotic femoral fractures group had no complications, and their bone healing was good. The use of plates rather than intramedullary fixation devices might have contributed to the high reoperation rate observed elsewhere [5]. In patients with AFF, intramedullary nail insertion should be the first choice in treatment. However, there are some cases in which antegrade intramedullary nail insertion will be difficult. In our case, retrograde nail insertion was useful for severe hip osteoarthritis.

We used a similar array of implants in both groups, although more adjuvants tended to be given to patients receiving antiresorptive therapy. In particular, more teriparatide was given postoperatively to patients in the AFF group. The use of teriparatide in patients with AFF has been reported to significantly shorten the postoperative recovery and reduce rates of delayed healing or nonunion [13]. And its efficacy in AFF has been proposed in a systematic review [14]. Thus, the use of teriparatide may be useful for the treatment of AFF.

Our study has some limitations. We had a limited number of Japanese patients. It is difficult to obtain a large sample in the study of a relatively rare injury. Complications were rare, and there were no significant differences between the two groups, and there is a possibility that this outcome differs from other races. Retrospective studies carry an inherent risk of observer bias, including the potential for missing data and an inability to control for confounding variables. We did not obtain functional outcomes for the patients, and we were unable to rigorously evaluate and compare the time to recovery between the two groups. It is worthwhile to note that, for this study, few similar correlational studies have been attempted; therefore, potential for further exploration is substantial. Future research on this topic should include a larger sample size and stratify patients according to different ethnicities if the sample size permits.

5. Conclusion

Atypical femoral shaft fractures are often seen in those treated with antiresorptive therapy; in this study, intramedullary nailing was chosen more often, but the time to bone healing was delayed compared with osteoporotic femoral fractures. There was no significant difference in complications rates, but iatrogenic femoral fractures occurred during intramedullary nail insertion, and plate fixation cases needed reoperation. Therefore, we should distinguish atypical femoral shaft fractures from osteoporotic femoral shaft fractures.

References

[1] E. Shane, D. Burr, B. Abrahamsen et al., "Atypical subtrochanteric and diaphyseal femoral fractures: second report of a task force of the American Society for Bone and Mineral Research," *Journal of Bone and Mineral Metabolism*, vol. 29, pp. 1–23, 2014.

[2] H. H. Soh, I. T. H. Chua, and E. B. K. Kwek, "Atypical fractures of the femur: effect of anterolateral bowing of the femur on fracture location," *Archives of Orthopaedic and Trauma Surgery*, vol. 135, no. 11, pp. 1485–1490, 2015.

[3] L.-P. Chen, T.-K. Chang, T.-Y. Huang, T.-G. Kwok, and Y.-C. Lu, "The correlation between lateral bowing angle of the femur and the location of atypical femur fractures," *Calcified Tissue International*, vol. 95, no. 3, pp. 240–247, 2014.

[4] Y. Zenke, S. Ikeda, F. Fukuda et al., "Study of atypical femoral fracture cases coupled in a multicenter study," *Journal of UOEH*, vol. 38, no. 3, pp. 207–214, 2016.

[5] J. Schilcher, "High revision rate but good healing capacity of atypical femoral fractures. A comparison with common shaft fractures," *Injury*, vol. 46, no. 12, pp. 2468–2473, 2015.

[6] S. De Das, T. Setiobudi, L. Shen, and S. De Das, "A rational approach to management of alendronate-related subtrochanteric fractures," *The Journal of Bone and Joint Surgery—British Volume*, vol. 92, no. 5, pp. 679–686, 2010.

[7] M. L. Prasarn, J. Ahn, D. L. Helfet, J. M. Lane, and D. G. Lorich, "Bisphosphonate-associated femur fractures have high complication rates with operative fixation trauma," *Clinical Orthopaedics and Related Research*, vol. 470, no. 8, pp. 2295–2301, 2012.

[8] D. P. Taormina, A. I. Marcano, R. Karia, K. A. Egol, and N. C. Tejwani, "Symptomatic atypical femoral fractures are related to underlying hip geometry," *Bone*, vol. 63, pp. 1–6, 2014.

[9] S. Sasaki, N. Miyakoshi, M. Hongo, Y. Kasukawa, and Y. Shimada, "Low-energy diaphyseal femoral fractures associated with bisphosphonate use and severe curved femur: a case series," *Journal of Bone and Mineral Metabolism*, vol. 30, no. 5, pp. 561–567, 2012.

[10] A. Giusti, N. A. T. Hamdy, O. M. Dekkers, S. R. Ramautar, S. Dijkstra, and S. E. Papapoulos, "Atypical fractures and bisphosphonate therapy: a cohort study of patients with femoral fracture with radiographic adjudication of fracture site and features," *Bone*, vol. 48, no. 5, pp. 966–971, 2011.

[11] J. C. Lo, S. Y. Huang, G. A. Lee et al., "Clinical correlates of atypical femoral fracture," *Bone*, vol. 51, no. 1, pp. 181–184, 2012.

[12] R. P. H. Meier, T. V. Perneger, R. Stern, R. Rizzoli, and R. E. Peter, "Increasing occurrence of atypical femoral fractures associated with bisphosphonate use," *JAMA Internal Medicine*, vol. 172, no. 12, pp. 930–936, 2012.

[13] N. Miyakoshi, T. Aizawa, S. Sasaki et al., "Healing of bisphosphonate-associated atypical femoral fractures in patients with osteoporosis: a comparison between treatment with and without teriparatide," *Journal of Bone and Mineral Metabolism*, 2014.

[14] G. I. Im and S. H. Lee, "Effect of teriparatide on healing of atypical femoral fractures: a systemic review," *Journal Bone Metabolism*, vol. 22, pp. 183–189, 2015.

2

Cost-Effectiveness Analysis of Total Hip Arthroplasty Performed by a Canadian Short-Stay Surgical Team in Ecuador

Michael Schlegelmilch,[1,2] Saifee Rashiq,[2,3] Barbara Moreau,[2] Patricia Jarrín,[4] Bach Tran,[5] and Anderson Chuck[3,5]

[1]*Faculty of Medicine and Dentistry, University of Alberta, Edmonton, AB, Canada*
[2]*Canadian Association of Medical Teams Abroad, Edmonton, AB, Canada*
[3]*Department of Anesthesiology and Pain Medicine, University of Alberta, Edmonton, AB, Canada*
[4]*Fundación Tierra Nueva, Quito, Ecuador*
[5]*Institute of Health Economics, Edmonton, AB, Canada*

Correspondence should be addressed to Saifee Rashiq; srashiq@ualberta.ca

Academic Editor: Allen L. Carl

Background. Few charitable overseas surgical missions produce cost-effectiveness analyses of their work. *Methods.* We compared the pre- and postoperative health status for 157 total hip arthroplasty (THA) patients operated on from 2007 to 2011 attended by an annual Canadian orthopedic mission to Ecuador to determine the quality-adjusted life years (QALYs) gained. The costs of each mission are known. The cost per surgery was divided by the average lifetime QALYs gained to estimate an incremental cost-effectiveness ratio (ICER) in Canadian dollars per QALY. *Results.* The average lifetime QALYs (95% CI) gained were 1.46 (1.4–1.5), 2.5 (2.4–2.6), and 2.9 (2.7–3.1) for unilateral, bilateral, and staged (two THAs in different years) operations, respectively. The ICERs were $4,442 for unilateral, $2,939 for bilateral, and $4392 for staged procedures. Seventy percent of the mission budget was spent on the transport and accommodation of volunteers. *Conclusion.* THA by a Canadian short-stay surgical team was highly cost-effective, according to criteria from the National Institute for Health and Care Excellence and the World Health Organization. We encourage other international missions to provide similar cost-effectiveness data to enable better comparison between mission types and between mission and nonmission care.

1. Background

In the past decade, osteoarthritis (OA) had the largest increase of associated disability adjusted life years (DALYs) globally and was the tenth leading cause of years of life lost due to a disability [1]. Recent world data suggest that deaths from rheumatic diseases are also increasing [2]. Total hip arthroplasty (THA) is the definitive treatment for end-stage degenerative hip disease, but many cultural and socioeconomic barriers to accessing THA, such as race, exist worldwide [3]. Individuals in low- and middle-income countries (LMICs) are disproportionately impeded by these barriers and are thus largely denied the opportunity to receive THAs. Given the dependence that many of them have on manual labor for subsistence, the inaccessibility of treatment can have a large economic impact.

Charitable donations to organizations that deliver medical and surgical care in LMICs are common in wealthier nations. In 2010, Canadian charities received more than $1.5 billion in donations to support medical work of all kinds, of which a subset is earmarked for short-stay surgical missions [4]. While all charities publish the ways in which donor funds are spent, very few provide cost-effectiveness analyses of their interventions.

The Canadian Association of Medical Teams Abroad (CAMTA) (http://www.camta.com), an Edmonton, Alberta, based charity, conducts annual orthopedic surgical missions to Ecuador to perform THAs in adults and miscellaneous complex orthopedic procedures in children. CAMTA's origins began with the direct observation of shortfalls in access to such care made by an informally constituted team of visiting health providers many years ago. It began operating in Ecuador in 2002, treating early onset hip osteoarthritis attributable to the failed detection or treatment of developmental dysplasia of the hip. It should be noted that CAMTA offers these specific interventions because they lie within the expertise of its members, not because they were prioritized by any assessment of local needs. CAMTA works in the hospitals of Fundación Tierra Nueva (FTN), a health and social welfare charity in Quito. It also provides some educational programing for Ecuadorian orthopedic surgeons. In parallel, it offers other capacity building initiatives not described here.

The purposes of this investigation were to calculate the cost effectiveness of the THA operations that CAMTA performs and to compare this with published cost-effectiveness data for other humanitarian surgical and nonsurgical programs.

2. Methods

Approval was obtained from the Health Research Ethics Board, Health Panel of the University of Alberta, to use data routinely collected for quality assurance purposes for this investigation.

FTN (http://www.fundaciontierranueva.org.ec) is a faith-based charity in Quito, Ecuador, that offers social assistance and health care to those who cannot afford to procure it privately. Examples of its activities include ambulatory care, obstetric services, child development support, mobile dental care, and support for those with disabilities. In addition, it operates an acute care hospital with a surgical suite. Here, local surgeons perform general surgery, gynecology, urology, and orthopedics (including THA but not pediatrics). In parallel, overseas surgical teams, of which CAMTA is one, perform specialty surgery on a short-stay basis on a rotating schedule. FTN is supported by a combination of charitable donations and remittances from the government for providing medically necessary services. FTN supplies CAMTA with clinic, operating, and recovery rooms, sterilizing facilities, postoperative beds, some nurses, social workers, administrative and maintenance personnel, laundry, utilities, and piped oxygen. It invoices CAMTA for these items. It charges consumable items at cost and provides the services of its personnel at their usual hourly rate. CAMTA provides all other personnel (surgeons, anesthetists, family physicians, most nurses, physiotherapists, translators, surgical equipment cleaners, and lay helpers) and all other consumables (drugs, dressings, surgical prostheses, and physiotherapy appliances). Personnel numbers are adjusted from year to year depending on workload. CAMTA receives and stores donations of some consumable items in Canada. These are transported in the personal luggage of its participants for each mission at no cost. A small number of items that are deemed mission critical and which are unavailable in Ecuador (principally a few specific anesthesia drugs) are purchased in Canada and transported in the same manner. The remaining necessary consumables are purchased locally. The proportion of supplies acquired locally varies from year to year, depending on the available quantity of donations.

2.1. Participant Selection. Patients who are referred from FTN primary care and who might, on clinical grounds, benefit from THA are identified during the year preceding each mission by a specific affiliated Ecuadorian orthopedic surgeon. This group is then means-tested by the Social Work Department of FTN according to its own criteria in order to confirm that they could not otherwise afford the cost of surgery and is then referred to CAMTA. FTN considers household size, total household income, and the number of children or others depending on the earning potential of the patient in order to determine eligibility for CAMTA services, seeking always to prioritize those in the greatest need. It demands at least some contribution from the recipient to the cost of the care it delivers, but this too is means-tested and might be as low as a dollar. (The cost of THA if obtained directly from FTN is $7750, comprising hospital costs of $3400 and prosthesis cost of $4350; about half of Ecuador's population is eligible to have that covered by social insurance, and a further 9% have private insurance, but such an outlay would be beyond the means of the remainder.)

Upon CAMTA's arrival, prospective candidates are screened for surgical appropriateness by Canadian surgeons. Patients are selected for surgery using the same clinical criteria as would have been applied in Canada. Anesthesiologists and family physicians then determine medical fitness for surgery, declining anyone in whom there is a high predictable risk of prolonged recovery or other complications. The costs of any necessary preoperative screening tests are nominally charged to the patient, but the costs of these are included in, not imposed in addition to, FTN's fee. In the event that the number of appropriate candidates exceeds the available surgical capacity in any mission year, surgical patients are selected based on the greatest financial need and most severe health burden. Those who are declined for this reason are invited to return the following year but are not prioritized. Here, we present an analysis of CAMTA's adult patients who underwent surgery from 2007 to 2011.

All patients underwent hip replacement via the posterolateral or lateral approach under spinal anesthesia and conscious sedation, with antibiotic prophylaxis and tranexamic acid administration. This is in keeping with prevailing practices in Canada. Allogeneic blood transfusion was administered as needed. Prophylaxis against deep vein thrombosis for the postdischarge period was provided. The vast majority of patients received uncemented titanium implants unless poor bone quality necessitated cemented implants. Patients were mobilized soon after surgery and discharged on crutches when they could climb a short flight of stairs, typically on postoperative day one. All patients were asked to return to see the affiliated local orthopedic surgeon at six weeks and three and six months. They were asked to return for follow-up with CAMTA one year later.

2.2. Health Outcomes. Duly validated Latin American Spanish language versions of two outcome instruments were administered. The SF-36 (Medical Outcomes Study 36-Item Short Form Health Survey) is a widely used instrument for quantifying self-reported quality of life in eight major

Table 1: 15D health state dimensions.

Each dimension is scored on a 5-point ordinal scale to best represent the respondent's present health status:
(i) Mobility
(ii) Vision
(iii) Hearing
(iv) Breathing
(v) Sleeping
(vi) Eating
(vii) Speech
(viii) Excretion
(ix) Usual activities
(x) Mental function
(xi) Discomfort and symptoms
(xii) Depression
(xiii) Distress
(xiv) Vitality
(xv) Sexual activity

Adapted from http://www.15d-instrument.net.

domains relating to health status [5]. All domains are scored on a scale from 0 to 100, which represent the worst to best possible health states. These results are summarized and presented as a physical component summary (PCS) and a mental component summary (MCS). It was administered preoperatively and at one year. Staged intervention patients were measured for outcomes after each surgery but only reported in this study after their final surgery. The mean of each of the eight domains was calculated each time point. These averages were used for cross-walking onto another instrument called the 15D for the purposes of determining a health utility score.

There were two separate instruments applied to assess patient outcomes during the study period: SF-36 and 15D. The SF-36 was applied pre-op and post-op for patients from 2007 and 2010 and pre-op in 2011. CAMTA began administering the 15D to patients at follow-up in 2012, for patients that received surgery in 2011 and so, in order to group patient data from all five mission years (2007–2011), we cross-walked the SF-36 from each patient onto the 15D. This method has been validated in patients with rheumatoid arthritis [6]. The 15D is a multiattribute utility instrument. Containing a profile of 15 dimensions, it provides a descriptive system of 31 billion discrete states (Table 1) [7, 8]. A set of utility weights of Finland and Denmark is used to generate the 15D score on a 0-1 scale, representing death to perfect health [9]. We rescaled the 15D single score onto a 0–100 scale to ease comparison between the 15D and SF-36. To cross-walk the SF-36, regression analysis was used to examine the relationship between the 15D utility score and 8 domain scores of the SF-36. Three statistical models were used and we found that an ordinary least squares (OLS) model outperformed Tobit and censored least absolute deviations models, as indicated by R-squared measure (0.79). Regression coefficients estimated in this OLS model were then selected for deriving utility scores in this study. Quality-adjusted life years (QALYs) gained were calculated based on the percent change in 15D scores for each surgery type over 1 year.

2.3. Costs. Costs are from the perspective of CAMTA and all of CAMTA's expenditures are precisely recorded to comply with its registered charity status. CAMTA's Canadian personnel donate their time and cover their own transportation and accommodation by securing donations, which are remitted to CAMTA. Other costs are defrayed by donations to the organization as a whole. During the study period, manufacturers donated most but not all surgical prostheses. We did not include, (but acknowledged) the opportunity costs of personnel who are not working elsewhere and the opportunity costs of not using the surgical and ward space for other uses. Half of CAMTA's patients are children, who were not subjects in this study. Costs attributable to the care of children were excluded from this analysis. All costs are in 2007 Canadian dollars.

2.4. Cost Effectiveness. The average cost of each surgery type was determined for unilateral, bilateral, and staged (two THAs in different years) THAs during the study period. Lifetime incremental QALYs gained were estimated with life expectancy tables and were discounted at a rate of 3.5% per year, in accordance with the NICE guidelines [10]. Lifetime QALYs gained and average cost per surgery were used to calculate a point estimate of the incremental cost-effectiveness ratio (ICER). Analyses were performed to determine the sensitivity of the ICER to the two largest categories of expenditures: personnel travel and accommodation and procurement of surgical prostheses.

2.5. Ethics and Data Storage and Management. Approval was obtained from the Health Ethics Review Board of the University of Alberta to use data which had been routinely collected as part of the mission years in question for this investigation. The data were stored in sealed boxes to which only senior CAMTA staff had access. Once transcribed onto electronic spreadsheets, they were encrypted and protected by password. Only anonymized data were used in the analysis.

3. Results

3.1. Enrolment and Demographics. During the five-year study, CAMTA operated on 157 adult patients receiving THA. The majority of patients were female (79%) with an average age of 49 years at the time of their first surgery and an average life expectancy of an additional 32 years, illustrating the comparative precocity of degenerative hip disease in Ecuador compared to Canada. Unilateral THAs comprised 79.6% (n = 125) of the total surgeries with 16.6% (n = 26) and 3.8% (n = 6) of patients receiving bilateral and staged THAs, respectively. Sixty-five patients (41.4%) were lost to follow-up at one year. Of the 92 patients with follow-up data, nearly a third had incomplete responses to the SF-36. There were no significant differences between patients who were included or lost to follow-up based on age or presurgery PCS or MCS score (Table 2).

3.2. Health Outcomes. Mean PCS scores improved from 34.2 to 45.6 (<0.001). No significant improvement in MCS scores was seen (p = 0.092). Health utility, measured by 15D

TABLE 2: Patient demographics for all patients in mission years 2007–2011.

	μ (SD) or n (%)		
	Enrolled	Lost to follow-up	p value
Participants	157	65	
Age	49.1 (10.6)	51.6 (14.8)	0.216
Presurgery PCS	33.9 (6.1)	35.4 (6.6)	0.166
Presurgery MCS	39.9 (8.2)	38.8 (10.2)	0.460
Gender (female)	124 (79.0)	59 (84.3)	0.352
Unilateral	125 (79.6)	65 (93.0)	0.011
Bilateral	26 (16.6)	4 (5.7)	0.025
Staged bilateral	6 (3.8)	1 (0.3)	0.133

scores, gained at one year (after the second surgery for staged patients) was the greatest for patients who received the staged intervention (14.1%; 0.141 QALYs), compared to bilateral (12.2%; 0.122 QALYs) and unilateral (10.3%; 0.103 QALYs) intervention.

3.3. Costs. The total mission costs for our study period were $1,107,996 CAD. The largest proportion of funds was allocated to transport and accommodation of personnel ($773,947; 70%). Even though the vast majority of the prosthetic joint component pieces were donated without charge, the purchase of the remainder made up the second largest cost at $231,687 (21%). The remaining costs were split between other medical supplies and drugs ($46,307; 4%) and fixed administrative costs (office supplies and equipment, legal and banking fees, and website maintenance) ($56,056; 5%). Mean cost per surgery was lowest for unilateral THA at $6,042, followed by bilateral THA at $7,229. Staged THAs required additional travel and OR costs and had a mean cost of $12,786 (Table 3).

3.4. Cost-Effectiveness and Sensitivity Analysis. The ICER for unilateral THAs was $4,443 and that for bilateral and staged THAs was $2,939 and $4,392, respectively (Table 3). Our sensitivity analysis indicates that removing the cost of prostheses would have decreased the ICER for unilateral THA by $1,031 (23%), by $955.17 (32%) for bilateral THA, and by $2,692 (61%) for staged procedures. If CAMTA had paid the full cost of prostheses, the ICER would have risen by $1,072.67 (24%) for unilateral THA, by $1,496.86 (51%) for bilateral surgery, and by $1,104.39 (25%) for staged surgery. Removing the cost of travel and accommodation for CAMTA personnel reduced the ICER 74% to $1,157 for unilateral, by 62% to $1,112 for bilateral, and by 78% to $952 for staged surgeries. In the hypothetical situation where all prostheses were donated free of cost, and excluding personnel costs, ICERs were $402, $234, and $200 for unilateral, bilateral, and staged surgeries, respectively (Table 4). Although we do not have data to propose an ICER for a scenario where Ecuadorian surgeons were performing the THA with prostheses acquired by CAMTA and donated, the final line of Table 4 may approximate this scenario. When no personnel costs were included but full prostheses costs were considered the ICER decreased by $2687.29 (60%) for unilateral, by $1131.52 (38%) for bilateral, and by $2843.42 (65%) for staged surgeries.

4. Discussion

We have shown that the mean lifetime cost per QALY for THA in our mission setting is between $2939 and $4442.77 and, depending on the classification of the costs of volunteer transport and accommodation, could be as low as $200.

Our outcomes are well below the threshold of £20,000/QALY ($32,000 CAD/QALY) for cost effectiveness, based on the NICE guidelines [11]. Another, more contextually appropriate, comparator of cost effectiveness uses national GDP. As recommended by World Health Organization, an ICER that is less than the GDP per capita is highly cost-effective [12]. The average GDP per capita in Ecuador during our study period was $4150 CAD [13]. This suggests that, by these definitions, bilateral THAs performed by CAMTA were highly cost-effective. Unilateral and staged interventions exceeded the WHO recommended benchmark by 7% and 6%, respectively.

Humanitarian surgical relief of congenital hand deformities in Honduras and cleft lip in India reported ICERs of $437/DALYs (Disability Adjusted Life Years, *not QALY*) and $247/DALYs, respectively [14, 15]. Orthopedic teams in Haiti ($362/DALYs) and Ecuador ($525/DALYs) and general or obstetrical surgical missions ($308/DALYs) in the Dominican Republic all report similar cost-effectiveness ratios [16–18]. A Médicines Sans Frontières evaluation of two surgical trauma hospitals in Nigeria and Haiti achieved ICERs of $172 and $223, respectively [19]. We reported our outcomes in QALYs gained because 15D is validated for that purpose [8]. In a systematic review of global surgical cost-effectiveness analyses, QALYs were more common, though less so in low- or middle-income countries [20]. Though these comparator studies reported DALYs, theoretical comparisons between QALYs and DALYs can be made, and occasionally QALYs gained will be close to or equal DALYs averted [21]. Although these two measures seek to quantify a similar experience, they are not necessarily reciprocal. The variance between QALY and DALY depends on age, disease duration, comorbid conditions, and the difference between quality of life and disability weights [21, 22]. Even while respecting the cautions that need to be exercised when comparing DALYs and QALYs, our findings are comparable.

An analysis of THAs in the UK reported an ICER of £2852 ($5225 CAD) [23]. However, these authors were able to account for the cost of revisions and complication management. This is a limitation of our study, as we could not account for costs of complications or revisions that CAMTA did not manage. This is a documented issue of many short-stay surgical missions and systematically leads to underestimated cost-effectiveness estimates [24]. We speculate that although complications occur, the rate is low and would not have a significant effect on our outcomes. In Western, tertiary level care settings, the complication rates for a THA 0.5% are in 15 years [23]. In one study of cleft palate repair by a short-stay surgical mission, the complication rate was 20 times greater than rates seen in the USA [25], but, to our knowledge, complication rates have not been compared for THAs.

In contrast, it is possible that for other reasons our study produced more conservative estimates of QALYs gained and

TABLE 3: Cost, incremental QALYs gained, and ICER for each surgery type.

Surgery	Mean cost ($CAD)	Mean incremental QALYs (95% CI)		ICER ($CAD/QALY)
		1 year	Lifetime	Lifetime
Unilateral ($n = 125$)	6,042.45 (5893.23–6191.67)	0.081 (0.06–0.11)	1.46 (1.40–1.52)	4,442.77 (4187.76–4697.78)
Bilateral ($n = 26$)	7,229.13 (6876.78–7581.49)	0.12 (0.07–0.16)	2.51 (2.39–2.63)	2,939.49 (2705.00–3173.99)
Staged ($n = 6$)	12,786.08 (11,473.35–14,098.81)	0.14 (0.00–0.29)	2.93 (2.76–3.10)	4,392.23 (3854.22–4930.24)

TABLE 4: Sensitivity analysis for cost of prostheses and of personnel travel and accommodation.

	ICER ($CAD/QALY) for lifetime		
	Unilateral	Bilateral	Staged
Actual	$4,442.77	$2,939.49	$4,392.23
No prostheses cost	$3,411.40	$1,984.32	$1,699.88
Full prostheses cost	$5,515.44	$4,436.35	$5,496.62
No personnel costs	$1,157.53	$1,112.35	$952.90
No personnel or prostheses costs	$402.74	$234.26	$200.68
No personnel with full prostheses costs	$1,755.48	$1,807.97	$1,548.81

overestimated ICERs. First, we were unable to measure the increased lifetime earnings and economic productivity that our patients could achieve after receiving a THA. Second, the quality of life benefits of increased survivability were not accounted for in our QALY calculations. Third, we are limited by attrition, which is a documented issue in the literature. International surgical missions report attrition rates ranging from 20% to 63% [24, 26]. Though we found no difference at baseline between those lost to follow-up and those who were not, we speculate that patients were more likely to be lost if they had favourable surgical outcomes, as they would feel no need to present to clinic. This is on the assumption that complication rates and all-cause mortality are lower than our rates of attrition which are nearly 30%. We assume this is not attributable to poor outcomes, given the previous discussion regarding estimates of complication rates.

Others have hypothesized that inefficiencies in process would produce cost-ineffective interventions when relief teams travel to a different country [16]. Our results suggest otherwise. The sensitivity analysis suggests a remarkably low ICER under circumstances where human resources and prostheses are entirely donated. A $200.68 donation could, in one such hypothetical scenario, procure one QALY for a patient with debilitating hip arthritis.

It is prudent to acknowledge that the perspective of analysis is from that of CAMTA and does not account for costs to patients or to the Ecuadorian health system or the opportunity costs of people and space used for this mission to operate. While CAMTA always welcomes the involvement of Ecuadorian trainees and medical staff in its cases, such involvement is self-initiated. CAMTA does not seek to actively build local capacity as part of its surgical care delivery (but has active parallel initiatives of this type which are not discussed here).

Ecuadorian practitioners are more than capable of performing THA and indeed do so in the very same hospital in which CAMTA operates. Why, then, is the mission needed at all? What would happen if it became impossible for CAMTA to return? We emphatically do not claim that the intermittent arrival of a large group of foreigners is the best way to deliver this care to those who need it, in Ecuador or, by extension, anywhere else, no matter how cost-effective it can be shown to be. Clearly, the optimal scenario would be the timely delivery of such care by local practitioners. What CAMTA brings to bear is essentially the deployment of a high concentration of resources and personnel in a short space of time. Vigorous debate can and must be had at all levels of governmental, professional, charitable, and public bodies about the best way to serve those who need health care of all kinds, in a manner that is accessible, sustainable, and of high quality. All we can hope to do here is to fuel that debate by attaching an approximate dollar value to the clinical results we have achieved.

Though the intrinsic clinical and logistical challenges of medical missions may push the task of outcome data collection out of mind, we concur with Bermudez (2010) in his plea for surgical missions to be evaluated using outcomes and not throughputs alone. Within its limits, our study calculates the quantitative benefit for the recipient from each dollar that CAMTA receives. We encourage medical charities of other types to provide similar information in order to provide the best comparative information to its current and potential donors.

Additional Points

Implication Statement. Total hip arthroplasty performed for low-income patients in Ecuador by a Canadian short-stay surgical team resulted in quality of life improvements with favourable cost effectiveness at $2,939 to $4,442 per Quality-Adjusted Life Year (QALY) gained.

Authors' Contributions

Michael Schlegelmilch contributed substantially to data analysis and manuscript writing. Saifee Rashiq conceived and designed the study and contributed substantially to data acquisition, data analysis, and manuscript writing. Barbara Moreau contributed substantially to data acquisition, reviewed the draft manuscript, and made important contributions to the final version. Patricia Jarrín reviewed the draft manuscript and made important contributions to the final version. Bach Tran and Anderson Chuck each made substantial contributions to data analysis and manuscript writing.

Acknowledgments

The authors acknowledge the assistance of Jaskaran Singh, Asha Olmstead, Karen Calhoun, Melissa Angyalfi, Jason Tong, and Tanya Atallah with data entry and of Marc Moreau, Arto Ohinmaa, and Ed Mason with the preparation of this manuscript.

References

[1] World Health Organization, *WHO Methods and Data Sources for Global Burden of Disease Estimates 2000–2011*, Periodical, 2013.

[2] GBD 2015 Mortality and Causes of Death Collaborators, "Global, regional, and national life expectancy, all-cause mortality, and cause-specific mortality for 249 causes of death, 1980–2015: a systematic analysis for the global burden of disease study 2015," *The Lancet*, vol. 388, pp. 1459–1544, 2016.

[3] L. S. M. Gomes, "THR in the young: South American perspective," *Bone and Joint*, 2012.

[4] M. Turcotte, "Charitable giving by canadians," *Canadian Social Trends*, vol. 17, 2012.

[5] J. Brazier, "The Short-Form 36 (SF-36) health survey and its use in pharmacoeconomic evaluation," *PharmacoEconomics*, vol. 7, no. 5, pp. 403–415, 1995.

[6] L. Linde, J. Sørensen, M. Østergaard, K. Hørslev-Petersen, and M. L. Hetland, "Health-related quality of life: Validity reliability, and responsiveness of SF-36, EQ-15D, EQ-5D, RAQoL, and HAQ in patients with rheumatoid arthritis," *The Journal of Rheumatology*, vol. 35, no. 8, pp. 1528–1537, 2008.

[7] S. I. Saarni, T. Härkänen, H. Sintonen et al., "The impact of 29 chronic conditions on health-related quality of life: A general population survey in Finland using 15D and EQ-5D," *Quality of Life Research*, vol. 15, no. 8, pp. 1403–1414, 2006.

[8] H. Sintonen, "The 15D instrument of health-related quality of life: properties and applications," *Annals of Medicine*, vol. 33, no. 5, pp. 328–336, 2001.

[9] K. Stavem, S. S. Frøland, and K. B. Hellum, "Comparison of preference-based utilities of the 15D, EQ-5D and SF-6D in patients with HIV/AIDS," *Quality of Life Research*, vol. 14, no. 4, pp. 971–980, 2005.

[10] National Institute for Health and Care Excellence, *Guide to the Methods of Technology Appraisal 2013*, Periodical, 2013.

[11] National Institution for Health and Care Excellence, *Departing from the Threshold*, Periodical, 2008.

[12] E. Marseille, B. Larson, D. S. Kazi, J. G. Kahn, and S. Rosen, "Thresholds for the cost–effectiveness of interventions: Alternative approaches," *Bulletin of the World Health Organization*, vol. 93, no. 2, pp. 118–124, 2015.

[13] GDP per Capita, *The World Bank*, 2016, https://data.worldbank.org/.

[14] K. K. Tadisina, K. Chopra, J. Tangredi, J. G. Thomson, and D. P. Singh, "Helping hands: a cost-effectiveness study of a humanitarian hand surgery mission," *Plastic Surgery International*, vol. 2014, Article ID 921625, 12 pages, 2014.

[15] B. Hackenberg, M. S. Ramos, A. Campbell et al., "Measuring and comparing the cost-effectiveness of surgical care delivery in low-resource settings: Cleft lip and palate as a model," *The Journal of Craniofacial Surgery*, vol. 26, no. 4, pp. 1121–1125, 2015.

[16] R. A. Gosselin, G. Gialamas, and D. M. Atkin, "Comparing the cost-effectiveness of short orthopedic missions in elective and relief situations in developing countries," *World Journal of Surgery*, vol. 35, no. 5, pp. 951–955, 2011.

[17] A. T. Chen, A. Pedtke, J. K. Kobs, G. S. Edwards Jr., R. R. Coughlin, and R. A. Gosselin, "Volunteer orthopedic surgical trips in Nicaragua: a cost-effectiveness evaluation," *World Journal of Surgery*, vol. 36, no. 12, pp. 2802–2808, 2012.

[18] J. P. Egle, A. McKendrick, V. K. Mittal, and F. Sosa, "Short-term surgical mission to the Dominican Republic: A cost-benefit analysis," *International Journal of Surgery*, vol. 12, no. 10, pp. 1045–1049, 2014.

[19] R. A. Gosselin and M. Heitto, "Cost-effectiveness of a district trauma hospital in Battambang, Cambodia," *World Journal of Surgery*, vol. 32, no. 11, pp. 2450–2453, 2008.

[20] A. J. Rios-Diaz, J. Lam, M. S. Ramos et al., "Global patterns of QALY and DALY use in surgical cost-utility analyses: A systematic review," *PLoS ONE*, vol. 11, no. 2, Article ID e0148304, 2016.

[21] F. Sassi, "Calculating QALYs, comparing QALY and DALY calculations," *Health Policy and Planning*, vol. 21, no. 5, pp. 402–408, 2006.

[22] M. R. Gold and P. Muennig, "Measure-dependent variation in burden of disease estimates: Implications for policy," *Medical Care*, vol. 40, no. 3, pp. 260–266, 2002.

[23] P. J. Jenkins, N. D. Clement, D. F. Hamilton, P. Gaston, J. T. Patton, and C. R. Howie, "Predicting the cost-effectiveness of total hip and knee replacement: a health economic analysis," *The Bone & Joint Journal*, vol. 95, no. 1, pp. 115–121, 2013.

[24] M. G. Shrime, A. Sleemi, and T. D. Ravilla, "Charitable platforms in global surgery:A systematic review of their effectiveness, cost-effectiveness, sustainability, and role training," *World Journal of Surgery*, vol. 39, no. 1, pp. 10–20, 2015.

[25] R. G. Maine, W. Y. Hoffman, J. H. Palacios-Martinez, D. S. Corlew, and G. A. Gregory, "Comparison of fistula rates after palatoplasty for international and local surgeons on surgical missions in ecuador with rates at a craniofacial center in the United States," *Plastic and Reconstructive Surgery*, vol. 129, no. 2, pp. 319e–326e, 2012.

[26] L. Bermudez, V. Carter, W. Magee Jr., R. Sherman, and R. Ayala, "Surgical outcomes auditing systems in humanitarian organizations," *World Journal of Surgery*, vol. 34, no. 3, pp. 403–410, 2010.

3

The Results of Hemivertebra Resection by the Posterior Approach in Children with a Mean Follow-Up of Five Years

Ramazan Erden Erturer,[1] Bekir Eray Kilinc,[2] Bahadir Gokcen,[1] Sinan Erdogan,[1] Kursat Kara,[1] and Cagatay Ozturk[1]

[1] *Department of Orthopedics, Istinye University, Istanbul, Turkey*
[2] *Orthopedics Clinic, Golhisar State Hospital, Burdur, Turkey*

Correspondence should be addressed to Bekir Eray Kilinc; dreraykilinc@gmail.com

Academic Editor: John P. Kostuik

Aim. To evaluate the radiologic and clinical results of patients who underwent deformity correction and stabilization for congenital spinal deformities using pedicle screws after hemivertebra resection. *Material and Method.* Nine patients, mean age 9.2, who underwent posterior hemivertebrectomy and transpedicular fixation for congenital spinal deformity and had longer than five years of follow-up were evaluated retrospectively. The hemivertebrae were located in the thoracic region in 4 patients and thoracolumbar transition region in 5 patients. The patients were evaluated radiologically and clinically in the postoperative period. *Results.* Mean length of follow-up was 64.2 months. The mean operating time was 292 minutes. The mean blood loss was 236 mL. The average hospitalization time was 7 days. The amount of correction on the coronal planes was measured as 31%. The mean segmental kyphosis angle was 45.7 degrees preoperatively and it was measured 2.7 degrees in the follow-up period. There were no statistically significant differences between the early postoperative period and final follow-up X-rays with respect to coronal and sagittal plane deformities. *Conclusion.* The ability to obtain a sufficient and balanced correction in the cases accompanied by long compensator curvatures that have a structural character in hemivertebra may require longer fusion levels.

1. Introduction

Vertebral anomalies may develop due to errors in formation or segmentation or a mixture of both. The type of the anomaly often determines the possibility of progression of the deformity. In particular, nonincarcerated and full segmented hemivertebrae may result in deformities that increase with growth. These deformities may be solely scoliotic or include kyphotic components. On the other hand, it is not possible to estimate the natural course for every case [1–3]. The primary goal in the treatment of congenital spinal deformities is to prevent the progression of the deformity and to provide a healthy growth of the spine. Correction of the already present deformity constitutes a part of the treatment plan in especially cases with severe degrees. Failure to intervene in patients who show a tendency towards progression may result in the formation of deformities which require long fusions and possess neurologic risks [2–5].

Numerous methods have been described for the treatment of congenital scoliosis. Among these hemivertebrae, excision is the only method that enables total correction of the deformity by eliminating the pathology and has predictable results [2, 3, 6]. However, it is a highly demanding technique and may cause neurological complications. While hemivertebra resection can be performed via an anterior-posterior combined approach, it is may be also completed with a posterior approach alone. The posterior-only procedure requires one less incision and it decreased the number of anterior approach-related complications [2].

The aim of this study was to present the results of average period of five-year follow-up in patients, diagnosed with congenital scoliosis and kyphoscoliosis and treated with transpedicular instrumentation and fusion methods after hemivertebra resection with the posterior approach.

2. Material and Method

Hemivertebra excisions through a single posterior approach, followed by short or long-segment fusion with transpedicular instrumentation, were performed in 9 children. All patients underwent surgery at our institution between May 2009 and September 2012. There were 4 girls and 5 boys. The mean age at time of surgery was 9.2 years (range, 6–13 years). Among these patients 8 had a single progressive hemivertebra and 1 had 2 progressive hemivertebrae. The hemivertebrae were located in the thoracic region (T3–T11) in 4 patients and thoracolumbar transition region (T12-L1) in 5 patients. Seven affected levels were scoliotic and 2 were kyphoscoliotic.

The diagnosis of hemivertebra was established by clinical, radiographic, CT, and MRI assessment. Standing full spine radiographs will allow the doctor to diagnose the type and severity of the congenital vertebral malformations and track the progression of the curvature over time. An MRI may be ordered to determine if there are spinal cord abnormalities.

Thorough physical, neurological, and radiologic examinations were performed for all patients, and additional systemic and organic anomalies were investigated. All patients underwent preoperative MRI, renal ultrasound, and echocardiography. Of the 8 patients, none had intraspinal anomaly and 1 showed associated anomalies in the genitourinary system.

Radiographic evaluations were made on the preoperative, postoperative, and follow-up standing posteroanterior and lateral radiographs. By using these radiographs, the angles of the curves were measured by the Cobb method. The results of measurements performed on the preoperative and follow-up radiographs were compared statistically. Statistical comparisons were performed with the Mann-Whitney U test. P values equal to or less than 0.05 were considered statistically significant.

3. Surgical Technique

Under general anesthesia, neuromonitoring was performed first; then the hemivertebra field was exposed using a posterior midline incision. One pair of pedicle screws was placed to each of the segments located one level above and below the hemivertebra. The pedicle screws located contralateral to the hemivertebra on the convex part were connected with the temporary rod. The hemivertebra lamina and pedicle were resected with a high speed burr. The spinal cord and the segmental root were protected. The excision was completed by resection of the hemivertebral body. The upper and lower vertebra endplates were abraded and prepared for fusion. An appropriately sized mesh cage was placed on the concave side of the deformity. The deformity was corrected by compression from the convex side aided by the pedicle screws and then checked by X-rays. Following appropriate correction, permanent rods were placed, and the system was locked (Figures 1(a) and 1(b)). For the correction of the deformity, four and more segments were included in the fusion field in three patients The procedure was completed after insertion of grafts to the posterior area. A body cast with femoral extension was applied before termination of anesthesia.

Table 1: Angular values of coronal and sagittal plane deformities preoperative, postoperative, and follow-up period.

	Cobb angle (coronal plane)	Segmental kyphosis angle (sagittal plane)
Preoperative	40.4° (32–68)	45.7° (12–52)
Postoperative	12.7° (5–18)	2.5° (2–6)
Follow-up period	12.5° (5–20)	2.7° (2–6)

4. Results

Mean length of follow-up was 64.2 (range, 54–97) months. The mean operating time was 292 minutes (range, 205–340 minutes). The mean blood loss was 236 mL (range, 180–300 mL). The average hospitalization time was 7 days (range, 5–11 days). Fusion was applied in 3 levels in 4 patients, 2 levels in 2 patients, 4 levels in 1 patient, 10 levels in 1 patient, and 11 levels in one patient. Mean scoliosis angle in scoliotic patients was 40.4 degrees (range, 32–68) before and 12.7 degrees after the operation. Mean segmental kyphosis angle was 45.7 (range, 12–52), which were measured as 2.5 and 2.7 after the operation, respectively (Table 1). There were statistically no significant differences between the early postoperative measurements and final follow-up radiographs with respect to coronal and sagittal plane deformities.

There were no intra- or postoperative neurologic complications, nor any cases of deep or superficial infections. There were no obvious pseudoarthrosis, decompensation, or implant failures at the final follow-up.

5. Discussion

Untreated hemivertebra, both full or semisegmented, can lead to serious spinal deformities. It is difficult to predict the natural course of hemivertebrae [1–3]. Generally hemivertebra with contralateral bars are accepted to carry the worst prognosis, followed by hemivertebra at two levels on the same side, single hemivertebra, and wedge vertebra [1].

In case of progressive deformity, nonsurgical methods such as bracing cannot prevent deformity progression. There is an agreement in the literature on the application of surgical treatment in progressive curves [5, 7].

In particular, nonincarcerated hemivertebrae may cause wide and rigid curves in adolescence when left untreated. The location of the hemivertebra is a significant factor in the progression of the deformity. The potential for progression of the curve was found to be higher in pathologies located in the thoracolumbar transition zone or the lumbar area [8]. Prophylactic hemivertebra treatment before the development of compensatory curves or before they possess a structural character is another suggested method. Kyphoscoliotic deformities that reach adulthood become much more difficult to treat problems and are associated with pain, functional insufficiency, and the development of neurologic deficits [8–10]. In our patients, we made the decision for surgery based on the size of the current deformity or its progression.

Various surgical methods have been described for the management of congenital spinal deformities. Among these

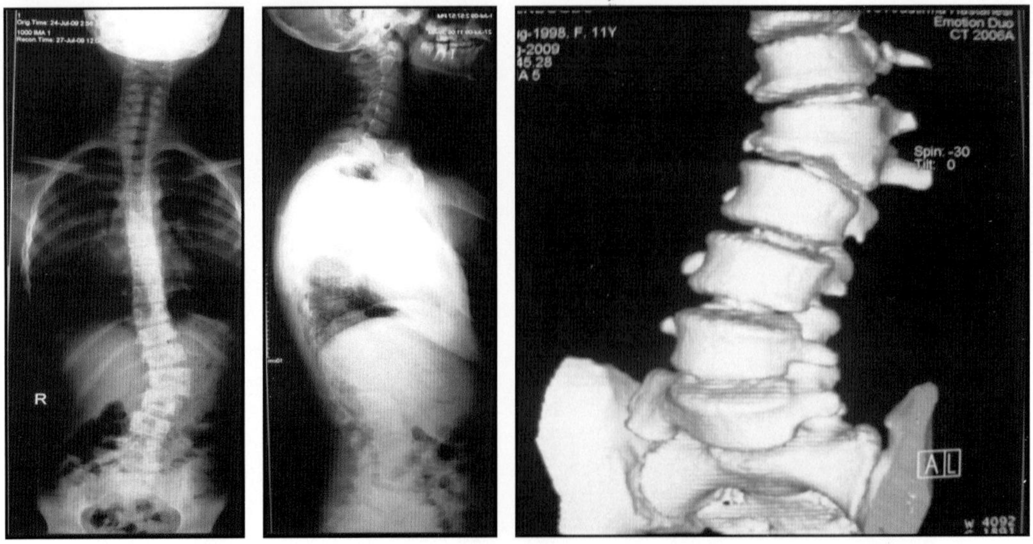

(a) A 10-year-old child L1 hemivertebrae AP-Lateral X-ray and 3D CT

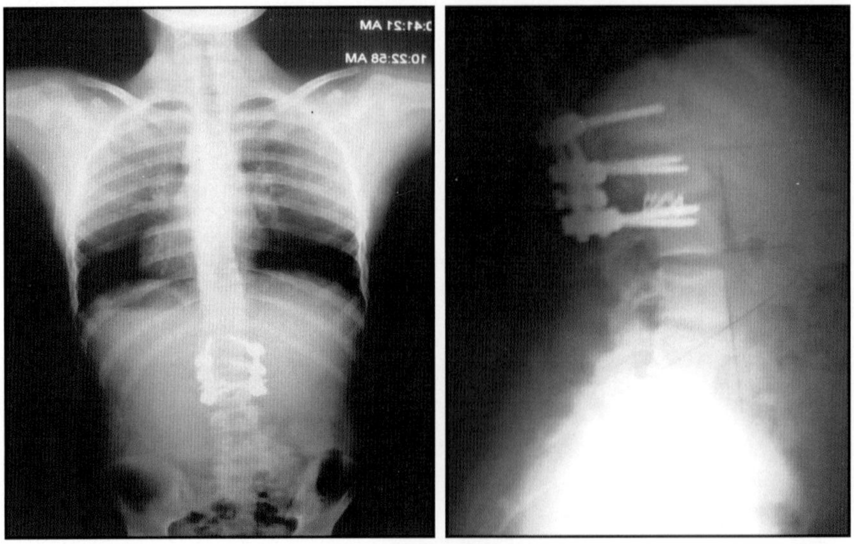

(b) Postoperative 4-year AP-Lateral X-ray

Figure 1

methods, posterior in situ arthrodesis, anterior and posterior hemiepiphysiodesis, and hemiarthrodesis provide a limited correction. The assessment and estimation of the results are difficult [3]. Although there are reports, which state that hemiepiphysiodesis can be applied successfully, especially in association with instrumented fusion techniques, it is impossible to correct the curves in patients who have developed rigid and structural curves [8, 11]. In a multicentric study, Yaszay et al. compared hemiepiphysiodesis or in situ fusion, instrumented fusion without hemivertebra excision, and instrumented hemivertebra excision. They found that although a higher rate of complications was seen with hemivertebra resection compared to the other two methods, better correction rates were achieved [12]. It is stated that the deformity can be progressively corrected using the recently developed growing rods techniques and may be used in selected patients; however, in a study on this topic, Elsebai et al. reported that complications developed in eight out of the 19 patients [13, 14].

On the other hand, hemivertebra excision is the only method that allows complete correction of the deformity by elimination of the pathology and yields predictable results. Royle first described hemivertebra excision in 1927, and recent studies have proven that it is a reliable and effective method in the treatment of congenital scoliosis [2–5, 15–18]. This method was initially described as the combination of the anterior and posterior approaches performed in one or two stages, yet operations via the posterior approach only have become more predominant recently [2, 3, 19, 20]. In 1991, Ruf and Harms introduced an innovative surgical technique of posterior hemivertebra resection with transpedicular instrumentation, which is especially suitable for early correction

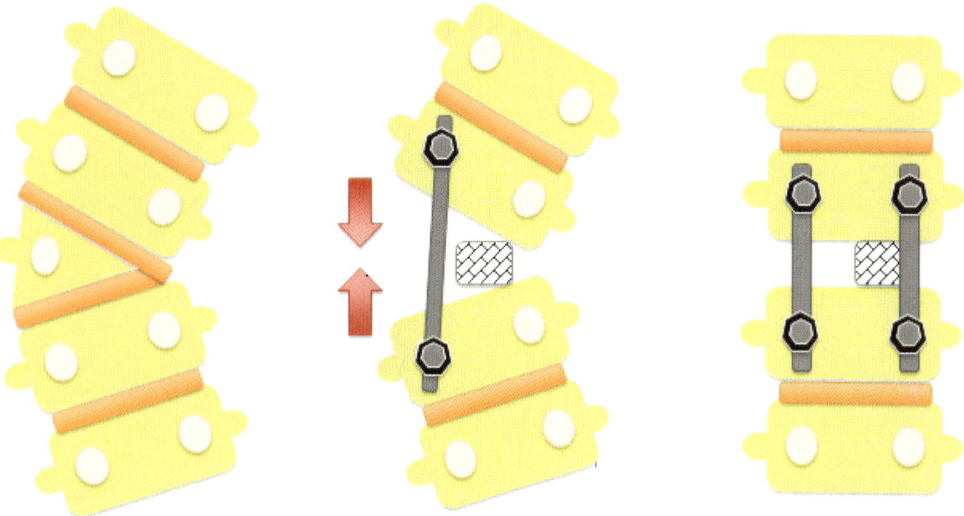

Figure 2: Correction of the coronal plan deformities using mesh cage after hemivertebra resection.

in very young children [3]. Either the combined approach or the posterior-only approach provides similar correction rates in the coronal and sagittal planes. In a comparative study, Mladenov et al. obtained similar results with respect to angular measurement, yet the complication rates were lower and the recovery periods were shorter in operations performed by the posterior approach only [4]. Jalanko et al. concluded as a result of their study that PL resection was technically more demanding and slightly faster method for hemivertebral resection. It had nearly as good correction rate as the AP-method but with more minor complications [7]. The posterior-only procedure requires one fewer incision and has decreased the number of anterior approach-related complications [2]. Ruf et al. listed that the advantages of hemivertebra resection by the posterior approach with simultaneous application of transpedicular instrumentation were excellent correction of the curve in the frontal and sagittal planes, early mobilization with high stability, no requirement for anterior access, and low neurologic risk [3, 6].

The average amount of correction in the sagittal and coronal planes we achieved after hemivertebra resection with the posterior-only approach is around 90%. This rate was 54% in the study by Nakamura et al. [20], 75% in the study by Aydogan et al. [19], and 77% in the study by Jalanko et al. [7].

Although there are concerns on the use of pedicle screws in children with growth potential, studies by Ruf et al. showed that the method did not show an adverse effect on the vertebral growth and did not result in any narrowing in the spinal canal. It is suggested that the number of levels included in the fusion site should be kept at a minimum, especially in patients with a high potential for growth. On the other hand, the risk of new deformity development increases in short fusions [3, 6]. Deformities that have developed due to hemivertebrae only and not associated with compensatory curves are amenable to correction by using short segment instrumentation. Therefore management of the deformity by appropriate timing becomes significant. Patients with severe curves in whom compensatory curves have developed require long fusions. In patients who do not have compensator curvature, the deformities could be corrected with short system instrumentation limited to one level above and one below the pathologic segment.

Previous studies have reported that various complications may develop after hemivertebra resection including infection, bleeding, temporary or permanent neurologic injuries, failed instrumentation or recurrence of the deformity [2, 5, 8, 16, 20]. The correction attained during the postoperative period remained stable in all patients, and none of the patients sustained any of the complications reported in the literature.

Previous studies have reported that operations performed by posterior surgery are technically more demanding, and the risk of developing neurologic complications is higher compared to combined surgery [2, 7, 8, 18]. Recent studies have shown significantly lower complications rates [6, 10, 13]. A clear view of the neural structures prior to correction maneuver is recommended to avoid neurologic complications [3]. Neuromonitoring was used routinely in all our cases. Complications such as hemorrhage, bleeding, infections, and recurrence of deformity associated with hemivertebra resection are rarely reported in the literature, but we have not encountered such a negative situation in our series (2-8).

When the fusion level is determined, the size of the curvature and the presence of the accompanying compensatory curvature become important. Correction of deformity should be attempted with a fusion that will take off the least segments (Figure 2). However, in cases of long thoracic or thoracolumbar spines or structural characterization of the compensatory curves, it may be necessary to apply long-segment fusion to correct the deformity (Figures 3(a), 3(b), and 3(c)). Therefore, surgical intervention in progressive cases should be performed at the earliest age.

There were no complications after operations performed under neuromonitoring. In addition to its contribution to fusion, the mesh cage inserted to the level undergoing

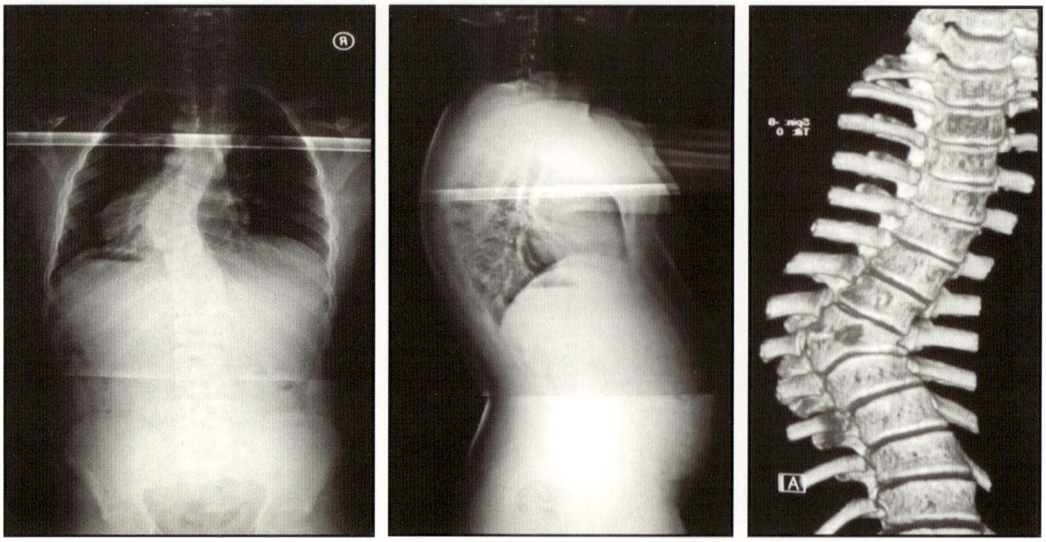

(a) 13-year-old female L1 hemivertebrae AP-Lateral X-ray and 3D CT

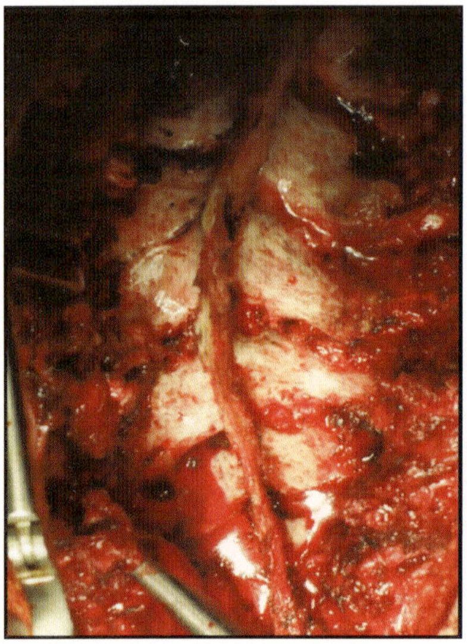

(b) Intraoperative view of the hemivertebrae

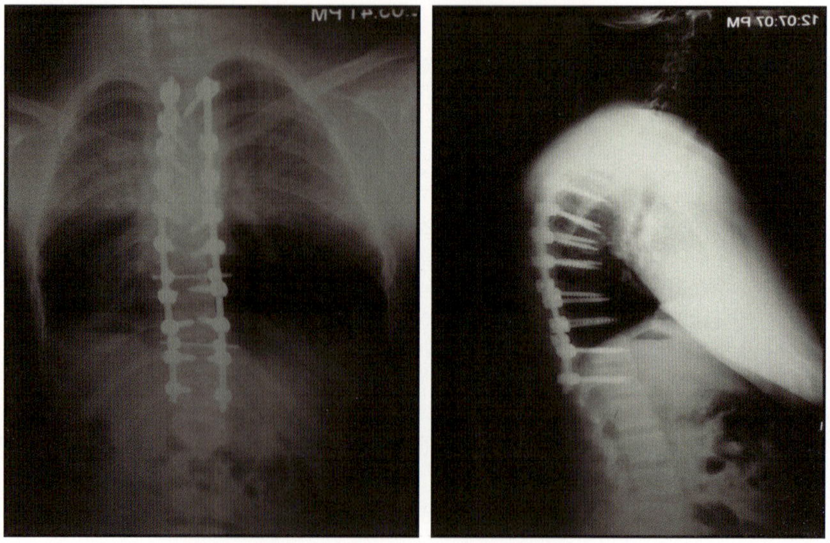

(c) Postoperative 3-year AP-Lateral X-ray

FIGURE 3

resection aids in the correction of the deformity by a lever effect. There were no significant recurrences in the coronal and sagittal plane deformities during the follow-up period. These results demonstrate that hemivertebra resection by a posterior approach with segmental posterior transpedicular instrumentation is an effective and safe treatment options in children with congenital spine deformities. Despite the five-year follow-up period, it is appropriate to reevaluate all of the patients at the end of the growth cycle to say that the deformity does not recur.

References

[1] M. J. McMaster and H. Singh, "Natural History of Congenital Kyphosis and Kyphoscoliosis. A Study of One Hundred and Twelve Patients," *The Journal of Bone & Joint Surgery*, vol. 81, no. 10, pp. 1367–1383, 1999.

[2] J. Zhang, W. Shengru, G. Qiu, B. Yu, W. Yipeng, and K. D. Luk, "The efficacy and complications of posterior hemivertebra resection," *European Spine Journal*, vol. 20, no. 10, pp. 1692–1702, 2011.

[3] M. Ruf and J. Harms, "Hemivertebra resection by a posterior approach: innovative operative technique and first results," *Spine*, vol. 27, no. 10, pp. 1116–1123, 2002.

[4] K. Mladenov, P. Kunkel, and R. Stuecker, "Hemivertebra resection in children, results after single posterior approach and after combined anterior and posterior approach: a comparative study," *European Spine Journal*, vol. 21, no. 3, pp. 506–513, 2012.

[5] D. C. Holte, R. B. Winter, J. E. Lonstein, and F. Denis, "Excision

of hemivertebrae and wedge resection in the treatment of congenital scoliosis," *The Journal of Bone & Joint Surgery*, vol. 77, no. 2, pp. 159–171, 1995.

[6] M. Ruf, R. Jensen, L. Letko, and J. Harms, "Hemivertebra Resection and Osteotomies in Congenital Spine Deformity," *Spine*, vol. 34, no. 17, pp. 1791–1799, 2009.

[7] T. Jalanko, R. Rintala, V. Puisto, and I. Helenius, "Hemivertebra resection for congenital scoliosis in young children: comparison of clinical, radiographic, and health-related quality of life outcomes between the anteroposterior and posterolateral approaches," *Spine*, vol. 36, no. 1, pp. 41–49, 2011.

[8] Y. Shono, K. Abumi, and K. Kaneda, "One-Stage Posterior Hemivertebra Resection and Correction Using Segmental Posterior Instrumentation," *Spine*, vol. 26, no. 7, pp. 752–757, 2001.

[9] R. B. Winter, J. H. Moe, and J. E. Lonstein, "Posterior spinal arthrodesis for congenital scoliosis. An analysis of the cases of two hundred and ninety patients, five to nineteen years old," *The Journal of Bone & Joint Surgery*, vol. 66, no. 8, pp. 1188–1197, 1984.

[10] S. Wang, J. Zhang, G. Qiu, S. Li, B. Yu, and X. Weng, "Posterior hemivertebra resection with bisegmental fusion for congenital scoliosis: more than 3 year outcomes and analysis of unanticipated surgeries," *European Spine Journal*, vol. 22, no. 2, pp. 387–393, 2013.

[11] A. Alanay, O. Dede, and M. Yazici, "Convex Instrumented Hemiepiphysiodesis with Concave Distraction: A Preliminary Report," *Clinical Orthopaedics and Related Research®*, vol. 470, no. 4, pp. 1144–1150, 2012.

[12] B. Yaszay, M. O'Brien, H. L. Shufflebarger et al., "Efficacy of hemivertebra resection for congenital scoliosis: a multicenter retrospective comparison of three surgical techniques," *Spine*, vol. 36, no. 24, pp. 2052–2060, 2011.

[13] H. B. Elsebaie, W. Kaptan, Y. El Miligui et al., "Anterior Instrumentation and Correction of Congenital Spinal Deformities Under Age of Four Without Hemivertebrectomy: a New Alternative," *Spine*, vol. 35, no. 6, pp. E218–E222, 2010.

[14] H. B. Elsebai, M. Yazici, G. H. Thompson et al., "Safety and efficacy of growing rod technique for pediatric congenital spinal deformities," *Journal of Pediatric Orthopaedics*, vol. 31, no. 1, pp. 1–5, 2011.

[15] N. D. Royle, "The operative removal of an accessory vertebra," *Med J Aust*, vol. 1, pp. 467-468, 1928.

[16] V. Deviren, S. Berven, J. A. Smith, A. Emami, S. S. Hu, and D. S. Bradford, "Excision of hemivertebrae in the management of congenital scoliosis involving the thoracic and thoracolumbar spine," *The Journal of Bone and Joint Surgery*, vol. 83, no. 4, pp. 496–500, 2001.

[17] B. C. Callahan, G. Georgopoulos, and R. E. Eilert, "Hemivertebral Excision for Congenital Scoliosis," *Journal of Pediatric Orthopaedics*, vol. 17, no. 1, pp. 96–99, 1997.

[18] W. Xu, S. Yang, X. Wu, and C. Claus, "Hemivertebra excision with short-segment spinal fusion through combined anterior and posterior approaches for congenital spinal deformities in children," *Journal of Pediatric Orthopaedics B*, vol. 19, no. 6, pp. 545–550, 2010.

[19] M. Aydogan, C. Ozturk, M. Tezer, C. Mirzanli, O. Karatoprak, and A. Hamzaoglu, "Posterior vertebrectomy in kyphosis, scoliosis and kyphoscoliosis due to hemivertebra," *Journal of Pediatric Orthopaedics B*, vol. 17, no. 1, pp. 33–37, 2008.

[20] H. Nakamura, H. Matsuda, S. Konishi, and Y. Yamano, "Single-stage excision of hemivertebrae via the posterior approach alone for congenital spine deformity: follow-up period longer than ten years," *Spine*, vol. 27, no. 1, pp. 110–115, 2002.

4

Pathology and Treatment of Traumatic Cervical Spine Syndrome: Whiplash Injury

Nobuhiro Tanaka,[1] Kivanc Atesok,[2] Kazuyoshi Nakanishi,[1] Naosuke Kamei,[1] Toshio Nakamae,[1] Shinji Kotaka,[1] and Nobuo Adachi[1]

[1]*Department of Orthopaedic Surgery, Institute of Biomedical & Health Sciences, Hiroshima University, Hiroshima, Japan*
[2]*Department of Orthopaedic Surgery, University of Alabama at Birmingham, Birmingham, AL, USA*

Correspondence should be addressed to Nobuhiro Tanaka; nobut@hiroshima-u.ac.jp

Academic Editor: John P. Kostuik

Traumatic cervical syndrome comprises the various symptoms that occur as a result of external force such as that of a traffic accident. In 1995, the Quebec Task Force on whiplash-associated disorders (WAD) formulated the Quebec classification, with accompanying clinical practice guidelines. These guidelines were in accordance with the stated clinical isolated or combined symptoms of the syndrome: neck pain, headaches, dizziness, numbness of head or face, eye pain, vision loss, double vision, tinnitus, hearing loss, nausea, and numbness and/or weakness of extremities. In recent years, cerebrospinal fluid hypovolemia or fibromyalgia has been recognized as a major notable cause of a variety of symptoms, although many clinical questions remain regarding the pathology of this syndrome. Therefore, its diagnosis and treatment should be conducted extremely carefully. While the Quebec classification and its guidelines are very useful for the normalization and standardization of symptoms of traumatic cervical syndrome, in the future, we would like to see the emergence of new guidelines that better address the diversity of this disease.

1. Introduction

Traumatic cervical syndrome is defined as the "biological and neurological consequences for the cervical spine and nervous system caused by neck trauma, and is a syndrome comprising various symptoms of the motor and nervous system [1] but also mental, neurological, as well as otological and visual balance dysfunction" [2, 3] (Table 1). The symptoms can include minor neck trauma without the so-called "whip" movement of the neck. "Whiplash injury," which has been traditionally diagnosed after a traffic injury, is pathologically incorrect and should not be used as part of clinical language, because it may cause various misunderstandings among communities and patients. Most injuries occur during a rear-end auto accident, but the injury can also result from a sports accident, physical abuse, or other trauma. Also Ferrari [4] noticed that whiplash is an example of illness induced by society, in general, and by physicians in particular. These symptoms may appear even in the absence of any visible injuries.

The report of the Quebec Task Force on whiplash-associated disorders in 1995 classified whiplash-associated disorders (WAD) into five grades based on symptoms and severity [2]. In this manuscript, we discuss the clinical signs of traumatic cervical syndrome which conform to the Quebec classification.

2. Quebec Classification

The Quebec classification includes neck symptoms and a range of neurological problems, as well as spine fractures or dislocations, and it is divided into 5 grades from 0 to IV [2] (Tables 2 and 3). Grades 0, I, and II correspond to the so-called "whiplash injury," and grades III and IV are classified as traumatic cervical spinal cord injury. Symptoms such as

Table 1: Neurological symptoms after whiplash injury [1].

Headaches	Migraine-type headache Tension-type headache Cervicogenic-type headache Temporomandibular joint derangement Greater occipital neuralgia Third occipital headache
Cognitive and psychological symptoms	Memory, attention, or concentration impairment Sleep disturbance Psychiatric disorders: anxiety, depression, phobic travel, anxiety, and posttraumatic stress disorder
Dizziness	Vestibular dysfunction Cervical origin Brainstem dysfunction
Visual symptoms	Blurred vision Reduced visual field Photophobia Disordered fusion Reading and driving difficulties Reduced accommodation
Paresthesias	Trigger points Brachial plexopathy Cervical radiculopathy Spinal cord compression
Weakness	Brachial plexopathy Cervical radiculopathy Spinal cord compression
Rare symptoms	Torticollis Tremor Transient global amnesia Hypoglossal nerve palsy Superior laryngeal nerve paralysis Cervical epidural hematoma Brainstem infarct Internal carotid and vertebral artery dissection Symptomatic Chiari malformation

Table 2: Clinical classification on whiplash-associated disorders proposed by the Quebec Task Force [2].

Grade	Clinical presentation
0	No complaint about neck pain No physical signs
I	Neck complaint of pain, stiffness, or tenderness No physical signs
II	Neck complaint Musculoskeletal signs including Decreased range of movement Point tenderness
II	Neck complaint Musculoskeletal signs Neurological signs including Decreased or absent deep tendon reflexes Muscle weakness Sensory deficits
IV	Neck complaint and fracture or dislocation

dizziness, tinnitus, headache, memory loss, swallowing, and temporomandibular joint pain can appear in any grade.

3. Clinical Symptoms

3.1. Neck Pain. Although symptoms of traumatic cervical syndrome vary from patient to patient (Table 1), neck pain and cervical discomfort are typical symptoms [1]. Deans et al. [6] reported that neck pain occurs in 65% of patients within 6 hours, 93% within 24 hours, and 100% within 72 hours after neck injury. Many factors can influence the extent and location of the injury, such as traffic accident specifics (speed, direction, and safety equipment) and the state of the victim's cervical spine. In addition to the constructional elements of the cervical spine such as muscles, intervertebral discs, and facet joints, the injury may be caused by neural elements including the spinal dorsal root ganglion, vertebral artery, and the sympathetic nervous system. Typical clinical characteristics of the injury include the patient not complaining of neck pain immediately after the accident, but then complaining of neck pain a few hours later or the next day. This time lag can be explained by synovitis of the facet joints, where the synovial tissue involved in the facet joint has been damaged by nonphysiological behavior during a collision, which may induce synovitis of the facet joint after several hours, leading to neck pain and a limited range of motion [7].

In general, traumatic cervical spine syndrome is not protracted, and many patients recover from the symptoms within a few weeks or months. However, some reports suggest that neck pain and headaches continue for several years in 20–40% of patients, with 3-4% of patients unable to return to work [8]. Radanov et al. [9] reported that 97% of chronic traumatic cervical syndrome patients have neck pain. Clinical conditions are usually complicated and enigmatic when the injury is chronic, while the potential exists for abnormally prolonged arthritis of the synovial membrane, cervical nerve root irritation of the posterior branches, and vestibular reflex abnormalities due to vestibular dysfunction, neck muscle tension, or fibromyalgia (see below), but details of the pathology remain unclear.

3.2. Headache. Headaches present as chronic symptoms in 70% of patients [8]. According to the headache classification proposed by the International Headache Society (2nd edition) [10] (Section 3.2.1), a cervicogenic headache is defined as a headache resulting from disorders of the cervical spine. The diagnostic criteria following the blockade of a cervical

Table 3: Clinical spectrum of whiplash-associated disorders as proposed by the Quebec Task Force [2].

Grade	Presumed pathology	Clinical presentation
I	Microscopic or multimicroscopic lesion Lesion is not serious enough to cause muscle spasm	Usually presents to a doctor more than 24 h after trauma
II	Neck sprain and bleeding around soft tissue (articular capsules, ligaments, tendons, and muscles) Muscle spasm secondary to soft tissue injury	Usually presents to a doctor in the first 24 h after trauma Nonspecific radiation to the head, face, occipital region, shoulder, and arm form soft tissues injuries Neck pain with limited range of motion due to muscle spasm
III	Injuries to neurologic system by mechanical injury or by irritation secondary to bleeding or inflammation	Presents to a doctor usually within a few hours after the trauma Limited range of motion combined with neurologic symptoms and signs

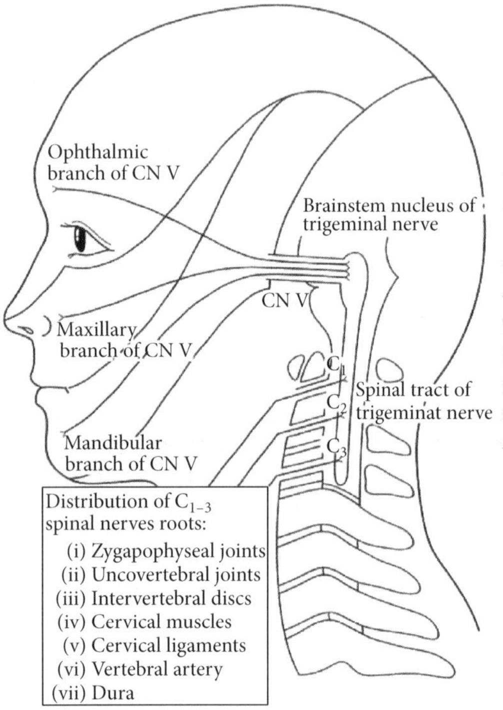

Figure 1: Schema of connection between upper spinal nerve roots and trigeminal nerve [5].

structure include referred pain from a source in the neck, perceived in the head and/or face, and evidence of a disorder or lesion within the cervical spine or soft tissues of the neck.

Some of the proposed trigger mechanisms of a cervicogenic headache are compression or inflammation of the C2 nerve root; referred pain of the first branch of the trigeminal nerve from C2 nerve root irritation trough anastomosis; emerging pain in the trigeminal nerve area caused by stimulation of the upper spinal nerve roots from the anatomical connection between the spinal trigeminal nucleus and dorsal horn at the C2-3 spinal level [5] (Figure 1); a tension headache due to entrapment of the occipital nerve after pericranial muscles constrict from cervical muscle strain or spasm. Many cervicogenic headaches are caused by movement of the neck, and pain is usually located in the occipital region, with persistent pain gradually increasing on an elapsed chronic course. Psychological factors such as fatigue, lack of sleep, stress, and depression are reported to influence cervicogenic headaches [7].

3.2.1. Diagnostic Criteria of Cervicogenic Headache [8]

(A) Pain, referred from a source in the neck and perceived in one or more regions of the head and/or face, fulfilling criteria (C) and (D)

(B) Clinical, laboratory, and/or imaging evidence of a disorder or lesion within the cervical spine or soft tissues of the neck known to be, or generally accepted as, a valid cause of headache (Tumors, fractures, infections, and rheumatoid arthritis of the upper cervical spine have not been validated formally as causes of headache but are nevertheless accepted as valid causes when demonstrated to be so in individual cases. Cervical spondylosis and osteochondritis are not accepted as valid causes for the fulfillment of criterion (B). When myofascial tender spots are the cause, the headache should be coded under 2, *tension-type headache.*)

(C) Evidence that the pain can be attributed to the neck disorder or lesion based on at least one of the following:

(1) Demonstration of clinical signs that implicate a source of pain in the neck (Clinical signs acceptable for criterion C1 must have demonstrated reliability and validity. The future task is the identification of such reliable and valid operational tests. Clinical features such as neck pain, focal neck tenderness, history of neck trauma, mechanical exacerbation of pain, unilaterality, coexisting shoulder pain, reduced range

of motion in the neck, nuchal onset, nausea, vomiting, and photophobia are not unique to a cervicogenic headache. These may be features of a cervicogenic headache, but they do not define the relationship between the disorder and the source of the headache.)

(2) Abolition of headache following diagnostic blockade of a cervical structure or its nerve supply using placebo or other adequate controls (Abolition of headache means complete relief of headache, indicated by a score of zero on a visual analogue scale (VAS). Nevertheless, acceptable as fulfilling criterion C2 is ≥90% reduction in pain to a level of <5 on a 100-point VAS.)

(D) Pain resolves within 3 months after successful treatment of the causative disorder or lesion

3.3. Vertigo. There are two types of dizziness: vertigo and planktonic, and physicians should be careful in their diagnosis of the symptoms, because brain-stem bleeding sometimes manifests itself as vertigo, when in fact it is mostly caused by an inner ear disorder. Planktonic dizziness is caused by craniocervical disorder (Chiari malformation, spinal cord tumor, etc.) or failure of the input system regarding the spinal cord. Dizziness originating from the cervical spine is collectively known as cervical vertigo, and it may be caused by circulatory failure of the vertebral artery, proprioceptor dysfunction of the cervical spine (nerve root or spinal cord disorders at C1—3), or cervical sympathetic nervous system disorders (Barré-Lieou syndrome). Hinoki [11] proposed a hypothesis in which the hypothalamus plays a fundamental role in explaining vertigo after injury. They reported that autonomic reflexes in patients with whiplash injury can be explained as being not only due to overexcitation of the cervical sympathetic nerves, but also due to the cervical and lumbar proprioceptors in producing vertigo.

3.4. Barré-Lieou Syndrome. Symptoms of Barré-Lieou syndrome include headache, dizziness, and other cervical sympathetic nervous system disorders, some of which can be classified as traumatic. Hypertension of the cervical sympathetic nerves and vertebral arterial circulatory disorders, stem failure, peripheral vestibular disorders, and psychogenic problems are caused mainly by stress. These symptoms are known as posterior cervical sympathetic syndrome, previously recognized as a syndrome associated with chronic cervical disease, but recently it often comprises a convenient but false diagnosis for atypical symptoms [12].

3.5. Numbness in Head and Face. Disruption of the trigeminal spinal nucleus, which conveys superficial facial perception along the C2-3 spinal level (see above), can lead to numbness or loss of sensation around the face in an "onion skin" distribution area, followed by a spinal cord lesion at the upper cervical spine [6].

3.6. Eye Symptoms. There are reports that eye symptoms emerge in 35% of traumatic cervical syndrome patients [13]. Eye pain due to trigeminal nerve stimulation, eye movement disorder (double vision) caused by oculomotor nerve disorders, visual deficit due to optic nerve disorders, and blepharoptosis due to sympathetic nervous system disorders are present.

3.7. Nausea and Vomiting. It is reported that nausea and vomiting are found in 17 to 29% of patients. Almost all cases have neck pain complications. Subsequently these symptoms persist for more than 6 months in 33% of patients [7].

3.8. Limb Symptoms. Numbness or muscle weakness of the upper extremities may appear as nerve root or spinal cord symptoms, although limb symptoms of traumatic cervical syndrome often do not produce any findings in imaging studies. Because there are few available laboratory procedures for these patients, appropriate treatment based on their pathophysiology is difficult to administer.

De Reuck [14] reported the usefulness of investigating motor evoked potentials (MEPs) in patients who had been suffering from grade II WAD for more than 6 months. They found that 13 patients had prolonged central (CMCT) and/or peripheral motor conduction times (PMCT) compared to normal values, and they recommended that MEP examination be performed in all patients with persistent pain even in the absence of objective neurological signs and nonsignificant changes on imaging. In our study, we also used electrophysiological examination using MEPs following transcranial magnetic stimulation for traumatic cervical syndrome patients, and we found significant elongation in PMCT and/or distal latencies following nerve stimulation at the cervical nerve root or Erb's point in 4 out of 11 patients who had limb symptoms without significant imaging abnormalities but with no obvious CMCT abnormalities [15]. These results may indicate potential nerve disorder in the cervical nerve root or brachial plexus in patients with traumatic cervical syndrome, even in those who develop symptoms of malaise without obvious muscle atrophy or electromyographic changes.

3.9. Other. The mechanisms of the following symptoms are unclear: ringing in the ears, hearing loss, insomnia, loss of concentration, fatigability, fever, memory loss, temporomandibular joint pain, and anginal-like chest pain (cervical angina).

4. CSF Hypovolemia

In Japan, some physicians have insisted that the cause of CSF hypovolemia is traumatic CSF leak, and they call this syndrome traumatic CSF hypovolemia [16]. CSF hypovolemia syndrome exhibits a variety of symptoms such as neck pain, visual deficit, double vision, dizziness, nausea, vomiting, ringing in the ears, hearing loss, and headaches. These symptoms resemble those of a whiplash injury, and some of them occur sporadically as traumatic cervical syndrome [17–19]. The diagnostic criteria of traumatic CSF leakage is defined as follows: (1) early vesicular radioisotope cisternography (RIC) accumulation (EVA); (2) promoted radioisotope (RI)

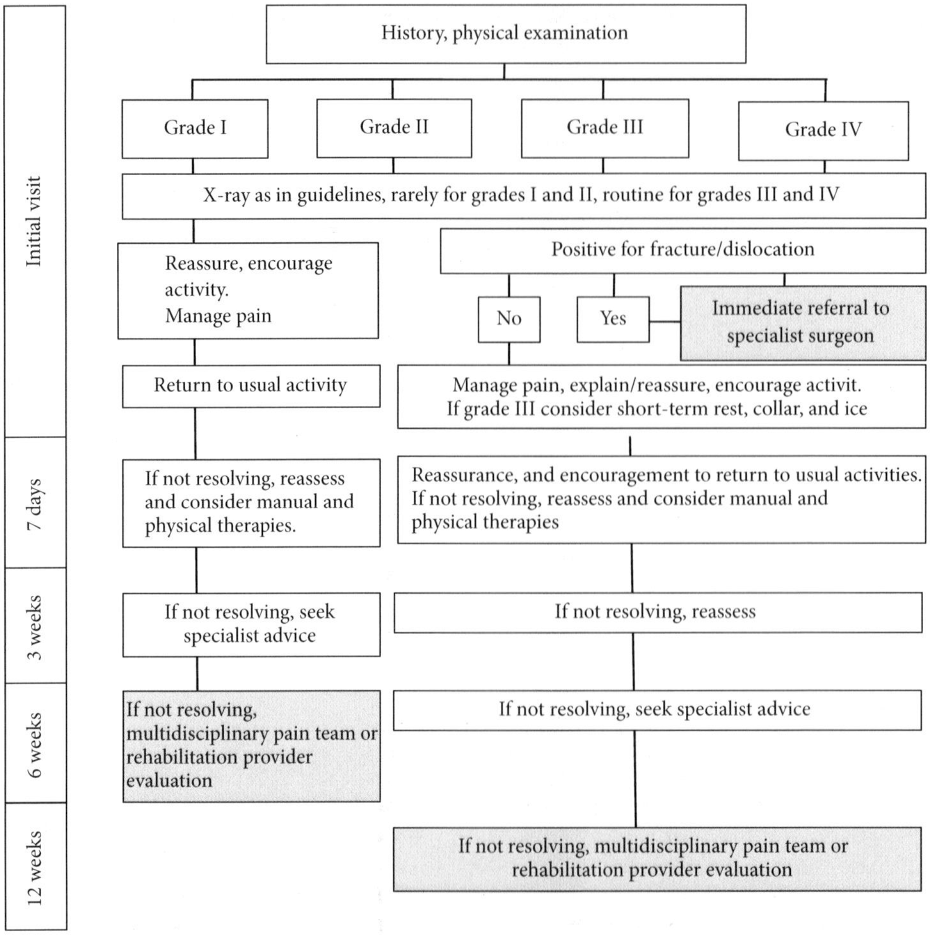

FIGURE 2: Clinical practice guidelines by Quebec Task Force on whiplash-associated disorders [2].

clearance from the spinal cavity; (3) presence of abnormal paraspinal RI accumulation (PSA) [20]. However, Hashizume et al. [21] reported that traumatic CSF leak was not observed on CT myelography findings in patients with WAD, in whom CSF leak was suspected when comparing the RIC. An epidural blood patch (EBP) is the therapy of choice in patients with chronic WAD with a suspected CSF leak. Treatment for traumatic cervical spine syndrome should be uniform and logically based on medical science, and invasive treatment such as EBP should be carefully performed only in selected patients. The association of a CSF leak with chronic WAD has never been established, although its symptoms may be reduced following treatment.

5. Fibromyalgia

Fibromyalgia is defined as a neurosensory disorder characterized by widespread muscle pain, joint stiffness, and fatigue, and there are almost no inflammatory findings or abnormalities which indicate organic disorders such as bone and joint diseases, neurodegenerative diseases, rheumatic diseases, or malignant tumors. Other common symptoms of fibromyalgia present with psychosomatic characteristics, such as irritability, sleep disorders, anxiety, depression, and the onset of this disease, are seen predominantly in women in their fifties.

Fibromyalgia is reported to occur as a result of cervical spine injury in 21.6% of patients [22]. Ferrari [23] prospectively examined 268 patients and he found 2 cases (0.8%) of fibromyalgia after acute whiplash injury. Although the etiology and development processes may relate to mental fatigue or physical trauma based on genetic predisposition, the relationship between spine injury and fibromyalgia remains unclear.

6. Clinical Practice for Quebec Guidelines

Clinical practice guidelines were established by the Quebec Task Force on whiplash-associated disorders [2] (Figure 2), to standardize the treatment and its duration based on the severity of symptoms. The final treatment evaluation regarding soft tissue repair is determined at 12 weeks after injury. However, as mentioned above, traumatic cervical syndrome has symptoms across diverse fields such as otolaryngology, neurology, neurosurgery, and internal medicine, as well as orthopaedic symptoms, and they overlap (functional anatomic factors), vary in duration (a time factor), and depend on the biological or social situation of the patient (individual factors). For treatment of WAD, clinicians should realise that expression of clinical symptoms is implicated in biopsychosocial model. WAD according to the Quebec classification can range from a muscle sprain to spinal cord contusions to a fractured vertebra. The latter two are rarer and can easily be detected. But, for the majority of cases, there are considerable cases who have pain with no visible cause. Therefore, the Quebec guidelines may not be applicable for all patients with traumatic cervical syndrome. Although the Quebec classification and its guidelines are very useful for standardization of the symptoms of traumatic cervical syndrome, more comprehensive guidelines are necessary to enable more accurate treatment responses to this diverse disease.

References

[1] D. C. Alpini, G. Brugnoni, and A. Cesarani, Eds., *Whiplash Injuries Diagnosis and Treatment*, Springer-Verlag, Italia, 2nd edition, 2014.

[2] W. O. Spitzer, M. L. Skvtn, L. R. Salmi et al., "Scientific monograph of the Quebec task force on whiplash-assciated disorders: redefining "whiplash"and its management," *Spine*, vol. 20, pp. 2–235, 1995.

[3] R. W. Teasell, "The clinical picture of whiplash injuries," in *Spine: State of the Art Reviews Vol 7 No3 Cervical Flexion-extension Whiplash Injuries*, R. W. Teasell and A. P. Shapiro, Eds., pp. 373–389, Hanley & Belfus, Philadelphia, Pa, USA, 1993.

[4] M. Ferrari, *The Whiplash Encyclopedia*, Jones Bartlett Learning, 2006.

[5] S. Haldeman and S. Dagenais, "Cervicogenic headaches: A critical review," *The Spine Journal*, vol. 1, no. 1, pp. 31–46, 2001.

[6] G. T. Deans, J. N. Magalliard, M. Kerr, and W. H. Rutherford, "Neck sprain-a major cause of disability following car accidents," *Injury*, vol. 18, no. 1, pp. 10–12, 1987.

[7] K. Endo, *Whiplash Injury Handbook*, Springer-Japan, Tokyo, Japan, 2006.

[8] M. Benoist and J.-P. Rouaud, "Whiplash: myth or reality?" *Joint Bone Spine*, vol. 69, no. 4, pp. 358–362, 2002.

[9] B. P. Radanov, G. Di Stefano, A. Schnidrig, and M. Sturzenegger, "Common whiplash: Psychosomatic or somatopsychic?" *Journal of Neurology, Neurosurgery & Psychiatry*, vol. 57, no. 4, pp. 486–490, 1994.

[10] Head Classification Committee of The International Headache Society, "The international classification of headache disorders," *Cephalagia 24 (suppll)*, vol. 9, no. 160, 2004.

[11] M. Hinoki, "Vertigo due to whiplash injury: a neuro-otological approach," *Acta Oto-Laryngologica Supplementum*, vol. 419, pp. 9–29, 1985.

[12] J. M. Perce, "Barre-Lieu "syndrome"," *Neurol Neurosurg Psychiatry*, vol. 75, no. 319, 2004.

[13] N. Bogduk, "Post whiplash syndrome.," *Australian Family Physician*, vol. 23, no. 12, pp. 2303–2307, 1994.

[14] J. De Reuck, "Motor evoked potentials in patients with chronic whiplash-associated disorder grade II," *Neurologia i Neurochirurgia Polska*, vol. 51, no. 5, pp. 372–374, 2017.

[15] Y. Oishi, N. Tanaka, and Y. Ito, "Electrical physiological study of traumatic cervical syndrome; using magnetic stimulation motor evoked potentials," *[in Japanese] The Journal of the Japanese Society and for Spine Surgery and Related Research*, vol. 15: 394, 2004.

[16] M. Shinonaga, "Diagnosis and treatment of low cerebrospinal fluid pressure headache," *Japan Medical Association*, vol. 136, pp. 2205–2208, 2008.

[17] G. Schaltenbrand, "Neuere Anschauungen zur Pathphysilgie de Liqurzirkulatin," *Zenteralbl Neurochir*, vol. 3, pp. 290–300, 1938.

[18] S. Chen, M. Hagiwara, and P. C. Roehm, "Spontaneous intracranial hypotension presenting with severe sensorineural hearing loss and headache," *Otology & Neurotology*, vol. 33, no. 8, pp. e65–e66, 2012.

[19] E. Moriyama, H. Terada, and S. Ishikawa, "Spinal cerebrospinal fluid leakage after motor vehicle accident - Two case reports," *Neurologia medico-chirurgica*, vol. 49, no. 7, pp. 306–309, 2009.

[20] The Committee for the Guideline of the Cerebrospinal Fluid Hypovolemia Workshop, "Guideline for diagnosis of cerebrospinal fluid hypovolemia," in *Cerebrospinal Fluid Hypovolemia Workshop*, Medical Review Co., Tokyo, Japan, 2007, 15–8.

[21] K. Hashizume, K. Watanabe, M. Kawaguchi, A. Fujiwara, and H. Furuya, "Comparison between computed tomography-myelography and radioisotope- cisternography findings in whiplash-associated disorders suspected to be caused by traumatic cerebrospinal fluid leak," *The Spine Journal*, vol. 37, no. 12, pp. E721–E726, 2012.

[22] D. Buskila, L. Neumann, G. Vaisberg, D. Alkalay, and F. Wolfe, "Increased rates of fibromyalgia following cervical spine injury: a controlled study of 161 cases of traumatic injury," *Arthritis & Rheumatism*, vol. 40, no. 3, pp. 446–452, 1997.

[23] R. Ferrari, "A prospective study of the 1-year incidence of fibromyalgia after acute whiplash injury," *RMD Open*, vol. 1, no. 1, Article ID e000007, 2015.

5

Spinopelvic Dissociation: Comparison of Outcomes of Percutaneous versus Open Fixation Strategies

Jeffrey M. Pearson,[1] Thomas E. Niemeier,[1] Gerald McGwin,[2] and Sakthivel Rajaram Manoharan[1]

[1]*Department of Orthopedic Surgery, University of Alabama at Birmingham, Birmingham, AL, USA*
[2]*Department of Epidemiology, University of Alabama at Birmingham, Birmingham, AL, USA*

Correspondence should be addressed to Thomas E. Niemeier; niemeier.te@gmail.com

Academic Editor: Yohan Robinson

Introduction. Spinopelvic dissociation injuries are historically treated with open reduction with or without decompressive laminectomy. Recent technological advances have allowed for percutaneous fixation with indirect reduction. Herein, we evaluate outcomes and complications between patients treated with open reduction versus percutaneous spinopelvic fixation. *Methods.* Retrospective review of patients undergoing spinopelvic fixation from a single, level one trauma center from 2012 to 2017. Patient information regarding demographics, associated injuries, and treatment outcome measures was recorded and analyzed. All fractures were classified via the AO Spine classification system. *Results.* Thirty-one spinopelvic dissociations were identified: 15 treated with open and 16 with percutaneous techniques. The two treatment groups had similar preoperative characteristics including spinopelvic parameters (pelvic incidence and lumbar lordosis). Compared to open reduction internal fixation, percutaneous fixation of spinopelvic dissociation resulted in statistically significantly lower blood loss (171 cc versus 538 cc; $p = 0.0013$). There were no significant differences in surgical site infections ($p = 0.48$) or operating room time ($p = 0.66$). *Conclusion.* Percutaneous fixation of spinopelvic dissociation is associated with significantly less blood loss. Treatment outcomes in terms of infection, length of stay, operative cost, and final alignment between the open and percutaneous group were similar.

1. Introduction

Spinopelvic dissociation or U type sacrum fracture is a rare injury that involves a transverse sacral fracture pattern and can be associated with a high rate of neurologic injury, up to 57% (Figure 1) [1–4]. In large case series, spinopelvic dissociative injuries account for only 2.9% of all pelvic ring traumas [5, 6]. Traditional treatment methods involving open reduction with internal fixation have been observed to have high rates of postoperative infections up to 14–16% [7–10]. In the last decade, percutaneous fixation (Figure 2) of these injuries has gained popularity with reported improved clinical outcomes [11, 12].

Herein, we critically evaluate results of spinopelvic dissociations treated with either percutaneous or open reduction. To our knowledge, this is the largest series of patients with spinopelvic dissociation treated surgically. We hypothesized that percutaneous fixation of spinopelvic dissociation using minimally invasive fusion from lumbar four or five to pelvis would result in shorter operative time, fewer postoperative transfusions, and decreased estimated blood loss while adequately reestablishing spinopelvic parameters.

2. Methods

A retrospective review was conducted on all operatively managed spinopelvic dissociations treated between January 2012 and March 2017 at a single, level one trauma center. Institutional review board approval was obtained. Inclusion criteria were patients over 18 years of age with diagnosed spinopelvic dissociation based on pelvic X-rays and CT scans. Patients with preoperative lower lumbar, sacral, or pelvic hardware were excluded. Patient characteristics and demographics

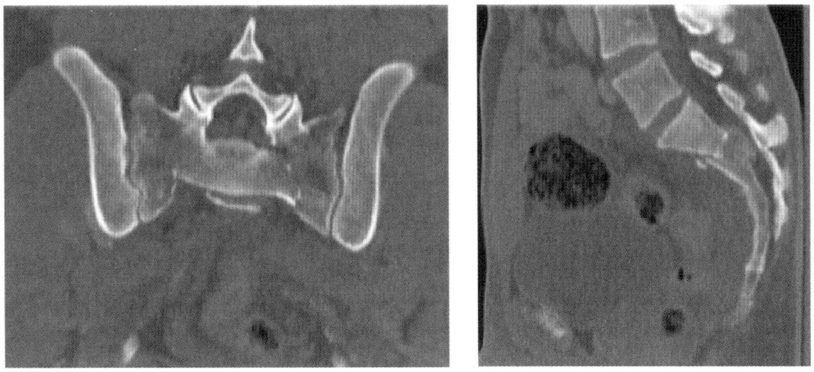

(a) (b)

Figure 1: Coronal (a) and midsagittal (b) preoperative CT scan. Note the bilateral sacral fractures with horizontal S2 fracture with a 37-degree kyphotic deformity.

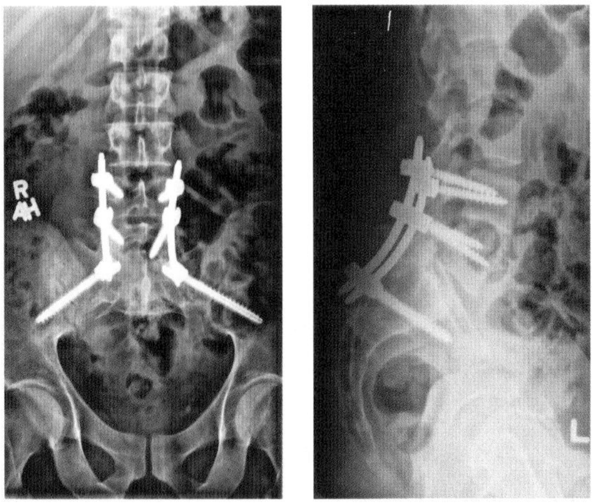

(a) (b)

Figure 2: AP (a) and lateral (b) radiographs of patient seen in Figure 1 at 16 months postoperatively treated with percutaneous fixation. Note the resolution of kyphotic deformity with consolidation of fracture lines.

were collected for all patients including age, gender, mechanism of injury, associated injuries, neurological injury, and tobacco use. The injuries were classified according to the Arbeitsgemeinschaft für Osteosynthesefragen (AO) sacrum classification. Pelvic X-rays were also subclassified based on modifiers M3 being anterior pelvic ring injury and M4 sacroiliac joint injury [13].

All surgeries were performed by fellowship-trained spine, orthopedic surgeons during this initial inpatient stay. The decision of open versus percutaneous fixation was nonrandomized and at the judgment of the attending surgeon. This was usually based on associated injuries such as soft tissue near a possible incision site, body habitus, and surgeon training. Younger trained surgeons tended to perform percutaneous procedures while older ones tended to perform traditional open reduction techniques. All percutaneous surgeries used indirect reduction and four or five percutaneous lumbar pedicle screws with iliac fixation as described by Wang et al. [11]. Percutaneous transsacral fixation was not used in any of the patients. Neurological dysfunction (cauda equina or sacral nerve root disruption) was treated with either laminectomies or fracture reduction with indirect decompression.

The surgical procedure began with standard spinal monitoring and general anesthesia. The patients were positioned prone on an open top table with large bumps under the thighs to accentuate an extension force on the legs. This high extension was our main reduction maneuver in the surgical procedure. Bilateral L5 pedicle screws were placed under fluoroscopic guidance with Jamshidi needles, and these were also used for the iliac fixation. Initial placement of the needle for iliac fixation was just ventromedial to the PSIS. From this point using a teardrop view, the Jamshidi needle was guided down between the inner and the outer tables of the pelvis. Following placement of the needle, inlet, outlet, and lateral views were obtained to ensure no violation of the sciatic notch.

In-hospital clinical outcomes were measured and included surgical site infection, transfusions within 72 hours postoperatively, operative time, and estimated blood loss.

Table 1: Preoperative patient characteristics.

	Open (n = 15)	Closed (n = 16)	p value
Age	44.86	37.87	0.3046
Gender	Male: 9 Female: 6	Male: 11 Female: 5	0.7160
Tobacco use	8 (53%)	8 (50%)	0.4589
Cauda equina	3 (20%)	3 (18%)	1.00

After discharge, patients were followed up at routine intervals as outpatients. Postoperative complications including hardware irritation and spinopelvic parameters (pelvic incidence and lumbar lordosis) were recorded for all patients. All patients were made weight bearing as tolerated unless other lower extremity fractures prohibited this.

Demographic, clinical, and outcome measures were compared between the fixation groups using Fisher's exact test and Student's t-test for categorical and continuous variables, respectively. p values ≤ 0.05 (two-sided) were considered statistically significant.

3. Results

Thirty-one patients with spinopelvic dissociation were identified at our institution from 2012 to 2017. The cohort consisted of 15 patients treated with open reduction and lumbopelvic fixation and 16 with indirect reduction and percutaneous lumbopelvic fixation. Age, sex, and tobacco use were similar between the two groups ($p > 0.05$) (Table 1). Outpatient follow-up was on average 7.8 months for the open group and 9.9 months for the closed group ($p = 0.50$). Both groups included three patients with preoperative symptoms of cauda equina.

Injury patterns were classified based on the AO sacrum classification system [13]. Our results can be found in Table 2. Fractures were classified as nondisplaced sacral U type variant (C0), sacral U type variant without posterior instability (C1), bilateral complete type B fractures without transverse fracture (C2), and displaced U type sacrum fracture (C3). In addition to these categories, fractures were also classified based on modifiers of anterior pelvic ring injury (M3) and sacroiliac joint injury (M4). Of the 15 open procedures, 5 were C0, 1 was C2, and 9 were C3. Of these 15, a total of 6 were M3 modifiers signifying anterior pelvic ring injury. Of the 16 percutaneous procedures, 8 were classified as C0 and 8 were C3. Five from the C0 percutaneous subgroup had M3 modifiers. Of the C3 group, 2 had an anterior ring injury (M3), 1 had a posterior sacroiliac joint disruption (M4), and a total of 2 had both modifiers (M3, M4). This information can be found in Table 2.

Associated injuries are shown in Table 3. The cohort of 31 patients included 18 (58%) with long bone fractures (8 in the open and 10 in the closed group) that prompted surgical treatment. Other associated injuries included closed head injuries (42%), acetabular fractures (39%), and other spine fractures (48%).

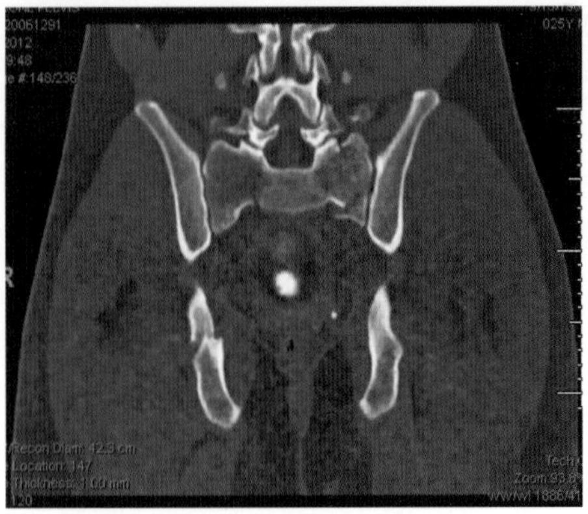

Figure 3: Preoperative coronal CT scan of a patient with spinopelvic dissociation.

Postoperative outcomes are shown in Table 4. Mean intraoperative blood loss was significantly higher ($p = 0.0013$) in the open reduction (538 cc) group in comparison to the percutaneous group (171 cc). Transfusions within 72 hours postoperatively were seen in seven patients (43%) treated with percutaneous fixation and in three patients (20%) treated with open reduction ($p = 0.25$). Average length of stay for the open group was 14.9 days and 17.5 days in the percutaneous group ($p = 0.57$). OR cost for the percutaneous procedure averaged at $83,705.80 per case and $63,963.13 for the open procedure ($p = 0.29$).

Postoperatively, spinopelvic radiographic parameters (lumbar lordosis and pelvic incidence) were similar between the two groups (Table 3). Average lumbar lordosis was 54.1 degrees in the open group and 53.8 degrees in the percutaneous group ($p = 0.96$). Pelvic incidence was 65.8 degrees in the open group and 64.7 degrees in the closed group ($p = 0.84$). No surgical site infections were seen in the percutaneous treatment cohort, whereas one infection was observed with the open reduction cohort ($p = 0.48$). A comparable amount in each group underwent hardware removal at a later date; 40% (6/15) in the open group and 31% (5/16) in the closed group underwent hardware removal ($p = 0.72$). Figures 3 and 4 show another example of patients in our cohort. This shows pre- and postoperative images for fixation with open reduction internal fixation.

4. Discussion

Modern technologic advances in orthopedic instrumentation have allowed for the adoption of percutaneous techniques to treat spinopelvic dissociation. Historic treatment with open reduction with lumbopelvic fixation of spinopelvic dissociation has been associated with a high infection rate [9, 10]. Schildhauer et al. observed an infection rate of 16% with open reduction and internal fixation of spinopelvic dissociations [8]. With current minimally invasive strategies, percutaneous instrumentation has been shown to have low rates of wound complication and decreased blood loss [12].

In the current study, we compared surgical as well as postoperative outcomes of open versus percutaneous fixation

TABLE 2: Fracture pattern classification. All fracture patterns were AO sacrum classification type C.

AO Spine	C0 (nondisplaced U type sacrum fracture)				C1 (alternative sacrum U type fracture without posterior instability)				C2 (bilateral complete type B injuries without transverse fracture)				C3 (displaced U type sacrum fracture)			
Modifiers	–	M3	M4	M3, 4	–	M3	M4	M3, 4	–	M3	M4	M3, 4	–	M3	M4	M3, 4
Open	5	2			0				1	1			9	3		
Closed	8	5			0				0				8	2	1	2

TABLE 3: Associated traumatic injuries.

	Open ($n = 15$)	Closed ($n = 16$)	Total ($n = 31$)
Traumatic brain injury	2 (13%)	1 (6%)	3 (10%)
Closed head injury	9 (60%)	4 (25%)	13 (42%)
Extremity fracture	8 (53%)	10 (63%)	18 (58%)
Anterior pelvic ring fracture	6 (40%)	11 (69%)	17 (55%)
Acetabulum fracture	4 (27%)	5 (31%)	9 (29%)
Thoracic injury	7 (47%)	10 (63%)	17 (55%)
Blunt abdominal injury	4 (27%)	6 (38%)	10 (32%)
Associated spine injury	6 (40%)	9 (56%)	15 (48%)

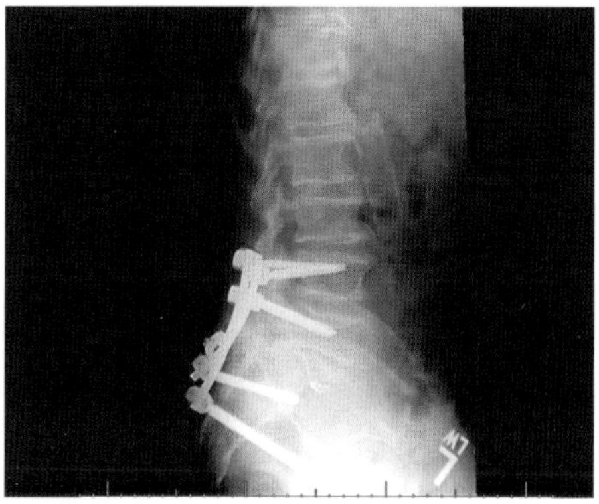

FIGURE 4: Postoperative films of patient treated with open reduction internal fixation of spinopelvic dissociation.

in a cohort of 31 patients. To our knowledge, this is the largest study to be reported on patients with spinopelvic dissociation treated surgically [9, 12, 14]. Through utilizing indirect reduction techniques as described by Nork et al., we were able to show satisfactory fracture reduction with equivalent (p = 0.96, 0.84) postoperative lumbar lordosis (LL) and pelvic incidence (PI) in both treatment groups [5, 15]. The limitation of our study is that spinopelvic measures were primarily evaluated compared to the actual reduction of the fracture site. Though there is individual variability in the spinopelvic parameters, studies have shown that it can be used as a surrogate of fracture reduction in the sagittal plane and the primary driver of clinical outcome [16].

In the current study, percutaneous fixation of spinopelvic dissociation showed a statistically lower intraoperative blood loss compared to open reduction internal fixation (171 cc versus 528 cc, $p = 0.0013$) and a lower rate of postoperative infections (1 versus 0, $p = 0.483$). Blood loss is difficult to analyze as a sole outcome when associated injuries are not taken into account. Aside from traumatic brain injury and closed head injury, the closed cohort had more associated injuries than the open group (Table 4). This discrepancy in preoperative patient characteristics likely explains the increased length of stay in our percutaneous group compared to the cohort. Despite the procedure being one that results in less blood loss and shorter operative time, the percutaneous patient population had more injuries on average than the open group, likely resulting in a longer hospital stay. Our results correlate with the literature seen with minimally invasive spine (MIS) that emphasized improved short-term clinical outcomes with percutaneous technology [17–20]. Meta-analysis by Phan and colleagues confirmed no excessive screw malposition, decreased infection, and decreased hospital stay with percutaneous spinal techniques [20]. Furthermore, given the severe nature of the trauma sustained by patients with spinopelvic dissociation, these patients are undergoing many procedures for various injuries such as long bone fractures. In settings such as this, the benefits of minimally invasive procedures cannot be overstated.

One surgical site infection was observed in the cohort. The patient was involved in an ATV accident and sustained a type C3, M3 (AO Spine classification) spinopelvic dissociation in addition to anterior pelvic ring disruption with 5 cm of pubic symphysis diastasis. Ten days after a combined anterior pelvic ring and open posterior spinopelvic fixation, the patient underwent debridement with retention of hardware. With prolonged IV antibiotics, the patient progressed to bony union without any further intervention.

Operative time was twenty-nine minutes shorter in the percutaneous group in comparison to the open group. While

Table 4: Postoperative outcomes on operatively treated patients. Note that blood loss was statistically significantly less in the percutaneous cohort.

	Open ($n = 15$)	Closed ($n = 16$)	p value
Pelvic incidence	65.8°	64.68°	0.8413
Lumbar lordosis	54.14°	53.81°	0.9568
Surgical site infection	1 (6.67%)	0 (0%)	0.4839
Transfusion post-op	3 (20%)	7 (43%)	0.2524
Operative time (minutes)	311	282	0.6665
Estimated blood loss (cc)	538	17	0.0013
Hardware removal	6 (40%)	5 (31%)	0.7160
Length of hospital stay (days)	14.91	17.45	0.5696
Length of follow-up (months)	7.75	9.93	0.5042
OR charges	$249,387.95	$347,205.22	0.1837
OR cost	63,963.13	$83,705.80	0.2922

this relationship does not meet statistical significance, it is of clinical and financial importance. Work by Macario estimates that operating room time per minute in US hospitals costs an average of $62 [21]. In review of our hospitals' cost data, we found that the total cost for the percutaneous group was greater ($p = 0.29$) than of the open treatment group. This increased cost is likely due to many factors such as using new percutaneous implants and intraoperative navigation; however, as itemized cost data were not available, we are unable to pinpoint an exact reason for the difference in cost. Further, we noted that there were decreased operative times in the percutaneous group despite the rising learning curve of the surgeon and the fluoroscopy staff.

Sacral laminectomy and decompression were performed only in patients who had focal compression of sacral nerve roots. In our study, 6 of the 31 displaying bowel and bladder dysfunction did not have decompression. Unlike cauda equina of the lumbar spine, neurological injuries secondary to sacral fractures are not considered neurologic emergencies requiring decompression within 48 hours. Schildhauer and colleagues showed that surgical timing did not correlate with clinical outcomes in patients with cauda equina secondary to spinopelvic dissociation [8]. This was confirmed by Lindahl et al. who additionally showed that laminectomy did not improve bladder or bowel function in patients who underwent decompression [22]. The role of open sacral decompression on ultimate outcome remains unclear and is beyond the scope of the current study. As shown earlier, the reduction of the fracture via percutaneous methods is comparable to that obtained with open reduction internal fixation. Figure 3 shows the pre- and postoperative imaging for a patient who underwent percutaneous fixation whereas Figure 4 shows the same imaging with an open reduction. As evidenced here, similar reduction can be obtained without the need for an invasive approach.

There are several limitations to this study including those inherent to a retrospective review. First and foremost, selection bias plays a role in all retrospective reviews. The decision to treat injuries, open versus closed, was based on the surgeon's preference and experience. Factors going into choosing which intervention a patient underwent are likely related to physician preference as well as body habitus, overall physiologic health, and underlying comorbidities. The majority of our patient selection was based on the age and training of the surgeon. The two younger physicians with more recent training tended to perform percutaneous techniques whereas the older physicians performed open reduction. The type of surgical skill necessary for both open and closed procedures varies as well. In the percutaneous procedure, one must master positioning of the Jamshidi needle in space while correlating this to the radiographic images. This type of procedure does not involve sacral laminectomy and the fine dexterity required in this aspect of an open approach. The patients reviewed were subject to care under several different surgeons and were nonrandomized to treatment groups. Unfortunately, the retrospective chart review did not include information on the soft tissue condition of the patients. This would have certainly affected the decision-making of the treating team had this been documented in the chart. Given the severe nature of the trauma sustained by these patients, it is inherently difficult to independently evaluate outcomes of a single procedure given their multisystem traumatic injuries. As Table 3 shows, the shear nature of the diversity of these patients and their extensive injuries makes a thorough comparison of these two patient groups difficult. Though it is a large series on an infrequently encountered injury, larger and better powered studies are required to further validate our results. We recognize the relatively short follow-up for this cohort and the need for longer studies to fully evaluate the effects of open versus closed surgical treatment in these patients.

In conclusion, percutaneous fixation of spinopelvic dissociation showed superior outcomes compared to open reduction internal fixation. Percutaneous fixation allowed for a statistically significant decrease in operative blood loss, while also showing a trend of decreasing the operating room time and surgical site infection. Though biomechanically triangular osteosynthesis is superior to stand-alone lumbopelvic fixation, clinically stand-alone fixation without the addition of iliosacral screws results in good outcomes in our series. Percutaneous fixation of spinopelvic dissociation is a less morbid and more expeditious method of pelvic stabilization compared to open reduction internal fixation.

References

[1] R. T. Bents, J. C. France, J. M. Glover, and K. L. Kaylor, "Traumatic spondylopelvic dissociation: A case report and literature review," *The Spine Journal*, vol. 21, no. 15, pp. 1814–1819, 1996.

[2] K. J. Gibbons, D. S. Soloniuk, and N. Razack, "Neurological injury and patterns of sacral fractures," *Journal of Neurosurgery*, vol. 72, no. 6, pp. 889–893, 1990.

[3] J. G. Bonnin, "Sacral fractures and injuries to the cauda quine," *The Journal of Bone & Joint Surgery*, vol. 27, pp. 113–127, 1945.

[4] R. Roy-Camille, G. Saillant, G. Gagna, and C. Mazel, "Transverse fracture of the upper sacrum: suicidal jumper's fracture," *Spine*, vol. 10, no. 9, pp. 838–845, 1985.

[5] S. E. Nork, C. B. Jones, S. P. Harding, S. K. Mirza, and M. L. C. Routt Jr., "Percutaneous stabilization of U-shaped sacral fractures using iliosacral screws: Technique and early results," *Journal of Orthopaedic Trauma*, vol. 15, no. 4, pp. 238–246, 2001.

[6] C. U. Dussa and B. M. Soni, "Influence of type of management of transverse sacral fractures on neurological outcome. a case series and review of literature," *Spinal Cord*, vol. 46, no. 9, pp. 590–594, 2008.

[7] C. Bellabarba, T. A. Schildhauer, A. R. Vaccaro, and J. R. Chapman, "Complications associated with surgical stabilization of high-grade sacral fracture dislocations with spino-pelvic instability," *Spine*, vol. 31, supplement 11, pp. S80–S88, 2006.

[8] T. A. Schildhauer, C. Bellabarba, S. E. Nork, D. P. Barei, M. L. Chip Routt Jr., and J. R. Chapman, "Decompression and lumbopelvic fixation for sacral fracture-dislocations with spino-pelvic dissociation," *Journal of Orthopaedic Trauma*, vol. 20, no. 7, pp. 447–457, 2006.

[9] M. A. König, S. Jehan, A. A. Boszczyk, and B. M. Boszczyk, "Surgical management of U-shaped sacral fractures: A systematic review of current treatment strategies," *European Spine Journal*, vol. 21, no. 5, pp. 829–836, 2012.

[10] A. J. G. Gribnau, P. B. V. Hensbroek, R. Haverlag, K. J. Ponsen, H. D. Been, and J. C. Goslings, "U-shaped sacral fractures: Surgical treatment and quality of life," *Injury*, vol. 40, no. 10, pp. 1040–1048, 2009.

[11] M. Y. Wang, S. C. Ludwig, D. G. Anderson, and P. V. Mummaneni, "Percutaneous iliac screw placement: description of a new minimally invasive technique," *Neurosurgical Focus*, vol. 25, no. 2, article E17, 2008.

[12] S. K. Williams and S. M. Quinnan, "Percutaneous lumbopelvic fixation for reduction and stabilization of sacral fractures with spinopelvic dissociation patterns," *Journal of Orthopaedic Trauma*, vol. 30, no. 9, pp. e318–e324, 2016.

[13] C. Bellabarba, G. D. Schroeder, C. K. Kepler et al., "The AOSpine sacral fracture classification," *Spine Journal*, vol. 6, supplement 1, p. s-0036, 2016.

[14] H.-D. Lee, C.-H. Jeon, S.-H. Won, and N.-S. Chung, "Global sagittal imbalance due to change in pelvic incidence after traumatic spinopelvic dissociation," *Journal of Orthopaedic Trauma*, vol. 31, no. 7, pp. e195–e199, 2017.

[15] M. P. Sullivan, H. E. Smith, J. M. Schuster, D. Donegan, S. Mehta, and J. Ahn, "Spondylopelvic dissociation," *Orthopedic Clinics of North America*, vol. 45, no. 1, pp. 65–75, 2014.

[16] R. A. Hart, M. I. Badra, A. Madala, and J. U. Yoo, "Use of pelvic incidence as a guide to reduction of H-type spino-pelvic dissociation injuries," *Journal of Orthopaedic Trauma*, vol. 21, no. 6, pp. 369–374, 2007.

[17] C. W. B. Peng, W. M. Yue, S. Y. Poh, W. Yeo, and S. B. Tan, "Clinical and radiological outcomes of minimally invasive versus open transforaminal lumbar interbody fusion," *Spine*, vol. 34, no. 13, pp. 1385–1389, 2009.

[18] R. J. Mobbs, P. Sivabalan, and J. Li, "Minimally invasive surgery compared to open spinal fusion for the treatment of degenerative lumbar spine pathologies," *Journal of Clinical Neuroscience*, vol. 19, pp. 829–835, 2012.

[19] A. G. Kulkarni, H. Bohra, A. Dhruv, A. Sarraf, A. Bassi, and V. M. Patil, "Minimal invasive transforaminal lumbar interbody fusion versus open transforaminal lumbar interbody fusion," *Indian Journal of Orthopaedics*, vol. 50, no. 5, pp. 464–472, 2016.

[20] K. Phan, P. J. Rao, and R. J. Mobbs, "Percutaneous versus open pedicle screw fixation for treatment of thoracolumbar fractures: Systematic review and meta-analysis of comparative studies," *Clinical Neurology and Neurosurgery*, vol. 135, pp. 85–92, 2015.

[21] A. Macario, "What does one minute of operating room time cost?" *Journal of Clinical Anesthesia*, vol. 22, no. 4, pp. 233–236, 2010.

[22] J. Lindahl, T. J. Mäkinen, S. K. Koskinen, and T. Söderlund, "Factors associated with outcome of spinopelvic dissociation treated with lumbopelvic fixation," *Injury*, vol. 45, no. 12, pp. 1914–1920, 2014.

6

Comparing Dorsal Tangential and Lateral Views of the Wrist for Detecting Dorsal Screw Penetration after Volar Plating of Distal Radius Fractures

Juan M. Giugale,[1] Mitchell S. Fourman,[1] Deidre L. Bielicka,[2] and John R. Fowler[1]

[1]*Department of Orthopaedic Surgery, University of Pittsburgh Medical Center, Pittsburgh, PA, USA*
[2]*Department of Orthopaedic Surgery, Rutgers-Robert Wood Johnson Medical Center, New Brunswick, NJ, USA*

Correspondence should be addressed to John R. Fowler; johnfowler10@gmail.com

Academic Editor: Panagiotis Korovessis

Background. The dorsal tangential (DT) view has been shown to improve the detection of dorsal screw perforation during volar distal radius fracture fixation. Here we performed a cadaveric imaging survey study to evaluate if the DT view was uniformly beneficial for all screws. *Methods.* Standardized placement of fixed-angle volar distal radius plates was performed on two cadavers. Fluoroscopic images depicting variable screw perforation of each of the four screw holes on the plate were generated. A 46-image survey was distributed at a large academic medical center. Respondents were asked to answer if the screw was perforating through the dorsal cortex in each image. Statistical analysis was performed using Fisher's exact test. A p value $< .05$ was considered significant. *Results.* The DT view offered a significantly more reliable determination of dorsal screw penetration than traditional lateral imaging for the radial-most screw at all degrees of perforation and the middle two screws at 2 mm of perforation. Residents and attendings had more accurate screw readings overall using the DT view. *Conclusions.* The DT view is superior to traditional lateral imaging in the detection of small amounts of dorsal perforation of the radial-most three screws of a fixed-angle volar plate.

1. Introduction

Although volar plate fixation has become the gold standard in the treatment of unstable distal radius fractures, extensor tendon irritation and rupture are known complications of this procedure. The etiology of extensor rupture is believed to relate to dorsal screw prominence in the majority of cases [1, 2]. Intraoperative lateral fluoroscopic films are typically used to assess screw depth after insertion. However, the presence of Lister's tubercle makes the distal radial cortex convex, not flat. A previous anatomic study showed that the height of Lister's tubercle ranges from 1.4 to 6.6 mm in relation to the radial border of the radius [3]. This implies that the screws radial and ulnar to Lister's tubercle can be proud several millimeters and still appear to be within the dorsal cortex on lateral fluoroscopic films. Prior work also examined the third extensor compartment floor through a limited dorsal approach after volar fixation and found that 12.5% of patients had dorsal screw prominence not identified on lateral fluoroscopic films [4].

The dorsal tangential view has recently received attention as an intraoperative fluoroscopic imaging technique that may better detect dorsal radius screw penetration [2, 5–7]. It has been shown to have a sensitivity of 95% for a dorsal screw protrusion of 1.0 mm when evaluated by two fellowship-trained orthopedic surgeons [7]. However, this technique has not been tested on multiple groups with variable fellowship and degree of training backgrounds.

Here we performed a cadaveric experiment and related survey study to compare the relative efficacies of the lateral and dorsal tangential (DT) views in the identification of dorsal screw prominence across training backgrounds. We hypothesized that the DT view is more effective than the lateral view in the detection of dorsal screw prominence at all experience levels.

2. Methods

All protocol elements were approved by the Committee for Oversight of Research and Clinical Training Involving

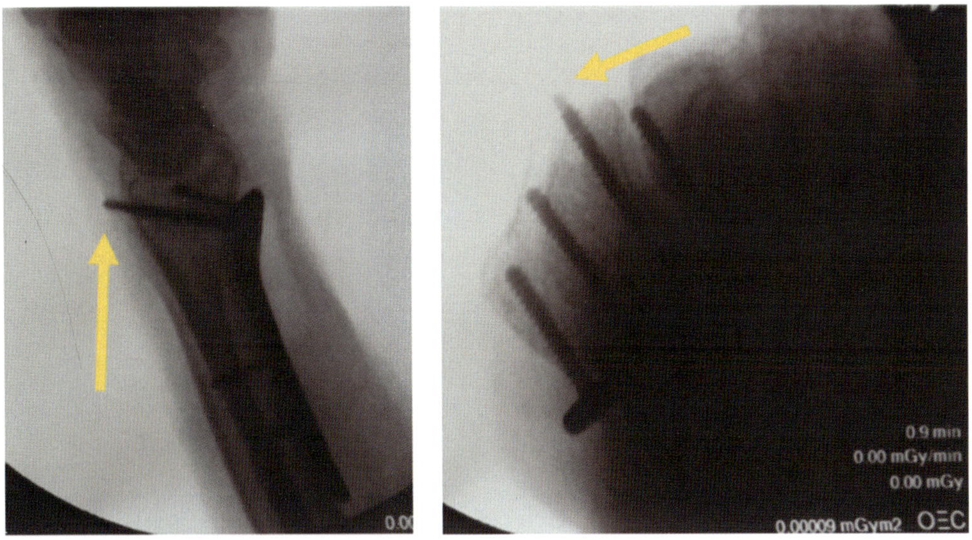

(a) (b)

FIGURE 1: Fluoroscopic (a) dorsal tangential and (b) traditional lateral views of third screw from the radial aspect of the plate with a 4 mm dorsal cortex protrusion, as presented during survey analysis. Yellow arrows denote the protruding screw.

Descents (CORID #587) at our institution. All procedures followed were in accordance with the ethical standards of the responsible committee on human experimentation (institutional and national) and with the Helsinki Declaration of 1975, as revised in 2008. A traditional volar approach to the wrist was performed on two fresh-frozen cadaveric forearms, permitting the placement of a fixed-angle distal radius plate (Stryker, Kalamazoo, MI) with 4 distal screw holes. Screws were inserted into each of the distal holes with their tips flush with the dorsal cortex, confirmed by visual inspection through a separate dorsal incision. Plate positioning and placement were performed by the senior investigator (JRF). A screw from a single hole was then removed and replaced with a longer screw, producing a collection of images with standardized single screw prominences of 0, 2, 4, or 6 mm. Lateral and DT fluoroscopic radiographs were obtained after each screw exchange (Figures 1(a) and 1(b)). A true lateral was obtained by rotating the image until the pisiform overlapped the distal pole of the scaphoid. To produce the DT view, the wrist was maximally flexed and the forearm was placed at a 15° inclination in relation to the axis of the mini-C arm radiographic beam.

A total of 46 images were digitized into high quality digital image files and randomized using an online survey platform (Kwiksurveys, Bristol, United Kingdom). Surveys were distributed to orthopedic surgery residents, fellows, and faculty. Instructions for each survey question asked the respondent to consider each image individually and determine if the screw had penetrated the dorsal cortex. All questions were in a binary yes/no format and asked the respondent to identify any screw protrusion in each successive image. Results were analyzed with GraphPad Prism 6.0 (LaJolla, CA) using Fisher's exact test for categorical data, as normality cannot by assumed given the limited sample size included in this study. In all cases, significance was defined as $p < .05$.

TABLE 1: Cohort and subgroup accuracy in the identification of screw prominence using either the DT or lateral views.

	Accuracy DT view	Accuracy lateral view	p value
Cohort ($n = 18$)	78.6%	62.4%	<.0001*
Attending ($n = 7$)	80.3%	65.6%	<.05*
Fellow ($n = 4$)	73.2%	65.8%	.39
Resident ($n = 7$)	80.2%	57.6%	<.0001*

*Statistical significance ($p < .05$).

3. Results

Completed responses were logged from a total of 18 respondents (7 faculty, 7 residents, and 4 fellows) out of a total of 52 faculty, fellows, and residents surveyed. A response was considered complete if it included answers to all questions. An additional five responses that failed to meet this criterion were removed from our sample size.

The overall accuracy of screw prominence across all-comers was significantly greater with the DT view (78.6%) compared to the lateral view (62.4%, $p < .0001$). Significant differences between DT and lateral view accuracy were also observed in the attending (80.3% versus 65.6%, $p < .05$) and resident (80.2% versus 57.6%, $p < .0001$) subgroups (Table 1). The composite sensitivity, specificity, and positive/negative predictive values of both groups were equivocal (Table 2).

The lateral view was unable to accurately identify 2 mm prominence at all screw positions (min accuracy 5.9 ± 8.3% at radial styloid screw versus 61.1% at ulnar corner screw) and

Table 2: Composite sensitivity and specificity of the lateral and DT views.

(a) Lateral view

		Actual screw prominence	
		Prominent	Not prominent
Survey response	Prominent	212	128
	Not prominent	8	22
		Sensitivity	96.4%
		Specificity	14.7%
		PPV	62.4%
		NPV	73.3%

(b) DT view

		Actual screw prominence	
		Prominent	Not prominent
Survey response	Prominent	274	71
	Not prominent	8	21
		Sensitivity	97.2%
		Specificity	22.8%
		PPV	79.4%
		NPV	72.4%

continued to be problematic at all screw prominence lengths at the radial styloid view (13 ± 1.8% at 4 mm and 49.4 ± 61.5% at 6 mm). However, more ulnar positions showed improved accuracy (Table 3). In contrast, the DT view had significantly stronger performance at the radial styloid screw at all screw prominences (78.1 ± 4.4% at 2 mm, 93.5 ± 6.3% at 4 mm, and 96.9 ± 4.4% at 6 mm). The worst accuracy in the DT group was in identifying a 2 mm prominence of the ulnar corner screw (50 ± 44.2%). Statistical comparison between views at each screw position and prominence could not be performed because of the reduced number of total views available.

4. Discussion

Extensor tendon rupture after volar plate fixation of distal radius fractures may occur secondary to screw prominence. The protuberance of Lister's tubercle can mask dorsal screw penetration on lateral fluoroscopic views. The dorsal tangential (DT) view has been proposed as a method that can more sensitively detect dorsal screw prominence compared to standard lateral radiographs. Our work suggests that the primary advantage of the DT view compared to traditional lateral fluoroscopic views is in the evaluation of small degrees (2 mm) of screw protrusion on the radial three screws on a fixed-angle volar plate. Larger magnitudes of screw protrusion further limit the benefit of the DT view to the single most-radial screw on the plate. Overall, the DT view was found to be more reliable than the lateral view by all experience cohorts but active clinical fellows. However, the sensitivity and specificity of both techniques were still equivocal.

Our findings appear to stand in contrast to existing work. Ozer et al. [7] compared four radiographic views (lateral, 45 degree supination, 45 degree pronation, and dorsal tangential views) to determine the most sensitive view to detect screw protrusion. The authors found that the dorsal tangential view was sensitive at detecting screw penetration into the 3rd and 4th compartment (both compartments ulnar to Listers tubercle) with a sensitivity of 88–98% for screws 1–3 mm proud. However, the sensitivity of the dorsal tangential view to 1–3 mm proud screws radial to Lister's tubercle was only 35–48%. In contrast, the results of this study noted an increased accuracy of the DT view compared to the lateral view in the evaluation of more radial screws (Table 3), while ulnar imaging was generally equivocal between both views.

This disagreement may be independent of the benefit of the DT view. Cadaveric work by Perry et al. [8] found that the central and slightly ulnar screws of more commonly used volar plate models were most likely to include the extensor pollicis longus tendon in their k-wire and screw trajectory. In an evaluation of 18 cadaveric arms, none of the most-radial or most-ulnar screw holes were associated with EPL interaction and were therefore not labeled by that study as "high risk." Further, the "at risk" central screws were also found to be more likely to penetrate their corresponding extensor compartments, a finding supported by other cadaveric and ultrasound studies [9, 10]. In our work, the DT view was superior to the lateral view in the identification of a 2 mm prominence of the two central screws of the plate used in our model. This small prominence has still been associated with tendon pathology, particularly in those screws that threaten the third or fourth dorsal compartments [10]. Based on this additional evidence, the benefit of the DT versus lateral view at the radial- or ulnar-most screw holes of any plate appears to be clinically irrelevant. Instead, the improved sensitivity of the DT view in the identification of a small amount of dorsal cortex perforation through central plate holes highlights its true clinical benefit.

While Wall et al. [11] demonstrated that unicortical distal radius screws spanning 75% of the bone offer a similar biomechanical construct to bicortical screw fixation, coronal shear injuries require bicortical fixation to optimize construct rigidity. In any fracture pattern that requires bicortical fixation, vigilance should be exercised to avoid dorsal screw prominence and the may be considered to ensure minimal screw penetration. Joseph and Harvey [12] used the DT view as a final fluoroscopic check prior to skin closure in 15 distal radius fractures with a coronal-split element and found that the DT view led to screw exchange in 26.6% of cases. In general, the DT view has been found to be a better "rule-out" indicator than "rule-in," with a negative predictive value of 97% but a sensitivity of only 67% [13]. Additional benefits of the DT view include reduced radiation exposure during evaluation, which is beneficial if using this technique for screw exchange prior to closure [14], as well as confirmation of adequate reduction of the sigmoid notch during fixation [15].

While the findings of this work appear to be largely supported by prior work, our study has several limitations. There is a small amount of unpreventable variability in positioning and obtaining the dorsal tangential and lateral fluoroscopic films. As demonstrated by Haug et al. [6], the accuracy of the dorsal tangential view decreases as inclination of the forearm

TABLE 3: Overall accuracy based on imaging technique and screw position and degree of prominence.

	1 (radial styloid)	2	3	4 (ulnar corner)
DT 0 mm	84.6% (1 image)			
Lat 0 mm	85.7% (1 image)			
DT 2 mm	78.1 ± 4.4%	100% (1 image)	79.5 ± 11.4%	50 ± 44.2%
Lat 2 mm	5.9 ± 8.3%	35.6 ± 49.01%	18.9% (1 image)	61.1% (1 image)
DT 4 mm	93.45 ± 6.3%	100% (1 image)	60 ± 56.6%	65.8 ± 40.0%
Lat 4 mm	13.0 ± 1.8%	75 ± 35.4%	100% (1 image)	83.3% (1 image)
DT 6 mm	96.9 ± 4.4%	100% (1 image)	75.2 ± 26.8%	78.9 ± 3.4%
Lat 6 mm	49.4 ± 61.5%	97.6 ± 4.1%	100% (1 image)	50.8 ± 61.7%

deviates from 15° relative to the axis of the fluoroscopic beam. We accepted this slight variability, recognizing that a similar deviation from optimal beam position would exist clinically. The aim of our cadaveric study was to better understand the utility of two different fluoroscopic views in identifying screw penetration. The true clinical impact of each screw is likely not to be equal and cannot be quantified by our study. It is therefore reasonable to postulate that variability between these two imaging techniques may not translate into a similar degree of difference clinically. This is important when considering the slight variability that may exist between plate manufacturers, although our findings suggest that radially placed holes, wherever their exact position, will still benefit from imaging from the dorsal tangential view. Further investigation is required to determine if the dorsal tangential view affects the rate of extensor tendon rupture clinically and if this complication leads to worse clinical outcomes. We must also assess intraobserver consistency to confirm that our findings are reproducible.

5. Conclusion

In a survey study based on measurements made using a cadaveric model, we found that the DT view is superior to the lateral view of the wrist in the identification of any degree of dorsal cortex perforation of the radial-most screw in a volar locking plate. Further, the DT view may also be superior to the lateral view in the detection of 2 mm screw prominence in central plate holes. Further work that utilizes an increased sample size and image quantity and considers additional plate types and hole configurations is required to validate the findings of this pilot work.

Ethical Approval

All procedures followed were in accordance with the ethical standards of the responsible committee on human experimentation (institutional and national) and with the Helsinki Declaration of 1975, as revised in 2008.

References

[1] L. M. Berglund and T. M. Messer, "Complications of volar plate fixation for managing distal radius fractures," *Journal of the American Academy of Orthopaedic Surgeons*, vol. 17, no. 6, pp. 369–377, 2009.

[2] K. Ozer and S. Toker, "Dorsal tangential view of the wrist to detect screw penetration to the dorsal cortex of the distal radius after volar fixed-angle plating," *Hand*, vol. 6, no. 2, pp. 190–193, 2011.

[3] W. Pichler, G. Windisch, G. Schaffler, R. Rienmüller, and W. Grechenig, "Computer tomography aided 3D analysis of the distal dorsal radius surface and the effects on volar plate osteosynthesis," *Journal of Hand Surgery: European Volume*, vol. 34, no. 5, pp. 598–602, 2009.

[4] E. C. Benson, A. DeCarvalho, E. A. Mikola, J. M. Veitch, and M. S. Moneim, "Two potential causes of EPL rupture after distal radius volar plate fixation," *Clinical Orthopaedics and Related Research*, no. 451, pp. 218–222, 2006.

[5] A. Brunner, C. Siebert, C. Stieger, A. Kastius, B.-C. Link, and R. Babst, "The dorsal tangential X-ray view to determine dorsal screw penetration during volar plating of distal radius fractures," *Journal of Hand Surgery*, vol. 40, no. 1, pp. 27–33, 2015.

[6] L. C. Haug, B. C. Glodny, Deml. et al., "A new radiological method to detect dorsally penetrating screws when using volar locking plates in distal radial fractures. The dorsal horizon view".

[7] K. Ozer, J. M. Wolf, B. Watkins, and D. J. Hak, "Comparison of 4 fluoroscopic views for dorsal cortex screw penetration after volar plating of the distal radius," *Journal of Hand Surgery*, vol. 37, no. 5, pp. 963–967, 2012.

[8] D. C. Perry, D. M. G. Machin, J. A. Casaletto, and D. J. Brown, "Minimising the risk of extensor pollicis longus Rupture following volar plate fixation of distal radius fractures: A cadaveric study," *Annals of the Royal College of Surgeons of England*, vol. 93, no. 1, pp. 57–60, 2011.

[9] W. Pichler, W. Grechenig, H. Clement, G. Windisch, and N. P. Tesch, "Perforation of the third extensor compartment by the drill bit during palmar plating of the distal radius," *Journal of Hand Surgery: European Volume*, vol. 34, no. 3, pp. 333–335, 2009.

[10] T. S. Sügün, N. Karabay, Y. Gürbüz, K. Özaksar, T. Toros, and M. Kayalar, "Screw prominences related to palmar locking plating of distal radius," *Journal of Hand Surgery: European Volume*, vol. 36, no. 4, pp. 320–324, 2011.

[11] L. B. Wall, M. D. Brodt, M. J. Silva, M. I. Boyer, and R. P. Calfee, "The effects of screw length on stability of simulated osteoporotic distal radius fractures fixed with volar locking plates," *Journal of Hand Surgery*, vol. 37, no. 3, pp. 446–453, 2012.

[12] S. J. Joseph and J. N. Harvey, "The dorsal horizon view: Detecting screw protrusion at the distal radius," *Journal of Hand Surgery*, vol. 36, no. 10, pp. 1691–1693, 2011.

[13] D. Ganesh, B. Service, B. Zirgibel, and K. Koval, "The Detection of Prominent Hardware in Volar Locked Plating of Distal Radius Fractures: Intraoperative Fluoroscopy Versus Computed Tomography," *Journal of Orthopaedic Trauma*, vol. 30, no. 11, pp. 618–621, 2016.

[14] L. Vaiss, S. Ichihara, D. G. H. Ramirez, S. Hendriks, P. Liverneaux, and S. Facca, "A comparative study about ionizing radiation emitted during radiological "skyline" view of the wrist in pronation versus supination," *European Journal of Orthopaedic Surgery and Traumatology*, vol. 25, no. 2, pp. 309–311, 2014.

[15] G. Klammer, M. Dietrich, M. Farshad, L. Iselin, L. Nagy, and A. Schweizer, "Intraoperative imaging of the distal radioulnar joint using a modified skyline view," *Journal of Hand Surgery*, vol. 37, no. 3, pp. 503–508, 2012.

Acetabular Debonding: An Investigation of Porous Coating Delamination in Hip Resurfacing Arthroplasty

Eric Robinson, Dani Gaillard-Campbell, and Thomas P. Gross

Midlands Orthopaedics & Neurosurgery, 1910 Blanding Street, Columbia, SC 29201, USA

Correspondence should be addressed to Dani Gaillard-Campbell; dani.gaillard@midorthoneuro.com

Academic Editor: Panagiotis Korovessis

Background. To date, there have been no published investigations on the cause of acetabular debonding, a rare failure phenomenon in metal-on-metal hip resurfacing where the acetabular porous coating delaminates from the implant while remaining well fixed to the pelvic bone. *Purposes.* This study aims to summarize the current understanding of acetabular debonding and to investigate the discrepancy in rate of debonding between two implant systems. *Patients and Methods.* To elucidate potential causes of debonding, we retrospectively analyzed a single-surgeon cohort of 839 hip resurfacing cases. Specifically, we compared rate of debonding and manufacturing processes between two implant systems. *Results.* Group 1 experienced significantly more cases of debonding than Group 2 cases (4.0% versus 0.0%, p value<0.0001). Implant manufacturing processes differed in surface coating, heat treatment, postmanufacturing treatment, and apex thickness. Debonded implants were more likely to have missed RAIL guidelines (p=0.04). *Conclusions.* We identified implant system, postoperative time, and acetabular component placement as variables contributing to rate of debonding. We recommend minimizing acetabular inclination angle according to RAIL guidelines. Further, we evaluated manufacturing differences between the two implant systems but did not have access to proprietary data to identify the cause of debonding. Both implants met ASTM standards, yet only the Group 1 implant debonded. This suggests the second implant had greater fatigue shear strength. Because the Group 2 implant achieved a more durable interface that did not debond, we suggest the ASTM F1160 standard for fatigue shear strength be increased to that achieved by its manufacturer. *Level of Evidence II.* A retrospective evaluation of prospectively collected data.

1. Introduction

After early enthusiasm in the 2000s [1, 2], hip resurfacing arthroplasty (HRA) fell into disfavor due to a high incidence of metallosis with poorly designed implants and at outlier centers [3]. HRA is more technically demanding than total hip arthroplasty (THA) and necessitates a separate, steeper learning curve. Available data suggest HRA performed by experienced resurfacing surgeons offers greater functional capacity and improved durability over THA [4–6]. Other advantages include superior hip stability [7–9], greater bone preservation leading to less-challenging revision surgeries [10–12], and lower 10-year all-cause mortality in matched patient populations when compared to THA [13].

To further improve the success and performance of HRA, research groups should evaluate failure modes of resurfacing systems and devise appropriate solutions. In 2012, the FDA presented a memorandum discussing safety and efficacy of metal-on-metal (MoM) hip implant systems [14]. This report identified common failure modes of MoM systems, but despite the substantial level of detail, the memorandum failed to mention a rare and poorly understood failure mode in MoM HRA implant systems, debonding of the porous titanium (Ti) coating from the cobalt (Co) chrome acetabular component.

Debonding occurs when shear forces applied at the bone-implant interface are too high, causing patches of porous coating to shear from the cup upon loading. Acetabular debonding has been investigated in a few, small case studies [15–17], but to date, no studies have been published reporting rates of debonding in a single, large cohort. Debonding presents an unusual failure mode that may illuminate flaws in implant design or manufacturing processes. The current paper presents a retrospective analysis of a single-surgeon

Table 1: Demographic information.

	Demographic Information		
	Group 1	Group 2	
Variable	Corin	Biomet	P-value
Number of Cases	371	728	–
Age (years)	53.8 ± 9.3	55.1 ± 8.2	0.0177∗
BMI	28.2 ± 5.2	27.9 ± 4.7	0.3371
Female gender (%)	32%	29.1%	0.3125
Preoperative Harris Hip Score	43.4 ± 10.3	45.6 ± 11.8	0.0024∗
Diagnosis (%)			
Osteoarthritis	74.1%	81.6%	0.00398∗
Osteonecrosis	11.9%	4.3%	0.0001∗
Dysplasia	7.5%	8.7%	0.5287
Legg Perthes	0.8%	1.7%	0.2585
Post Trauma	0.3%	0.3%	0.9840
Rheumatoid Arthritis	1.1%	2.3%	0.1499
Slipped Capital Epiphysis	0.5%	1.0%	0.4654
Other	3.8%	0.3%	0.0001∗

∗ represents significance.

database with over 5000 HRA cases. We compared the rate of debonding as a unique failure between the two different HRA implant systems used in our practice: the Corin Cormet 2000 and Biomet M2a Magnum-ReCap™ systems. The purpose of this paper was twofold: (1) to summarize the current literature and present a hypothetical mechanism of debonding failure and (2) to evaluate any discrepancy in rate of debonding between the two implant systems by investigating differences in the implant manufacturing and testing processes.

2. Methods

2.1. Patients and Follow-Up Method. The senior author (TPG) maintains a prospective database (OrthoVault, Columbia, SC) of more than 5000 HRA procedures. This surgeon has performed HRA since 1991, and therefore, none of these cases are from his initial learning curve. The current study analyzes 839 consecutive procedures between January 2001 and December 2007, with a minimum 10-year follow-up. Approvals for this study and report were obtained from the Institutional Review Board of Lifepoint Health Providence Hospitals in Columbia, South Carolina. In this study, we compare two similar implants with respect to a single failure mechanism: late acetabular component loosening. The first cohort (Group 1) comprised 329 Corin Cormet devices implanted between 2001 and 2004. The second group (Group 2) consisted of 510 Biomet Magnum™ cases performed between 2004 and 2007. The two groups were demographically similar, although Group 2 was slightly older (p value=0.01) with a higher preoperative clinical score (p value=0.0024), on average (Table 1). Group 2 had more patients with posttrauma HRA (2.7% versus 0.3%, p=0.009). Further, Group 1 had a higher proportion of patients with osteonecrosis (11.2% versus 4.1%, $p < 0.0001$), although no HRA cases with a diagnosis of osteonecrosis reported acetabular debonding.

2.2. Implant Systems. The senior author used these two implant systems in a consecutive fashion. Between March 2001 and December 2004, the hybrid cemented Corin Cormet 2000 system (Corin, Cirencester, UK) was employed as a part of a multicenter United States FDA trial. Between December 2004 and December 2007, Biomet devices comprised a cemented ReCap™ femoral component and an uncemented Magnum™ acetabular component (Biomet, Warsaw, Indiana) and were used in an off-label fashion for total hip resurfacing.

Both groups employed similar hybrid MoM HRA implants, and each cohort had a minimum follow-up of 10 years. Similarities between the two acetabular components (Table 2) include a cast, high-carbon (>0.2%) CoCr substrate shot blasted with alumina grit and then coated with plasma-sprayed, unalloyed Ti. The coverage arcs are similar between these two implants, but the Group 2 implant arc is 4° less for each implant size on average. There are also several, notable differences in the manufacturing processes of these two devices. The Group 1 implant [24] is double heat-treated, and an additional layer of hydroxyapatite (HA) is plasma sprayed onto the Ti layer. Two sets of relatively thick antirotation fins at the equator imbed into the ischium and pubis during impaction. The Group 2 implant system is not heat-treated and does not have an HA layer. There are four pairs of smaller, thinner fins evenly spaced around the circumference of the implant. Implant dimensions are roughly sketched in Figure 1.

Several details, including those of the porous coating processes, are proprietary and not known to us. Average bead size was only available for the Cormet device [25]. Pore size range, but not mean pore size, was available for the Biomet

Table 2: Comparison of acetabular component design and manufacturing processes.

	Corin Cormet 2000	**Biomet M2a-Magnum**
Acetabular Diameter Difference (Outer-Inner Diameter)	6-8 mm [18]	6 mm [19]
Bulk alloy	CoCrMo [18, 20]	CoCrMo [19]
Carbon content	"High" [4, 5], 0.2-.35% [18]	"High" [21], 0.23-.28% [19]
Surface coating*	Dual plasma spray (Ti+ HA) [18]	Plasma spray (Ti) [19]
Heat treatment*	Yes [18]	No [19]
Manufacturing process*	Cast [21] with hot isostatic pressing and solution annealing [18]	As cast [21]
Roughening of cast implant	Honed with a shotblast of alumina grit [22]	Honed with a shotblast of alumina grit [19]
Sphericity	3.8 μm [21], <10 μm [18]	1.9 μm [21], 5 μm [19]
Surface roughness	0.030 um [21]	0.031 um [21]
Equator/peripheral thickness	4 mm [23], 5.6 mm [21], 4.2 mm (our measurement)	3 mm [19], 3.4 mm [21], 3 mm (our measurement)
Apex thickness*	3 mm [23]	6 mm [19]
Coverage arc for implants with bearing size 40-56mm	160-166^0 [20]	156-162^0 [19]
Radial clearance	97.67 μm (Medium) [21], 75-200 μm [22]	120.93 μm (High) [21], 75-150 μm [19]

*Bold with asterisks represents difference.

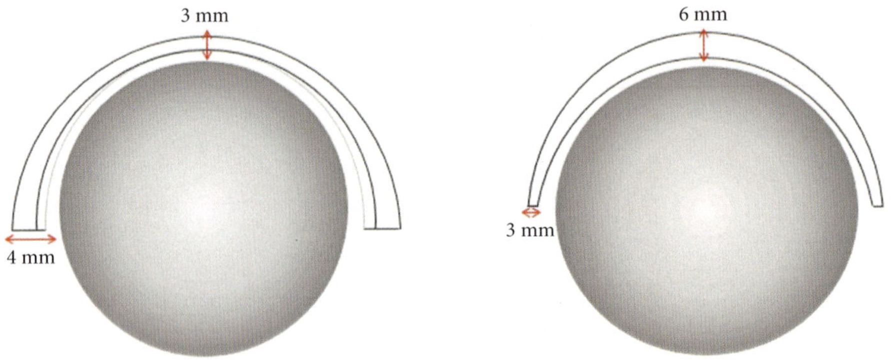

FIGURE 1: Implant design sketches. Corin (left) and Biomet (right) cup dimensions shown, with the gray sphere representing the femoral head.

Magnum [19]. We were unable to find time to fixation for either device.

2.3. Procedure. All procedures were performed using a posterior approach as described previously [26]. Before 2009, acetabular components were positioned with an acetabular inclination angle (AIA) under 55°, based on research by De Smet [27].

2.4. Clinical and Radiographic Analysis. Office or remote follow-up was requested at 6 weeks, 1 and 2 years, and every other year thereafter. A clinical questionnaire, radiographs, and a physical examination testing range-of-motion and strength were performed at each visit. After 1 year, physical examinations were no longer done routinely on remote follow-ups. The OrthoVault database (Midlands Orthopaedics & Neurosurgery, Columbia, South Carolina) supported our collection and analysis of demographic, clinical, and radiographic data for all patients.

Patient questionnaires facilitated the collection of information necessary for calculating the following clinical scores: Harris hip score (HHS) [28], University of California, Los Angeles (UCLA) activity score [29], and visual analogue scale (VAS) pain score for normal and worst days [30]. HHS determines clinical outcome; UCLA activity scores measure activity level on a scale from 1 to 10, for which 10 represented the highest level of activity; VAS pain scores rate the level of pain from 0 to 10, with zero representing no pain and 10 representing maximum levels of debilitating pain.

Both supine and standing anterior-posterior pelvis and lateral radiographs are taken and analyzed for component position, shifting, and radiolucencies by the senior author at each follow-up interval and upon request. We determine the acetabular inclination angle (AIA) on a standing pelvis radiograph by measuring the angle formed by two straight lines: one parallel to flat face of the acetabular component and the other tangential to the precipice of both ischial tuberosities. We measured all radiographs using InteleViewer (InteleRAD, Chicago, IL, USA).

2.5. Statistical Methods. The significance level α was defined as 0.05 for all statistical analyses in this study. A paired, two-tailed Student's T-test was used to calculate the significant difference between average preoperative and postoperative numerical outcomes within and between study groups. When comparing two population proportions, a two-sample Z-test was used. Kaplan-Meier survivorship curves were plotted to evaluate implant survival among different groups. Log-rank and Wilcoxon tests were performed to calculate significant differences between survivorship curves. Curves and survivorship statistical tests were generated using XLSTAT (New York, NY).

TABLE 3: Acetabular failures by category.

Type	Corin	Biomet	P-value
# Cases	371	728	–
(1) Late Loosening	15 (4.0%)	2 (0.3%)	<0.0001∗
Debonding	13 (3.5%)	0 (0.0%)	<0.0001∗
Intact Coating	0 (0.0%)	2 (0.3%)	0.3125
Unknown	1 (0.3%)	0 (0.0%)	0.1615
(2) Early Loosening	2 (0.5%)	8 (1.1%)	0.3576
(3) AWRF	4 (1.1%)	4 (0.5%)	0.3271

∗ indicates significance.

3. Results

In Group 1, there was a significantly higher rate of late acetabular component loosening, as well as loosening categorized as debonding; cup loosening characterized as debonding is confirmed intraoperatively. Both groups had a minimum of 10 years' follow-up, at which point Kaplan-Meier (KM) implant survivorship was 96.0% and 97.2%, respectively ($p=0.0008$) (Figure 2). With debonding as an endpoint, 10-year Group 1 implant survivorship was 97.8% and Group 2 implant survivorship was 100% ($p<0.0001$).

Table 3 lists the incidence of acetabular failure modes; definitions and descriptions of each failure mode are detailed in Table 4. Debonding only presented in Group 1, occurring at a mean of 9.7 years (range 4 to 14 years). The surgeon identified debonding intraoperatively at revision surgery, and this was confirmed by the surgical assistance and implant company representative; the implant coating appeared delaminated from the implant bulk material and well fixed in the pelvic

Table 4: Acetabular failure descriptions.

Failure Category	Description
1. Late acetabular loosening	Thought to represent initial implant integration with subsequent failure of attachment. We divide late loosening into three subtypes for more detailed analysis
1a. Debonding of the porous coating	The main mode of interest in the current study. In these cases, initial fixation is achieved through bone ingrowth. At some point beyond 2 years, the well-fixed, porous layer from the component substrate "debonds", causing subsequent implant loosening. The patients typically have excellent function prior to loosening with no change in acetabular component position on radiographs. They will then present with a 2-3-month prodrome of mild symptoms without radiographic findings before a sudden acute worsening of symptoms and an inability to bear weight on the affected leg. Loosening is then obvious radiographically with shifting of the acetabular component into a markedly steeper position. Intraoperative findings include a grossly loose acetabular component with a section of porous coating debonded from the implant substrate. This contiguous "sheet" of plasma spray coating, usually 20 to 30% of the total surface, is seen to be well fixed to the surrounding bone. The remainder of the porous coating remains attached to the implant and has no apparent bone ingrowth. There is a mild amount of metallosis and reactive fluid with no soft tissue mass. There is no fibrous pseudomembrane.
2b. Loosening with intact porous coating	Rarely occurs after 2 years without debonding. These cases may represent cases of initial fibrous ingrowth with radiographically stable implants for at least 2 years and subsequent loss of fibrous fixation. They present with late onset of chronic pain and late change in radiographic AIA. They have acceptable metal ion levels (<10 μm/L) and small collections of serosanguinous fluid, with no significant metallosis, soft tissue masses, or muscle destruction. We exclude cases of AWRF (described below) from this group. Intraoperatively, the acetabular component is either grossly loose or easily detached with a tamp. There is a thin 2-3 mm fibrous membrane present, and the adjacent bone is typically quite hard.
3c. Status of porous coating unknown	Cases that have failed beyond 2 years and were revised elsewhere; therefore, we cannot categorize the mode of failure or status of the implant coating.
2. Early acetabular loosening	Occurs before 2 years and is thought to be due to failure of bone ingrowth into the acetabular component, which can present with an acute cup spinout or a gradual symptomatic shift. In both types, the component usually shifts into a more steeply inclined position. The porous coating is found intact, and in early cases, blood may be encountered where the soft tissue dissection from the original operation has not yet completely healed. In the later cases of gradual shift, there is usually a fibrous layer with serous fluid. Black Ti metallosis is rarely seen. We have not observed AWRF before 2 years.
3.Adverse wear-related failure (AWRF)	Caused by inadequate coverage arc [15, 31]. The relationship of AWRF to component bearing size, coverage arc, and implant AIA on standing radiographs was elucidated in our 2013 RAIL paper [31], which describes a safe zone for placing all cup sizes with a 99% confidence level. When these current study cases were performed, the importance of cup position was not yet appreciated. Therefore, a small percentage of AWRF occurred due to acetabular component malposition. These failures present with progressive chronic pain, usually after 5 years postoperatively. If routine blood metal ion testing at 2 years is undertaken, as recommended by DeSmet [15], these cases can be discovered before the patients become symptomatic and when soft tissue damage is minimal. Initially, radiographs are unremarkable except for unacceptably steep AIA (according to RAIL). Progressive femoral neck narrowing and lysis can occur in late cases. 3D studies show large fluid collections and soft tissue masses. Extensive grey tissue staining, milky tan fluid, and inflammatory soft tissue masses are encountered at revision. Usually, some metallic filled lysis is present. Bone loss is typically much less prominent than soft tissue inflammation. Component loosening is rare. We have never seen significant muscle destruction in HRA AWRF. In our experience, tissue inflammation in THA due to trunnion corrosion may be more severe with low ion levels and should be considered separately from HRA pure bearing wear. We emphasize that the tissue destruction seen in MoM THA cases cannot be considered equivalent to AWRF in HRA.

TABLE 5: Clinical and radiographic data.

Clinical and Radiographic Data			
	Group 1	Group 2	
Variable	Corin	Biomet	P-value
n	**371**	**728**	–
Clinical Data			
Harris Hip Score (Post-Op)	93.6 ± 14.6	96.7 ± 7.6	0.0001∗
UCLA Score	6.6 ± 2.1	7.2 ± 2.0	0.0001∗
VAS Pain: Regular Day	0.6 ± 1.6	0.3 ± 0.9	0.001∗
VAS Pain: Worst Day	1.7 ± 2.6	1.4 ± 2.2	0.03∗
Mean Cobalt	2.6 ± 3.7	1.7 ± 1.8	0.0001∗
Mean Chromium	1.7 ± 2.3	1.1 ± 1.3	0.0001∗
Radiographic Data			
Acetabular Inclination Angle (°)	45.6 ± 7.2	45.1 ± 11.7	0.6504
Radiolucency	4 (0.01%)	0 (0.00%)	0.005∗
Osteolysis	3 (0.01%)	2 (0.00%)	0.200

∗ indicates significance.

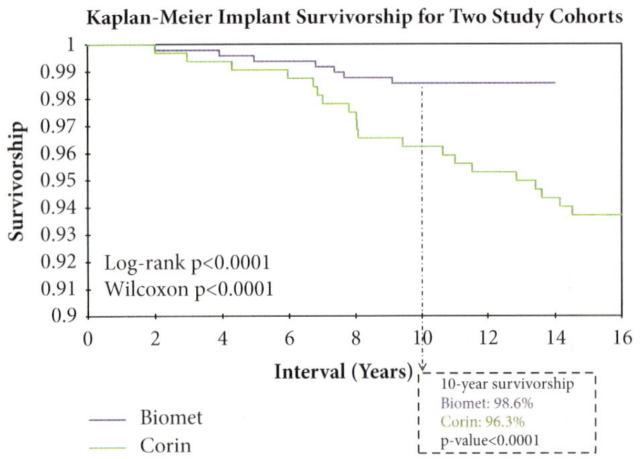

FIGURE 2: Kaplan-Meier implant survivorship for two study cohorts. Kaplan-Meier implant survivorship analysis using late acetabular failure as an endpoint. All cases in both groups have a minimum of 10 years' follow-up. At 10 years, survivorship is 97.2% for Biomet and 96.0% for Corin (p=0.0008). Late acetabular failure is defined as failure of acetabular component >2 years. Results of the log-rank test (p value <0.0001) and Wilcoxon test (p value <0.0001) show significant difference in the occurrence of late acetabular failures between the two implant groups.

bone. The surgical team only recorded where debonding occurred in three cases (23% of debonding cases). Of these, delamination was reported to have occurred on the outer edges of the cup. Amount of delamination ranged from 33 to 90% of the acetabular porous coating. Other acetabular failure modes, such as failure of ingrowth, AWRF, and late loosening with intact porous coating, were not different between the two groups (p value=0.2, p value=0.5, and p value=0.3, respectively). One Group 1 patient had revision surgery elsewhere, and therefore we categorized their failure as "unknown" loosening.

Figure 3 presents the number of late acetabular failure cases for Group 1 implant systems, dependent on time since

TABLE 6: Acetabular position data.

	Debonded Corin	ALL Corin	ALL Biomet
# Met RAIL	4/13 (30.8%)	133/227 (58.6%)	265/506 (52.4%)
Avg AIA	48.0 ± 8.6	44.2 ± 7.3	45.1 ± 11.7

surgery. Two Group 1 acetabular failures occurred before 2 years (0.5% of total cases) with all other acetabular failures occurring thereafter (5.1%). Failures occurred at a mean of 8.5 years. There were no differences between the time since surgery and rate of late failure. There was no statistical difference between date of HRA surgery and rate of late failure, although we observed most instances of Group 1 debonding were from cases performed in 2002. Manufacturers often use outside suppliers to perform porous coating. Unfortunately, the manufacturer would not provide us with vendor information for failed implants. Therefore, we investigated failure rate of implants from specific time periods; we could not establish any correlation. Group 2 implants failed late at 7 and 8 years. Clinical data (Table 5) indicate a higher postoperative HHS and UCLA activity score for Group 2 (HHS p value<0.0001, UCLA p value<0.0001), as well as lower VAS pain scores on regular and worst days (regular p value<0.0001, worst p value=0.0315). Radiographic data indicate a lower instance of radiolucency (p value<0.005) in Group 2 (Table 5). No debonding cases presented radiolucency. Nine debonding cases (69.2% total debonding cases) presented AIA over the relative acetabular inclination limit (RAIL) [32] on their earliest postoperative radiographs, as compared to 94 or 227 measured radiographs (41.4%) from Group 1 (p=0.04) (Table 6).

4. Discussion

We investigated a poorly understood failure phenomenon in which the porous coating debonds from the acetabular component. Several centers have published case studies

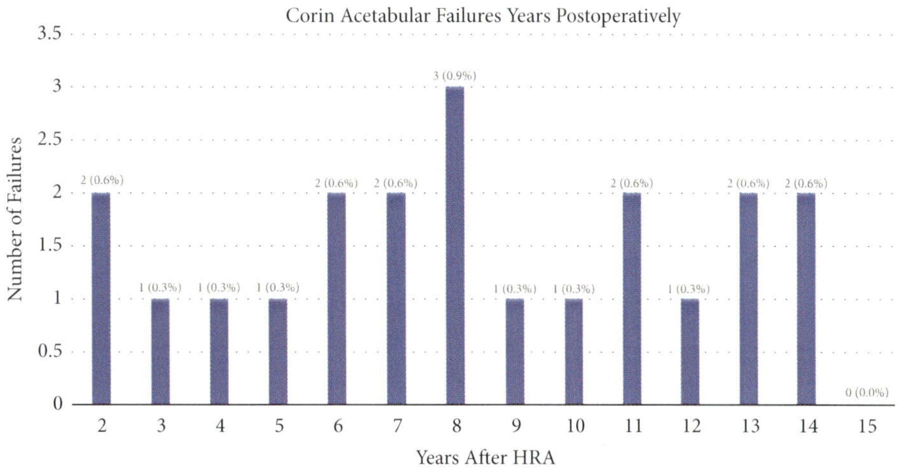

FIGURE 3: Corin late acetabular failure distribution over postoperative time. Figure 3 presents a distribution of Corin acetabular failures over postoperative time. Callouts show number of failures and percentage of the entire cohort (371 cases). Two cases failed before 2 years postoperatively (0.5% of cases) and are considered failure of ingrowth.

on debonding [15–17]. However, our group is the first to analyze a large clinical database and report rate of acetabular component debonding in two implant systems.

We prospectively recorded details of all complications and failures in our database. For this study, we considered only acetabular failure modes, which include late loosening (>2 years), early loosening ($\leq$2 years), early cup shift ($\leq$2 years), and AWRF (Table 4). Results of the log-rank test (p value=0.0001) and Wilcoxon test (p value=0.0001) revealed implant choice as a significant factor in late acetabular failure, with 13 cases of Group 1 debonding out of 371 total surgeries (3.5%) (Figure 2). Group 2 presented 2 instances of late acetabular failure out of 728 surgeries (0.3%); during revision surgery, the surgeon (TPG) did not classify either of these complications as debonding.

Herein, we retrospectively analyzed clinical data routinely collected as part of standard care. We did not perform retrieval analyses on delaminated implants, although it would be beneficial in understanding where and how extensively debonding occurs. Debonding was confirmed intraoperatively during revision surgery by three professionals familiar with the surgery and product. All debonding patients reported abrupt onset of pain and presented a sudden cup shift on recent X-rays. Most recent metal ion levels prior to loosening were within optimal range, and the mean did not vary significantly from nonloosened cases (4.2 ± 2.7 μg/L, and 2.6 ± 3.7 μg/L, respectively; p value=0.1107). However, moderate metallosis was present intraoperatively in cases revised by the primary surgeon. All cases of debonding presented after 4 years postoperatively. Debonded cups met RAIL in only 30.8% of cases, as compared to 58.6% of all Group 1 cups (p=0.04). However, there was no difference in average AIA or number of cases above the RAIL between Group 1 and Group 2. Thus, cup position may contribute, but is not the sole cause, of debonding. Age, BMI, sex, diagnosis, and postoperative activity did not influence risk of debonding. We identified implant system, postoperative time, and AIA as factors that contribute to risk of debonding.

The available literature comprises three case studies on cup debonding in HRA [15–17] and three in THA [33–35]. These case studies suggest that debonding occurs when shear forces applied at the bone-implant interface are too high, causing patches of porous coating to shear from the cup upon loading. Delport *et al.* [15] found the surface coating of the debonded implant well fixed into the pelvis bone at revision surgery and reported signs of metallosis, although they did not publish metal ion values. Our group primarily performs HRA, and we have thus not encountered debonding in THA. However, we know four case studies on delamination [33–35]. Each group noted significant osteolysis and metallosis in their debonding cases. Amount of porous coating debonding ranged from 60 to 100% of the cup surface.

Manley *et al.* [36] found that the fatigue shearing strength of bead-sintered coating-substrate interfaces was similar to or less than that between coating and bone. An *in vivo* study found shearing strength at the bone-implant interface was between 4.25 and 7.81 MPa for plasma-sprayed, porous Ti coatings [31]. An *in vitro* analysis [24] of Ti porous coat-substrate interfaces found static shear strength to be greater than 20 MPa, on average; this same report showed the coating can withstand fatigue shear forces of 10 MPa for at least 10^7 cycles, per the ASTM F1160 standard [14].

Corin reported static shear strength for the surface-substrate interface of the Cormet cup as 20.9 MPa in a batch of 5, but the standard deviation was 4.1 MPa [14]. Corin also completed shear fatigue strength testing on six samples for 10 million cycles at 10 MPa with no failures. Hot isostatic pressing (HIP) treatment of the Group 1 component may influence the bonding between the porous coat and substrate since HIP removes carbides. HIP may introduce residual stresses into the two materials, as the modulus of elasticity of the porous coat is one-third that of the substrate; however, it has been shown that HIP can increase the strength of adhesion between coat and substrate if done after the PVD process [37, 38].

Although we evaluated differences in implant design and manufacturing processes, we cannot be sure which design features caused Group 1 implants to debond significantly more than Group 2 cups. As described, Corin uses double heat treatment, HIP, and solution annealing, while Biomet does not. A study by Daniel *et al.* concluded that implants with double heat treatment present more wear and osteolysis [39]. With more information on the manufacturing process, we could know whether Corin's HIP introduces residual stresses into the implant, depending on which stage it is performed [37, 38]. Corin uses HA in their acetabular component coating, while Biomet does not; this may contribute to greater bone ingrowth and a stronger lock between bone and the implant surface [40]. In some accounts [21], sphericity between the components differs significantly. Lastly, the Biomet acetabular component has a thicker cup apex at 6 mm compared to Corin cups at 4 mm. Increased apex thickness prevents deformation during impaction, and thus, the Group 2 device may accumulate less damage intraoperatively [41]. We did not record the location of implant debonding in most cases, so we lack the information to identify a consistent pattern. However, of the cases that we did record details of debonding, we identified that delamination usually occurred on the outer edges of the cup and that 33 to 90% of the porous coating had detached from the implant and remained well fixed in the bone.

We hypothesize that debonding occurs at a higher rate in implants with a lower fatigue shear strength, and therefore, the ASTM F1160 testing standard for fatigue shear strength needs to be increased. Microfractures accumulate during daily and strenuous activity while osteocytes remodel bone and repair these microfractures [42]. However, the torsional strain and fatigue shearing stress transmit to the implant, which has no inherent repair capabilities. Thus, despite the greater shear strength at the substrate-coating interface, the bone-coating interface does not accumulate fatigue strain [43, 44]. Inelastic mismatch strain between the surface film and bulk material may also contribute to debonding of the coating [1, 40].

A primary limitation of this study stems from using these resurfacing devices in a consecutive fashion. Group 1 has a follow-up of 13 to 15 years, while the Group 2 is 10 to 13 years out from surgery. However, most acetabular failures occur before 10 years postoperatively (Figure 3). Additionally, to minimize this follow-up bias, we provide an additional comparison of all late loosening between the two groups that occurred before 10 years (2.2% of Group 1 cases, 0.3% of Group 2 cases, p value=0.002). Secondly, many details of the implant manufacturing processes are proprietary, and therefore another limitation is our lack of enough detailed information to identify the exact cause of debonding. Another limitation is our classification of debonding as a binary "yes or no"; detailing the mechanism or extent of debonding will require a future retrieval analysis study. However, the primary purpose of this study was to identify whether rate of debonding varied between implant brands and if there were any differences in the manufacturing processes. Lastly, the Corin group had fewer cases with posttraumatic HRA and was more diagnosed with osteonecrosis. However, no cases with osteonecrosis or posttraumatic HRA debonded.

5. Conclusion

This paper presents a retrospective analysis of a single-surgeon cohort, an implant manufacturer comparison, and a literature review of acetabular debonding, a rare and poorly understood failure mode. In debonding, bone ingrows into the implant initially, but late loosening occurs when the plasma porous coat on the outer face of the acetabular cup becomes detached from the bulk implant and remains fixed to the pelvic bone. Acetabular component position seems to have some influence; we recommend surgeons align acetabular cups according to the RAIL guidelines. Furthermore, the Group 1 acetabular cup failed from debonding at a rate of 3.5% while the Group 2 cup did not delaminate. We identified postoperative time, AIA, and implant type as risk factors for debonding. The differences in manufacturing processes and design (Table 2) for the Group 1 implant likely contribute to its high rate of debonding. According to the current available literature, debonding of the porous coat occurs due to accumulation of microfractures at the coating-substrate interface. Therefore, we believe that a fatigue failure test may be more relevant to this failure mode than a static test. We suggest that the ASTM F1160 standard for fatigue shear strength be increased to minimize the chance that implant coatings will debond even after years of vigorous activity.

Abbreviations

HRA: Hip resurfacing arthroplasty
THA: Total hip arthroplasty
MoM: Metal-on-metal
Ti: Titanium
Co: Cobalt
Cr: Chromium
PVD: Physical vapor deposition
HA: Hydroxyapatite
AWRF: Adverse wear-related failure
HHS: Harris hip score
UCLA: University of California Los Angeles
VAS: Visual analog scale
AIA: Acetabular inclination angle
KM: Kaplan-Meier
RAIL: Relative acetabular inclination limit
HIP: Hot isostatic pressing.

Acknowledgments

This study was paid in full by the primary surgeon (Thomas P. Gross). This research was funded by the senior author and Midlands Orthopaedics & Neurosurgery. The authors do not report any other funding sources or financial support.

References

[1] K. Corten, R. Ganz, J.-P. Simon, and M. Leunig, "Hip resurfacing arthroplasty: current status and future perspectives," *European Cells and Materials*, vol. 21, pp. 243–258, 2011.

[2] H. C. Amstutz and M. J. Le Duff, "Background of metal-on-metal resurfacing," *Proceedings of the Institution of Mechanical Engineers, Part H: Journal of Engineering in Medicine*, vol. 220, no. 2, pp. 85–94, 2006.

[3] S. Williams, I. Leslie, G. Isaac, Z. Jin, E. Ingham, and J. Fisher, "Tribology and Wear of Metal-on-Metal Hip Prostheses: Influence of Cup Angle and Head Position," *The Journal of Bone and Joint Surgery-American Volume*, vol. 90, no. Suppl 3, pp. 111–117, 2008.

[4] P. E. Beaulé, "Surface arthroplasty of the hip: A review and current indications," *Seminars in Arthroplasty*, vol. 16, no. 1, pp. 70–76, 2005.

[5] H. C. Amstutz, P. E. Beaulé, F. J. Dorey, M. J. Le Duff, P. A. Campbell, and T. A. Gruen, "Metal-on-metal hybrid surface arthroplasty: two to six-year follow-up study," *The Journal of Bone & Joint Surgery—American Volume*, vol. 86, no. 1, pp. 28–39, 2004.

[6] M. M. Innmann, S. Weiss, F. Andreas, C. Merle, and M. R. Streit, "Sports and physical activity after cementless total hip arthroplasty with a minimum follow-up of 10 years," *Scandinavian Journal of Medicine & Science in Sports*, vol. 26, no. 5, pp. 550–556, 2016.

[7] T. P. Gross and F. Liu, "Current status of modern fully porous coated metal-on-metal hip resurfacing arthroplasty," *The Journal of Arthroplasty*, vol. 29, no. 1, pp. 181–185, 2014.

[8] H. C. Amstutz, L. E. Wisk, and M. J. Le Duff, "Sex as a Patient Selection Criterion for Metal-on-Metal Hip Resurfacing Arthroplasty," *The Journal of Arthroplasty*, vol. 26, no. 2, pp. 198–208, 2011.

[9] S. S. Jameson, D. J. Langton, S. Natu, and T. V. F. Nargol, "The Influence of Age and Sex on Early Clinical Results After Hip Resurfacing. An Independent Center Analysis," *The Journal of Arthroplasty*, vol. 23, no. 6, pp. 50–55, 2008.

[10] D. W. Howie, "Metal-on-metal resurfacing versus total hip replacement-the value of a randomized clinical tria," *Orthopedic Clinics of North America*, vol. 36, p. 135, 2005.

[11] H. Amstutz, M. Le Duff*, and P. Campbell, "10 Years of Experience with Metal-On-Metal Hybrid Hip Resurfacing: A Review of 1000 Conserve Plus," *The Journal of Arthroplasty*, vol. 23, no. 2, p. 318, 2008.

[12] T. P. Gross, "Outcomes after revision of metal-on-metal hip resurfacing arthroplasty," *The Journal of Arthroplasty*, vol. 29, no. 9, pp. 219–223, 2014.

[13] A. R. Kendal, D. Prieto-Alhambra, N. K. Arden, A. Carr, and A. Judge, "Mortality rates at 10 years after metal-on-metal hip resurfacing compared with total hip replacement in England: Retrospective cohort analysis of hospital episode statistics," *BMJ*, vol. 347, 2013.

[14] Corin Group, "Corin Cormet 2000 FDA executive summary," Tech. Rep., 2012.

[15] H. P. Delport, B. Van Backle, and J. De Schepper, "Debonding of the acetabular porous coating in hip resurfacing arthroplasty a case report," *Acta Orthopædica Belgica*, vol. 77, no. 1, pp. 125–127, 2011.

[16] M. A. Jacobs, T. Bhargava, J. M. Lathroum, and M. W. Hungerford, "Debonding of the Acetabular Porous Coating in Hip Resurfacing Arthroplasty," *The Journal of Bone and Joint Surgery-American Volume*, vol. 91, no. 4, pp. 961–964, 2009.

[17] R. Ray, E. B. Goudie, and P. Gaston, "Debonding of the acetabular porous coating of a hip resurfacing arthroplasty: A case report," *Hip International*, vol. 22, no. 2, pp. 230–232, 2012.

[18] PMA P050016, *PMA P050016 Cormet 2000 Hip Resurfacing System*, Gaithersburg, 2007.

[19] B. Orthopedics, "M2a-magnum™ large metal articulation: design rationale," Tech. Rep., 2009.

[20] Corin Group, "Corin metal-on-metal: a clinical overview," Tech. Rep., 2011.

[21] C. Heisel, J. A. Kleinhans, M. Menge, and J. P. Kretzer, "Ten different hip resurfacing systems: Biomechanical analysis of design and material properties," *International Orthopaedics*, vol. 33, no. 4, pp. 939–943, 2009.

[22] Orthopaedic and Rehabilitation Devices Advisory Panel, "Metal-on-metal implant systems," Tech. Rep., 2012.

[23] P. Campbell, P. E. Beaulé, E. Ebramzadeh et al., "Erratum: The John Charnley award: a study of implant failure in metal-on-metal surface arthroplasties," *Clinical Orthopaedics and Related Research*, vol. 469, no. 9, p. 2657, 2011.

[24] Corin Cormet 2000 Hip Resurfacing System Premarket Approval, 2000.

[25] Corin, Corin Cormet 2000 FDA Executive, 2012.

[26] M. D. Gaillard and T. P. Gross, "Reducing the failure rate of hip resurfacing in dysplasia patients: a retrospective analysis of 363 cases," *BMC Musculoskeletal Disorders*, vol. 17, no. 1, 2016.

[27] K. A. Desmet and C. Van Der Straeten, "The Interpretation of Metal Ion Levels in Unilateral and Bilateral Hip Resurfacing," in *Clinical Orthopaedics and Related Research*, 2012.

[28] W. Harris and W. J. Maloney, "Endosteal errosion in association with stable uncemented femoral components," in *The Journal of bone and joint surgery*, vol. 72, pp. 1025–1034, 1990.

[29] C. A. Zahiri, T. P. Schmalzried, E. S. Szuszczewicz, and H. C. Amstutz, "Assessing activity in joint replacement patients," *The Journal of Arthroplasty*, vol. 13, no. 8, pp. 890–895, 1998.

[30] J. Scott and E. C. Huskisson, "Graphic representation of pain," *PAIN*, vol. 2, no. 2, pp. 175–184, 1976.

[31] V. I. Kalita, A. I. Mamaev, V. A. Mamaeva et al., "Structure and shear strength of implants with plasma coatings," *Inorganic Materials: Applied Research*, vol. 7, no. 3, pp. 376–387, 2016.

[32] F. Liu and T. P. Gross, "A safe zone for acetabular component position in metal-on-metal hip resurfacing arthroplasty: Winner of the 2012 HAP Paul award," *The Journal of Arthroplasty*, vol. 28, no. 7, pp. 1224–1230, 2013.

[33] A. R. Hsu, Z. Vaughn, and J. I. Huddleston, "Early catastrophic failure of a porous-coated acetabular cup due to bead shedding. A case report," *Hip International*, vol. 19, no. 4, pp. 392–395, 2009.

[34] Ł. Łapaj, J. Markuszewski, T. Rybak, and M. Wierusz-Kozłowska, "Debonding of porous coating of a threaded acetabular component: Retrieval analysis," *Journal of the Mechanical Behavior of Biomedical Materials*, vol. 17, pp. 107–111, 2013.

[35] P. Ylinen, "Acetabular cup loosening - Peeling off of the plasma-sprayed porous coating in 2 cases," *Acta Orthopaedica*, vol. 67, no. 5, pp. 508–510, 1996.

[36] M. T. Manley, G. Kotzar, L. S. Stern, and A. Wilde, "Effects of repetitive loading on the integrity of porous coatings," *Clinical Orthopaedics and Related Research*, vol. 217, pp. 293–302, 1987.

[37] A. Abdel-Samad, E. Lugscheider, K. Bobzin, and E. Maes, "Technology C. The influence of hot isostatic pressing on plasma sprayed coatings properties," *Surface and Coatings Technology*, pp. 10–14, 2006.

[38] W. N. Capello, J. A. D'Antonio, J. R. Feinberg, M. T. Manley, and M. Naughton, "Ceramic-on-Ceramic Total Hip Arthroplasty: Update," *The Journal of Arthroplasty*, vol. 23, no. 7, pp. 39–43, 2008.

[39] J. Daniel, H. Ziaee, A. Kamali, C. Pradhan, T. Band, and D. J. W. McMinn, "Ten-year results of a double-heat-treated metal-on-metal hip resurfacing," *The Journal of Bone & Joint Surgery (British Volume)*, vol. 92, no. 1, pp. 20–27, 2010.

[40] Y. C. Tsui, C. Doyle, and T. W. Clyne, "Plasma sprayed hydroxyapatite coatings on titanium substrates. Part 1: Mechanical properties and residual stress levels," *Biomaterials*, vol. 19, no. 22, pp. 2015–2029, 1998.

[41] Z. M. Jin, S. Meakins, M. M. Morlock et al., "Deformation of press-fitted metallic resurfacing cups. Part 1: Experimental simulation," *Proceedings of the Institution of Mechanical Engineers, Part H: Journal of Engineering in Medicine*, vol. 220, no. 2, pp. 299–309, 2006.

[42] K. L. Ong, M. T. Manley, and S. M. Kurtz, "Have contemporary hip resurfacing designs reached maturity? A review.," *The Journal of Bone & Joint Surgery*, vol. 90, pp. 81–88, 2008.

[43] Y. Liao, E. Hoffman, M. Wimmer, A. Fischer, J. Jacobs, and L. Marks, "CoCrMo metal-on-metal hip replacements," *Physical Chemistry Chemical Physics*, vol. 15, no. 3, pp. 746–756, 2013.

[44] A. Lynn and D. DuQuesnay, "Hydroxyapatite-coated Ti–6Al–4V," *Biomaterials*, vol. 23, no. 9, pp. 1937–1946, 2002.

8

Standardised Warfarin Reversal Expedites Time to Theatre for Fractured Neck of Femur Surgery and Improves Mortality Rates: A Matched Cohort Study

Thomas S. Moores, Benjamin D. Chatterton, Matthew J. Walker, and Phillip J. Roberts

Department of Trauma and Orthopaedics, Royal Stoke University Hospital, Stoke-on-Trent, Staffordshire, UK

Correspondence should be addressed to Matthew J. Walker; matthewjohnwalker1987@googlemail.com

Guest Editor: Sumon Nandi

Background. This study aims to evaluate outcomes for warfarinised hip fracture patients and compare them with a matched nonwarfarinised group, before and after the introduction of national hip fracture guidelines in the United Kingdom. *Methods.* A retrospective cohort study of 1743 hip fracture patients was undertaken. All patients admitted taking warfarin were identified. These patients were then matched to nonwarfarinised patients using nearest neighbour propensity score matching, accounting for age, sex, hip fracture type, and Nottingham Hip Fracture Score. A pre-guideline group (no standardised warfarin reversal regimen) and a post-guideline group (standardised regimen) were identified. Outcomes assessed included time to INR less than 1.7, time to theatre, length of stay, and 30-day and 1-year mortality. *Results.* Forty-six warfarinised hip fracture patients were admitted in the pre-guideline group (mean age 80.5, F:M 3:1) and 48 in the post-guideline group (mean age 81.2 years, F:M 3:1). Post-guideline patients were reversed to a safe operative INR level within 18 hours of admission, decreasing the time to first dose vitamin K ($p<0.001$). 70% of warfarinised patients were operated upon within 36 hours, compared to 19.6% with no regimen ($p<0.05$). After anticoagulation reversal protocol, thirty-day mortality decreased from 15.2% to 8.3% and 1-year mortality from 43.5% to 33% for warfarinised patients, which is comparable to nonwarfarinised matched patients. There was no significant change in the length of stay pre- and post-guideline for both groups of patients. *Conclusions.* Proactive anticoagulant management and expedient surgery reduces morbidity and mortality when managing this surgically challenging subset of hip fracture patients.

1. Introduction

1.1. Background and Rationale. An estimated 1% of the United Kingdom (UK) population take warfarin [1] for conditions including atrial fibrillation, venous thromboembolic disease (deep vein thrombosis or pulmonary embolism), cerebrovascular disease, or following cardiac valve surgery [2]. It is estimated that 3.2% of hip fracture patients are admitted taking warfarin [3]; this figure is anticipated to increase in accordance with the predicted rising hip fracture incidence [4] in the UK. There are an estimated 80,000 hip fracture cases per year in the UK [5], and therefore approximately 2500 hip fracture patients will be admitted taking warfarin each year [3]. Traditionally, these patients were considered at high risk, due to the increased risk of bleeding and associated perioperative complications. This subset of hip fracture patients poses a surgical challenge, with UK National Institute of Health and Care Excellence (NICE) guidance [4] focusing upon holistic multidisciplinary patient care, including safely optimising anticoagulation and other comorbidities to undergo emergency surgery [4]. This strategy decreases morbidity and mortality for all hip fracture patients [6–8]. Although no agreed national guidelines exist for the reversal of warfarin in the UK, the use of standardised reversal regimens has been shown to be beneficial in-patient optimisation and reduces their delay to theatre [9, 10]. This, combined with national incentivised “Best Practice” tariff (BPT) [11] and NICE guidelines on holistic care for hip fracture patients [4], has reduced mortality and morbidity [12, 13].

Warfarin is a vitamin K antagonist derived from coumarin [14]. Options to reverse its effect include oral vitamin K, intravenous vitamin K at either high or low dosages, dose omission, and blood products, including fresh frozen plasma (FFP) or prothrombin complex concentrates (PCC) [9, 10, 15–17]. Oral vitamin K takes up to 48 hours to be effective. Blood products have a limited window of effectiveness, need to be used in conjunction with vitamin K, and have additional problems of cost and adverse reactions [9, 10]. Intravenous vitamin K is advocated if surgery can be delayed beyond 12 hours; otherwise blood products may have a role [18–20] to reach a safe operative INR [21, 22]. Seventy-seven percent of delays to theatre beyond 48 hours in hip fracture patients are the result of poorly controlled medical comorbidity or pending investigations [23, 24]. Anticoagulation reversal accounts for 11% of comorbidity related delays [24], which is associated with increased 30-day mortality [4, 7, 25, 26]. Outcomes for warfarinised patients have been recently reported by Lawrence et al., showing that after controlling for prognostic factors such as age, ASA, and AMTS, warfarin therapy at the time of hip fracture is associated with increased time to surgery, length of stay, and increased mortality [27]. However, there has been no analysis against a matched group of patients who were not anticoagulated with warfarin on admission.

1.2. Objectives. We hypothesised that the introduction of our standardised regimen for the reversal of anticoagulation in fractured neck of femur patients would expedite their surgery and possibly reduce subsequent length of stay and post-operative mortality. The aims of this study were to evaluate outcomes for warfarinised patients admitted with a hip fracture before and after the introduction of a standardised reversal regimen for warfarin, compared to matched non-warfarinised patients. The measurable outcomes chosen were time to theatre, length of stay, and post-operative mortality.

2. Patients and Methods

2.1. Study Design. This study was a retrospective analysis of prospectively collected matched data. A search through our institution's database was performed on all patients admitted to our institution between the 1st of January 2008 and 28th February 2012 with a hip fracture. A list of patients admitted between these dates for whom the primary International Classification of Diseases-10 (ICD-10) diagnosis code for their spell corresponded to hip fracture (S72.0, fracture of neck of femur; S72.1, pertrochanteric fracture; S72.2, sub-trochanteric fracture) was generated [28]. These patients were cross-referenced with our institutions admissions database to ensure that the data were accurate. This was further cross-referenced with our institutions National Hip Fracture Database (NHFD) records for all hip fracture patients input onto the National Audit Programme [12]. No patients were excluded. The key outcomes assessed included time to first dose of vitamin K and International Normalized Ratio (INR) less than 1.7 (this is our centres agreed safe operative level by surgeons and anaesthetists), time to theatre, length of stay, and 30-day and 1-year mortality. The time to INR of less than 1.7 is taken from time of admission to the time of publication of the laboratory published results on the electronic pathology system for all cases.

2.2. Identification of Patients. From the generated hip fracture patient list, comorbidities were recorded on our institutions' admissions database, which allowed us to identify all patients admitted on warfarin for any reason. These patients were assigned to the "warfarinised" arm of the study. This cohort continued with their warfarin therapy long-term following surgery. The generated hip fracture patient list was also the source of the matched nonwarfarinised patients. This cohort were assigned to the "matched" arm of the study. Post-operatively, the matched cohort were given the standard prophylactic regimen of 4 weeks daily subcutaneous dalteparin as venous thromboembolic event (VTE) prophylaxis.

Warfarinised patients were divided into a pre-guideline and post-guideline group, with the introduction of the BPT of April 2010 being the delineation between these groups. The pre-guideline group included all warfarinised patients between 1st January 2008 and 31st March 2010, whilst the post-guideline group included all patients between 1st April 2010 and 28th February 2012. The pre-guideline group were not treated with a standardised warfarin reversal protocol and received variable amounts of intravenous vitamin K, at variable times based on the clinical judgement of the clinical team. The post-guideline group received a standardised protocol of low dose 2mg intravenous vitamin K every 6 hours from admission until their INR was less than 1.7.

Electronic patient records were used to establish patient demographics, Nottingham Hip Fracture Score, admission date, time to theatre, discharge date, and date of death for each patient, allowing calculation of 30-day and 1-year mortality. The fracture pattern was obtained from the patient's ICD-10 primary diagnosis code [28]. These were categorised as (i) intracapsular fracture and (ii) extracapsular and sub-trochanteric fractures and cross-referenced with the admission database and PACS (Picture Archiving and Communication System) radiological software. Theatre and anaesthetic databases were accessed for timings to theatre, operation type, and ASA grade. The time to theatre was calculated from time of admission in the Emergency Department to the time the patient entered the anaesthetic room in hours. Timings to theatre were categorised as (i) less than 36 hours, (ii) 36-48 hours, (iii) greater than 48 hours, and (iv) no operation. These categories have been devised because the BPT target for time to theatre is less than 36 hours, and the NICE target is less than 48 hours, allowing comparison of our data with the National Hip Fracture Database (NHFD). Length of stay was expressed in days and is the time from admission in A&E to discharge from orthopaedic care and relates to their acute hospital spell. Thirty-day mortality was calculated by including patients who had died on any day up to and including day 30 following admission, and for 1-year mortality calculation patients who died up to and including 365 days from their day of admission were included in the analysis.

2.3. Statistical Analysis

2.3.1. Patient Matching. The pre-guideline and post-guideline warfarinised cohorts were matched separately with nonwarfarinised patients using a "one to one nearest neighbour model" of propensity score matching for the variables of age (years), sex, fracture type, and Nottingham Hip Fracture Score [29]. Patient matching was necessary to compare outcomes for patients admitted on warfarin versus those who were not anticoagulated. Once each warfarin case had been matched to a nonwarfarin case, that patient was eliminated from any further matching to avoid duplication of patients and allow direct comparison of outcomes for these patients.

2.3.2. Outcomes. Data were collated in Microsoft Excel 2010, and data analysis was performed using SPSS Statistics for Windows (version 22.0, IBM Corp., Armonk, NY, 2013) and the statistical package R (R version 3.0.2 (2012-09-25)) [30]. Descriptive statistics were used to describe the study population, with independent samples t-tests used to analyse continuous variables and chi-squared test used to analyse categorical variables. Statistical significance was assumed if $p<0.05$. For the pre-guideline and post-guideline groups their matched nonwarfarinised cases were compared for any difference in age, sex, fracture type, and Nottingham Hip Fracture Score (NHFS). Kaplan-Meier survival curves were used to compare survival between warfarinised and nonwarfarinised patients in the pre-guideline and post-guideline groups. Additionally, a further analysis of survival comparing warfarinised patients from the pre-guideline group to warfarinised patients in the post-guideline group was undertaken, with patient death being the survival outcome in both cases. This was calculated from day of admission to date of death or date of final follow-up. Chi-squared analysis was used to compare the survival curves between the two groups, with a p value of less than 0.05 ($p<0.05$) being considered significant.

3. Results

3.1. Study Population. A total of 1743 patients were initially identified from electronic patient records, 786 from the pre-guideline group and 957 from the post-guideline group. In the pre-guideline group 46 patients (5.9%) were admitted taking warfarin (33 females, 13 males), with a mean age of 80.5 years (±7.6 years, range 61-93 years). There were 26 intracapsular hip fractures and 20 extracapsular hip fractures, and the mean NHFS predicted a 9.2% (±6.5%) 30-day operative mortality. In the post-guideline group 48 patients (5.0%) were admitted taking warfarin (32 females, 16 males), with a mean age of 81.2 years (±8.0 years, range 62-100 years). There were 28 intracapsular hip fractures and 20 extracapsular hip fractures, and the mean NHFS predicted a 7.2% (±3.7%) 30-day operative mortality. Each patient was matched for age, sex, fracture type, and NHFS; there was no significant difference in these variables between warfarinised or nonwarfarinised patients in the pre-guideline group. In the post-guideline group there was no statistical difference between variables except in NHFS. The nonwarfarinised matched group had a mean NHFS of 9.8% (±7.6%) for 30-day operative mortality; this was statistically significant compared to the mean 7.2% for the warfarinised controls ($p=0.04$). This data is summarised in Table 1.

3.2. Comparison of Warfarinised Groups Pre- and Post-Guideline. Comparing the demographics of the two warfarinised groups showed no statistical difference in age ($p=0.641$), in sex 3:1 female ($p=0.901$) to male ($p=0.743$) ratio, or between extracapsular ($p=1.000$) and intracapsular ($p=0.960$) fractures. There was a statistically significant difference ($p=0.006$) between mean NHFS of 9.2 (±6.5) and 7.2 (±3.7), for pre-guideline and post-guideline groups, respectively.

3.3. Warfarin Reversal Management to Safe Operative Level. As shown in Table 1, the mean admission INR was 2.6 and 2.5 for the pre-guideline and post-guideline warfarinised groups, respectively. In the pre-guideline group there was no standardised reversal regimen, and each patient received different treatment. Patients received either no treatment or intravenous vitamin K, with doses ranging from 1mg to 10mg. The mean time from admission to administering the first dose of intravenous vitamin K was 13.07 hours (± 7.07), with a range of 1-28 hours after admission.

In the post-guideline group all patients received the same standardised reversal regimen with a mean time to 1st dose vitamin K of 3 hours; comparing this to the pre-guideline group of 13.07 hours, this result was statistically significant (please see Table 2).

3.4. Time to Theatre. As shown in Table 3, there was a mean delay to theatre of 70.36 hours (± 61.9 hours) from admission for the warfarinised patients, pre-guideline. The mean time to theatre for the matched pre-guideline nonwarfarinised patients was significantly lower, 44 hours ($p=0.03$). In the post-guideline patients who were on warfarin, there was a mean time to theatre of 46 hours (± 37.927 hours). The mean time to theatre for those not taking warfarin was 43 hours ($p=0.755$).

In the pre-guideline group of patients taking warfarin, 19.6% were operated upon in less than 36 hours compared to 45.7% of the nonwarfarinised group at the same time. Following the introduction of a local warfarin reversal protocol and incentivised guidelines, 70.8% of patients taking warfarin were operated upon within 36 hours, which is comparable to the 77% of nonwarfarinised patients at the same time. Prior to the introduction of national guidelines giving the 36 [18] and 48-hour [19] targets, there were no specific targets, but the NHFD reported outcomes for surgery within 48 hours [26]. Therefore, comparing the pre-guideline groups, 28.3% of warfarinised patients and 65.2% of nonwarfarinised patients were operated upon within 48 hours. After national targets were introduced, these figures improved to 77.1% of warfarinised patients and 85.4% of nonwarfarinised patients having surgery within the 48-hour target. Since the introduction of a local warfarin reversal protocol there has been a statistically significant decrease in

Table 1: Summary of study population demographics for propensity score matched cohorts pre- and post-guidelines. (M: male, F: female, IC: intracapsular, EC: extracapsular; comparing warfarin cases column relates to the warfarin cases pre- and post-guideline; * p < 0.05 is statistically significant.)

		Pre-Guideline			Post-guideline			P-Value
		Case	Matched	P-value	Case	Matched	P-value	Comparing warfarin cases
Total		46	46/786		48	48/957		
Age years	Mean	80.5 (±7.6)	80.5 (+/- 7.4)	0.97	81.2 (+/- 8.0)	81.3 (+/- 8.3)	0.97	0.641
	Range	61-93	61-93		62-100	62-104		
Sex (%)	M	13 (28.3)	14 (30.4)	0.89	16 (33.3)	17 (35.4)	0.92	0.743
	F	33 (71.7)	32 (69.6)	0.93	32 (66.7)	31 (64.6)	0.9	0.901
NHFS		9.2 (+/- 6.5)	8.9 (+/- 5.2)	0.86	7.2 (+/- 3.7)	9.8 (+/- 7.6)	*0.04	*0.006
Fracture Type (%)	IC	26 (57)	26 (57)	1.0	28 (58)	28 (58)	1.0	0.960
	EC	20 (43)	20 (43)	1.0	20 (42)	20 (42)	1.0	1.0
INR on Admission	Mean	2.6 (+/-0.9)			2.5 (+/- 1.0)			0.87
	Range	1.2-5.1			1.4-4.9			

Table 2: A comparison of pre- and post-guideline time to first dose of 2mg intravenous vitamin K from admission.

		Pre-Guideline	Post-Guideline	P Value
Time to 1st dose Vitamin K (Hours)	Mean	13.07 (+/-7.07)	3.00 (+/-1.11)	*<0.001
	Range	1-28	2-6	

time to theatre for 36 hours (p=0.039) and 48 hours (p=0.041) when comparing the two warfarinised groups.

3.5. Length of Stay. The mean length of stay was 5.1 and 1.6 days less for the nonwarfarinised matched patients in the pre- and post-guideline groups, respectively (p=0.10 and 0.22). Following the introduction of the local warfarin protocol, the length of stay increased by 5 days; however, this was not statistically significant (p=0.408) (Table 4).

3.6. Mortality. Referring to Table 5, in the pre-guideline group, 30-day mortality for the warfarinised and nonwarfarinised patients was 15.2% and 8.7%, respectively (p=0.34). One-year mortality was 43.5% and 26.1% for the warfarinised and matched nonwarfarinised patients, respectively (p=0.15). There was a mean follow-up of 54 months allowing Kaplan-Meier analysis and chi-squared analysis of the difference between the two curves (see Figure 1).

In the post-guideline group, 30-day mortality for the warfarinised and nonwarfarinised patients was 8.3% and 6.2%, respectively (p=0.63). One-year mortality was 33.3% and 33.3%, respectively, for the warfarinised and matched nonwarfarinised patients (p=1.00). There was a mean follow-up of 38 months allowing Kaplan-Meier analysis and chi-squared analysis of the difference between the two curves (see Figure 2). There was no statistical difference in long-term survival between warfarinised and nonwarfarinised patients (p=0.992). There was also no significant difference in long-term survival between pre- and post-guideline warfarinised patients (p=0.67) and between pre- and post-guideline matched patients (p=0.43)

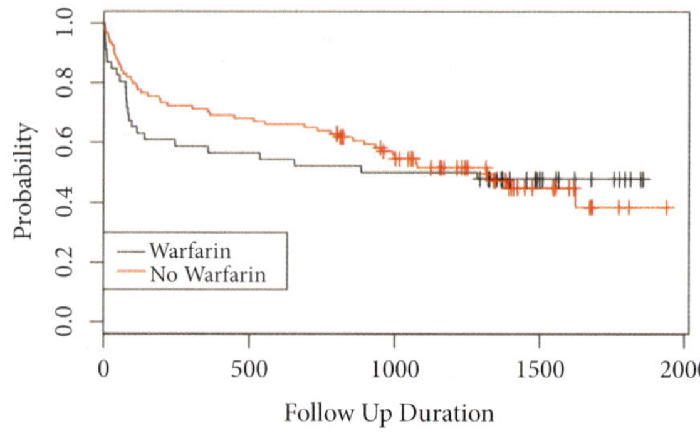

Figure 1: Kaplan-Meier curve of pre-guideline matched warfarinised and nonwarfarinised patients during 54-month follow-up (follow-up duration in days).

4. Discussion

The NHFD has shown that introduction of national guidelines has had a significant beneficial effect on outcomes for all hip fracture patients [12]. However, they do not

Table 3: A comparison of time to theatre between pre- and post-guideline, and warfarinised and matched patients.

		Pre-Guideline			Post-Guideline			Odds Ratio (95% CI) Pre- and Post-Guideline		P Value
		Case	Matched	P-value	Case	Matched	P-value	Comparing Warfarin Cases	Comparing Matched Cases	Comparing warfarin cases
Time to Theatre (Hours)	Mean (SD)	70.4 (61.93)	44.2 (40.97)	*0.039	46 (37.97(	42.5 (80.90)	0.79			*0.036
	Range	13-307	9-183		12-183	13-571				
Time to Theatre (Hours) n (%)	<36	9 (19.6)	21 (45.7)	*0.024	34 (70.8)	37 (77.1)	0.279	7.83 (2.96-20.70)	4.50 (1.76-11.51)	*0.039
	36-48	4 (8.7)	9 (19.6)		3 (6.3)	4 (8.3)				*0.041
	<48	13 (28.3)	30 (28.3)	*0.002	37	41 (85.4)	0.12	6.47 (2.50-16.72)	3.83 (1.24-11.78)	<0.001
	>48	25 (54.3)	14 (30.4)		11 (22.9)	5 (10.4)				*0.047
	No op	8 (17.4)	2 (4.3)		0 (0)	2 (4.2)				

Table 4: A comparison of pre- and post-guideline length of stay between warfarinised and nonwarfarinised matched patients.

		Pre-Guideline			Post-Guideline			Change in LOS		P Value	
		Case	Matched	P Value	Case	Matched	P Value	Case	Matched	Comparing Warfarin Cases	Comparing Matched Cases
Length of Stay (Days)	Mean (SD)	17.3 (14.2)	13.2 (9.4)	0.10	22.4 (39.7)	14.8 (15.1)	0.22	5.1	1.6	0.408	0.53

Table 5: A comparison of pre- and post-guideline mortality % at 30 days and at 1 year for warfarinised patients and nonwarfarinised matched patients.

		Pre-Guideline				Post-Guideline				Hazard Ratio (95% CI)		P Value
		Case	Matched	P Value	Hazard Ratio (95% CI)	Case	Matched	P Value	Hazard Ratio (95% CI)	Comparing Warfarin Cases	Comparing Matched Cases	Comparing Warfarin Cases
Mortality (%)	30-Day	15.2	8.7	0.34	1.81 (0.14-5.90)	8.3	6.2	0.63	1.36 (0.44-4.16)	0.97 (0.48-1.96)	1.42 (0.76-1.96)	0.299
	1 Year	43.5	26.1	0.15	1.70 (1.34-2.15)	33.3	33.3	1.0	0.96 (0.75-1.24)	1.16 (0.65-2.07)	0.86 (0.41-1.78)	0.312

identify specific subsets of high-risk patients who may benefit from specific optimisation, for example, warfarinised patients requiring an anticoagulation reversal protocol to ensure national targets are met. Patients admitted with a hip fracture requiring emergency surgery whilst being anticoagulated with warfarin pose a challenging surgical dilemma. Our findings suggest that having a warfarin reversal protocol as part of preoperative optimisation has significantly reduced the time to theatre for this challenging subset of patients. The majority of warfarinised patients (77%) are undergoing their emergency surgery within the national targets, which has likely contributed to a reduced length of stay and decreased 30-day and 1-year mortality [4, 11].

Reviewing the NHFD reveals that the average age for hip fracture patients is 80 years, with a 3:1 female to male ratio [4]. Our pre-guideline cases had a mean age of 80.5 with 71.7% being female, which is consistent with the NHFD audit demographic data. In the post-guideline group the mean age was slightly higher at 81.2 years, with 33% of patients being male; this differs from the NHFD population, with males known to have poorer outcomes following hip fracture [31]. The national average life expectancy in 2010 was 79 years for males and 83 years for females [32], with our cohort having their hip fracture at approximately this age and the age range for the cohorts reaching 93 years and 100 years in the pre- and post-guideline groups, respectively. These patients would have a high mortality risk due to their age and comorbidities even prior to the additional increase in mortality risk associated with hip fracture, which is an independent clinical risk factor [33]. A comparable distribution is seen when comparing the type of fracture to that recorded in the NHFD (57% intracapsular types, 40% extracapsular types, and 3% unknown) [12].

The previously reported proportion of patients taking warfarin admitted with a hip fracture is reported as a minimum of 3.2% [3]. This was higher in our study population,

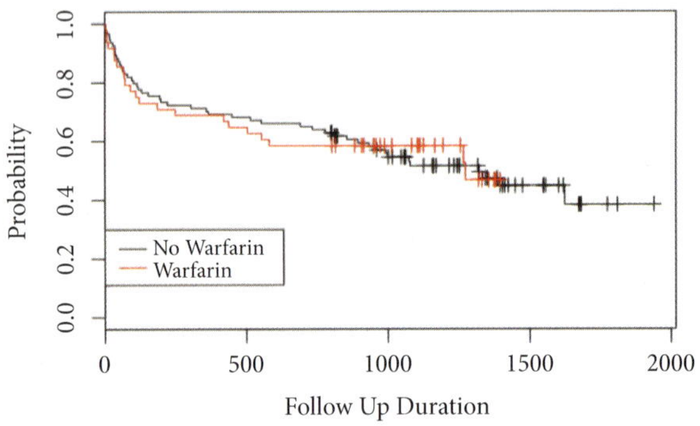

FIGURE 2: Kaplan-Meier curve of post-guideline matched warfarinised and nonwarfarinised patients during 58-month follow-up (follow-up duration in days).

being 5.9% and 5.0% for pre- and post-guideline groups, respectively. As patients live longer, they have an increased risk of developing comorbidities requiring warfarin therapy to reduce their embolic relative risk [3, 17]. Our warfarinised patients were older than those seen in Ashouri et al.'s population, which may explain our higher proportion of warfarinised patients [3].

The biggest delay in warfarin reversal was the time to the first dose of vitamin K. Without a protocol this was poorly addressed with a mean time to first dose of 13 hours. This significantly reduced to 3 hours ($p<0.001$) after protocol introduction, with all patients INR being in a safe operative range within 24 hours of admission. It is well reported that the early hip fracture surgery is associated with improved outcomes, with national guidance suggesting surgery within 48 hours [4, 7, 8, 11]. Indeed, recent studies have suggested that outcomes deteriorate when surgery is delayed beyond 12 hours [6]. Repeated low dose intravenous vitamin K is appropriate to achieve surgery within 36 hours [9], but if surgery within 12 hours was necessary to improve outcomes, then blood products would need to be considered [18]. The use of FFP and PCC is unreported in hip fracture literature and should be given with caution and on haematology advice, due to potential complications including Transfusion Related Acute Lung Injury (TRALI), anaphylaxis, blood borne infections (HIV and Hepatitis B), and allo-immunisation [34, 35].

Length of stay has fallen since the introduction of the national guidelines but was greater for warfarinised patients compared to their matched controls in both the pre- and post-guideline groups. In the pre-guideline group the delay in preoperative reversal of warfarin contributed, with delayed surgery being associated with increased length of stay, morbidity including pressure sores and respiratory infections, and mortality [7], to complications not seen in our cohort.

The NHFD reports on 30-day and 1-year mortality, but there is no long-term mortality data. For our cohorts we have mortality data reported at final follow-up of mean 54 months and 34 months in the pre- and post-guideline groups, respectively. Mortality at 30 days and 1 year was higher in the pre-guideline warfarinised group (15.2% and 43.5%) compared to their matched cases (8.7% and 26.1%). This supports the proposition that delays to theatre and poor preoperative warfarin anticoagulation reversal are associated with poorer outcomes in warfarinised patients compared to their matched cases [7, 8, 31]. Chatterton et al. reported post-mortem data for deaths within 30 days with pneumonia being the commonest cause of death [13]. Given the delays to theatre preoperatively (mean 70 hours), warfarinised patients were at high risk for pneumonia secondary to poor lung ventilation because of immobility, posture, opiate medications, and pain. Following the introduction of the warfarin reversal protocol and national incentivised guidelines, 30-day mortality for the warfarinised and nonwarfarinised patients had reduced to 8.3% and 6.2%, respectively ($p=0.63$), which is comparable to the NHFD data [12]. Reversing the INR rapidly and safely has meant that 77% of patients were operated upon within 48 hours, which is known to improve outcomes [7, 8, 32, 36]. One-year mortality was 33.3% in both the warfarinised and matched nonwarfarinised patients (Figure 2), with no difference between mortality curves ($p=0.992$). Long-term follow-up is rare for hip fracture patients, and the Kaplan-Meier curves demonstrate that mortality is greatest in the first year followed by mortality plateaus with no difference (pre-guideline $p=0.776$, post-guideline $p=0.992$) between the warfarinised and nonwarfarinised curves by 54 and 38 months of follow-up, respectively.

The strengths of this study design include the case matching to enable comparison between outcomes in warfarinised and nonwarfarinised hip fracture patients. Matching was utilised to address the issues of confounding in the design phase of the study. The method of matching used a one to one nearest neighbour model [29], which allows direct analysis of treatment of anticoagulation reversal compared to those not anticoagulated at admission. Limitations include the patient list being generated utilising the ICD-10 codes for hip fracture [28]. This should not have affected our study because hip fracture coding in the UK has not changed since 1995 [37], predating our study period. In addition, a systematic review of 32 studies has shown that discharge coding accuracy levels are sufficiently robust for research use [38]. Furthermore, our data was cross-referenced with multiple sources to confirm accuracy. Due to the retrospective nature of this study we were also unable to obtain specific data on post-operative complications including wound issues, thrombotic events, or pressure sores.

This matched cohort study of a surgically challenging subset of hip fracture patients shows poorer outcomes for warfarinised patients than a matched cohort of nonwarfarinised patients. Implementing a proactive warfarin reversal policy coupled with national incentivised care standards facilitates rapid surgery, improving holistic care and 30-day and 1-year mortality. Intravenous vitamin K is safe to achieve surgery within 36 hours; however if surgery within 12 hours could improve outcomes further, then blood products may be required, an area that requires further research.

by the senior author of this paper. The collected and processed data used for the statistical calculations are on a spreadsheet in the possession of all authors. Both the database and spreadsheet can be accessed on request.

Disclosure

Level of evidence is level III.

Acknowledgments

The authors are grateful to the Clinical Coding Department and Anaesthetic Department theatre analyst at their institution for assistance with data collection for this study.

References

[1] M. Marzolini and H. A. Wynne, "Should patients manage their own oral anticoagulation therapy?" *Reviews in Clinical Gerontology*, vol. 12, no. 4, pp. 275–281, 2003.

[2] M. Sudlow, R. Thomson, B. Thwaites, H. Rodgers, and R. A. Kenny, "Prevalence of atrial fibrillation and eligibility for anticoagulants in the community," *The Lancet*, vol. 352, no. 9135, pp. 1167–1171, 1998.

[3] F. Ashouri, W. Al-jundi, A. Patel, and J. Mangwani, "Management of Warfarin Anticoagulation in Patients with Fractured Neck of Femur," *Haem*, p. 194628, 2011.

[4] National Institute for Health and Care Excellence, "Hip Fracture: The management of hip fracture in adults (2011)," CG124. London. (date last accessed November 2014) https://www.nice.org.uk/guidance/CG124.

[5] Health Episode Statistics. Primary diagnosis: 4 character, S72.0–S72.2. (date last accessed 16 August 2014) http://www.hes-online.org.uk/Ease/servlet/ContentServer?siteID=1937&categoryID=214.

[6] C. P. Bretherton and M. J. Parker, "Early surgery for patients with a fracture of the hip decreases 30 day mortality," *The Bone & Joint Journal*, vol. 97, no. B(1), pp. 104–108, 2015.

[7] T. Shiga, Z. Wajima, and Y. Ohe, "Is operative delay associated with increased mortality of hip fracture patients? Systematic review, meta-analysis, and meta-regression," *Canadian Journal of Anesthesia*, vol. 55, no. 3, pp. 146–154, 2008.

[8] L. Moja, A. Piatti, V. Pecoraro et al., "Timing matters in hip fracture surgery: patients operated within 48 hours have better outcomes. A meta-analysis and meta-regression of over 190,000 patients," *PLoS ONE*, vol. 7, no. 10, Article ID e46175, 2012.

[9] T. S. Moores, A. Beaven, A. E. Cattell, C. Baker, and P. J. Roberts, "Preoperative warfarin reversal for early hip fracture surgery," *Journal of Orthopaedic Surgery*, vol. 23, no. 1, pp. 33–36, 2015.

[10] A. Leonidou, R. Rallan, N. Cox, J. Pagkalos, and J. Luscombe, "Comparison of different warfarin reversal protocols on surgical delay and complication rate in hip fracture patients.," *Journal of Orthopaedic Surgery (Hong Kong)*, vol. 21, no. 2, pp. 142–145, 2013.

[11] Department of Health Payment by Results team, "Best Practice Tariff," (last accessed December 2014). http://www.dh.gov.uk/health/2012/02/confirmation-pbr-arrangements/.

[12] Royal College of Physicians, "National Hip Fracture Database annual report 2014," London: RCP, 2014. http://www.nhfd.co.uk/20/hipfractureR.nsf/vwcontent/2014reportPDFs/$file/NHFD2014ExtendedReport.pdf?OpenElement.

[13] D. B. Chatterton, T. S. Moores, A. Cattell et al., "Cause of death and factors associated with early in-hospital mortality after hip fracture: An eight-year retrospective cohort study of 4426 patients," *The Bone & Joint Journal*, vol. 97B, pp. 246–251, 2015.

[14] D. S. Whitlon, J. A. Sadowski, J. W. Suttie, and J. A. Sadowski, "Mechanism of Coumarin Action: Significance of Vitamin K Epoxide Reductase Inhibition," *Biochemistry*, vol. 17, no. 8, pp. 1371–1377, 1978.

[15] R. Bansal and D. K. Watson, "Surgical delay in acute admissions on warfarin: Are we doing enough?" *International Journal of Clinical Practice*, vol. 59, no. 11, pp. 1283–1288, 2005.

[16] R. H. White, T. McKittrick, R. Hutchinson, and J. Twitchell, "Temporary discontinuation of warfarin therapy: Changes in the international normalized ratio," *Annals of Internal Medicine*, vol. 122, no. 1, pp. 40–42, 1995.

[17] M. Al-Rashid and M. J. Parker, "Anticoagulation management in hip fracture patients on warfarin," *Injury*, vol. 59, no. 11, pp. 1283–1288, 2005.

[18] British Committee for Standards in Haematology, "BTTF. Guidelines for the use of fresh-frozen plasma, cryoprecipitate and cryosupernatant," The British Society for Haematology; 2004.

[19] H. G. Watson, T. Baglin, S. L. Laidlaw, M. Makris, and F. E. Preston, "A comparison of the efficacy and rate of response to oral and intravenous Vitamin K in reversal of over-anticoagulation with warfarin," *British Journal of Haematology*, vol. 115, no. 1, pp. 145–149, 2001.

[20] J. Ansell, J. Hirsh, E. Hylek, A. Jacobson, M. Crowther, and G. Palareti, "Pharmacology and management of the vitamin k antagonists: american college of chest physicians evidence-based clinical practice guidelines," *CHEST*, vol. 133, no. 6, pp. 160–198, 2008.

[21] T. T. Horlocker, D. J. Wedel, H. Benzon et al., "Regional Anesthesia in the Anticoagulated Patient," *Regional Anesthesia and Pain Medicine*, vol. 28, no. 3, pp. 172–197, 2003.

[22] C. Kearon and J. Hirsh, "Management of anticoagulation before and after elective surgery," *The New England Journal of Medicine*, vol. 336, no. 21, pp. 1506–1511, 1997.

[23] C. P. Charalambous, S. Yarwood, C. Paschalides et al., "Factors delaying surgical treatment of hip fractures in elderly patients," *Annals of the Royal College of Surgeons of England*, vol. 85, pp. 117–119, 2003.

[24] M. P. Fantini, G. Fabbri, M. Laus et al., "Determinants of surgical delay for hip fracture," *The Surgeon*, vol. 9, no. 3, pp. 130–134, 2011.

[25] Scottish Intercollegiate Guidelines Network, "Guideline 111. Management of hip fracture in older people. A national clinical guideline," 2009. (last accessed December 2014) https://www.sign.ac.uk/assets/sign111.pdf.

[26] C. G. Moran, R. T. Wenn, M. Sikand, and A. M. Taylor, "Early Mortality after hip fracture: is delay before surgery important?" *Journal of Bone and Joint Surgery*, vol. 87, no. 3, pp. 483–498, 2005.

[27] J. E. Lawrence, D. M. Fountain, D. J. Cundall-Curry, and A. D. Carrothers, "Do Patients Taking Warfarin Experience Delays to Theatre, Longer Hospital Stay, and Poorer Survival After Hip Fracture?" *Clinical Orthopaedics and Related Research*, vol. 475, no. 1, pp. 273–279, 2017.

[28] World Health Organisation, "International Statistical Classification of Diseases and Related Health Problems 10th Revision," (date last accessed 16 August 2014) http://apps.who.int/classifications/icd10/browse/2010/en.

[29] P. C. Austin, "An introduction to propensity score methods for reducing the effects of confounding in observational studies,"

Multivariate Behavioral Research, vol. 46, no. 3, pp. 399–424, 2011.

[30] R Core Team, "R: A language and environment for statistical computing. R Foundation for Statistical Computing, Vienna, Austria, 2013," (accessed December 2014) http://www.R-project.org/.

[31] F. Hu, C. Jiang, J. Shen, P. Tang, and Y. Wang, "Preoperative predictors for mortality following hip fracture surgery: a systematic review and meta-analysis," *Injury*, vol. 43, no. 6, pp. 676–685, 2012.

[32] Office for National Statistics, "Mortality in England and Wales: Average Life Span," Published December 2012. (date last accessed December 2014) http://www.ons.gov.uk/ons/dcp171776_292196.pdf.

[33] S. A. Frost, N. D. Nguyen, J. R. Center et al., "Excess mortality attribuitable to hip fracture: a relative Survival analysis," *Bone*, vol. 56, pp. 23–29, 2013.

[34] S. MacLennan and L. M. Williamson, "Risks of fresh frozen plasma and platelets," *The Journal of Trauma*, vol. 60, pp. S46–S50, 2006.

[35] S. Travis, R. Wray, and K. Harrison, "Perioperative anticoagulant control," *British Journal of Surgery*, vol. 76, no. 11, pp. 1107-1108, 1989.

[36] C. L. Daugaard, H. L. Jorgensen, T. Riis, J. B. Lauritzen, B. R. Duus, and S. Van Der Mark, "Is mortality after hip fracture associated with surgical delay or admission during weekends and public holidays? A retrospective study of 38,020 patients," *Acta Orthopaedica*, vol. 83, no. 6, pp. 609–613, 2012.

[37] S. Balasegaram, A. Majeed, and H. Fitz-Clarence, "Trends in hospital admissions for fractures of the hip and femur in England, 1989-1990 to 1997-1998," *Journal of Public Health*, vol. 23, no. 1, pp. 11–17, 2001.

[38] E. M. Burns, E. Rigby, R. Mamidanna et al., "Systematic review of discharge coding accuracy," *Journal of Public Health*, vol. 34, no. 1, pp. 138–148, 2012.

9

Evidence of Negative Effects of Defect Size and Older Patient Age by Quantitative CT-Based 3D Image Analysis in Ultraporous Beta-Tricalcium Phosphate Grafted Extremity Bone Defects at One Year

Timothy A. Damron and Kenneth A. Mann

SUNY Upstate Medical University, Syracuse, New York, USA

Correspondence should be addressed to Timothy A. Damron; damront@upstate.edu

Academic Editor: Allen L. Carl

Introduction. Synthetic bone graft materials are commonly used to fill defects after curettage of benign bone lesions. Ultraporous beta tricalcium phosphate (TCP) is a popular synthetic compound used in this situation. Prior clinical studies based on plain X-ray analysis suggest incorporation of TCP is incomplete, even when combined with bone marrow (BMA). *Purpose*. The purpose was to analyze volumetric CT-based changes in defects grafted with TCP with/without BMA in a completed prospective RCT to objectively determine (1) relationship between size and age versus TCP incorporation and (2) whether there is an advantage to addition of BMA. *Methods*. Twenty-one patients with CT scans at ≥1 year follow-up available for digital analysis (TCP=10, TCP w/BMA =11) form the study population. CT image stacks were evaluated by creating volumetric masks using MIMICS imaging software for total defect, graft remaining, and graft incorporated volumes graft incorporation endpoints. *Results*. Overall, there was significant (p=0.0029) negative correlation ($r^2 = 0.38$) between defect size and ratio of incorporated bone to defect size. This relationship remained strong ($r^2 = 0.56$) particularly for defects > 20 cc but not for smaller defects. Bone width was also a significantly related factor ($r^2 = 0.94$), with less graft incorporation in larger bone sites, in part likely due to the linear relationship between defect size and bone width. Relationship with age was complex and closely tied to defect volume. For larger defect volumes, younger patients were more successful at graft incorporation. Although age itself was not an independently significant factor, as defect volume increased, advanced age more negatively impacted new bone formation. *Conclusions*. Larger size defect and affected bone and advancing age appear to be important negative factors in synthetic graft incorporation. Results showed no advantage to addition of BMA to TCP.

1. Introduction

Defects created after curettage of benign bone tumors may be filled with autologous, allograft, or synthetic graft materials [1, 2]. In our prior use of the synthetic bone graft substitute ultraporous beta-tricalcium phosphate (TCP), the material performed well with the addition of local blood alone, but there was radiographic evidence of graft material that had not fully incorporated after a year or longer [3]. Although prolonged persistence of unincorporated TCP may serve as a potential stress riser, no adverse effects were observed in that study, and subsequent reports on its use have also been promising [4–6].

The addition of bone marrow aspirates to the TCP material has been suggested to enhance incorporation. In our completed randomized prospective clinical study, we were unable to show a significant difference in radiographic incorporation for TCP combined with bone marrow aspirate (TCP-BMA) compared to TCP alone [4]. However, both groups showed qualitative evidence of progressive TCP incorporation over time. No quantitative analysis of the CT scans from that study has been reported.

Despite the potential of allowing more detailed analysis of bone defect healing, CT scans have been underutilized for assessing the incorporation of graft materials. Most of the recent usage has been in the areas of spine, periodontal, and foot/ankle procedures [5–16]. The only bone defect study in which CT scans have been utilized is the aforementioned prospective clinical evaluation of TCP, but the analysis was performed in an arguably subjective fashion by radiology interpretation [4]. No detailed quantitative CT analysis was performed.

The purpose of this study was to use a quantitative CT-based volumetric imaging analysis approach for a detailed quantitative subanalysis of the previously reported larger prospective study comparing the use of TCP alone to TCP with BMA as bone fillers after curettage of benign lesions. Our hypotheses were that TCP incorporation into new bone would proceed at the greatest rate in (1) smaller defects in smaller bones, (2) younger patients, and (3) those that received BMA and that (4) evidence of *cortical* bone healing would be identified beyond filling of the *medullary* defect.

2. Methods

Under an IRB-approved prospective randomized controlled clinical trial design study, patients (age 4-65) undergoing surgery by the first author (TAD) at a single institution (SUNY Upstate Medical University) to remove benign bone lesions via curettage were randomized to two treatment groups. Accrual began in 2004 and was all follow-up was completed during calendar year 2009. Patients with active infection, bone marrow disorders, other contraindications to use of supplemental bone marrow aspiration, those with posttraumatic defects, those who preferred autologous or allogeneic graft material alone (without synthetic filler) and those who declined follow-up were excluded. One group underwent curettage and grafting with ultraporous beta tricalcium phosphate (TCP, Vitoss, Orthovita, Inc.) alone and the other group underwent curettage and grafting with TCP and BMA (TCP/BMA) [4].

For the purposes of this study, the CT scans provided the outcome variables based upon the mentioned quantitative CT-based volumetric imaging analysis. Of the 55 patients who completed the randomized prospective trial, CT scans were obtained in 34 patients at approximately one year postoperatively. Five of those patients also had CT scans at 2 years and 1 patient at 3 years. However, due to the transition to completely digital imaging over the time course of this study, twenty patients (11 male / 9 female) with twenty-one lesions had one or more CT scans available for digital analysis (TCP=10, TCP/BMA =11 lesions) and form the basis of this study. Clearly, potential bias is introduced by the exclusion of those CT scans that were unable to be retrieved for digital analysis, but without access, the quantitative analysis was simply not able to be performed. In order to minimize the potential for additional bias, all remaining subjects were included for analysis.

During surgery, the lesion was first curetted completely. In cases of more aggressive lesions, extended curettage was accomplished, consisting of extension of the intralesional margin by high speed burr in all cases and use of adjunctive argon beam coagulation in some. During curettage, decompression of the proximal and/or distal medullary cavity, where feasible, was done in order to ensure that the lesion was eliminated and to enhance healing. Morsellized grains of TCP were compacted into the defect to fill it. The graft material was impacted with bone tamps into the periphery of the defect until it was firmly compacted. Then, more graft was added and impacted in an identical fashion. This was done until the defects were completely filled and the surface of the graft material was flush with the surface of the cortical bone overlying the defect. Those in the TCP/BMA group underwent the same procedure but also underwent bone marrow aspiration. The bone marrow aspirate was harvested with a standard bone marrow aspiration needle from the anterior iliac crest in volumes of 2-3 cc aliquots per pass. The aspiration needle was repositioned through a single point of insertion in the skin for each pass within the ilium. The ratio of BMA to TCP ranged from 1:3 to 1:2 [4]. The bone marrow was mixed with the TCP before the insertion into the defect in an identical fashion as previously described. Prophylactic internal fixation was performed to maintain bone stability and minimize the risk of fracture during defect healing in six of the 21 lesions.

Each patient was managed using the same postoperative guidelines based on anatomic location, size and characteristics of the lesion. For subjects with upper extremity lesions, upper body activities including but not limited to throwing, lifting, and strength training were restricted for 6 weeks postoperatively and until the patient lacked noticeable tenderness or pain in addition to radiographic evidence of some healing of the defect. Most of the patients with lesions in the lower extremity were asked to be toe-touch weight-bearing with axillary crutches for the first 6 weeks postoperatively. This was followed by slow resumption of complete weight bearing activities once the pain and tenderness subsided and radiographic analysis revealed signs of healing. Lower extremity lesion patients were allowed to return to usual activities, including impact activities, 3 months postoperatively under normal circumstances.

CT scans were obtained at approximately 1 year using a Siemens Sensation 16 scanner (Siemens AG, Erlnagen, Germany). For five patients, a second series of scans were obtained at approximately 2 years postop for clinical follow-up purposes. In one case, a third scan was obtained at 3 years postop, also for clinical reasons. The CT scan protocols were based on standard of care for the particular skeletal location and ranged from 100 to 120 kV (median: 120 kV) with 33 to 198 mAs (median: 91mAs), inplane resolution of 0.17 to 0.91mm (median: 0.48mm), and scan spacing of 0.7 to 1.0mm (median: 0.8mm). Slice thickness was 1mm for all scans.

Quantitative CT-based volumetric imaging analysis was as follows. Digital image sets were imported into MIMICS image processing software (Materialise, Plymouth, MI) to identify and segment the defect region into un-remodeled TCP graft material (TCP), newly formed bone tissue (NB), and the surrounding original bone (Figure 1). TCP was distinguished by high radiodensity compared to surrounding bone. The new bone (NB), occupying space between the original bone and TCP, was distinguished by the bony margin between new and existing bone. Masks were created for these three regions using a combination of gray scale thresholding and manual identification (Figure 1). The masked regions

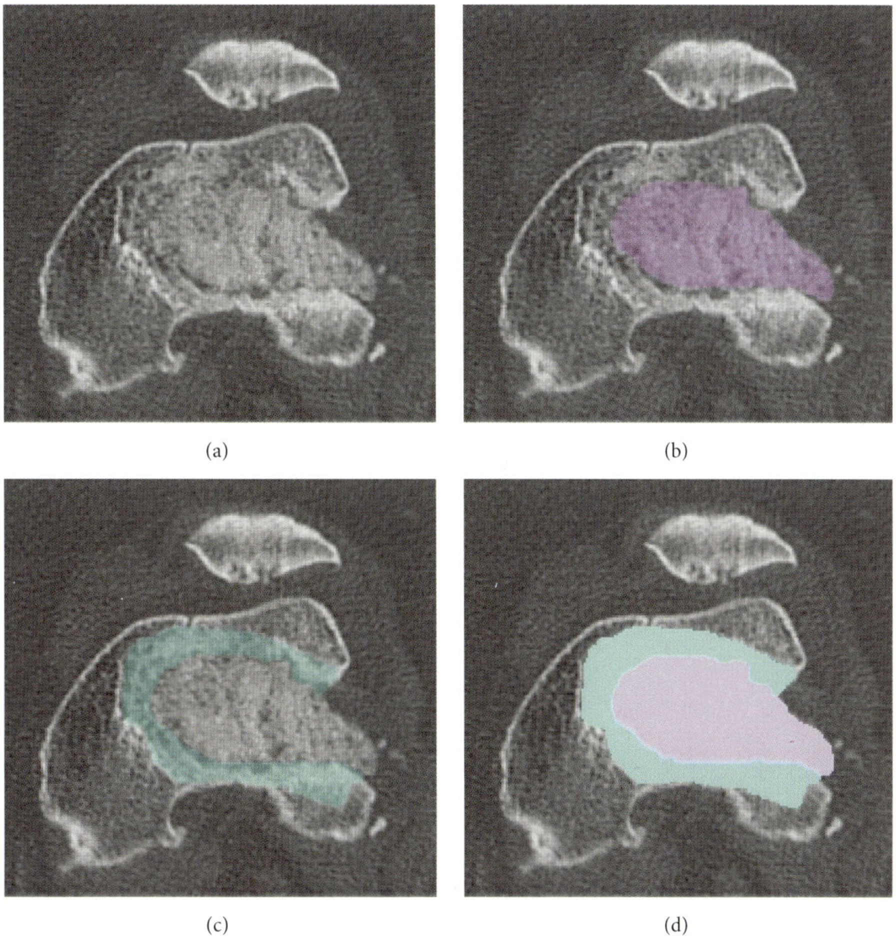

FIGURE 1: Axial section of distal femur with defect filled by TCP (a). The mask of the TCP (b) and new bone (c) are identified and combined (d).

were built into three-dimensional volumetric objects from which the volume (cc) of TCP remaining (TCP) and TCP incorporated into new bone (NB) growth was determined (Figures 2 and 3). The total volume of the original defect (DV) was assumed to be the sum of these two values (NB + TCP). The new bone fraction (NB/DV) was used to assess TCP graft incorporation.

Bone width (mm) was measured at the midpoint of the defect. This was measured medial-lateral in the coronal plane at the proximal-distal midpoint for long bones. In the clavicle, it was measured cephalocaudad in the coronal plane located at the midportion of the lesion mediolateral. As expected, DV was closely related to size of the bone. (Figure 4)

The size of the remaining cortical defect was determined by fitting an ellipse to the cortical defect in the 3D image and measuring the lengths of the major and minor axis. The average of the major and minor axis lengths was divided by the bone diameter in the region, resulting in the cortical defect fraction (CDF).

To determine if TCP incorporation was greatest in smaller defects at one year after surgery, a linear regression model was used with new bone fraction (NB/DV) as the dependent variable and original defect volume (DV) as the independent variable. To determine if TCP incorporation was related to the size of the bone being grafted, another linear regression model was used with NB/DV as the dependent variable and bone width as the independent variable. To determine if incorporation of TCP into new bone would be greater in younger patients, a linear regression model was used with the new bone (NB) as the dependent variable, and age, DV, and the interaction between age and DV (age∗DV) as independent variables. To determine if the amount of new bone was dependent on use of BMA, an analysis of covariance was used with use of BMA as an independent variable, and DV as the covariate.

3. Results

Participants had a mean age of 22 years with a range from 4 to 66 years at time of 1 year CT. Nine patients (ten lesions) had been randomized to receive TCP alone while 11 patients (11 lesions) had been randomized to receive TCP with BMA. The 21 bone lesions were located in the proximal femur (N=4), distal femur (N=5), fibula (N=3), tibia (N=2), humerus (N=2), clavicle (N=2), metacarpal (N=1), proximal phalanx

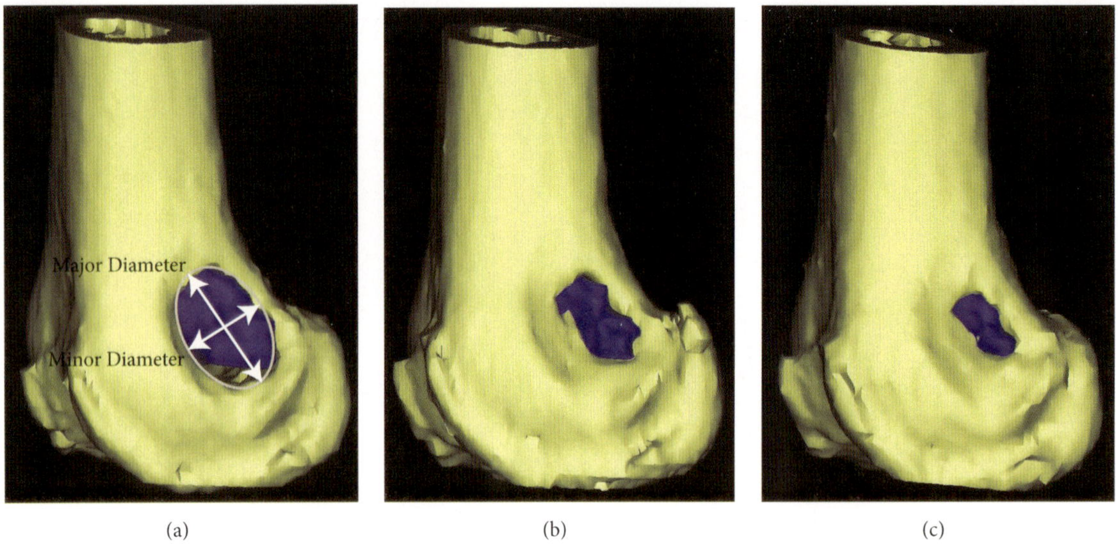

FIGURE 2: A 3D reconstruction of the example shown in Figure 1 at 1 year (a), 2 years, (b) and 3 years (c) postoperatively. The TCP is shown in dark blue. The new bone formation is not shown for clarity. The major and minor diameter of the cortical defect are shown (a).

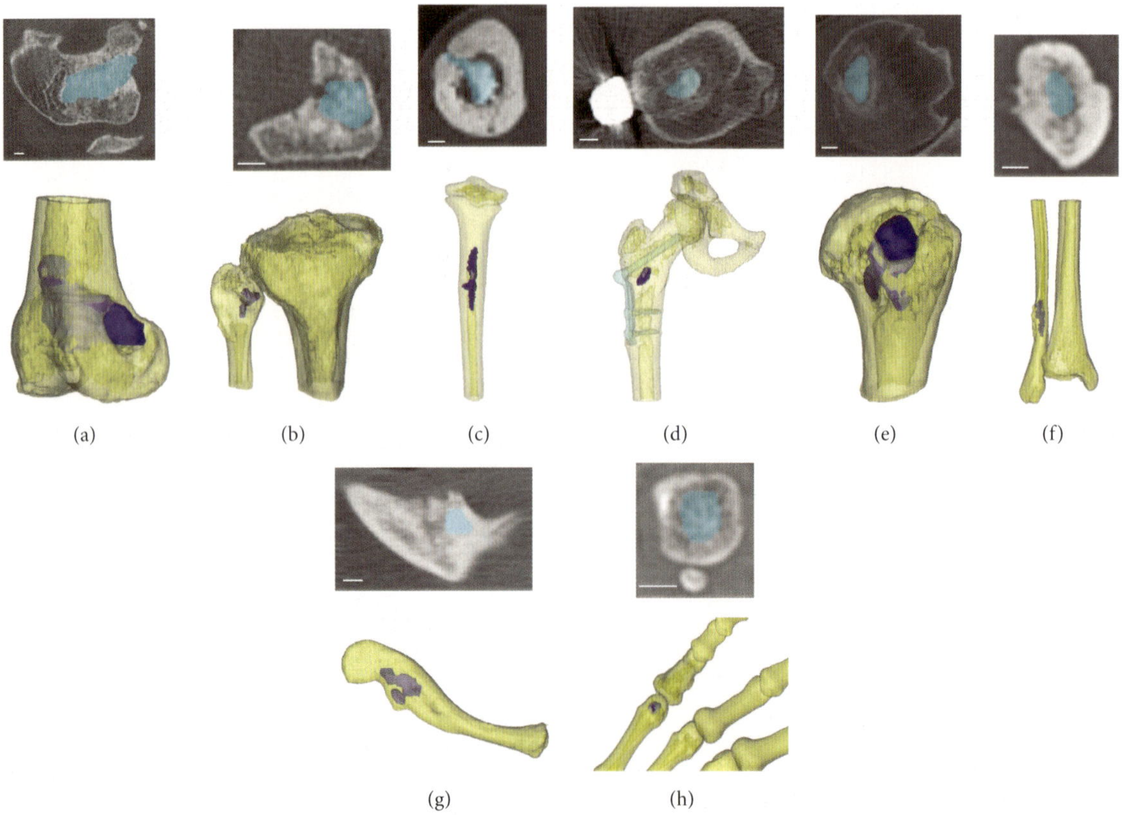

FIGURE 3: Representative axial CT and 3D reconstructed images of remaining TCP (blue) at 1-year postop for distal femur (a), proximal fibula (b), proximal tibia (c), proximal femur (d), proximal humerus (e), distal fibula (f), clavicle (g), and metacarpal (h).

(N=1), and middle phalanx (N=1). The two phalangeal lesions were from the same patient.

Summary statistics for the 21 skeletal defects are shown in Table 1. Defect volume ranged from 0.12 cc to almost 100 cc with median volume of 8 cc. New bone fractions (NB/DV) ranged from 0.54 to 1.0 with a mean of 0.76, indicating that on average 76% of the defect volume was replaced with new bone. The cortical defect fraction (CDF) ranged from 0 to 0.67 with a median of 0.15. Five of the defects had no remaining cortical defect at 1 year.

TABLE 1: Descriptive statistics for 21 bone lesions.

Parameter	Mean	Median	Std Dev	Min	Max
Patient Age	22.3	16	18.3	4	66
Original Defect Volume (DV, mm^3)	23520	8006	31390	107	94490
New Bone Volume (NB, mm^3)	15480	7025	18780	66	58220
Remaining TCP Volume (mm^3)	8037	1570	13010	0	41910
New Bone Fraction (NB/DV)	0.76	0.76	0.13	0.54	1.0
Cortical Defect Diameter Major (mm)	11.2	7.7	15.0	0	62.0
Cortical Defect Diameter Minor (mm)	5.4	2.2	6.7	0	22.2
Cortical Defect Fraction (CDF)	0.21	0.15	0.20	0	0.67

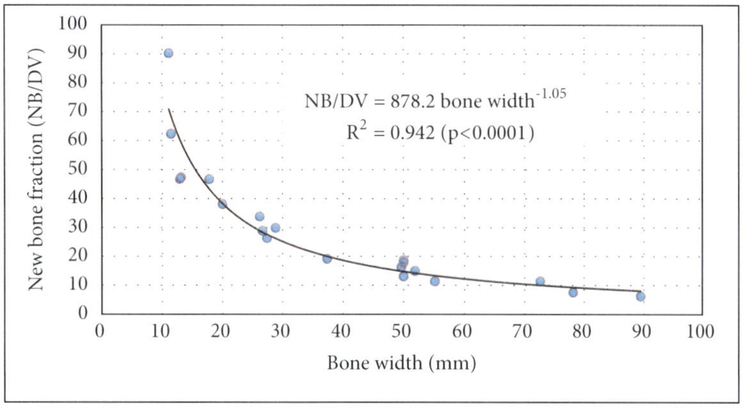

FIGURE 4: Initial defect volume (cc) as a function of bone width.

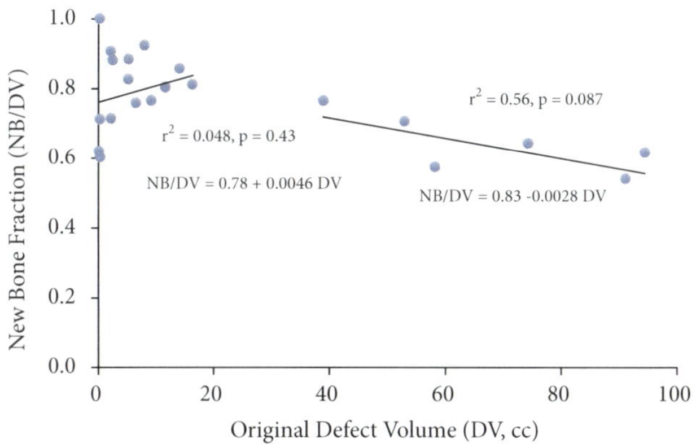

FIGURE 5: The new bone fraction (NB/DV) was greater for small defect volumes (DV). Overall, there was a significant decrease (p=0.0029) in NB/DV with increasing DV (r^2=0.38). When separated into smaller (<20cc) and larger defect volume groups (>20cc), there was a trend towards decreased new bone fraction in the >20cc group.

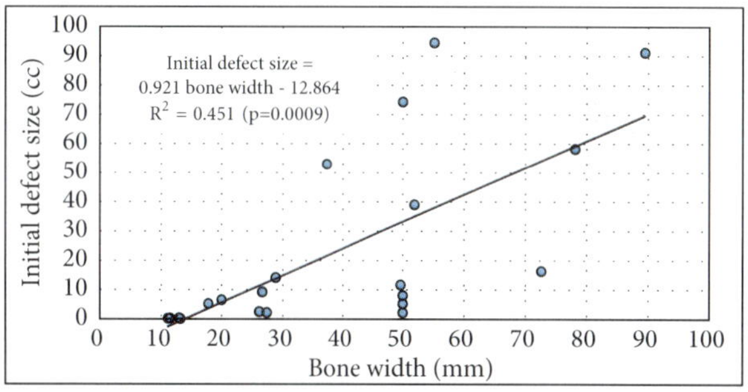

FIGURE 6: New bone fraction (NB/DV) was inversely proportional to bone width.

Analyzed overall, there was significant (p=0.0029) negative correlation (r^2 = 0.38) between the fraction of new bone (NB/DV) and the original defect volume (DV) (Figure 5). However, when defects less than and greater than 20 cc size were analyzed separately, this relationship was not quite as clear. The same inverse linear relationship between NB/DV and DV held true for DV greater than 20 cc with an even stronger correlation coefficient (r^2=0.56), although the fewer numbers (n = 6) in this subset analysis did not allow statistical significance (p = 0.09). Although in the subset analysis for defects less than 20 cc there appeared to be a positive relationship between NB/DV and DV, the relationship was weak and not significant (r^2 = 0.048, p = 0.43). The large amount of scatter in the NB/DV for the small defects is due to the division between two small numbers as DV approaches zero. For the remainder of the analyses, new bone volume (NB) was used as the primary dependent variable.

In part likely due to the linear relationship between defect size and bone size (Figure 4), NB/DV was highly related to the bone size (Figure 6). The largest lesions were in the distal femurs and proximal tibias, and the smallest lesions were in the phalanges, metacarpal, and clavicle.

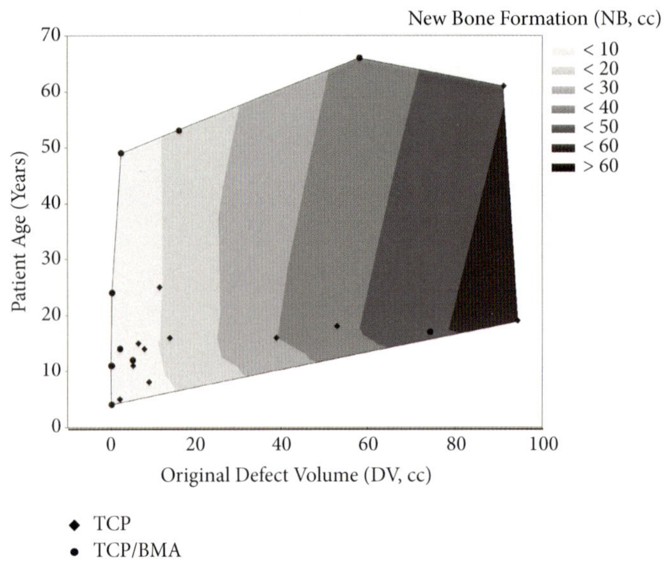

FIGURE 7: A contour plot of the influence of patient age and original defect volume (DV) on new bone formation (NB). Using a multiple regression model, patients with larger DV had higher NB ($p<0.0001$). Increasing age coupled to increasing DV (age∗DV) had reduced NB ($p=0.0003$). NB is TCP/BMA data (diamonds) and TCP data (filled circles) are shown.

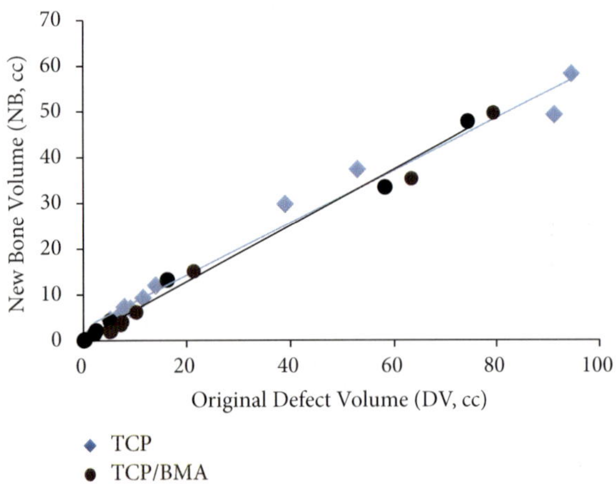

FIGURE 8: New bone volume (NB) as a function of original defect volume (DV) for the TCP and TCP/BMA groups. Linear regression lines through the two groups are also shown.

For larger defect volumes, younger patients were more successful at incorporation (Figure 7). Using a linear regression model, the defect volume ($p<0.0001$) was a strong positive predictor, and the interaction term (Age∗DV) ($p=0.0003$) was a strong negative predictor of new bone formation (or incorporation). Age itself was not a significant factor ($p=0.50$).

There was no statistically significant difference in new bone formation (NB) between TCP alone and TCP with BMA groups ($p=0.27$). Additionally, the slope of the NB versus DV relationship was not different for the two groups ($p=0.29$) (Figure 8). The two groups were not significantly different with respect to fractional cortical defect ratio (CDF) ($p=0.576$).

Evidence of cortical bone healing identified beyond filling of the medullary defect was impossible to evaluate in subjects with only one CT scan. However, in the anecdotal and very small subset of five patients with CT scans at a second and third time point, qualitative evidence suggesting progressive medullary new bone formation and cortical bone healing was observed (Figure 9).

4. Conclusions

Synthetic alternatives to autogenous and allogeneic bone graft fillers continue to be developed and explored [1, 2, 17–19]. Variability in rates of graft incorporation exist between materials, with calcium sulfate products thought to resorb rather quickly and hydroxyapatite to persist indefinitely [3, 19–22]. Tricalcium phosphate has an intermediate pattern of graft incorporation, which has led to frequent clinical usage [1–12, 14–16, 23]. In our completed prospective clinical trial from which the CT scans in this study were derived, no significant difference was detected in bone graft incorporation parameters between patients with benign curetted defects randomized to receive either ultraporous beta-TCP alone or combined with autogenous iliac crest bone marrow [4]. Numerous additional clinical studies have evaluated the use of ultraporous beta-TCP for other indications, including trauma and spinal fusion [7, 9–12, 14–18, 24–29]. None have established clearly whether there is a benefit to the addition of BMA to the TCP. However, none have utilized the more detailed quantitative CT based volumetric analysis described herein.

The main impetus behind the prospective randomized study had been to determine if the addition of bone marrow to ultraporous beta-TCP would improve parameters of graft incorporation [4]. A prior retrospective study suggested that use of this graft material mixed with only local blood incorporated more slowly than was desirable [3]. Since prolonged graft persistence of other graft materials, such as

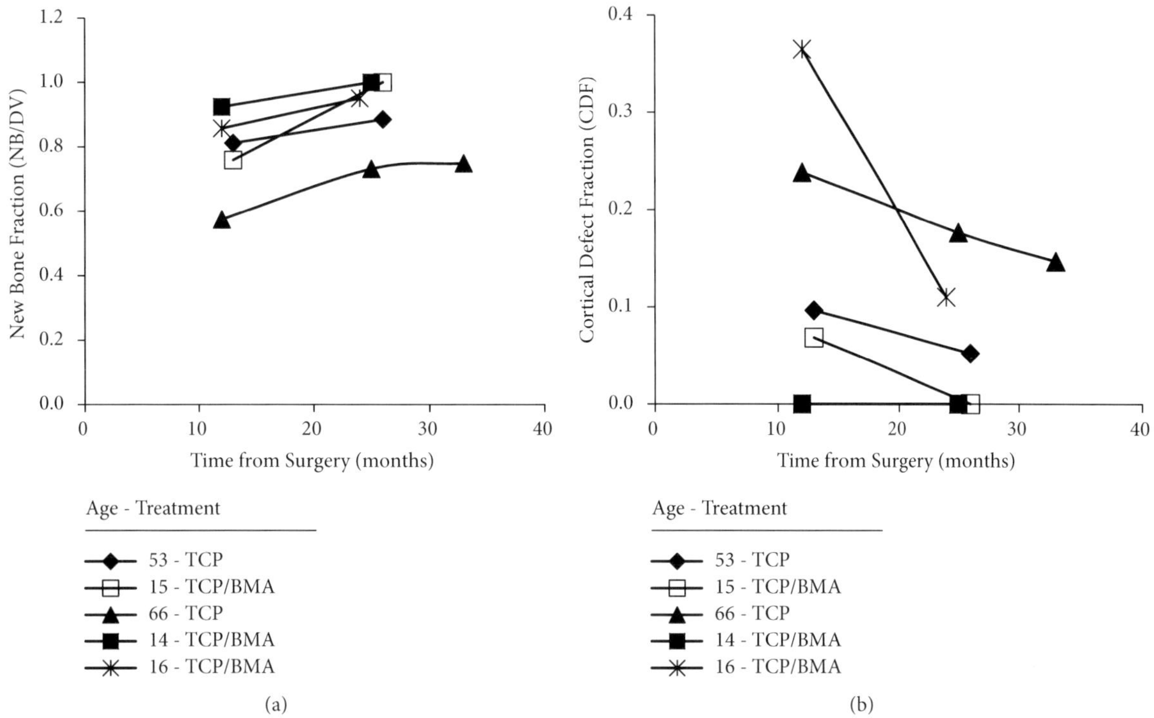

FIGURE 9: Medullary new bone fraction (a) and cortical defect fraction (B) as a function of months of healing for the five patients with more than one serial CT scan. Note that progressive improvement in medullary NB formation (incorporation) occurred in all of the five patients (a) and progressive decrease in cortical defect fraction (defect graft incorporation) occurred in four out of the five patients (b).

hydroxyapatite, served as stress risers and resulted in late fractures, the addition of bone marrow was hypothesized to improve graft incorporation, as it has been shown to do in the laboratory [30–32]. However, neither the previously reported study with qualitative radiographic analysis nor the current quantitative CT analysis based results support this hypothesis [4]. Potential explanations for this lack of difference, apart from simple lack of a true difference, are numerous. First, the number of CT scans available for the current analysis were much smaller even than those available for the larger parent study due to a transition to digital images. Second, the surgical technique used for the study may have contributed to blurring the differences. In all study patients the adjacent intramedullary canal was penetrated surgically in order to allow access to adjacent bone marrow. Additionally, the amount of bone marrow aspirate may have been suboptimal to afford a healing advantage to the bone marrow group [4].

With respect to whether quantitative analysis would be able to delineate differences in graft incorporation between groups suggested by earlier nonquantitative studies to be different (e.g., age and size of the defect), the results were more fruitful but complex. Based on the current results, graft incorporation was correlated in part with the size of the original curetted defect. Overall, this was a significant linear inverse relationship, but when separated out into a subset analysis of defects larger than or smaller than 20 cc, only the larger defects held true to this relationship. Even more notable than the relationship with defect size was the strong negative relationship of graft incorporation to bone width (and hence medullary bone size). Defects in larger bones had lower graft incorporation in this CT based analysis. On one hand, this may seem counterintuitive if one theorizes that a larger medullary surface area provides more medullary cancellous bone and vascularity to stimulate healing. On the other hand, if the bone graft incorporates by creeping substitution at a relatively linear rate, as it seems to in the presented cases, the absolute size of the defect would mean that indeed smaller bones with smaller defects would result in a high fraction of bone healing at any given time postoperatively.

The relationship with age was complex and closely tied to defect volume. For larger defect volumes, younger patients were more successful at graft incorporation. Although age itself was not an independently significant factor in our regression model, as defect volume increased, advanced age had more of a negative impact on new bone formation.

This series is unable to provide definitive evidence of cortical healing with Vitoss as only five patients had serial CT scans. However, on those scans we did observe gradual healing over time. Based on the limited subset analysis, this evidence has to be considered anecdotal at best.

One finding that appears to contradict reports in the literature is that for many of the currently reported lesions, graft incorporation remained incomplete, even after one year of follow-up. Others have reported complete bone graft incorporation in between 6 and 9 months with ultraporous beta-TCP or similar beta-TCP compounds, but these reports have been based upon qualitative means of evaluation rather than CT [5, 6]. The current quantitative analysis and CT images also clearly show that the graft incorporation and trabeculation occurs from the periphery to the center, in a centripetal fashion, rather than the reverse, as has been suggested [6].

Limitations of this study include use of small amounts of bone marrow relative to the TCP graft material, poor statistical power, loss of ability to analyze some early study images collected prior to current digital imaging techniques, and presence of hardware artifact in patients who had simultaneous internal fixation. The ultraporous beta-TCP product used in this study has been recommended to be used in a 1:1 ratio of bone marrow to TCP, far greater than the ratio of between 1:2 and 1:3 employed in this study. The original power analysis for this study suggested an 80% power to show a 25% difference with the number of patients enrolled, but our attrition rate for the CT was 39%, hampering our statistical power. Weaknesses acknowledged, this study remains unique in its method of utilizing quantitative volumetric CT analysis of bone graft incorporation. Future study designs evaluating efficacy of bone grafting materials should consider inclusion of CT analysis of this sort in order to better elucidate the many remaining questions surrounding graft incorporation.

Disclosure

This research was presented in a preliminary fashion as a poster at the 2011 Annual Meeting of the Orthopaedic Research Society (http://www.ors.org/Transactions/57/1433.pdf).

Acknowledgments

This study was supported by an institutional research grant from Vitoss, Inc. (original manufacturer of Vitoss), with the first author (Timothy A. Damron) as Principal Investigator. The PI has received other institutional research grants from both Stryker, Inc. (current owner of Vitoss), and Wright Medical, Inc. (manufacturer of competitive product (Prodense). The PI is also currently a paid consultant to the Orthopedic Advisory Council for BoneSupport (associated with another competitive product, Cerament). This study was originally supported by institutional research support to the PI's institution by Vitoss, Inc. No further research support is currently being provided by Stryker, Inc. (current manufacturer of Vitoss). In addition, the authors acknowledge the contribution of Mickey Daugherty, MD, to the early phase of this work.

References

[1] M. Jäger, M. Herten, U. Fochtmann et al., "Bridging the gap: bone marrow aspiration concentrate reduces autologous bone grafting in osseous defects," *Journal of Orthopaedic Research*, vol. 29, no. 2, pp. 173–180, 2011.

[2] T. A. Damron, "Use of 3D β-tricalcium phosphate (Vitoss®) scaffolds in repairing bone defects," *Nanomedicine*, vol. 2, no. 6, pp. 763–775, 2007.

[3] C. J. Anker, S. P. Holdridge, B. Baird, H. Cohen, and T. A. Damron, "Ultraporous β-tricalcium phosphate is well incorporated in small cavitary defects," *Clinical Orthopaedics and Related Research*, no. 434, pp. 251–257, 2005.

[4] T. A. Damron, J. Lisle, T. Craig, M. Wade, W. Silbert, and H. Cohen, "Ultraporous β-tricalcium phosphate alone or combined with bone marrow aspirate for benign cavitary lesions," *The Journal of Bone & Joint Surgery—American Volume*, vol. 95, no. 2, pp. 158–166, 2013.

[5] C. Van Hoff, J. B. Samora, M. J. Griesser, M. K. Crist, T. J. Scharschmidt, and J. L. Mayerson, "Effectiveness of ultraporous β-tricalcium phosphate (vitoss) as bone graft substitute for cavitary defects in benign and low-grade malignant bone tumors.," *American journal of orthopedics (Belle Mead, N.J.)*, vol. 41, no. 1, pp. 20–23, 2012.

[6] H. J. Siegel, R. C. Baird III, J. Hall, R. Lopez-Ben, and P. H. Lander, "The outcome of composite bone graft substitute used to treat cavitary bone defects," *Orthopedics*, vol. 31, no. 8, p. 754, 2008.

[7] M. Thaler, R. Lechner, M. Gstöttner, C. Kobel, and C. Bach, "The use of beta-tricalcium phosphate and bone marrow aspirate as a bone graft substitute in posterior lumbar interbody fusion," *European Spine Journal*, vol. 22, no. 5, pp. 1173–1182, 2013.

[8] C. W. DiGiovanni, J. Baumhauer, S. S. Lin et al., "Prospective, randomized, multi-center feasibility trial of rhPDGF-BB versus autologous bone graft in a foot and ankle fusion model," *Foot & Ankle International*, vol. 32, no. 4, pp. 344–354, 2011.

[9] J. H. Park, C. G. Choi, S. R. Jeon, S. C. Rhim, C. J. Kim, and S. W. Roh, "Radiographic analysis of instrumented posterolateral fusion mass using mixture of local autologous bone and b-TCP (polybone®) in a lumbar spinal fusion surgery," *Journal of Korean Neurosurgical Society*, vol. 49, no. 5, pp. 267–272, 2011.

[10] S. Acharya, S. Kumar, A. Srivastava, and R. Tandon, "Early results of one-level cervical discectomy and fusion with stand-alone cervical cage and bone marrow soaked tricalcium phosphate," *Acta Orthopædica Belgica*, vol. 77, no. 2, pp. 218–223, 2011.

[11] P. G. Kumar, J. A. Kumar, N. Anumala, K. P. Reddy, H. Avula, and S. N. Hussain, "Volumetric analysis of intrabony defects in aggressive periodontitis patients following use of a novel composite alloplast: A pilot study," *Quintessence International*, vol. 42, no. 5, pp. 375–384, 2011.

[12] N. Epstein, "Efficacy of posterior cervical fusions utilizing an artificial bone graft expander, beta tricalcium phosphate," *Surgical Neurology International*, vol. 2, no. 1, p. 15, 2011.

[13] K. Nagahama, M. Kanayama, D. Togawa, T. Hashimoto, and A. Minami, "Does alendronate disturb the healing process of posterior lumbar interbody fusion? A prospective randomized trial," *Journal of Neurosurgery: Spine*, vol. 14, no. 4, pp. 500–507, 2011.

[14] S. Bansal, V. Chauhan, S. Sharma, R. Maheshwari, A. Juyal, and S. Raghuvanshi, "Evaluation of hydroxyapatite and beta-tricalcium phosphate mixed with bone marrow aspirate as a bone graft substitute for posterolateral spinal fusion," *Indian Journal of Orthopaedics*, vol. 43, no. 3, pp. 234–239, 2009.

[15] N. Zwetyenga, S. Catros, A. Emparanza, C. Deminiere, F. Siberchicot, and J. Fricain, "Mandibular reconstruction using induced membranes with autologous cancellous bone graft and HA-βTCP: animal model study and preliminary results in patients," *International Journal of Oral and Maxillofacial Surgery*, vol. 38, no. 12, pp. 1289–1297, 2009.

[16] N. E. Epstein, "Beta tricalcium phosphate: observation of use in 100 posterolateral lumbar instrumented fusions," *The Spine Journal*, vol. 9, no. 8, pp. 630–638, 2009.

[17] N. E. Epstein, "A preliminary study of the efficacy of beta tricalcium phosphate as a bone expander for instrumented posterolateral lumbar fusions," *Journal of Spinal Disorders & Techniques*, vol. 19, no. 6, pp. 424–429, 2006.

[18] R. J. Linovitz and T. A. Peppers, "Use of an advanced formulation of β-tricalcium phosphate as a bone extender in interbody lumbar fusion," *Orthopedics*, vol. 25, no. 5, pp. s585–s589, 2002.

[19] S. Larsson, "Calcium phosphates: What is the evidence?" *Journal of Orthopaedic Trauma*, vol. 24, no. 1, pp. S41–S45, 2010.

[20] B. K. B. Tay Vikas, V. Patel, and D. S. Bradford, "Calcium sulfate- and calcium phosphate-based bone substitutes mimicry of the mineral phase of bone," *Orthopedic Clinics of North America*, vol. 30, no. 4, pp. 615–623, 1999.

[21] F. Zhang, J. Chang, J. Lu, K. Lin, and C. Ning, "Bioinspired structure of bioceramics for bone regeneration in load-bearing sites," *Acta Biomaterialia*, vol. 3, no. 6, pp. 896–904, 2007.

[22] D. K. Resnick, A. Nanda, and E. C. Benzel, "Vitoss bone substitute," *Neurosurgery*, vol. 50, no. 5, pp. 1162–1164, 2002.

[23] S. Becker, O. Maissen, and I. Ponomarev, "Osteopromotion with a plasmatransglutaminase on a ss-TCP ceramic," *Journal of Materials Science: Materials in Medicine*, 2007.

[24] T. A. Russell and R. K. Leighton, "Comparison of autogenous bone graft and endothermic calcium phosphate cement for defect augmentation in tibial plateau fractures. A multicenter, prospective, randomized study," *The Journal of Bone & Joint Surgery*, vol. 90, no. 10, pp. 2057–2061, 2008.

[25] A. R. Vaccaro, P. G. Whang, T. Patel et al., "The safety and efficacy of OP-1 (rhBMP-7) as a replacement for iliac crest autograft for posterolateral lumbar arthrodesis: minimum 4-year follow-up of a pilot study," *The Spine Journal*, vol. 8, no. 3, pp. 457–465, 2008.

[26] T. Lerner, V. Bullmann, T. L. Schulte, M. Schneider, and U. Liljenqvist, "A level-1 pilot study to evaluate of ultraporous β-tricalcium phosphate as a graft extender in the posterior correction of adolescent idiopathic scoliosis," *European Spine Journal*, vol. 18, no. 2, pp. 170–179, 2009.

[27] L. Dai and L. Jiang, "Single-Level Instrumented Posterolateral Fusion of Lumbar Spine With β-Tricalcium Phosphate Versus Autograft," *The Spine Journal*, vol. 33, no. 12, pp. 1299–1304, 2008.

[28] L. Dai and L. Jiang, "Anterior cervical fusion with interbody cage containing β-tricalcium phosphate augmented with plate fixation: a prospective randomized study with 2-year follow-up," *European Spine Journal*, vol. 17, no. 5, pp. 698–705, 2008.

[29] A. L. Jones, R. W. Bucholz, M. J. Bosse et al., "Recombinant human BMP-2 and allograft compared with autogenous bone graft for reconstruction of diaphyseal tibial fractures with cortical defects. A randomized, controlled trial," *The Journal of Bone & Joint Surgery—American Volume*, vol. 88, no. 7, pp. 1431–1441, 2006.

[30] S. Becker, O. Maissen, P. Igor, S. Thierry, B. Rahn, and W. Ingo, "Osteopromotion by a β-tricalcium phosphate/bone marrow hybrid implant for use in spine surgery," *The Spine* 31, no. 1, pp. 11–17, 2006.

10

Timing of Frontal Plane Trunk Lean, Not Magnitude, Mediates Frontal Plane Knee Joint Loading in Patients with Moderate Medial Knee Osteoarthritis

Freyja Hálfdanardóttir,[1] **Dan K. Ramsey**,[2] **and Kristín Briem**[1]

[1]*Faculty of Medicine, School of Health Sciences, University of Iceland, Saemundargata 2, 101 Reykjavík, Iceland*
[2]*Department of Health Professions Education, D'Youville College, 220 Koessler Administration Building (KAB), 320 Porter Ave, Buffalo, NY 14201, USA*

Correspondence should be addressed to Kristín Briem; kbriem@hi.is

Academic Editor: Allen L. Carl

The purpose of this study was to examine the influence of trunk lean and contralateral hip abductor strength on the peak knee adduction moment (KAM) and rate of loading in persons with moderate medial knee osteoarthritis. Thirty-one males (17 with osteoarthritis, 14 controls) underwent 3-dimensional motion analysis, strength testing of hip abductors, and knee range of motion (ROM) measures, as well as completing the knee osteoarthritis outcome score (KOOS). No differences were found between groups or limbs for gait cycle duration, but the osteoarthritis group had longer double-limb support during weight acceptance ($p < 0.001$) and delayed frontal plane trunk motion towards the stance limb ($p < 0.01$). This was reflected by a lower rate of loading for the osteoarthritis group compared to controls ($p < 0.001$), whereas no differences were found for peak KAM. Trunk angle, contralateral hip abductor strength, and BMI explained the rate of loading at the involved knee ($p < 0.001$), an association not found for the contralateral knee or control knees. Prolonged trunk lean over the stance limb may help lower peak KAM values. Rate of frontal plane knee joint loading may partly be mediated by the contralateral limb's abductor strength, accentuating the importance of bilateral lower limb strength for persons with knee osteoarthritis.

1. Introduction

Osteoarthritis (OA), knee OA in particular, is a large and growing public health concern. Notable increases in estimated years lived with disability owing to OA has been observed over the last 15 years [1] with concomitant activity limitations projected to increase [2]. Moreover the economic burden associated with knee OA is expected to rise concurrently with the ageing population, resulting in increased demand for primary and revision knee joint arthroplasty [3]. Therefore, emphasis has been focused on investigating whether conservative biomechanical modalities mediate disease progression [4, 5].

Frontal plane trunk movements have recently garnered increased attention, with evidence suggesting patients with severe medial compartment OA exhibit greater ipsilateral peak trunk lean as opposed to persons with less severity [6]. This may be an effective strategy for mediating pain relief [7], evoked by redirecting the ground reaction force more laterally and lowering medial compartment load as inferred by lower external knee adduction moments (KAM) observed among healthy controls [8–10] and persons with medial knee OA [11] during gait. Perhaps this may be an effective strategy, particularly for persons with mild to moderate knee OA, to attenuate KAM magnitudes similar to that of the uninvolved knee and/or controls, despite varus deformity [12–14].

It is during the first 10% of the gait cycle when transitioning from double- into single-limb support and weight acceptance (from initial contact (IC) of the stance limb until contralateral toe-off) when the first peak KAM typically occurs [15]. Yet the rate of loading throughout weight acceptance (WA), as reflected by the positive slope of the KAM profile, has been associated with medial knee joint degeneration, independent from the peak and KAM impulse [16]. Frontal plane pelvic stability and, thereby, trunk and hip joint motion are regulated by the hip abductor muscles. Effective control of hip and pelvis frontal plane movement calls for good eccentric control, not just of the hip abductors on the affected side but also on the contralateral side for stabilizing the pelvis prior to IC. The rate and magnitude of knee loading during WA may therefore be in part mediated by contralateral hip abductor strength, which has not been well studied. While recent studies have investigated the relationship between hip abductor function and gait parameters, none report an association between contralateral hip abductor strength, neuromuscular activation patterns, or ipsilateral peak KAM magnitudes after accounting for body size [17, 18]. A recent meta-analysis on studies of hip strength in people diagnosed with symptomatic knee OA demonstrated weaker isometric and isokinetic hip abduction strength [19]. Contralateral hip abductor strength would affect control of contralateral pelvic drop during stance, and greater pelvic drop has been shown to increase knee adduction moments [20]. Better understanding of the relationship between hip strength, trunk lean, and knee joint loading in people with knee OA may help clinicians design targeted rehabilitation programs for those affected by knee OA. Therefore, the purpose of this study was to examine whether frontal plane knee joint loading was related to temporal-spatial parameters and to determine whether contralateral hip abductor strength mediates loading in addition to trunk lean. We hypothesized that greater trunk lean would be evident in persons with symptomatic moderate medial compartment OA compared to matched controls, and that either ipsilateral or contralateral hip abductor strength might be inversely associated with loading parameters at the index knee of OA patients during the WA phase of gait.

2. Materials and Methods

Data for this cross-sectional laboratory study were collected during baseline measurements of patients who had been referred by orthopedic specialists for a fitting and trial treatment with an unloader (valgus) brace [21]. Due to limited number of female patients at the clinic who were inclined to try an unloader brace, a decision was made to include only males in this study. Seventeen male patients (aged 40–60 years) with confirmed medial knee OA, Kellgren Lawrence (KL) grade 2 or 3 radiographic changes [22], and clinical history of pain and functional impairments fulfilled the inclusion criteria. In cases where bilateral radiographic knee OA was diagnosed, the more symptomatic knee denoted the affected one. Patients were excluded if they had joint replacement surgery, periarticular fracture, osteotomy, knee ligament reconstruction, or arthroscopic surgery to any lower limb joint within 6 months of the study. Exclusion criteria also included radiologically confirmed OA in the ankle or hip joints, intra-articular corticosteroid or viscosupplementation injection to either knee joint within 3 months of study participation, or any musculoskeletal or neurological impairment, dermatological or circulatory problems in the lower extremities that might affect ambulation. Fourteen asymptomatic male subjects were recruited from the university community to serve as controls (CTRL) and were matched to the OA cohort by age (to within 5 years), weight (to within 5 kilograms), and height (to within 5 centimeters).

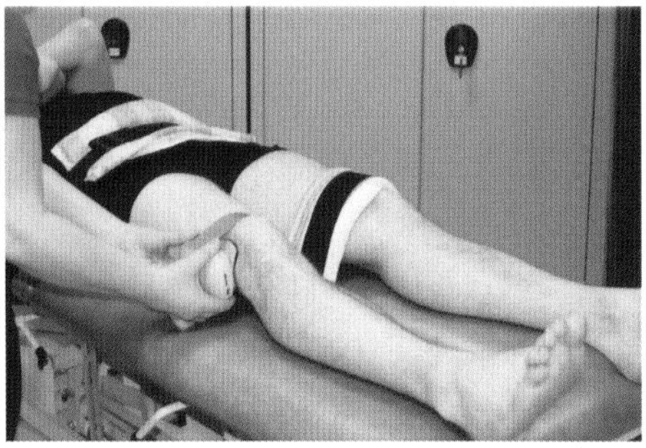

Figure 1: Isometric strength testing of hip abductors. Straps at pelvis and contralateral limb, as well as fixating hand-held dynamometer.

The protocol of this study was approved by the National Bioethics Committee and Data Protection Authority (VSNb2011100025/03.07). Participants signed an informed consent form and then completed the knee osteoarthritis outcome score (KOOS) questionnaire [23, 24]. Passive knee joint range of motion (ROM) was measured bilaterally from full extension to flexion by a single physical therapist with over 10 years of clinical experience. The same physical therapist also conducted hip abductor isometric strength testing with a hand-held dynamometer (Lafayette Manual Muscle Tester, Lafayette, USA) placed 5 cm proximal to the lateral femoral condyle with participants laying supine [25]. Straps were used to secure the pelvis and each lower limb during strength testing (Figure 1). After a single, submaximal practice trial, participants performed three maximal trials of 5 s duration, separated by 15 s of rest. The strongest trial was used for analysis, normalized by the participant's body mass index (BMI).

During motion capture, kinematic and kinetic data were collected at 100 Hz as participants walked across the lab floor at a brisk self-selected pace wearing their own comfortable low top walking shoes. Data were collected until 5 successful foot strikes per foot on force plate were obtained. A total of 47 retroreflective markers were used during three-dimensional gait analysis using 8 Oqus 300 infrared cameras (Qualisys AB, Gothenburg, Sweden) synchronized with two AMTI force plates (American Management Technology, Inc., Watertown, USA), embedded into the lab floor. Markers were placed over specific anatomic landmarks of participants in order to define proximal and distal trunk, pelvis, thighs, shanks, and feet as rigid segments, while clusters of 4-5 markers per segment were used for tracking purposes during walking trials (Figure 2). A static measurement was used to define segments and joint centers based on anatomical markers, as well as the relative position of tracking markers and each participant's body mass. Markers were autotracked and labeled using Qualisys Track Manager software while commercial software (Visual3D™, C-Motion, Germantown, USA) was used for further data processing.

Marker and force data were low-pass-filtered using a Butterworth filter with a cut-off frequency at 6 and 20 Hz, respectively. A model template was applied to define body

Table 1: Group mean (SD) and range of values for age, BMI, passive range of knee joint motion (ROM), abductor muscle strength, and scores for each subscale of KOOS.

	CTRL	OA
Age (years)	49.7 (7.4); 40–65	50.4 (6.2); 40–59
BMI (kg/m^2)	27.1 (7.4); 22.7–32.8	28.3 (3.1); 23.0–34.6
INV strength (kg/BMI)	1.05 (0.29); 0.42–1.64	1.04 (0.28); 0.72–1.69
UN strength (kg/BMI)	1.07 (0.27); 0.63–1.60	1.05 (0.25); 0.77–1.81
INV ROM (degrees)	140.2 (5.3); 133–150	127.3 (10.2); 107–139*†
UN ROM (degrees)	139.5 (4.1); 134–147	133.8 (9.6); 106–148
KOOS-pain	98.9 (2.2); 94–100	64.1 (16.6); 33–94*
KOOS-symptoms	95.3 (6.2); 82–100	68.3 (15.7); 46–96*
KOOS-ADL	99.4 (1.1); 97–100	71.8 (17.4); 43–97*
KOOS-sports/rec	98.9 (2.1); 95–100	31.5 (22.1); 0–80*
KOOS-QOL	96.9 (6.3); 81–100	38.4 (16.3); 6–63*

BMI: body mass index; INV: involved side; UN: uninvolved side; ROM: passive range of motion; ADL: activities of daily living. *Significant difference between groups ($p < 0.001$). †Significant difference between knees ($p < 0.01$).

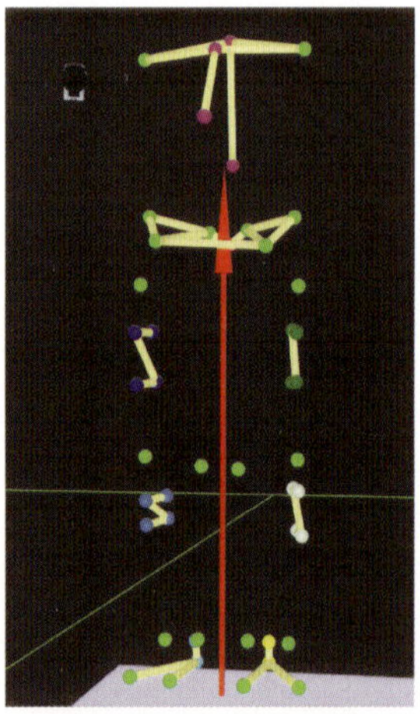

Figure 2: Marker setup used for creating the model. Anatomic markers in bright green. Tracking markers in various colors.

segments and their local reference systems, as well as joint centers. Rigid-body analysis and inverse dynamics post-processing were conducted to obtain kinematic variables between segments of the lower limbs based on an x-y-z Cardan ordered sequence. Frontal plane trunk motion was calculated with respect to the lab's coordinate system, in order to derive trunk position without the influence of pelvic tilt. Joint moments for the lower limbs were derived by inverse dynamics, resolving the joint moment into the proximal segment, using the software default settings for normalization to body mass (Nm/kg). Specific gait events (IC and TO) were defined by utilizing a force plate data threshold of 15 N, and those events then used for analysis related to the gait cycle, examining trunk lean during stance and specifically at the end of WA. Rate of loading (slope of the moment curve) was calculated as the change in frontal plane external knee joint moment from IC to the first peak KAM over time (seconds) [16]. Data were exported into Microsoft Excel and SPSS statistical software for data compilations and further analysis.

Of OA participants, the knee that was affected was on the left in 8 and on the right in 9 participants, and while 10 participants had unilateral involvement, 7 had some degree of radiographic OA (KL 1–3) on the medial or lateral compartment of the uninvolved side. These baseline data were collected prior to initiation of brace use and are the basis of this investigation. Half of the CTRL group was randomly allocated with a left "involved" and half with a right "involved" knee.

Independent t-tests were used to identify group differences in age, BMI, knee ROM, and KOOS. Multivariate analysis was used to identify differences between limbs and groups for strength and temporal-spatial values, trunk lean during WA, and knee joint loading (first peak KAM and rate of loading). A mixed stepwise regression analysis was applied for each group, with loading rate of the KAM during WA being the dependent variable. An initial multiple regression was run to assess the influence of contralateral hip abductor strength values and ipsilateral trunk lean on loading rate at the index knee, also including height and body mass based on biomechanical rationale [17, 26, 27]. Significant predictors of the loading rate were then entered into a sequential multiple linear regression model to determine individual contributions to the explained variance of the dependent variable. Level of significance was set at $p < 0.05$.

3. Results

No differences were found for mean age, height, mass, BMI, or strength between groups (Table 1). A significant deficit of knee ROM was evident on the involved side of OA participants as reflected by a group by limb interaction ($F = 11.824$, $p = 0.002$). Moreover, the CTRL group scored significantly higher on all KOOS subscales than the OA group, reflecting expected differences in self-reported knee related symptoms, functional abilities, and quality of life ($p < 0.001$).

No differences were found for mean (SD) walking speed ($p = 0.316$), between OA (1.58 (0.22) m/s) and CTRL (1.65 (0.16) m/s) groups. Duration of stance and swing for each

TABLE 2: Mean (SD) duration (s) and proportion (%) that participants of each group spent in stance versus swing and specifically during weight acceptance (WA) during each limb's gait cycle (GC).

	CTRL	% GC	OA	% GC
Inv stance	0.62 (0.04)	59.4 (1.7)†	0.66 (0.06)	62.9 (2.3)†
Uninv stance	0.62 (0.04)	59.9 (1.5)†	0.66 (0.06)	63.1 (2.7)†
Inv swing	0.42 (0.03)	40.6 (1.7)†	0.39 (0.04)	37.1 (2.3)†
Uninv swing	0.41 (0.03)	40.1 (1.5)†	0.38 (0.04)	36.9 (2.7)†
Inv WA	0.10 (0.02)	9.3 (1.5)*	0.14 (0.03)	13.0 (2.7)*
Uninv WA	0.10 (0.02)	9.9 (1.4)*	0.13 (0.03)	12.9 (2.6)*

Inv: involved limb; Uninv: uninvolved limb. Significant differences between groups for relative proportion of gait cycle (% GC) spent in stance versus swing († interaction of group by phase; $p < 0.001$). Significant group difference for WA as % GC (* main effect; $p < 0.001$).

TABLE 3: Mean (SD) values of the first external peak knee adduction moment (PKAM) and rate of loading during loading response at each knee.

	CTRL	OA
Inv PKAM ($Nm*kg^{-1}$)	0.72 (0.19)	0.74 (0.34)
Uninv PKAM ($Nm*kg^{-1}$)	0.74 (0.19)	0.75 (0.26)
Inv loading rate ($(Nm*kg^{-1})*s^{-1}$)	7.68 (2.78)*	5.92 (2.99)*
Uninv loading rate ($(Nm*kg^{-1})*s^{-1}$)	7.89 (2.79)*	5.65 (2.07)*

Inv: involved limb; Uninv: uninvolved limb. Significant group difference for rate of loading (* main effect; $p = 0.019$).

limb's gait cycle (GC) is presented in Table 2 as duration (time (sec)) and relative to the GC (% GC). No differences were found between groups for GC duration and both groups demonstrated interlimb symmetry. However, the OA group demonstrated prolonged stance and a shortened swing phase compared to controls (interaction; $F = 20.283$, $p < 0.001$) and the difference in stance was mostly due to a significantly longer double-limb support phase during WA ($F = 15.323$, $p < 0.001$).

No main effects of group or limb and no interaction with respect to the magnitude of the first peak KAM were found, but for rate of loading a significant main effect of group was found due to differences ($F = 6.205$; $p = 0.019$; Figure 3 and Table 3).

A significant interaction was seen due to group differences in the magnitude of trunk lean at the beginning but not at the end of WA ($F = 7.136$; $p = 0.012$, Figure 3). Post hoc tests revealed that at IC the CTRL group had already initiated trunk lean towards the stance limb (mean (SD) 1.4° (1.4°)), whereas the OA group's trunk position was vertical (0.0° (1.0°); $p < 0.001$). This was further reflected in an earlier transition of CTRL group from a lean towards the stance limb, moving towards the contralateral limb during midstance, which happened at a mean (SD) of 59 (17)% of the stance phase compared to a significantly delayed transition at 71 (21)% of stance for OA participants ($F = 10.186$; $p = 0.004$, Figure 3). The overall group difference in mean peak trunk lean values was only 0.15° (n.s.).

Multiple regression analysis demonstrated that a model that included ipsilateral frontal plane trunk angle at the end of WA, contralateral hip abductor strength, and BMI as independent variables best explained the rate of loading at the index knee. The resulting model demonstrated significance ($F(3, 13) = 15.486$, $p < 0.001$, adjusted $R^2 = .731$) and indicated that each factor added significantly to the model

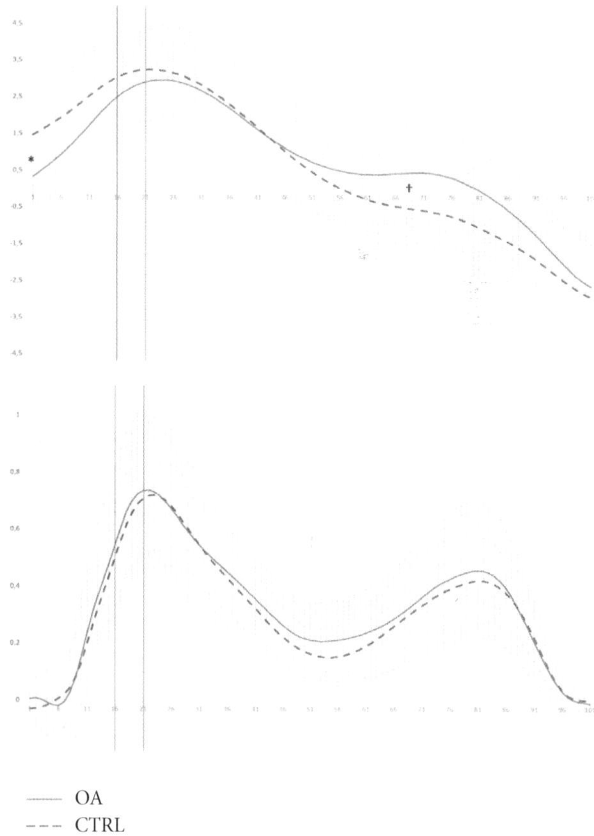

FIGURE 3: Mean frontal plane trunk angle (degrees), above, and frontal plane knee moment (Nm/kg), below, during the stance phase of the gait cycle (normalized to 101 data points). Trunk angle values are positive for leaning towards the stance side and negative for leaning towards the swing side. Vertical lines indicate end of each group's WA. Significant group difference of trunk angle at IC (* $p < 0.001$) and timing of trunk lean transition († $p < 0.01$).

towards lowering the rate of loading (trunk angle (Beta = .635; $p = 0.001$), contralateral hip strength (Beta = .722; $p < 0.001$), and BMI (Beta = .590; $p = 0.001$)). The same model was not successful in predicting ipsilateral PKAM ($p = 0.067$) or in predicting loading rate ($p = 0.455$) or PKAM ($p = 0.333$) on the contralateral side of OA participants or at either knee of controls ($p > 0.5$ for both).

4. Discussion

The main results of the study demonstrated that persons with moderate medial knee OA exhibit different movement patterns for frontal plane trunk lean compared to healthy controls. This strategy may assist in maintaining the KAM for this group to levels similar to that of controls during walking. Moreover, the rate of frontal plane knee joint loading during WA may be mediated, in part, by the contralateral limb's abductor strength.

Self-reported measures reflected distinct group differences in symptoms, function, and quality of life as was expected between the knee OA group and healthy controls, whereas other parameters including body size and hip abductor strength were not different. The OA group had a predominantly unilateral involvement with significant ROM deficits of the involved knee. However, although the group demonstrated clear differences in gait patterns when compared with CTRL group, interlimb differences were not evident for temporal-spatial parameters, trunk lean, or knee joint loading values within the OA group.

When temporal-spatial values were observed, the prolonged stance of OA participants was mostly due to a longer WA period, during which a transition is being made from double- to single-limb support. This is in agreement with previous reports [28] and could reflect a pain avoidance strategy by trying to shorten the time in single stance, as this would be the period where the GRF vector is directed more medially and involves greater loading onto the medial compartment than during double stance. The OA group maintained double stance until the first peak KAM while controls were at that point in single stance. Notably, peak KAM values did not capture kinetic differences between the two groups, whereas the rate of loading did. The rate of loading has been implicated in a more rapid rate of degeneration [16]. In addition to a slightly (n.s.) slower gait speed, a significantly prolonged WA for the OA group was coupled with delayed transition of trunk motion, whereby trunk lean towards the stance limb generally started after the initiation of the double stance period. This may represent a more cautious transition of weight and explain the slower rate of loading at the knee seen in the OA group. This, in turn, may contribute to maintaining the first peak KAM to lower values than what might otherwise have been the case for the OA group and thereby positively influence pain levels.

The magnitude of trunk lean has typically been reported as the peak value of the frontal plane motion, with the peak typically being less than 1° greater than that found at the first peak KAM of the knee and occurring somewhat later [13]. Peak values of trunk lean were similar to those previously shown for OA cohorts [6, 13, 29]. Group differences found at IC represent the altered timing of frontal plane trunk motion and were not found at the end of WA or for peak values (Figure 3). This is in accordance with the findings of Hunt et al., where differences in peak frontal plane trunk lean were only found between the group with severe OA and others (with mild or moderate OA and controls) [6]. A position of greater trunk lean at the end of WA was associated with a slower rate of frontal plane knee joint loading at the involved knee in our OA group. As noted previously, this likely reflects the effects of prolonged period of double stance during WA.

Intuitively one might expect that hip abductor strength deficiencies, which are recognized in the OA population [19], would result in less eccentric control, a more rapid contralateral pelvic drop with a resulting greater rate of loading onto the contralateral limb during WA. The results of the present study support this, as greater hip abductor strength on the uninvolved side was an independent predictor of lower rates of frontal plane knee joint loading of the affected knee in the OA group. A cross-sectional study of an OA cohort [30] showed a strong positive association between higher hip abductor strength and better functional performance. A recent systematic review [31] found that strengthening programs for hip abductor muscles improved strength and self-reported scores whereas no change in peak KAM values occurred. Investigating possible effects of hip strengthening exercise on frontal plane knee joint loading rate may cast a light on this relationship.

All participants were male with K-L grade 2 and 3, which may limit the external validity of the study, as sex dependent biomechanical differences are recognized during gait [32] and findings might differ for those with more severe OA (K-L grade 4) [6]. An "a priori" power analysis was not performed, but the observed power for the interactions found was 73% for trunk angle and greater than 90% for temporal-spatial parameters. The secondary regression analysis may suffer from the low number of participants, in particular for the control group, but nonetheless statistical significance was achieved for the affected side of the OA group.

5. Conclusion

In order to maintain KAM levels near normal levels, persons with moderate knee OA may benefit from strategies that lower the rate of knee joint loading. Part of this strategy may be achieved by prolonged double stance during WA and altered timing, not degree, of frontal plane trunk motion to affect the magnitude of knee joint loading. Strength of hip abductors may influence their ability to maintain a prolonged trunk position over the stance limb and provide eccentric control while lowering the pelvis prior to contralateral WA, which may also assist in slowing down the rate of loading and controlling peak KAM values.

Authors' Contributions

All authors have made substantial contributions to the study and the manuscript.

Acknowledgments

Financial support was received from the Icelandic Physiotherapy Association. The authors would like to thank orthopedic surgeons at Orkuhúsið Orthopedic Center for assistance with recruitment. Einfríður Árnadóttir, radiologist at Röntgen Orkuhúsið, graded radiographic changes.

References

[1] C. Global Burden of Disease Study, "Global, regional, and national incidence, prevalence, and years lived with disability for 301 acute and chronic diseases and injuries in 188 countries, 1990–2013: a systematic analysis for the global burden of disease study 2013," *Lancet*, vol. 386, no. 9995, pp. 743–800, 2015.

[2] J. M. Hootman and C. G. Helmick, "Projections of US prevalence of arthritis and associated activity limitations," *Arthritis & Rheumatism*, vol. 54, no. 1, pp. 226–229, 2006.

[3] S. Kurtz, K. Ong, E. Lau, F. Mowat, and M. Halpern, "Projections of primary and revision hip and knee arthroplasty in the United States from 2005 to 2030," *The Journal of Bone & Joint Surgery*, vol. 89, no. 4, pp. 780–785, 2007.

[4] L. K. Caldwell, L. L. Laubach, and J. A. Barrios, "Effect of specific gait modifications on medial knee loading, metabolic cost and perception of task difficulty," *Clinical Biomechanics*, vol. 28, no. 6, pp. 649–654, 2013.

[5] M. Simic, R. S. Hinman, T. V. Wrigley, K. L. Bennell, and M. A. Hunt, "Gait modification strategies for altering medial knee joint load: a systematic review," *Arthritis Care & Research*, vol. 63, no. 3, pp. 405–426, 2011.

[6] M. A. Hunt, T. V. Wrigley, R. S. Hinman, and K. L. Bennell, "Individuals with severe knee osteoarthritis (OA) exhibit altered proximal walking mechanics compared with individuals with less severe OA and those without knee pain," *Arthritis Care & Research*, vol. 62, no. 10, pp. 1426–1432, 2010.

[7] D. J. Bechard, T. B. Birmingham, A. A. Zecevic, I. C. Jones, J. R. Giffin, and T. R. Jenkyn, "Toe-out, lateral trunk lean, and pelvic obliquity during prolonged walking in patients with medial compartment knee osteoarthritis and healthy controls," *Arthritis Care & Research*, vol. 64, no. 4, pp. 525–532, 2012.

[8] J. Favre, J. C. Erhart-Hledik, E. F. Chehab, and T. P. Andriacchi, "General scheme to reduce the knee adduction moment by modifying a combination of gait variables," *Journal of Orthopaedic Research*, vol. 34, no. 9, pp. 1547–1556, 2016.

[9] T. A. Gerbrands, M. F. Pisters, and B. Vanwanseele, "Individual selection of gait retraining strategies is essential to optimally reduce medial knee load during gait," *Clinical Biomechanics*, vol. 29, no. 7, pp. 828–834, 2014.

[10] J. C. Van Den Noort, I. Schaffers, J. Snijders, and J. Harlaar, "The effectiveness of voluntary modifications of gait pattern to reduce the knee adduction moment," *Human Movement Science*, vol. 32, no. 3, pp. 412–424, 2013.

[11] M. Simic, M. A. Hunt, K. L. Bennell, R. S. Hinman, and T. V. Wrigley, "Trunk lean gait modification and knee joint load in people with medial knee osteoarthritis: The effect of varying trunk lean angles," *Arthritis Care & Research*, vol. 64, no. 10, pp. 1545–1553, 2012.

[12] N. Foroughi, R. Smith, and B. Vanwanseele, "The association of external knee adduction moment with biomechanical variables in osteoarthritis: a systematic review," *The Knee*, vol. 16, no. 5, pp. 303–309, 2009.

[13] M. A. Hunt, T. B. Birmingham, D. Bryant et al., "Lateral trunk lean explains variation in dynamic knee joint load in patients with medial compartment knee osteoarthritis," *Osteoarthritis and Cartilage*, vol. 16, no. 5, pp. 591–599, 2008.

[14] K. Mills, M. A. Hunt, and R. Ferber, "Biomechanical deviations during level walking associated with knee osteoarthritis: a systematic review and meta-analysis," *Arthritis Care & Research*, vol. 65, no. 10, pp. 1643–1665, 2013.

[15] J. Perry, *Gait Analysis: Normal and Pathological Function*, SLACK, Thorofare, NJ, USA, 1992.

[16] D. C. Morgenroth, J. R. Medverd, M. Seyedali, and J. M. Czerniecki, "The relationship between knee joint loading rate during walking and degenerative changes on magnetic resonance imaging," *Clinical Biomechanics*, vol. 29, no. 6, pp. 664–670, 2014.

[17] C. O. Kean, K. L. Bennell, T. V. Wrigley, and R. S. Hinman, "Relationship between hip abductor strength and external hip and knee adduction moments in medial knee osteoarthritis," *Clinical Biomechanics*, vol. 30, no. 3, article no. 3905, pp. 226–230, 2015.

[18] D. J. Rutherford, C. Hubley-Kozey, and W. Stanish, "Hip abductor function in individuals with medial knee osteoarthritis: Implications for medial compartment loading during gait," *Clinical Biomechanics*, vol. 29, no. 5, pp. 545–550, 2014.

[19] M. Deasy, E. Leahy, and A. I. Semciw, "Hip strength deficits in people with symptomatic knee osteoarthritis: A systematic review with meta-analysis," *Journal of Orthopaedic & Sports Physical Therapy*, vol. 46, no. 8, pp. 629–639, 2016.

[20] C. Dunphy, S. Casey, A. Lomond, and D. Rutherford, "Contralateral pelvic drop during gait increases knee adduction moments of asymptomatic individuals," *Human Movement Science*, vol. 49, pp. 27–35, 2016.

[21] F. Hálfdanardóttir, *Proximal Effects of Unloader Bracing for Medial Knee Osteoarthritis: Analyses of Muscle Activation and Movement Patterns of Hip and Trunk During Walking*, p. 68, Faculty of Medicine, University of Iceland, Reykjavík, Iceland, 2015.

[22] J. H. Kellgren and J. S. Lawrence, "Radiological assessment of osteo-arthrosis," *Annals of the Rheumatic Diseases*, vol. 16, no. 4, pp. 494–502, 1957.

[23] K. Briem, "Reliability, validity and responsiveness of the icelandic version of the knee injury and osteoarthritis outcome score (KOOS)," *Laeknabladid*, vol. 98, no. 7-8, pp. 403–407, 2012.

[24] E. M. Roos, H. P. Roos, L. S. Lohmander, C. Ekdahl, and B. D. Beynnon, "Knee injury and osteoarthritis outcome score (KOOS)—development of a self-administered outcome measure," *Journal of Orthopaedic & Sports Physical Therapy*, vol. 28, no. 2, pp. 88–96, 1998.

[25] Y.-H. Pua, T. W. Wrigley, S. M. Cowan, and K. L. Bennell, "Intrarater test-retest reliability of hip range of motion and hip muscle strength measurements in persons with hip osteoarthritis," *Archives of Physical Medicine and Rehabilitation*, vol. 89, no. 6, pp. 1146–1154, 2008.

[26] M. A. Hunt and K. L. Bennell, "Predicting dynamic knee joint load with clinical measures in people with medial knee osteoarthritis," *The Knee*, vol. 18, no. 4, pp. 231–234, 2011.

[27] R. F. Moyer, T. B. Birmingham, B. M. Chesworth, C. O. Kean, and J. R. Giffin, "Alignment, body mass and their interaction on dynamic knee joint load in patients with knee osteoarthritis," *Osteoarthritis and Cartilage*, vol. 18, no. 7, pp. 888–893, 2010.

[28] J. L. Astephen, K. J. Deluzio, G. E. Caldwell, and M. J. Dunbar, "Biomechanical changes at the hip, knee, and ankle joints

during gait are associated with knee osteoarthritis severity," *Journal of Orthopaedic Research*, vol. 26, no. 3, pp. 332–341, 2008.

[29] E. Esfandiari, M. Kamyab, H. R. Yazdi, N. Foroughi, and M. A. Sanjari, "The immediate effect of lateral wedge insoles, with and without a subtalar strap, on the lateral trunk lean motion in patients with knee osteoarthritis," *Geriatric Orthopaedic Surgery and Rehabilitation*, vol. 4, no. 4, pp. 127–132, 2013.

[30] M. A. Tevald, A. Murray, B. A. Luc, K. Lai, D. Sohn, and B. Pietrosimone, "Hip abductor strength in people with knee osteoarthritis: a cross-sectional study of reliability and association with function," *The Knee*, vol. 23, no. 1, pp. 57–62, 2016.

[31] G. E. Ferreira, C. C. Robinson, M. Wiebusch, C. C. D. M. Viero, L. H. T. Da Rosa, and M. F. Silva, "The effect of exercise therapy on knee adduction moment in individuals with knee osteoarthritis: a systematic review," *Clinical Biomechanics*, vol. 30, no. 6, pp. 521–527, 2015.

[32] A. Phinyomark, S. T. Osis, B. A. Hettinga, D. Kobsar, and R. Ferber, "Gender differences in gait kinematics for patients with knee osteoarthritis," *BMC Musculoskeletal Disorders*, vol. 17, no. 1, article no. 157, 2016.

11

Management of Subtrochanteric Proximal Femur Fractures

Christopher Jackson, Mina Tanios, and Nabil Ebraheim

Department of Orthopedic Surgery, University of Toledo Medical Center, Toledo, OH 43614-5807, USA

Correspondence should be addressed to Nabil Ebraheim; nabil.ebraheim@utoledo.edu

Academic Editor: Allen L. Carl

Subtrochanteric femur fractures are an uncommon injury in orthopedics, but when they are encountered they may present difficulties in management. The purpose of this paper is to examine the recent literature on the epidemiology, classification, initial evaluation, and definitely treatment for these injuries. These will assist the physician to determine the optimal treatment strategy and avoid potential surgical complication.

1. Introduction

Fractures of the proximal femur is a very important topic in the field of orthopedic surgery, but much of that attention is placed on fractures of the femoral neck and intertrochanteric areas. An additional area that must be well understood is the subtrochanteric (ST) region of the femur, which is defined as the proximal femoral shaft located within 5 cm of the lesser trochanter (Figure 1). This area experiences high levels of stress and fractures to this area can result in significant complications and poor clinical outcomes if not managed properly.

2. Epidemiology and Risk Factors

The overall incidence rate of fractures of the proximal femur is found to be approximately 230 per 100,000 patients with approximately 5-10% of these fracture occurring within the ST region [1, 2]. Overall the incidence has been estimated to be approximately 15-20/100,000. In terms of age, many studies have found that ST femur fractures occur in a bimodal distribution. One study delineated that approximately two-thirds of all ST fractures occur in patients older than 50 years of age with another 25% occurring in patients aged 17-50 [4]. In terms of gender, females have been found to be at high risk for ST femur fractures with up to a 33% higher incidence rate compared to males [2, 4]. In addition to age and gender, other elicited risk factors include low total bone mineral density, diabetes mellitus, and the use of bisphosphonate medications for the treatment of osteoporosis [5, 6]. The influence of bisphosphonates on the development of atypical femur fractures has garnered significant attention recently with elevated risk with prolongation of therapy, most notably after 5-10 years of treatment [1, 7]. Despite this risk, the overall protection from typical femoral neck and intertrochanteric fractures generated by bisphosphonate use appears to outweigh the increased risk for atypical ST fractures [7]. Overall, due to the prevalence of this injury in the field of orthopedic trauma and with no apparent changes in the incidence in these fractures since 1996 [2] it is prudent for the orthopedic surgeon to have a good understanding of the anatomy of the ST region, presentation, initial work-up, preoperative management, operative stabilization, and postoperative care.

3. Anatomy and Biomechanics

As mentioned before the ST area of the proximal femur is defined as the proximal femur that lies 5 cm distal to the lesser trochanter. The primary structural support to this area is the femorale calcar which is a posteromedial structure that begins just distal to the lesser trochanter and travels proximal to support the posteroinferior femoral neck. Early biomechanical studies found that this section of bone can experience up to 1200 N of force within the ST area with standing and gait [8].

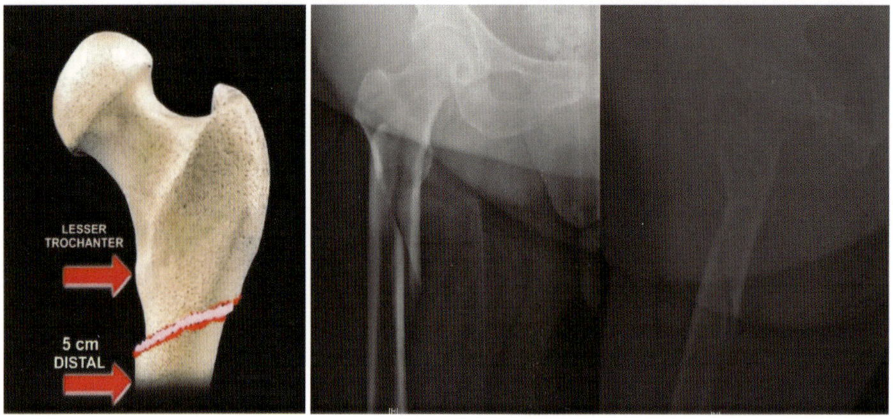

FIGURE 1: Anatomy of the subtrochanteric area of the femur: the subtrochanteric area of the femur is defined as the area 5 cm distal to lesser trochanter.

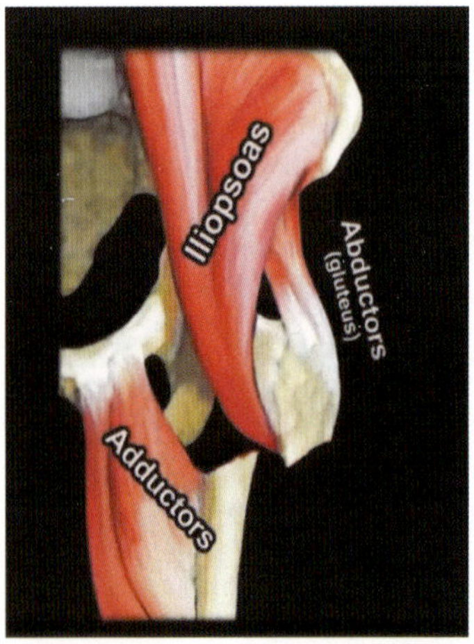

FIGURE 2: Subtrochanteric fracture deformity: The typical deformity of the subtrochanteric femur fracture is one of external rotation and abduction of the proximal segment and adduction of the distal segment.

These forces are important because while these force can be tolerated in young healthy bone they may overpower weaker osteoporotic bone. In addition to the static forces placed on the proximal femur, this region experiences increased stress secondary to the multiple muscular attachments in the region, which include the lateral hip abductors, medial hip adductors, the iliopsoas, and short external rotators. These muscular attachments have been shown to increase stresses around the hip and proximal femur [9]. In addition to the stresses applied to the ST region, these multiple muscle groups produce predictable deformities patterns that must be understood in order to achieve a proper reduction. The classic deformity that occurs in ST femur fractures is proximal segment abduction, external rotation, and flexion caused by the pull of the gluteus medius, gluteus minimus, the short external rotators, and iliopsoas and adduction of the distal fragment by the gracilis and adductor muscle groups. (Figure 2)

4. Presentation: History and Physical Examination

Typically, patients will present in 1 of 2 scenarios. The first one will be a younger patient following a high energy mechanism of injury such as an MVA or fall from height. The patient will usually have multiple injuries and the first priority should be determining whether the patient requires ATLS and volume resuscitation. The second common situation is an elderly patient following a low mechanism of injury which will typically present with an isolated fracture. Following ATLS protocols or in the situation of a low energy MOI, a thorough history should be taken. This should include the MOI, pain, ability to ambulate, the presence of neurologic or vascular symptoms, and the presence of prodromal hip pain or contralateral hip pain. Medication histories should be taken looking for the use of bisphosphonates and the length of therapy.

Examination of the affected lower extremity will reveal a shorted and externally rotated extremity. Injuries are typically closed but examination of the skin should be through as open femur fractures represent extremely serious injuries with significant soft tissue damage. Neurovascular examination should be performed and deficits should be worked up appropriately. Finally, a history of another joint or extremity pain followed by a skeletal survey to rule out other musculoskeletal injuries should be performed.

5. Imaging and Classification

Initial imaging of the patient with a suspected ST fracture includes an AP pelvis and full-length femur films. These initial imagings will allow for proper injury identification and classification of the fracture. Typical findings will be the proximal fragment resting in abduction, external rotation, and flexion with the distal fragment in adduction. The fracture will also typically be in a long oblique orientation with varying amounts of comminution. In the setting of a history of prolonged bisphosphonate use with or without contralateral hip and thigh pain, the surgeon should attempt

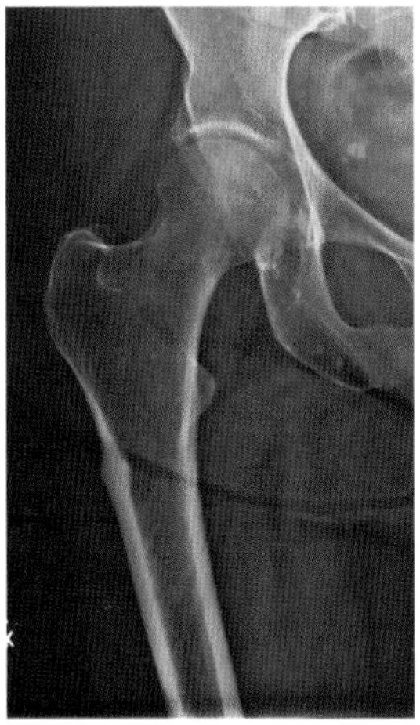

FIGURE 3: Atypical subtrochanteric femur fracture: Initial identification of atypical subtrochanteric femur fractures can be identified by characteristic lateral cortical thickening.

to identify atypical fracture patterns associated with bisphosphonates. Recently the American Society for Bone and Mineral Research developed criteria for the identification of atypical ST femur fractures. Common radiographic features of atypical ST femur fractures include transverse fracture patterns with minimal comminution, lateral cortical thinking, and a posteromedial spike in the setting of a low energy injury (Figure 3). The importance of identifying atypical fractures associated with bisphosphonates is the fact that there is a high incidence of bilateral fractures, recommendations for discontinuation of bisphosphonate and conversion to teriparatide, and the need for prophylactic fixation of lateral insufficiency fractures to prevent completion of the fracture [10, 11]. These recommendations come from the overserved improvement in patients with hip pain and lateral cortical thickening with protected weight bearing and conversion from bisphosphonate treatment to teriparatide and lack of improvement with similar treatment in patients with documented radiolucent lines in the lateral cortex. Advanced imaging modalities, such as CT or MRI, can be performed in cases with equivocal plain radiographs to identify occult cortex lucencies. These imaging modalities should also be used to tract the treatment of the stress fractures [3, 10]. Overall several different classification systems have been developed including the Russell-Taylor classification which is based on the presence of lesser trochanter comminution and fracture extension into the piriformis fossa which helped to guide treatment prior to the development of trochanteric start point intramedullary nails. The AO classification system also has a classification system describing fracture morphology and mechanism.

6. Emergency Department Management

After performing a history, physical examination, and imaging modalities, initial treatment should always begin with any required resuscitative measures as indicated by ATLS protocols. Following stabilization and ruling out other injuries, the patient may be placed in skeletal traction. Skeletal traction through the use of a distal femoral pin has been shown to restore length of the affected extremity and improve preoperative pain scores [12]. Finally, medical optimization with the assistance of internal medicine/geriatrics has been found to improve inpatient mortality, long-term mortality, and length of stay [13].

7. Definitive Management: Nonoperative

Due to the high morbidity and mortality associated with nonoperative management, there are only a few instances where it is acceptable. First the patient in extremis with a high risk of mortality from anesthesia or other medical conditions should avoid surgical treatment. Secondly, hospice patients with minimal discomfort may be treated nonoperatively. However, numerous benefits, such as improved mobility, decrease of pain, and improving the care provided by care givers by the definitive fixation, should be thoroughly discussed with all individuals involved in the medical decision-making process before proceeding with nonoperative management [14].

8. Definitive Management: Intramedullary Nailing

Overall, the use of intramedullary fixation has become the gold standard for the treatment of ST femur fractures (Figure 4). Overall, intramedullary nailing has been shown to decrease operative time, fixation failure, and hospital length of stay when compared to extramedullary devices [15]. Wiss et al. examined 95 acute ST femur fractures and found average time to union to be 25 weeks with 7 complications including 1 nonunion and 6 malunions [16]. Similar results were found by Shah et al. who examined 51 ST fractures treated with intramedullary nailing and found good results with 1 delayed union in a pathologic fracture secondary to malignancy and 1 case of failure of fixation. This study also revealed overall Harris hip scores of 90.1 at 12 months [16]. Despite the apparent success of intramedullary nailing, slight nuances to the techniques of the procedure have been found to improve outcomes, including the nail starting point, proximal screw orientation, and length of the nail.

In terms of the proximal entry point for an anterograde intramedullary nailing, the surgeon has a choice of a piriformis start point and a greater trochanteric start point. Advantages of the piriformis start point include reduction of the incidence of varus malreduction and medial cortex injury with reaming [17]. Disadvantages are difficulty in obtaining a proper start point in obese patients, patients with hypertrophic short external rotators, or greater trochanter overhang. Additional excessive anterior placement of the starting point by as little as 6 mm can increase the risk of anterior cortical blowout [18]. Finally, there is concern for the proximity of the piriformis start point to the cervical vessels of the medial femoral circumflex artery. The second starting point is the trochanteric start point. Advantages include protecting more of the soft tissue structures around the hip and easier placement [19]. However there is a greater concern

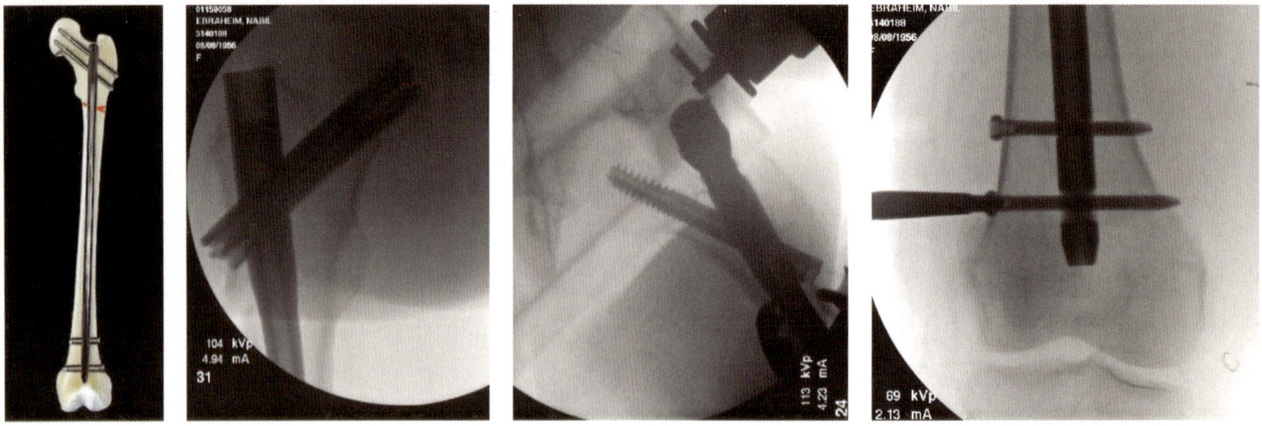

Figure 4: Intramedullary fixation of a subtrochanteric femur fracture: This diagram illustrates and provides radiographs of an example of intramedullary fixation of a subtrochanteric femur fracture. Proximal fixation is achieved through the use of cephalomedullary screws and distally with locked interlock screws.

for varus malreduction and vast changes in the “ideal” start point based on patient anatomy [3, 20]. Overall the ideal start point must be chosen based on unique patient and fracture characteristics including body habitus, bony anatomy of the proximal femur, and fracture lines into the greater trochanter or basicervical region.

The next technical aspect of anterograde femoral nailing is the proximal screw orientation. For more proximal diaphyseal femoral fractures the crossed proximal screws are used. However this type of construct only provides stabilization through bony contact at the entry site and cortical contact at the interlocking bolt sites. The development of reconstruction nail designs allows for additional fixation via forces between the cephalomedullary screw and the femoral neck and head preventing varus and flexion deformities [21]. In addition to orientation of the screws, the number of screws has been examined. Grisell et al. examined two different two-proximal screw constructs: one with parallel screws into the femoral head and neck and one with crossed screws. This study determined that the axial stiffness was greater in the cross screw construct [22]. In addition, studies have also shown two distal interlock screws provide greater stability than one [21].

Final aspects to intramedullary nailing include nail length, nail size, and nail material. In terms of nail length, the standard of care is full-length intramedullary nails. This is supported by biomechanical studies revealing weak constructs and peri-implant fractures when comparing long and short intramedullary devices [23]. In terms of implant diameter and material, biomechanical studies have shown that larger proximal diameter implants made of stainless steel provided greater fracture stability in rotation, shear, and axial motion over smaller diameter titanium implants [7]. Overall, long intramedullary nailing of ST femur fractures has been shown to provide great outcomes with limited complications.

9. Definitive Treatment: Plating

Aside from intramedullary nailing, numerous methods of open reduction and internal fixation of ST femur fractures are available. The most successful type of plating involves the use of 95-degree fixed angle blade plates (Figure 5). Despite some studies revealing moderately good results with fixed angle plating with nonunion rates of approximately 0-10% with times to union of approximately 5 months [2, 24], more recent studies have found less appealing results [25]. These recent changes in outcomes, coupled with the high degree of difficulty in applying this fixed angle devices and decreased infection rates, higher union rates, and shorter operative times with intramedullary nailing, have led to decreased use in 95-degree fixed angle plates [14, 25]. Another form of fixed angle plating includes proximal femoral locking plates (Figure 6). These systems have been shown to have better biomechanical properties than blade plate constructs. However recent studies have also shown poor results including high malunion/nonunion rates and subsequent reoperation rates close to 35% [14, 26]. Finally 135-degree compression plates, commonly used for intertrochanteric hip fractures, have been shown to have failure of fixation upwards of 56%

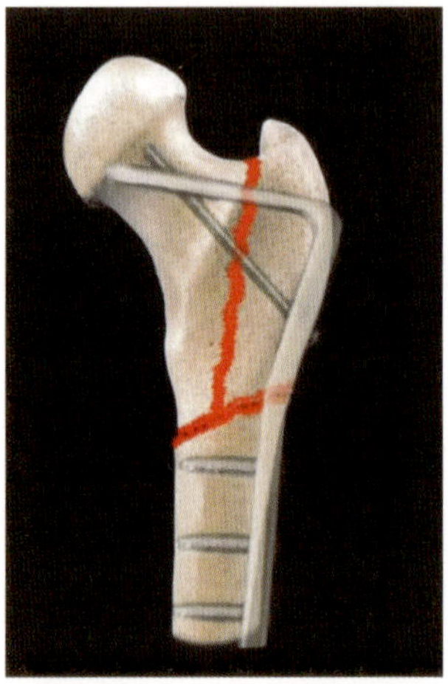

Figure 5: Extramedullary fixation of subtrochanteric femur fractures: This diagram illustrates the use of a 95-degree blade plate construct for the treatment of subtrochanteric femur fractures.

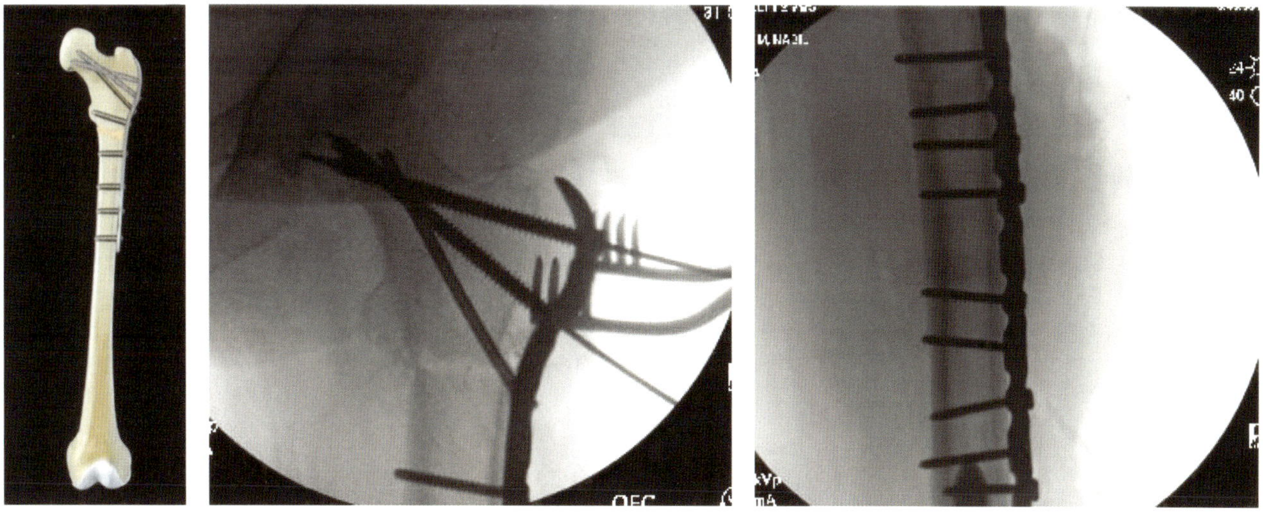

Figure 6: Extramedullary fixation of subtrochanteric femur fractures: This diagram illustrates and provides radiographs of the use of a proximal femoral locking plate construct for the treatment of subtrochanteric femur fractures.

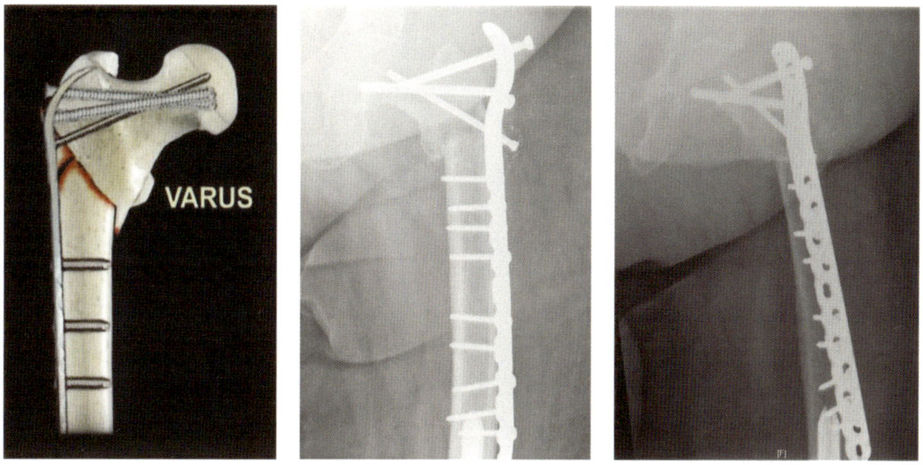

Figure 7: Varus collapse of subtrochanteric femur fractures: This diagram illustrates and provides a radiographic example of a subtrochanteric fracture varus nonunion.

and therefore have been abandoned in the surgical treatment of ST femur fractures [21].

Despite poorer results of open reduction and internal fixation with fixed angle constructs when compared to intramedullary nailing, open plating may still have a prominent role in the acute treatment of ST femur fractures. One study by Robertson et al. showed a large improvement in malunion rates (27% versus 0%) when provisional plating of ST femur fractures was performed prior to intramedullary nailing in fractures that required an open reduction. In addition there was no increase in operative time or blood loss when comparing all cases that required open reduction between the two study groups [15].

10. Complications

The complications of surgical treatment of ST femur fractures are similar to the complications for other types of proximal femur fractures, including mortality, nonunion, malunion, and infection. In terms of mortality rates, ST fracture 1-year mortality rates in elderly patients are similar to rates for femoral neck and IT fractures of approximately 9.5% at 30 days, 27% at 1 year, and up to 60% at 4 years [22, 27]. Interestingly, it appears that patients with atypical proximal femur fractures associated with bisphosphonates have a decreased mortality rate at 4 years when compared to typical ST fracture patterns [27].

In terms of malunion and nonunion rates, the main cause appears to be inability to obtain anatomic reductions intraoperatively. Development of improper reductions can be the result of improper starting points, especially too lateral with the trochanteric starting point, or lack of direct visualization, instrumentation, or provisional plate fixation prior to intramedullary nail insertion. In addition to increased rates of nonunion, excessive varus and flexion of the proximal segment can cause detrimental changes to gait mechanics. In general, the typical failure will result in a varus deformity (Figure 7) and these complications are typically treated with exchange intramedullary nailing or fixed angle plate constructs with or without bone grafting [14].

In terms of infection, both deep and superficial surgical site infections can occur following operative treatment of ST femur fractures. Typically superficial soft tissue infections can be treated conservatively with antibiotic alone. In terms of deep infections, they may be approached with surgical irrigation and debridement with antibiotics in an attempt to allow the fracture to heal prior to implant removal. However, should the patient be found to have a persistent infected nonunion, removal of the implant is needed followed by temporary fixation with an antibiotic intramedullary device followed by antibiotics until the infection has been effectively treated [14].

11. Summary

ST femur fractures are a less common type of hip fracture but can occur in both young and elderly patients after both high- and low-energy mechanisms of injury. While initial evaluation and treatment involve resuscitation and modalities such as skeletal traction, very rarely should treatment not proceed to surgical fixation. In terms of fixation, intramedullary nailing is the gold standard of treatment and can be performed safely for both typical and atypical ST fractures. However there are many technical aspects to intramedullary nailing that a surgeon must consider. While fixed angle constructs can be used for initial treatment of fixation, these methods are more commonly utilized for ST femoral malunion/nonunion treatment.

References

[1] R. M. Dell, A. L. Adams, D. F. Greene et al., "Incidence of atypical nontraumatic diaphyseal fractures of the femur," *Journal of Bone and Mineral Research*, vol. 27, no. 12, pp. 2544–2550, 2012.

[2] J. W. Nieves, J. P. Bilezikian, J. M. Lane et al., "Fragility fractures of the hip and femur: incidence and patient characteristics," *Osteoporosis International*, vol. 21, no. 3, pp. 399–408, 2010.

[3] P. N. Streubel, A. H. W. Wong, W. M. Ricci, and M. J. Gardner, "Is there a standard trochanteric entry site for nailing of subtrochanteric femur fractures?" *Journal of Orthopaedic Trauma*, vol. 25, no. 4, pp. 202–207, 2011.

[4] A. C. Ng, M. T. Drake, B. L. Clarke et al., "Trends in subtrochanteric, diaphyseal, and distal femur fractures, 1984-2007," *Osteoporosis International*, vol. 23, no. 6, pp. 1721–1726, 2012.

[5] B. Abrahamsen, P. Eiken, and R. Eastell, "Subtrochanteric and diaphyseal femur fractures in patients treated with alendronate: A register-based national cohort study," *Journal of Bone and Mineral Research*, vol. 24, no. 6, pp. 1095–1102, 2009.

[6] N. Napoli, A. V. Schwartz, L. Palermo et al., "Risk factors for subtrochanteric and diaphyseal fractures: the study of osteoporotic fractures," *The Journal of Clinical Endocrinology & Metabolism*, vol. 98, no. 2, pp. 659–667, 2013.

[7] C. S. Roberts, A. Nawab, M. Wang, M. J. Voor, and D. Seligson, "Second generation intramedullary nailing of subtrochanteric femur fractures: A biomechanical study of fracture site motion," *Journal of Orthopaedic Trauma*, vol. 16, no. 4, pp. 231–238, 2002.

[8] J. C. Koch, "The laws of bone architecture," *American Journal of Anatomy*, vol. 21, no. 2, pp. 177–298, 1917.

[9] M. Nordin and V. H, Basic biomechanics of the musculoskeletal system. Lippincott Williams Wilkins.n,.

[10] F. Feldman, "Atypical diaphyseal femoral fractures-new aspects," *Skeletal Radiology*, vol. 41, no. 1, pp. 75–81, 2012.

[11] A. Shah and M. Shah, "Functional outcomes of subtrochanteric femur fractures treated by intramedullary proximal femur nail," *International Journal of Orthopaedics*, vol. 3, no. 2, pp. 876–881, 2017.

[12] D. B. Bumpass, W. M. Ricci, C. M. McAndrew, and M. J. Gardner, "A prospective study of pain reduction and knee dysfunction comparing femoral skeletal traction and splinting in adult trauma patients," *Journal of Orthopaedic Trauma*, vol. 29, no. 2, pp. 112–118, 2015.

[13] K. V. Grigoryan, H. Javedan, and J. L. Rudolph, "Ortho-geriatric care models and outcomes in hip fracture patients: a systematic review and meta-analysis," *Journal of Orthopaedic Trauma*, vol. 28, no. 3, 2014.

[14] K. J. Koval, N. Rezaie, and R. S. Yoon, "Subtrochanteric Femur Fractures," in *In Proximal Femur Fractures*, pp. 101–112, Springer, Cham, 2018.

[15] R. Robertson, M. Tucker, and T. Jones, "Provisional Plating of Subtrochanteric Femur Fractures Before Intramedullary Nailing in the Lateral Decubitus Position," *Journal of Orthopaedic Trauma*, vol. 32, no. 4, pp. e151–e156, 2018.

[16] D. A. Wiss and W. W. Brien, "Subtrochanteric fractures of the femur: Results of treatment by interlocking nailing," *Clinical Orthopaedics and Related Research*, no. 283, pp. 231–236, 1992.

[17] D. Nicolaou and J. T. Watson, "Nailing proximal femur fractures: How to choose starting point and proximal screw configuration," *Journal of Orthopaedic Trauma*, vol. 29, no. 4, pp. S22–S27, 2015.

[18] K. D. Johnson, A. F. Tencer, and M. C. Sherman, "Biomechanical factors affecting fracture stability and femoral bursting in closed intramedullary nailing of femoral shaft fractures, with illustrative case presentations," *Journal of Orthopaedic Trauma*, vol. 1, no. 1, pp. 1–11, 1987.

[19] C. M. Ansari Moein, M. H. J. Verhofstad, R. L. A. W. Bleys, and C. Van Der Werken, "Soft tissue injury related to choice of entry point in antegrade femoral nailing: Piriform fossa or greater trochanter tip," *Injury*, vol. 36, no. 11, pp. 1337–1342, 2005.

[20] R. F. Ostrum, A. Marcantonio, and R. Marburger, "A critical analysis of the eccentric starting point for trochanteric intramedullary femoral nailing," *Journal of Orthopaedic Trauma*, vol. 19, no. 10, pp. 681–686, 2005.

[21] D. W. Lundy, "Subtrochanteric femoral fractures," *Journal of the American Academy of OrthopaedicSurgeons* , vol. 15, no. 11, pp. 663–671, 2007.

[22] N. S. Horner, K. Samuelsson, J. Solyom et al., "Implant-Related Complications and Mortality After Use of Short or Long Gamma Nail for Intertrochanteric and Subtrochanteric Fractures: A Prospective Study with Minimum 13-Year Follow-up," *JBJS Open Access*, vol. 2, no. 3, p. e0026, 2017.

[23] W. J. Kraemer, T. C. Hearn, J. N. Powell, and N. Mahomed, "Fixation of segmental subtrochanteric fractures: A biomechanical study," *Clinical Orthopaedics and Related Research*, no. 332, pp. 71–79, 1996.

[24] C. Kinast, B. R. Bolhofner, J. W. Mast, and R. Ganz, "Subtrochanteric fractures of the femur. Results of treatment with the 95o condylar blade-plate," *Clinical Orthopaedics and Related Research*, no. 238, pp. 122–130, 1989.

[25] W. W. Brien, D. A. Wiss, V. Becker, and T. Lehman, "Subtrochanteric femur fractures: A comparison of the zickel nail, 95° blade plate, and interlocking nail," *Journal of Orthopaedic Trauma*, vol. 5, no. 4, pp. 458–464, 1991.

[26] C. A. Collinge, R. Hymes, M. Archdeacon et al., "Unstable proximal femur fractures treated with proximal femoral locking plates: A retrospective, multicenter study of 111 cases," *Journal of Orthopaedic Trauma*, vol. 30, no. 9, pp. 489–495, 2016.

[27] M. Kharazmi, P. Hallberg, J. Schilcher, P. Aspenberg, and K. Michaëlsson, "Mortality after atypical femoral fractures: A cohort study," *Journal of Bone and Mineral Research*, vol. 31, no. 3, pp. 491–497, 2016.

12

Minimally Invasive Plate Osteosynthesis for Proximal Humerus Fractures: A Retrospective Study Describing Principles and Advantages of the Technique

Riccardo Luigi Alberio, Matteo Del Re, and Federico Alberto Grassi

Department of Orthopedics and Traumatology, University of East Piedmont, Hospital "Maggiore della Carità", Via Mazzini 18, Novara, Italy

Correspondence should be addressed to Riccardo Luigi Alberio; riccardo.alberio@gmail.com

Academic Editor: Allen L. Carl

Background. The aim of this study was to evaluate the clinical and radiographic results after minimally invasive plate osteosynthesis (MIPO) for proximal humerus fractures. Potential advantages of this approach include the easier exposure of the greater tuberosity and the limited surgical dissection around the fracture site. *Materials and Methods.* From October 2011 to March 2016, thirty-nine patients (32 women, 7 men) with a mean age of 64.9 years (range: 48–80) were surgically treated with the MIPO technique for proximal humeral fractures. According to Neer classification, there were 12 two-part, 24 three-part, and 2 four-part fractures and 1 two-part fracture-dislocation; the AO/OTA system was also used to categorize the fractures. The Constant-Murley (CMS) and the Oxford Shoulder (OSS) Scores were used to evaluate shoulder function. *Results.* Thirty-four patients were available for clinical and radiographic evaluation at a mean follow-up of 31.8 months (range: 12–54 months). All fractures healed and no postoperative complications occurred. Full recovery of pretrauma activities was reported by 27 patients, while 7 patients presented mild functional limitations. The mean absolute CMS was 75.2 (range: 55–95), the mean normalized CMS was 90.5 (range: 69–107), and the mean OSS was 43.7 (range: 31–48). The only statistically significant correlation was found between the female gender and lower absolute CMS and OSS. Radiographic evaluation revealed varus malunion in 4 cases and valgus malunion in 1 case, while incomplete greater tuberosity reduction was detected in 4 cases. All malunions were related to inadequate reduction at time of surgery and not to secondary displacement. *Conclusions.* MIPO for proximal humeral fractures is an effective and safe surgical procedure. The limited tissue dissection allows minimizing the incidence of nonunion, avascular necrosis, and infection. The technique is not easy, requires experience to achieve mastery, and should be reserved for selected fracture patterns. In our experience, the main advantage of this approach consists in the direct access to the greater tuberosity, thus facilitating its anatomic reduction and fixation.

1. Introduction

The incidence of proximal humerus fractures is increasing for two main reasons that reflect the bimodal distribution of these injuries. On one side, progressive aging of the population is associated with a rise in low energy injuries, particularly among women over 60 with osteopenia. On the other side, the wide participation in sport activities and the reduced mortality in traffic accidents are related to a growing rate of high-energy fractures requiring treatment [1, 2].

Owing to the wide variety of anatomo-clinical conditions, treatment options for proximal humeral fractures vary considerably. Surgical treatment is usually performed for displaced and/or unstable fractures with the goal of restoring normal anatomy as well as allowing early shoulder rehabilitation. Several procedures can be adopted for fracture fixation, but plating remains the most popular method of osteosynthesis. Undoubtfully, the introduction of locking plates has led to a great improvement in clinical outcomes and has widened indications for internal fixation, but the rate of failures and complications is still considerable.

While for fractures of the surgical neck many surgeons prefer nailing to plating, three- and four-part fractures are mainly treated with locking plates. Even in severe fracture patterns, plating is widely performed and this trend has reduced the rate of anatomic shoulder replacement performed for fractures [3, 4].

Open reduction and internal fixation through the deltopectoral approach may require extensive soft tissues dissection and strong deltoid retraction, particularly for gaining adequate access to the greater tuberosity [5, 6]. To overcome these drawbacks, a minimally invasive, deltoid-splitting approach has been adopted for plating proximal humeral fractures.

The minimally invasive plate osteosynthesis (MIPO) technique facilitates the exposure of the greater tuberosity and allows respecting vascularity and soft tissues around the fracture, thus preserving better conditions for bone healing [7–9]. However, this approach exposes the patient to an increased risk of axillary nerve injury if compared to the traditional deltopectoral approach [10, 11].

In this retrospective study, we report the clinical experience achieved in a consecutive series of 39 patients treated with MIPO technique for proximal humeral fracture.

2. Materials and Methods

From October 2011 to March 2016, thirty-nine patients were surgically treated with the MIPO technique for displaced proximal humerus fractures by a single surgeon at a single institution. In this clinical series, neither a treatment protocol nor inclusion/exclusion criteria were preventively established. The MIPO technique was performed for fractures in which reduction and plating had reasonable chances of success without exposing the anteromedial aspect of the proximal humerus. Fractures with wide diastasis between fragments, high-energy injuries with relevant soft tissue interposition between bone fragments, four-part fractures (excluding valgus impacted), and articular (head-splitting or severely impacted) fractures were not considered suitable for the MIPO technique. These lesions were either plated through a deltopectoral approach or treated with shoulder arthroplasty.

This series included 32 women and 7 men, with a mean age of 64.9 years (range: 48 to 80 years) at the time of injury. The dominant arm was involved in 24 cases (61.5%).

The mechanism of injury was a fall from standing height in 21 patients (53.8%), a traffic accident in 10 patients (25.6%), a sport accident in 5 patients (12.8%), and a fall from great height in 3 patients (7.7%).

All the patients underwent radiographic examination of the shoulder before surgery and a CT-scan of the shoulder was performed in 14 patients (35.9%) to better define the fracture pattern. According to Neer's criteria, the series included 12 two-part, 24 three-part, and 2 four-part fractures and 1 two-part fracture-dislocation. Fractures were also classified according to the AO/OTA system, as reported in Table 1.

Time span between trauma and surgery averaged 7,25 days, with a range of 2 to 17 days.

At the latest follow-up, clinical evaluation of the patients was performed using the absolute and normalized Constant-Murley Score (CMS) [12, 13] and the Oxford Shoulder Score (OSS) [14]. Radiograms of the shoulder (A-P view in internal and external rotation) were also taken to detect avascular necrosis (AVN), nonunion, malunion, implant malposition, and screws perforation.

Table 1: Classification of the fractures according to AO/OTA system.

AO/OTA		n
A	1	1
	2	0
	3	4
B	1	15
	2	15
	3	0
C	1	3
	2	1
	3	0

Mann–Whitney U test (SPSS 10.0) was used to compare functional outcomes with nonparametric statistical variables. P values less than 0,05 were considered statistically significant.

2.1. Surgical Technique. All patients are operated under general anesthesia in the beach-chair position. The affected limb overhangs the edge of the table and the patient's head is firmly secured with tape. The C-arm image intensifier is placed on the opposite side in order to visualize the fractured humerus with minimal obstacle for the surgeon.

Reduction of surgical neck fractures is attempted by closed manipulation before starting the procedure. The skin incision begins at the anterolateral corner of the acromion and extends 5 cm distally in line with the proximal humerus (Figure 1). The deltoid muscle is split along the anterior rafe and the subacromial bursa is removed. The cord-like axillary nerve is palpated on the deep surface of the deltoid approximately 2-3 cm below the inferior end of the wound.

Strong nonabsorbable sutures are placed in the rotator cuff at the bone-tendon junction for facilitating humeral head and tuberosities reduction. One or two 2 mm K-wires can be inserted in the humeral head and used as joysticks for helping fragment realignment. Head reduction can be maintained by inserting two additional K-wires in a position not interfering with plate implantation.

Using the insertion handle, the plate (Philos, DePuy Synthes, Solothurn, Switzerland) is slid along the humeral surface under the deltoid muscle and the axillary nerve. The plate should be seated just lateral to the bicipital grove and kept in contact with bone. In case of three- or four-part fractures, the greater tuberosity must be previously reduced and laid under the plate. In its final position, the superior edge of the plate should be 1 cm below the top of the greater tuberosity to avoid subacromial impingement.

A second skin incision is started at the level of the first diaphyseal screw hole of the insertion handle and extended distally according to the number of diaphyseal screws needed (Figure 1). After having aligned the inferior end of the plate with the humeral shaft, temporary fixation of the plate is

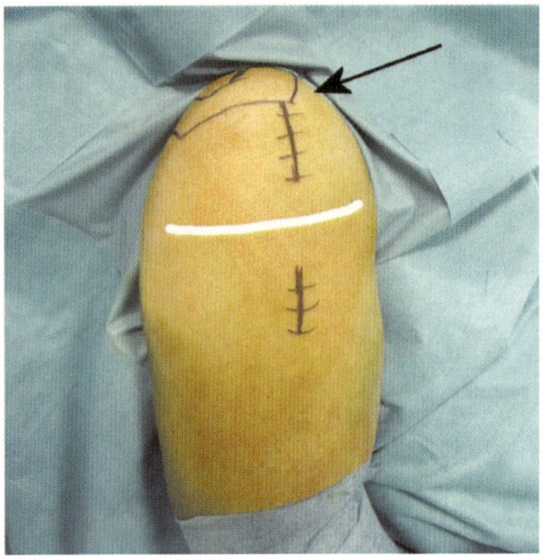

Figure 1: Surgical field of a right shoulder showing the two skin incisions performed for the MIPO technique. The proximal incision starts at the anterolateral corner of the acromion (arrow) and is approximately 5 cm long; the length of the distal incision varies according to the number of diaphyseal screws implanted. The white line shows the level and course of the axillary nerve.

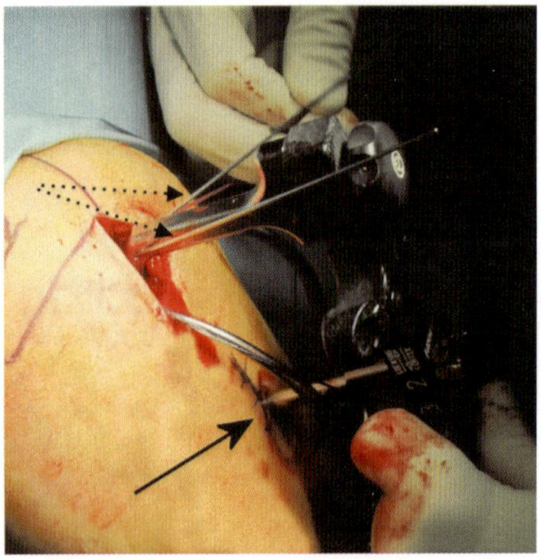

Figure 2: Insertion handle of the Philos plate with two 1.6 mm K-wires (dotted arrows) inserted in the humeral head for temporary fixation of the proximal fragment(s). Sleeve system (arrow) for insertion of bicortical locking or nonlocking screws in the humeral shaft.

performed by inserting two 1.6 mm K-wires in the humeral head through holes in the aiming device.

The reduction is checked with the image intensifier and a nonlocking bicortical screw is inserted in the humeral shaft using the sleeve system of the insertion handle (Figure 2). This step allows improving the alignment of the shaft with the head by taking advantage of the shape of the plate.

After having inserted four angular stable screws in the humeral head and one or two angular stable screws in the shaft, the insertion handle is removed. Additional screws can be inserted in the humeral head by abducting the arm in order to gain access to the inferior epiphyseal holes of the plate without jeopardizing the axillary nerve.

Fixation can be augmented by passing strong nonabsorbable sutures through the rotator cuff and anchoring them into the peripheral holes of the plate.

After wound closure, the arm is placed in a sling. Assisted passive elevation of the shoulder to 90° (hand to the top of the head) in the supine position is immediately started. The patient can also mobilize the upper limb gently for personal care and clothing as pain permits.

If X-rays taken at three weeks do not show any worrisome finding, the patient is encouraged to perform light activities of daily living and active elevation of the shoulder without resistance. The sling is gradually abandoned, but it is recommended to wear it for protection when out in public.

Further clinical and radiographic evaluations are carried out six weeks and three months after surgery. During this period, stretching and strengthening exercises are performed under the supervision of a physiotherapist to gradually improve shoulder function.

3. Results

Thirty-four patients were available for clinical and radiographic evaluation at a mean follow-up of 31.8 months (range: 12 to 54 months). Four patients declined to show up for logistical problems, while one patient was untraceable. All dropouts (12.8%) were women; therefore the last follow-up population included 27 female and 7 male patients with a mean age of 64.8 years (range: 48 to 80 years).

No intraoperative complications occurred. In one patient, hardware removal had to be performed three months after fixation, because the plate was not adherent to the bone surface and caused subacromial impingement during rehabilitation (Figure 3). The fracture healed uneventfully without secondary displacement.

At follow-up, the mean absolute CMS was 75.2 (range: 55-95) and the normalized one was 90.5 (range: 69-107) (Table 2). Pain was absent in 23 patients (67.6%), mild in 10 (29.4%), and moderate in one patient (3%).

Complete return to preinjury activity level was reported by 27 patients (79.4%), while 7 patients (20.6%) had some degree of functional impairment.

Active ROM showed no restriction in 19 patients (55.9%). Mild, moderate, and severe loss of shoulder motion were observed in 9 (26.5%), 3 (8.8%), and 3 (8.8%) patients, respectively.

The mean OSS was 43.7 (range: 31 to 48). In 30 patients (88.2%) the score was higher than 40, indicating an excellent subjective outcome, and in 3 patients (8.8%) it ranged from 35 to 40, revealing a mild subjective functional disability (Table 2).

Radiographic evaluation at follow-up did not show any case of AVN, nonunion, or screw perforation (Figure 4). Mild to moderate varus malunion of the humeral head was observed in 4 (11.8%) patients and valgus malunion in one (3%). Nonanatomical reduction of the greater tuberosity was evident in 4 (11.8%) patients. All malunions were not subsequent to secondary displacement, but were related to incomplete fracture reduction at the time of surgery (Figure 5).

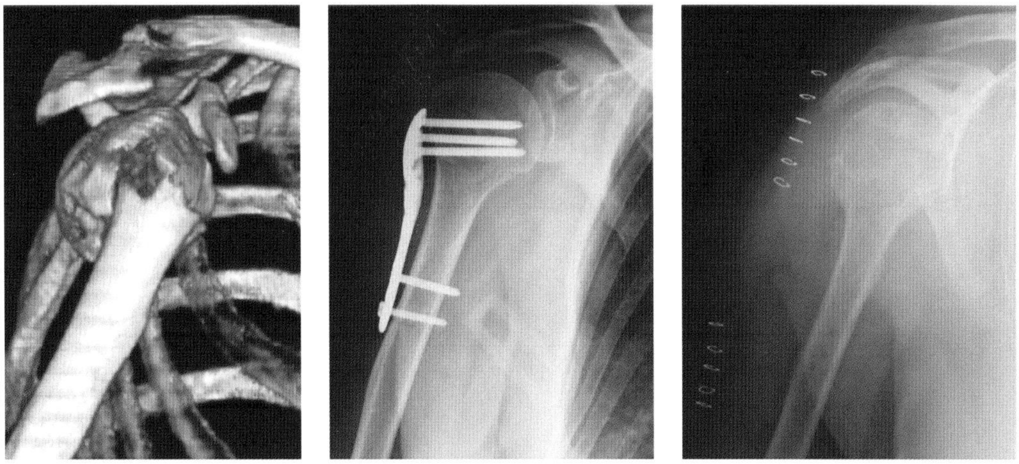

(a) (b) (c)

FIGURE 3: (a) Two-part varus nonimpacted fracture of the surgical neck (AO/OTA type A3) in a 57-year-old woman. (b) Postoperative radiogram: the plate was not flush with the bone surface and caused painful impingement during rehabilitation. (c) Three months after fixation the plate was removed; the fracture healed uneventfully.

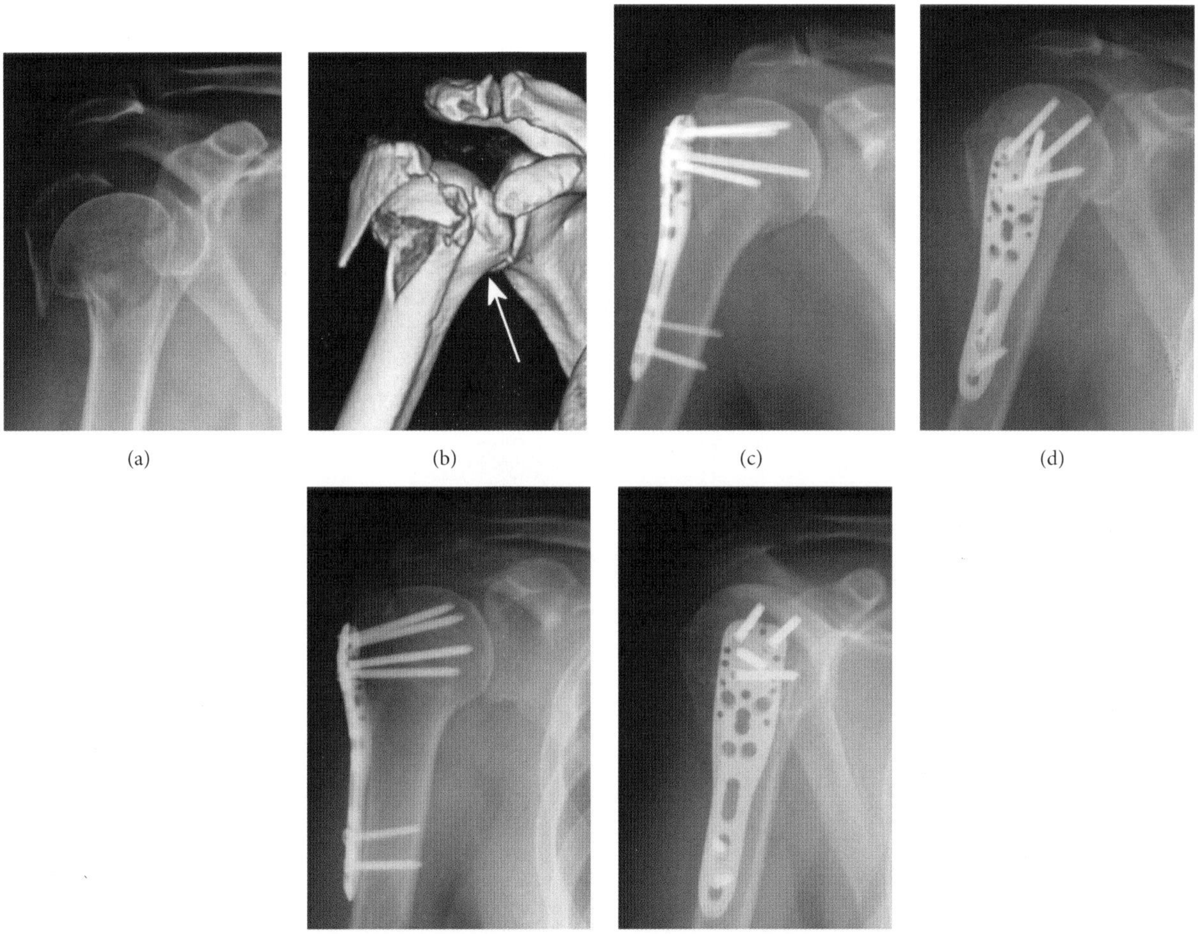

(a) (b) (c) (d)

(e) (f)

FIGURE 4: (a)-(b) Three-part valgus impacted fracture with severe displacement of the articular segment in a 48-year-old woman (AO/OTA type C2); the lesser tuberosity was in continuity with the shaft (arrow). (c)-(d) Postoperative radiograms in external (c) and internal (d) rotation showing anatomical reduction of the fracture. (e)-(f) The same radiographic views three months after surgery demonstrating union with no secondary displacement.

TABLE 2: Clinical data and outcome scores of patients evaluated at follow-up.

	Gender/Age	Fracture Type		F/U (months)	Malunion	Constant Score		Oxford Shoulder Score
		Neer	*AO/OTA*			*Absolute*	*Normalized*	
1	F/75	3-p	B2	54		85	107	48
2	F/55	3-p	B1	52	Tuberosity	83	100	45
3	F/77	3-p	B2	51		62	78	37
4	M/53	3-p	B2	50		89	98	47
5	F/60	3-p	B1	49		83	100	48
6	M/59	4-p	C1	49	Tuberosity	81	90	47
7	F/64	2-p	B2	47		66	81	41
8	F/57	2-p	A3	47		67	80	41
9	F/57	3-p	B1	44	Tuberosity	80	96	48
10	F/77	3-p	C1	43		59	74	40
11	F/55	3-p	B1	39	Tuberosity	78	93	37
12	F/69	2-p	A3	39		73	90	48
13	M/71	3-p	B1	37		72	83	45
14	M/52	2-p disl.	A1	37		95	105	48
15	M/62	2-p	A3	33		91	104	48
16	F/80	2-p	B2	32		77	97	43
17	F/77	3-p	B2	30	Varus	64	81	42
18	M/69	2-p	B2	29		83	95	48
19	F/66	3-p	B2	27		66	81	45
20	F/73	2-p	B2	26	Valgus	55	69	40
21	F/71	2-p	A3	25	Varus	67	84	31
22	F/50	3-p	B2	24		73	86	45
23	M/73	3-p	B1	23		87	101	48
24	F/52	2-p	B2	23		76	91	39
25	F/70	2-p	B1	23		59	72	41
26	F/75	3-p	B1	22		79	100	48
27	F/72	3-p	B2	21	Varus	77	97	44
28	F/71	2-p	B2	19		83	105	47
29	F/69	3-p	B1	16		77	95	42
30	F/72	3-p	B1	15	Varus	59	74	43
31	F/64	3-p	B1	15		72	88	40
32	F/49	2-p	B2	15		78	92	42
33	F/48	3-p	C2	13		85	101	44
34	F/60	3-p	B1	12		77	92	47
						75.2	**90.5**	**43.7**

Statistical analysis revealed a significant correlation between female gender and worse absolute CMS and OSS (Table 3). Functional scores did not correlate either with age (cut-off 70 years) or with fracture pattern. Worse outcomes were observed in patients with malunion, but differences in CMS and OSS with the rest of the patients were not statistically significant (Table 4).

TABLE 3: Correlation between clinical scores and gender.

	Constant Score		**Oxford Shoulder Score**
	Absolute	***Normalized***	
Female $n = 27$	72,59	89,04	42,81
Male $n = 7$	85,43	96,57	47,29
	$\boldsymbol{p = 0{,}003^*}$	$p = 0{,}089$	$\boldsymbol{p = 0{,}006^*}$

4. Discussion

Progressive aging of population is the most important factor contributing to the increasing incidence of proximal humeral fractures in highly developed countries [1, 2]. Most of these lesions can be successfully treated by conservative means,

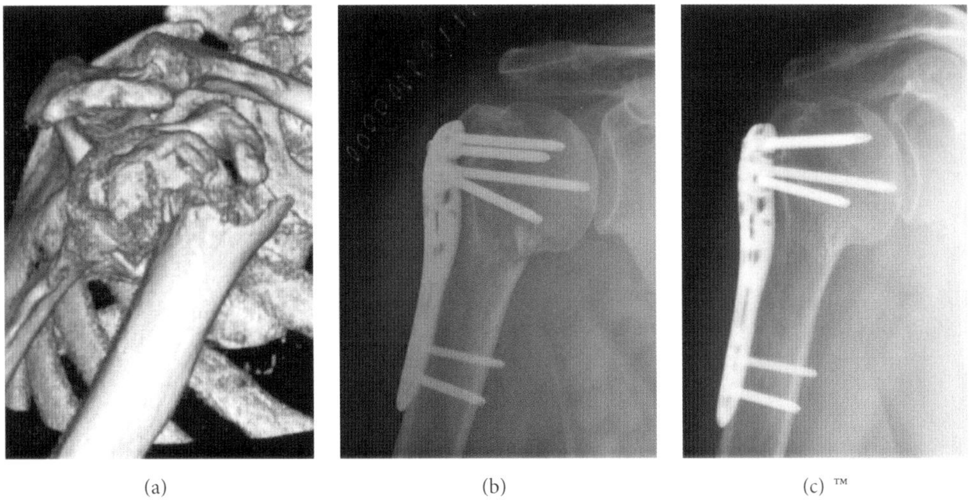

FIGURE 5: (a) Two-part varus nonimpacted fracture of the surgical neck (AO/OTA type A3) in a 71-year-old woman. (b) Anatomical reduction was not achieved at time of surgery: postoperative radiogram showed mild varus angulation of the humeral head. (c) One year after surgery fracture was healed without any aggravation of the varus.

TABLE 4: Correlation between clinical scores and malunion.

	Constant Score		**Oxford Shoulder Score**
	Absolute	***Normalized***	
No malunion $n = 25$	76,56	91,84	44,4
Malunion $n = 9$	71,56	87,11	41,89
	p = 0,312	*p = 0,284*	*p = 0,218*

but in many cases surgical treatment is required and several options are available.

Internal fixation with locking plates is widely performed, but the rate of complications and revisions is still high. Two different meta-analyses showed that the incidence of complications after this procedure is around 45% and that more than 13% of the patients undergo reoperation for different reasons, with the most common being loss of reduction and screw perforation [5, 15].

When plating a fracture of the proximal humerus, there are two conflicting goals to pursue: the first one is to achieve an anatomical reduction and a stable fixation of the bone fragments; the second one is to minimize surgical damage on soft tissues and vascularization. In fact, poor reduction and inadequate fixation almost inevitably lead to shoulder function with unsatisfactory clinical results. Conversely, extensive surgical dissections can compromise the healing process, increasing the risk of avascular necrosis (AVN), nonunion, loss of reduction, screw perforation, and infection.

The MIPO technique has been adopted to overcome these challenges in some fracture patterns. The transdeltoid approach facilitates exposure of the greater tuberosity without the need for retracting vigorously the deltoid or violating the rotator cuff. Therefore, the fracture site can be adequately exposed and reduction can be achieved with minimal impairment of the healing process.

The distal extension of the anterosuperior approach is insidious, specifically if compared to the deltopectoral access. No patient of this series required an uninterrupted incision to expose the upper part of the humerus or an inferior exposure to the humeral shaft. However, some authors recommend an extended transdeltoid approach for plating proximal humeral fractures. Extreme care and attention must be paid to isolate and protect the axillary nerve at the level of the mid-deltoid. In our opinion, the extended deltoid-splitting approach might be adopted as backup plan in case of need, but should be avoided whenever possible.

Since limited exposure of the metaphyseal region is achieved with the MIPO technique, it is preferable to perform the surgical procedure within few days from injury. This is because the formation of early fibrous callus in the proximal humerus might hinder fragment reduction. In this series of patients, the average time span between trauma and surgery was one week, an adequate interval to perform MIPO without encountering obstacles to reduction caused by the interposition of organized fibrous tissue. When surgery is delayed for more than two weeks, this potential problem should be taken into account, particularly when a relevant gap between fragments is present at the metadiaphyseal level.

Studies comparing the minimally invasive approach with the traditional deltopectoral approach reported better functional outcomes, lower surgical time, lower blood loss, shorter hospital stay, and faster fracture healing for the former [9, 16–18].

Numerous studies reported clinical outcomes and complications of the MIPO technique for fractures of the proximal humerus [19–27]. The average absolute CMS of these studies is 75.1 points, a value that matches the average score of 75.2 measured in our series of patients. Table 5 summarizes the most relevant data reported in previous studies dealing with the MIPO technique.

TABLE 5: Comparison of clinical results and complications reported with the MIPO technique.

Authors	Patients (*n*)	Mean age (years)	F/U (months)	Implant	Absolute Constant Score	Complications and failures
Acklin et al. (2013)	124	62	18	Philos	75	4 injuries of the ventral branch of axillary nerve (without clinical implications) 8 AVN 7 screw perforation
Jung et al. (2013)	38	72.4	18	Philos	75.7	1 injury of axillary nerve (axonotmesis) 1 fixation failure 1 plate impingement 1 superficial wound infection
Sohn et al. (2014)	62	57	37	Philos	80 (2-part) 74 (3-part) 62 (4-part)	3 plate impingement 1 screw perforation 5 varus malunion 1 greater tuberosity migration
Koljonen et al. (2015)	40	63	17.8	Philos	75	1 fixation failure with screws perforation 1 varus malunion
Chen et al. (2015)	27	67.3	20.8	Philos	89.4	1 screw perforation
Falez et al. (2015)	76	68.5	12	Philos	71	7 plate impingement 5 varus malunion 3 screw perforation 1 AVN 2 greater tuberosity resorption 1 greater tuberosity migration
Gönç et al. (2016)	31	58.4	12	Philos	73.2	2 temporary nerve injury (1 axillary, 1 radial) 1 deep infection 3 screw perforation 1 AVN 2 varus malunion
Park et al. (2014)	21	61	20.8	Periarticular PH-LP	79.4 (6 months) 82.7 (1 year)	1 delayed union 1 axillary nerve injury 1 screw perforation
Barco et al. (2012)	23	62	36	NCB-PH	64	2 deep infection 3 malunion (2 varus, 1 greater tuberosity) 3 screw perforation
Average	49.1	63.5	21.4		75.1	
Current study	34	64.8	31.8	Philos	75.2	9 malunion (4 varus, 1 valgus, 4 greater tuberosity) 1 plate impingement

In this series of patients, a significant difference in clinical results was detected according to gender: women showed worse outcomes than men not only in terms of absolute CMS, as could be expected, but also with regard to the OSS. However, it must be highlighted that this difference might be biased by the small sample size and the numerical disparity among the two groups (27 women versus 7 men).

The MIPO technique should not be considered an easy procedure and the surgeon must pay particular attention to avoid axillary nerve injuries. The use of the insertion handle might be helpful for this purpose, since this instrument facilitates sliding of the plate on the bone surface. No iatrogenic nerve injuries occurred in this series of patients, but other authors reported an incidence of this severe complication between 3,1% and 4,7% [19, 20, 25, 26].

The minimally invasive approach has the advantage of respecting indirect bone healing, thanks to a surgical exposure aimed at preserving fracture haematoma. This condition accelerates the healing process and allows an early removal of the plate when needed. In this clinical series, one

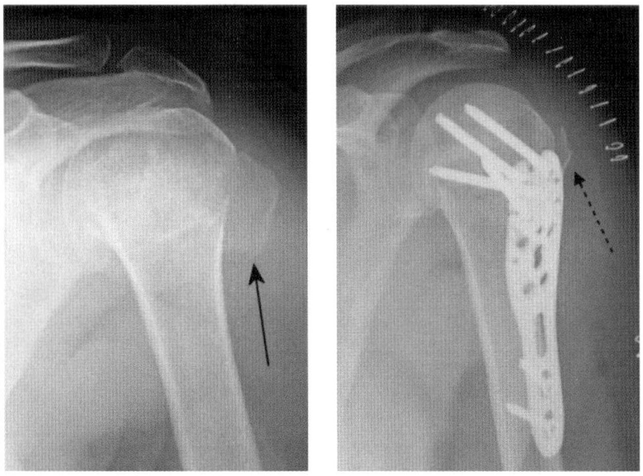

(a) (b)

FIGURE 6: (a) Three-part varus impacted fracture with posterior displacement of the greater tuberosity (arrow) in a 55-year-old woman (AO/OTA type B1). (b) Nonanatomical reduction of the greater tuberosity (dotted arrow). The distortion of the normal bone morphology was minimal and did not influence the clinical outcome.

patient required plate removal three months after fixation because of plate malpositioning and the fracture healed uneventfully. Other authors reported higher percentage of hardware removal for the same reason [11, 24], highlighting the importance of precise plate positioning to prevent subacromial impingement.

No secondary displacements were observed in the postoperative period and screws position was not a critical factor for maintaining reduction achieved at time of surgery. Even though several authors highlighted the importance of placing an inferior screw to support the medial calcar, this aspect does not seem essential with the MIPO technique. The handle of this specific system does not have a hole for the insertion of an oblique calcar screw, in order to avoid the risk of iatrogenic damage to the axillary nerve.

In our opinion, the short time required for fracture healing is the main factor that decreases the risk of fixation failure, even when anatomical reduction is not achieved. In case of osteoporotic bone, adequate calcar support might also be accomplished by some degree of shortening that can provide contact and impaction between head and shaft. Metaphyseal shortening should not exceed 2 cm; otherwise tuberosity reduction might be troublesome.

Malunion is the most frequent complication reported in literature [21, 23, 24] as well as in this study. It is mainly due to incomplete fracture reduction at the time of fixation, but it may also result from secondary displacement of bone fragments in the postoperative period, particularly in osteoporotic bone. In our experience, all malunions were caused by inadequate fracture reduction at the time of surgery. Varus malunion of the humeral head occurred in 11.8% of the patients and correlated with worse clinical outcomes, even though the difference was not statistically significant. It has been stated that only varus angulations greater than 20° correlate with poor clinical outcomes [22]. Malunion (nonanatomical reduction) of the greater tuberosity was observed in 11.8% of the patients as well, but the distortion of normal anatomy was negligible and did not compromise the clinical results (Figure 6).

The absence of AVN is consistent with the results of other studies [20–23] and the highest reported incidence of this complication after the MIPO technique is 8.2% [19]. Fixation through the deltopectoral approach is associated with higher rates of AVN [5, 15], but it should be underlined that the occurrence of this complication is greatly conditioned by the fracture type. Even though the minimum follow-up in this study is one year, it is still too early to exclude the risk of this complication for some patients conclusively.

Screw perforation can be caused by inaccurate length measurements during surgery, but it can occur later as a consequence of fixation failure, humeral head collapse, or tuberosity resorption. In literature, high rates of screws perforation have been reported by many authors [19, 25–27], but no case was observed in this study. The MIPO technique might be helpful in containing the risk of screw perforation, but prevention relies primarily on a careful selection of patients and a meticulous surgical procedure with optimal fluoroscopic intraoperative control.

The limitations of this study include the retrospective design and the limited number of patients. Moreover, inclusion criteria were not based on specific fracture patterns; the MIPO technique was indicated and performed by a single experienced shoulder surgeon, whose subjective evaluation of the lesion was critical in decision making. Current classification systems of proximal humeral fractures do not provide significant discrimination criteria for choosing between plating with MIPO or standard open technique. However, some fractures were not considered suitable for MIPO because it was felt that the limited surgical exposure could not allow adequate reduction or fixation. In our opinion, the MIPO technique should not be performed in case of wide diastasis between fragments, particularly after high-energy trauma, in presence of a "free floating" (not impacted) head fragment and in fractures where there might be the necessity to move from fixation to shoulder replacement intraoperatively.

Several options are now available for the surgical management of proximal humeral fractures, ranging from percutaneous pinning to reverse shoulder arthroplasty, but currently available literature cannot be used to derive any standardized, evidence-based treatment algorithm [28]. Significant variation in surgical practice is often indicative of a lack of scientific data and consensus in the medical community regarding optimal treatment.

The MIPO technique allows to achieve satisfactory clinical outcomes with a low complication rate, but success of treatment is also influenced by the individual level of surgical expertise. The procedure is not easy and the learning curve is clearly steeper for low-volume trauma surgeons and for severe fracture patterns. Minimal exposure of the fracture site, respect of the rotator cuff, easy access to the greater tuberosity, and reliable fixation allowing early rehabilitation are some of the advantages worth mentioning. The MIPO technique should be indicated after an accurate evaluation of the lesion by means of reproducible, high quality imaging studies. If plating is the selected treatment option and the fracture pattern requires a wide exposure for reduction, or if the surgeon does not feel confident with this approach, then the deltopectoral approach should be preferred.

Ethical Approval

The present study was performed in accordance with the ethical standards of the institutional research committee and with the 1964 Helsinki declaration as revised in 2000.

References

[1] T. Lind, K. Kroner, and J. Jensen, "The epidemiology of fracture of proximal humerus," *Archives of Orthopaedic and Trauma Surgery*, vol. 180, pp. 285–287, 1989.

[2] C. Bahrs, S. Tanja, B. Gunnar et al., "Trends in epidemiology and patho-anatomical pattern of proximal humeral fractures," *International Orthopaedics*, vol. 38, no. 8, pp. 1697–1704, 2014.

[3] C. Gerber, C. M. Werner, and P. Vienne, "Internal fixation of complex fratures of the proximal humerus," *The Journal of Bone and Joint Surgery*, vol. 86, pp. 848–855, 2004.

[4] D. Karataglis, S. I. Stavridis, G. Petsatodis, P. Papadopoulos, and A. Christodoulou, "New trends in fixation of proximal humeral fractures: A review," *Injury*, vol. 42, no. 4, pp. 330–338, 2011.

[5] R. C. Sproul, J. J. Iyengar, Z. Devcic, and B. T. Feeley, "A systematic review of locking plate fixation of proximal humerus fractures," *Injury*, vol. 42, no. 4, pp. 408–413, 2011.

[6] D. Krappinger, N. Bizzotto, S. Riedmann, C. Kammerlander, C. Hengg, and F. S. Kralinger, "Predicting failure after surgical fixation of proximal humerus fractures," *Injury*, vol. 42, no. 11, pp. 1283–1288, 2011.

[7] C. Gerber, A. G. Schneeberger, and T.-S. Vinh, "The arterial vascularization of the humeral head. An anatomical study," *The Journal of Bone & Joint Surgery*, vol. 72, no. 10, pp. 1486–1494, 1990.

[8] J. Smith, G. Berry, Y. Laflamme, E. Blain-Pare, R. Reindl, and E. Harvey, "Percutaneous insertion of a proximal humeral locking plate: an anatomic study," *Injury*, vol. 38, no. 2, pp. 206–211, 2007.

[9] P. Hepp, J. Theopold, C. Voigt, T. Engel, C. Josten, and H. Lill, "The surgical approach for locking plate osteosynthesis of displaced proximal humeral fractures influences the functional outcome," *Journal of Shoulder and Elbow Surgery*, vol. 17, no. 1, pp. 21–28, 2008.

[10] C. M. Robinson, L. Khan, A. Akhtar, and R. Whittaker, "The extended deltoid-splitting approach to the proximal humerus," *Journal of Orthopaedic Trauma*, vol. 21, no. 9, pp. 657–662, 2007.

[11] G. Röderer, J. Erhardt, M. Graf, L. Kinzl, and F. Gebhard, "Clinical results for minimally invasive locked plating of proximal humerus fractures," *Journal of Orthopaedic Trauma*, vol. 24, no. 7, pp. 400–406, 2010.

[12] C. R. Constant and A. H. G. Murley, "A clinical method of functional assessment of the shoulder," *Clinical Orthopaedics and Related Research*, no. 214, pp. 160–164, 1987.

[13] F. A. Grassi and M. S. Tajana, "The normalization of data in the Constant-Murley score for the shoulder. A study conducted on 563 healthy subjects," *La Chirurgia degli Organi di Movimento*, pp. 88-65, 2003.

[14] J. Dawson, R. Fitzpatrick, and A. Carr, "Questionnaire on the perceptions of patients about shoulder surgery," *The Journal of Bone & Joint Surgery (British Volume)*, vol. 78, no. 4, pp. 593–600, 1996.

[15] C. Thanasas, G. Kontakis, A. Angoules, D. Limb, and P. Giannoudis, "Treatment of proximal humerus fractures with locking plates: a systematic review," *Journal of Shoulder and Elbow Surgery*, vol. 18, no. 6, pp. 837–844, 2009.

[16] S. Chiewchantanakit and P. Tangsripong, "Locking plate fixation of proximal humeral fracture: Minimally invasive vs. standard delto-pectoral approach," *Journal of the Medical Association of Thailand*, vol. 98, no. 2, pp. 196–200, 2015.

[17] T. Lin, B. Xiao, X. Ma, D. Fu, and S. Yang, "Minimally invasive plate osteosynthesis with a locking compression plate is superior to open reduction and internal fixation in the management of the proximal humerus fractures," *BMC Musculoskeletal Disorders*, vol. 15, no. 1, article 206, 2014.

[18] K. Liu, P.-C. Liu, R. Liu, and X. Wu, "Advantage of minimally invasive lateral approach relative to conventional deltopectoral approach for treatment of proximal humerus fractures," *Medical Science Monitor*, vol. 21, pp. 496–504, 2015.

[19] Y. P. Acklin, K. Stoffel, and C. Sommer, "A prospective analysis of the functional and radiological outcomes of minimally invasive plating in proximal humerus fractures," *Injury*, vol. 44, no. 4, pp. 456–460, 2013.

[20] S.-W. Jung, "Indirect reduction maneuver and minimally invasive approach for displaced proximal humerus fractures in elderly patients," *Clinics in Orthopedic Surgery*, vol. 5, no. 1, pp. 66–73, 2013.

[21] H.-S. Sohn and S.-J. Shin, "Minimally invasive plate osteosynthesis for proximal humeral fractures: Clinical and radiologic outcomes according to fracture type," *Journal of Shoulder and Elbow Surgery*, vol. 23, no. 9, pp. 1334–1340, 2014.

[22] P. A. Koljonen, C. Fang, T. W. Lau, F. Leung, and N. W. Cheung, "Minimally invasive plate osteosynthesis for proximal humeral fractures," *Journal of Orthopaedic Surgery*, vol. 23, no. 2, pp. 160–163, 2015.

[23] H. Chen, X. Hu, H. Tang, G. Yang, and M. Xiang, "Minimal Invasive Percutaneous Osteosynthesis for Elderly Valgus Impacted Proximal Humeral Fractures with the PHILOS," *BioMed Research International*, vol. 2015, Article ID 971216, 2015.

[24] F. Falez, M. Papalia, A. Greco et al., "Minimally invasive plate osteosynthesis in proximal humeral fractures: one-year results of a prospective multicenter study," *International Orthopaedics*, vol. 40, no. 3, pp. 579–585, 2016.

[25] U. Gönç, "Minimally Invasive Plate Osteosynthesis with PHILOS-plate for Proximal Humerus Fractures," *Acta Orthopaedica et Traumatologica Turcica*, 2016.

[26] J. Park and S. Y. Jeong, "Complications and outcomes of minimally invasive percutaneous plating for proximal humeral fractures," *Clinics in Orthopedic Surgery*, vol. 6, no. 2, pp. 146–152, 2014.

[27] R. Barco, I. Barrientos, C. Encinas, and S. A. Antuña, "Minimally invasive poly-axial screw plating for three-part fractures of the proximal humerus," *Injury*, vol. 43, no. 2, pp. S7–S11, 2012.

[28] H. H. G. Handoll and S. Brorson, "Interventions for treating proximal humeral fractures in adults," *Cochrane Database of Systematic Reviews*, vol. 11, p. CD000434, 2015.

13

Osseointegrated Transcutaneous Device for Amputees: A Pilot Large Animal Model

Brian T. Grisez, Andrew E. Hanselman, Karim W. Boukhemis, Trapper A. J. Lalli, and Brock A. Lindsey

Department of Orthopaedics, West Virginia University, PO Box 9196, Morgantown, WV 26506-9196, USA

Correspondence should be addressed to Brock A. Lindsey; blindsey@hsc.wvu.edu

Academic Editor: Allen L. Carl

Traditional above-the-knee amputation prosthetics utilize a stump-socket interface that is well-known for skin/socket problems, sitting difficulty, disuse osteopenia, and increased work of ambulation. As a result, we evaluated a novel osseointegrated transcutaneous implant in a large animal. The implant was designed to promote osseointegration at the bone-implant interface and minimize complications. As proof of concept, four Dorset sheep underwent a two-stage surgery for forelimb placement of an osseointegrated transcutaneous implant utilizing Compress® technology (Biomet, Inc., Warsaw, IN). Two sheep received a long anchor plug (90 mm long x 9 mm in diameter) and two received a short anchor plug (46 mm long x 9 mm in diameter). Sixteen weeks after the initial surgery, the operative limbs, along with the attached implant, underwent radiographic and histological analysis for osseointegration. Periprosthetic fractures occurred in the two animals that received the longer internal prosthesis; one healed with splinting and the other animal underwent a second surgical procedure to advance the amputation site more proximal. No fractures occurred in the shorter internal prosthesis group. There was no histological evidence of infection and none of the transcutaneous adapters failed. Bone-implant osseointegration was demonstrated in two of three limbs that underwent histological analysis. This unique implant demonstrated osseointegration without transcutaneous adapter failure, all while displaying minimal infection risk from the outside environment. Although it involved short-term follow-up in a limited number of animals, this pilot study provides a platform for further investigation into the valid concept of using Compress® technology as an endo-exo device.

1. Introduction

Above-the-knee amputations have traditionally utilized a stump-socket interface for prosthetic attachment and ambulation. Unfortunately, this type of prosthetic design is associated with numerous problems. Skin changes (i.e., ulcerations, cysts, and contact dermatitis), increased energy expenditure during ambulation, disuse osteopenia, and sitting difficulty are the substantial issues [1, 2]. These factors, in turn, may lead to limited activity levels and decreased autonomy by amputees [3].

Osseointegrated transcutaneous femoral prosthetics were developed in the 1990s to address these problems [4]. Based on the work of Per-Ingvar Brånemark, who coined the term "osseointegration" with the development of dental implants, the basic prosthetic design consists of an internal intramedullary component, a transcutaneous component, and a detachable external prosthesis [5]. In comparison with stump-socket fixation, these devices have been shown to improve limb control and sensory perception, decrease oxygen consumption with ambulation, improve sitting comfort, and allow more efficient prosthetic donning and doffing [6]. Unfortunately, the transcutaneous nature and design of these implants predispose the amputee to infection, bone fracture, bone loss due to stress shielding, and implant failure [7, 8].

Currently, there are only a few osseointegrated transcutaneous prosthetic systems in use for humans and none of these systems are approved for general use in the United States. The current implant designs, although successful in their own ways, have substantial room for improvement, specifically in regard to the success of the osseointegration, the balance between the amount of bone stock required for implantation and removal of the implant, and the sturdiness of the transcutaneous component. As a result, we believe that large animal models are the appropriate first step in evaluation of a novel implant system utilizing Compress® technology (Biomet Inc., Warsaw, IN). In 2003, the Food and Drug Administration (FDA) approved the Compress® technology for use in limb-salvage procedures; this device provides a constant compressive load across the bone-implant interface. This design may act as a seal for the intramedullary canal, limiting ascending infection from the outside, while allowing for shorter working femoral length and preserving more bone stock if removal is necessary, all while avoiding stress shielding completely [9].

The overall goal of our study was to evaluate a unique osseointegrated transcutaneous implant utilizing Compress® technology and test it using a large animal model. Specifically, we wanted to use this pilot study as a proof-of-concept for acquisition of data that would help us further this research. The specific aims of this study include displaying the ability to surgically implant this novel design, evaluating the bone implant/interface by histology showing potential for complete osseointegration, minimizing infection risk, and obtaining robustness of the transcutaneous adapter without failure.

2. Materials and Methods

2.1. Implant Design. A novel intraosseous transcutaneous prosthesis was developed utilizing Compress® technology (Figure 1). It consisted of a proximal intramedullary anchor plug equipped with transverse, bicortical pins to provide rotational stability. The anchor plug was continuous with a Compress® titanium spindle with plasma sprayed titanium porous surface at the bone interface that provided approximately 600 pounds of force (*lbf*) across the bone-implant interface, in order to promote osseointegration. Compression was accomplished through the use of Belleville washers and a locking nut within the prosthesis itself. The internal mechanism of the spindle also contained a silicone gasket to make the seal from the internal prosthesis and medullary canal air and water tight. The spindle/anchor plug device allowed connection to a transcutaneous adapter. This sisal polished cobalt chrome adapter communicated with the outside environment to allow attachment of different external prostheses. Based on the results of prior studies [10, 11], the spindle and transcutaneous adapter were constructed to be smooth and highly polished, in an attempt to promote epithelialization of the skin-implant interface and limit abscess formation creating a stable stoma at the skin-implant interface.

2.2. Animal Surgery. Institutional Animal Care and Use Committee (*IACUC*) approval was obtained prior to study initiation. Four three-year-old, skeletally mature, female Dorset sheep (*Archer Farms, Inc., Darlington, MD*) (*average weight = 120 lbs*) underwent a two-stage implant procedure. The first stage consisted of surgical amputation of the forelimb at the distal radius, placement of the Compress® internal prosthesis, polyethylene cap, and closure of the soft-tissue envelope over a polyethylene spacer with an extraction hole distally for removal of the spacer percutaneously (Figures 1 and 2). Six weeks later, a second surgical procedure consisted of externalization of the coupling device through the formation of a transcutaneous portal, removal of the polyethylene spacer, and attachment of the transcutaneous prosthesis (Figures 1 and 2). The forelimb of the sheep was chosen due to its vertical alignment, compared to the hindlimb, thus more closely mimicking the forces experienced by the human femur during stance and movement. Two sheep (*1A and 1B*) received a longer anchor plug (*90 mm*) and two sheep (*2A and 2B*) received a shorter anchor plug (*46 mm*). This change was made because the size and bow of the forelimb contributed to the fractures experienced in the first group. Preoperative and intraoperative anesthesia consisted of xylazine (*0.02-0.2 mg/kg, IV*), ketamine (*7mg/kg, IV*), diazepam (*0.3 mg/kg, IV*), and isoflurane (*5% induction and 1.5-4% maintenance, inhalation*). Preoperative analgesia consisted of lidocaine (*2%, 8-10mL, SQ*) and bupivacaine (*up to 15 mL, SQ*). Postoperative analgesia consisted of fentanyl (*50 micrograms/hr, transdermal*) immediately postoperatively and morphine (*up to 10 mg daily, IM*) and butorphanol (*up to 20 mg, SQ or IV*). Other drugs included excenel (*2.2 mg/kg, SQ*) preoperatively and for three days postoperatively, vitamin B complex (*5mL, SQ*) for four days postoperatively, omeprazole (*1.0 mg/kg, PO*) for seven days postoperatively, probiotics (*1.0 mg/kg, PO*) for three days postoperatively, and kaopectate (*4oz, PO*) for three days postoperatively.

2.3. Postoperative Animal Care. During the six-week period between the first and second procedures, the animals were casted and limitation of weightbearing was attempted to limit rotational stress on the device until osseointegration began to occur at the bone spindle interface. However, nearly all animals used the experimental forelimb almost immediately. After the second surgical procedure, the animals were allowed to bear weight as tolerated. Throughout the duration of the study, animals were housed at a local research farm equipped to maintain large animals. Daily care was provided by staff trained in this particular species, with veterinarian care provided as needed. Daily assessment from the start of the study included ambulation ability, use of the prosthesis, bone fracture, and implant failure. Clinical assessment for infection included presence of fever, warmth or swelling of the limb, draining of purulent material from the wound after the first surgery and observation of frank pus and necrotic tissue at the time of the second surgery. Ten weeks after the second stage, or sixteen weeks from the first stage, the sheep were euthanized (*Pentobarbital/Euthasol/Fatal-Plus, 100 mg/kg, IV*) and their operative limbs were harvested.

2.4. Limb Analysis. Plain film radiographic images of the harvested limbs with the retained internal prostheses were performed immediately after euthanasia. The limbs with implanted prosthesis were soaked in 10% neutral buffered formalin for 72 hours, then wrapped in formalin-dampened gauze, and sent to the Histomorphometry and Molecular Analysis Core at University of Alabama at Birmingham for histological processing. Here, they were embedded in polymethyl methacrylate (*PMMA*) and cut into four quadrants

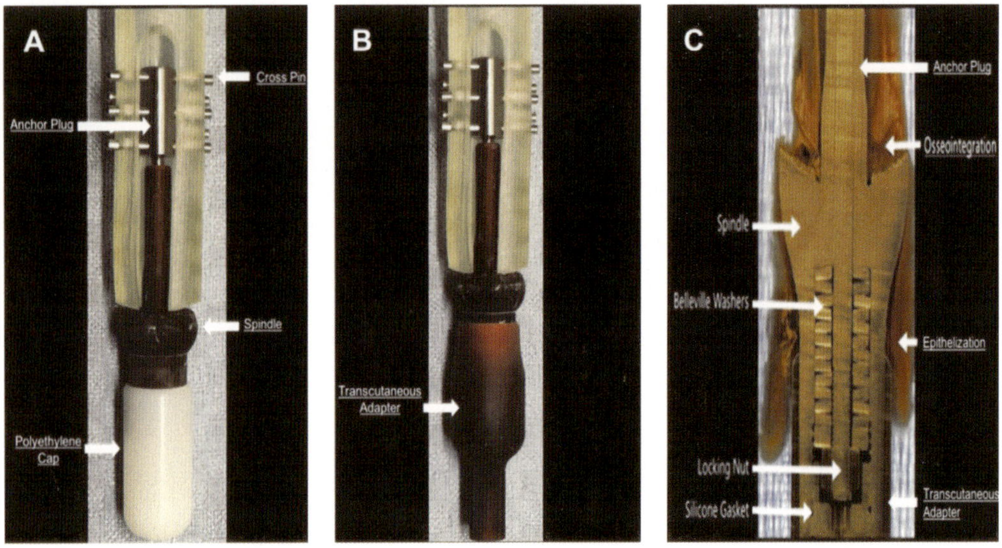

(a) (b) (c)

FIGURE 1: (a) During the first procedure, the spindle and anchor plug are implanted. A cap is placed over the spindle and the soft tissues are closed to allow for provisional healing. (b) The cap is removed at the second surgery and the taper fit transcutaneous adapter is applied. (c) A cross section of the implant demonstrating the compression mechanism. Compression of the spindle against the bone is generated by tightening of the anchor plug locking nut against the Belleville washers. The anchor plug is secured proximally by cross pins (not shown). A silicone gasket fits within the distal end of the spindle to deter bacterial migration proximally into the canal. The taper fit transcutaneous adapter is attached over the distal aspect of the spindle.

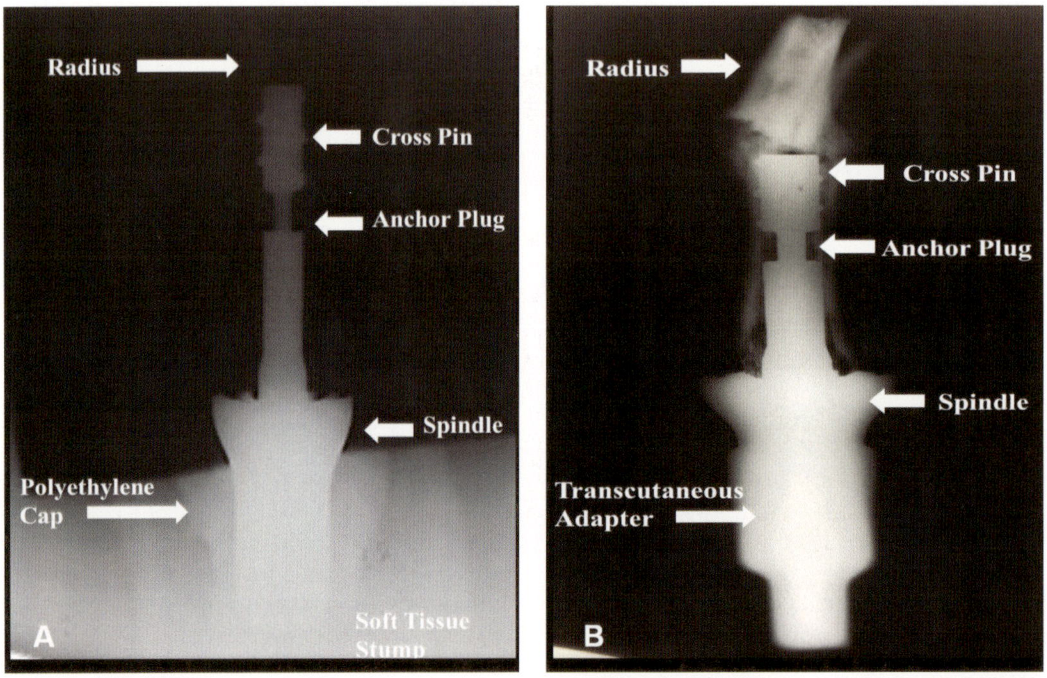

(a) (b)

FIGURE 2: Radiographic images of the staged implant procedure. (a) Implant of spindle components with polyethylene cap and primary wound closure (b) Removal of polyethylene cap which is replaced with a tapered-fit transcutaneous adapter.

TABLE 1: Results overview.

Sheep	Infection	Fracture	Implant Failure	Osseointegration
1A	Yes	Yes	No	n/a
1B	No	Yes	No	Yes
2A	No	No	No	Yes
2C	No	No	No	No

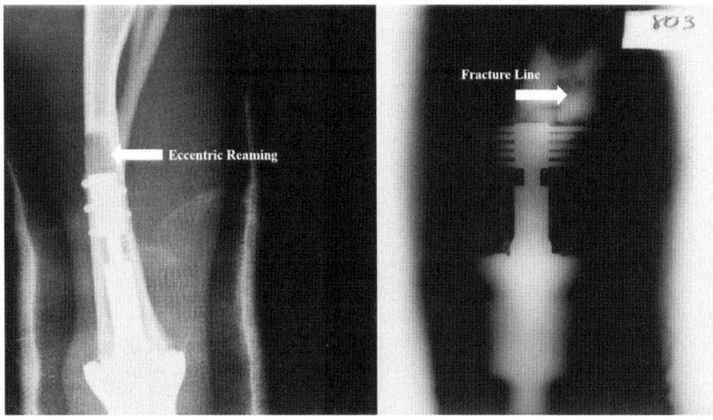

FIGURE 3: Two animals sustained fractures of their radius after the first surgery. It was presumed that eccentric reaming (left) due to the bow of the radius created a stress riser and resultant spiral type fracture (right)

along their longitudinal and transverse axes in a 90°-90° fashion using an EXAKT diamond band saw. One approximately 100 um section was then prepared from each quadrant using the EXAKT grinding system and stained with methylene blue/basic fuchsin stain (*hematoxylin and eosin-like stain*). They were specifically evaluated for infection *(assessing for inflammation at the interface*), osseointegration at the bone-spindle interface (*defined as >50% surface area of the bone with contact to the spindle*), and epithelialization at the skin-implant interface.

3. Results (Table 1)

Sheep 1A received the longer anchor plug (*90 mm*). Seventeen days after the first stage surgical procedure, the animal sustained a spiral type fracture proximal to the implant (Figure 3). Although casted after the initial surgery, the animal was full weight bearing immediately after surgery and did not show any signs of splinting or lameness of the limb prior to the fracture. Three days later, a second surgical amputation was performed moving the internal prosthesis more proximal toward the shoulder (*humerus*) using the same prosthesis because of a custom design. An autoclave was not available at the time of the surgery and the implant could not be sterilized. Six weeks later, the second stage procedure was performed to externalize the internal prosthesis. At that time, abscess formation was appreciated in the soft tissue surrounding the extramedullary portion of the implant. It appeared to be a deep infection with extraosseous involvement. We continued with the externalization procedure and postoperatively treated the animal with an antibiotic (*enrofloxacin*) for six weeks. Upon conclusion of the study, there was no clinical evidence of infection; no wound culturing was performed at the time of the initial infection or at the completion of the study. Since we deviated from the original research protocol by performing a revision of the first stage, we only performed gross histological analysis of the limb after euthanasia. This analysis demonstrated good evidence of epithelialization along the skin-implant interface with minimal downgrowth (Figure 4). No osseous histological analysis was completed on this animal because of such gross deviation from the protocol and it was felt that any further analysis would potentially skew any observations or results.

Sheep 1B received the longer anchor plug (*90 mm*) (Figure 5(a)). Similar to Sheep 1A, the animal sustained a spiral type fracture proximal to the implant 13 days after the second stage procedure. Unlike Sheep 1A, the implant was retained and the limb was splinted providing rotational control, as well as complete nonweightbearing of the limb (Figure 5(b)). After the limb was harvested, histological analysis revealed bone-implant osseointegration in all four quadrants (Figure 5(c)). Due to the unique surface design of the Compress® spindle base (*a solid structure with macro- and microtexture*), osseointegration is deemed complete with bony onlay at the spindle within the microtexture of the implant. Although this process takes years to complete, histological evidence of bony apposition is consistent with the process of osseointegration occurring. No osseointegration will occur along the anchor plug as this is a smooth surface and acts as a traction bar between the femur and the spindle.

No infection was appreciated clinically or histologically. Figure 5(d) demonstrates the animal weightbearing without restriction on the transcutaneous adapter after the second surgery.

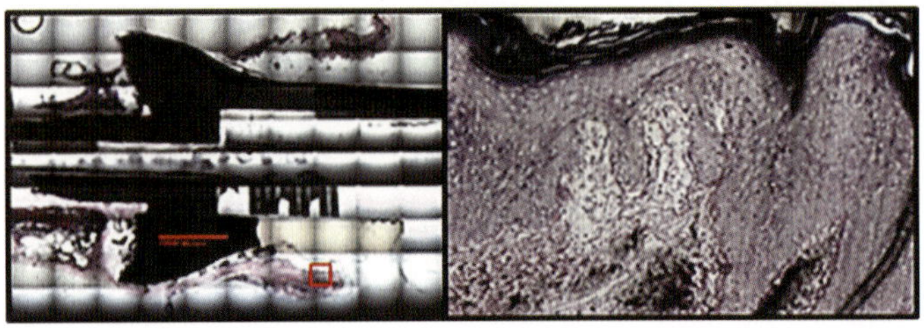

FIGURE 4: This figure shows the transcutaneous adaption of the skin epithelialization at the implant-skin interface (Sheep 1A).

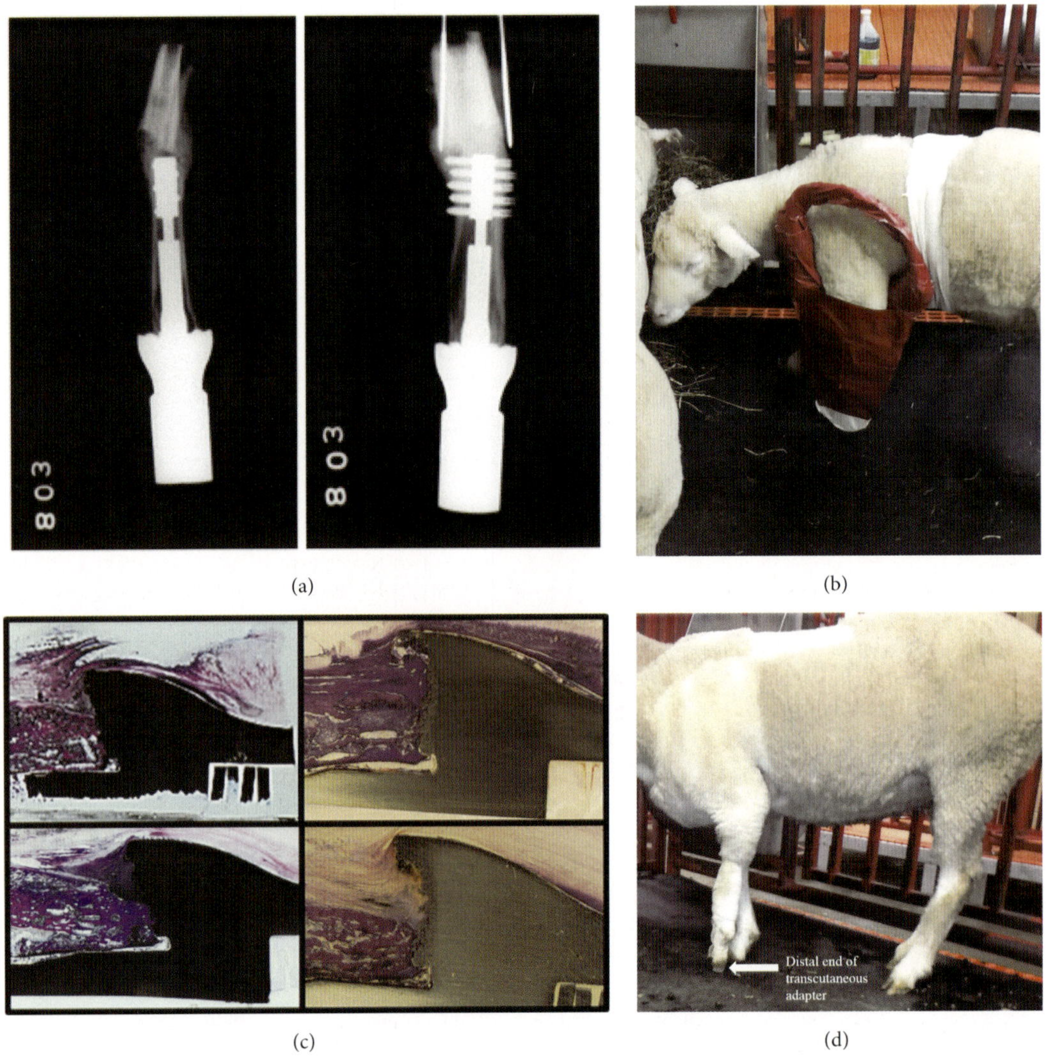

(a) (b) (c) (d)

FIGURE 5: (a) This figure shows radiographs of the implant in Sheep 1B. (b) This figure displays the splinted extremity of the fractured animal, Sheep 1B. (c) This figure demonstrates histological analysis of the osseointegration at all four quadrants in Sheep 1B. (d) This photograph taken after the second surgery demonstrates the animal weight bearing without restriction on the transcutaneous adapter.

Sheep 2A received the shorter internal implant (*46 mm*) (Figure 6(a)). No fractures or implant failure occurred; no infection was detected clinically or histologically. Osseointegration was appreciated on histological analysis in all four bone-implant quadrants (Figure 6(b)).

Sheep 2B received the shorter internal implant (*46 mm*) (Figure 7(a)). During the initial operative procedure, a drill bit broke due to surgeon error during implantation of a transverse pin; consequently, we were unable to place a pin at that site. No fractures occurred and no infection was detected clinically or histologically. Osseointegration was not appreciated on histological analysis in three of the four bone-implant quadrants; although bony down-growth toward the spindle interface is apparent (Figure 7(b)).

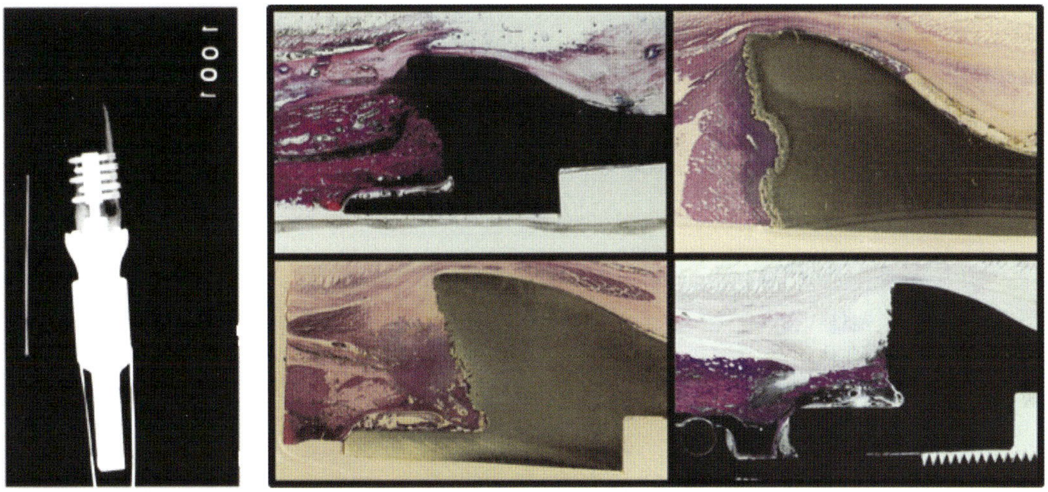

(a) (b)

Figure 6: (a) This figure shows radiographs of the implant in Sheep 2A. (b) Histological analysis of Sheep 2A demonstrating osseointegration at all four quadrants.

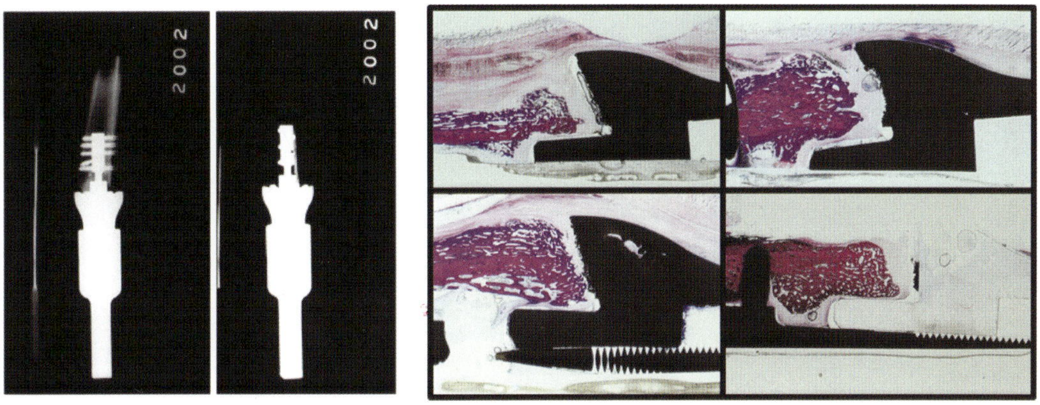

(a) (b)

Figure 7: (a) This figure shows radiographs of the implant in Sheep 2B. (b) Histological analysis of Sheep 2B demonstrating tenuous osseointegration in the lower left hand quadrant but only bony encroachment toward the spindle base in the other three quadrants without fulminant osseointegration.

4. Discussion

The aim of our pilot study was to develop a unique osseointegrated transcutaneous implant utilizing Compress® technology and test it in a small number of large animals over a short time period for acquisition of data that would help us develop a platform to continue this research. Specifically, we wanted the implant to demonstrate the potential for complete osseointegration at the bone-implant interface, display limited infection risk from the outside environment, and contain a stout enough transcutaneous adapter to prevent implant failure. Two of three limbs that underwent histology demonstrated bone-implant interface osseointegration in all four quadrants. In one limb that did not demonstrate bony apposition at the implant interface, an intraoperative surgeon error resulted in a reduction in the number of transverse pins that normally provide rotational control and increased stability. Modifying the anchor plug (from 10 mm to 9mm) to decrease the diameter created a ridge for the drill bit to catch causing it to break, which produced a significant amount of torque on the implant.

The two animals with the longer implant sustained fractures. One had a revision wherein the internal prosthesis was placed in the humerus and one healed after application of a splint that restricted weightbearing and provided rotational control. No fractures were observed in the shorter implant group. No evidence of transcutaneous adapter implant failure was observed in any of the animals. We believe the fractures occurred because of a distinct bow in the animal's radius, which did not allow a straight anchor plug of 90 mm to be implanted without some eccentric reaming of the cortical bone (Figure 3). This reaming created a stress riser and as we could not limit the animal's weightbearing, the bone fractured. Future studies could involve a time period of weight bearing restriction postoperatively as part of the established protocol.

No histological evidence of acute infection, presence of acute inflammatory cells (*polymorphonuclear neutrophils*), abscess formations, or bacteria was noted by histology (*Sheep 1B, 2A, and B*). Although some chronic inflammatory cells were noted, this was likely a mild foreign body reaction, which was consistently noted in all the specimens analyzed. One animal demonstrated clinical abscess formation prior to the second stage procedure. However, this complication was likely related to revision surgery since the same internal device was used and unable to be resterilized appropriately, which would logically lead to a higher infection risk. This infection was deep and appeared to be extraosseous in nature. Despite a contaminated environment, there were also no superficial infections. The infection responded well to antibiotic treatment and, even after being off antibiotics, the transcutaneous stoma showed no signs of infection.

Creating a stable stoma around the implant is an important feature in the development of a successful transcutaneous device. Aschoff et al. reported early device designs that utilized a porous transdermal component that was plagued with issues including skin irritation, patient discomfort, hypergranulation, and infection [10, 11]. Pendegrass and colleagues have done extensive investigation into implant-skin interface healing. Common reasons for failure at this interface include marsupialization, avulsion, and infection. Their work has indicated that smooth surfaces improve keratinocyte adhesion and if dermal, not epithelial, attachment occurs and epithelial down growth is prevented [12, 13]. The histology from our implant shows epithelialization of the skin around the transcutaneous adaptor with a stable stoma and minimal down growth at the implant, skin/air/interface. Although this device has maintained the idea of a stable stoma concept with no epidermal integration into the device itself, others (Pitkin et al.) have utilized titanium based pylons that have had some success in feline animal studies which shows some promise [14]. However, no large animal or human studies have been published as of yet.

There are few research groups implanting human devices throughout the world and advancements in this field in the United States have started to gain momentum; most studies use animal models. One study by Drygas et al. evaluated a Siberian husky implanted with bilateral tibial prostheses. The implant comprised a titanium intramedullary stem and a porous tantalum outer sleeve, inserted in a press-fit manner. One limb experienced aseptic loosening at 14 months and required reimplantation; however, the animal was able to walk, trot, and run 26 months postoperatively [15]. Although this study is important, it evaluated the prostheses in tibiae which does not readily translate to the more vertical alignment of the human leg. We chose the sheep model because of similarities to humans in both body weight and bone remodeling capabilities [16, 17]. As stated earlier, the forelimb of the sheep was chosen due to its vertical alignment and its ability to more closely mimic the forces experienced by the human femur [18].

Currently, the greatest contribution to development of an osseointegrated implant for amputees in the US has come from the University of Utah and the Veterans' Affairs Salt Lake City Health Care System. To date, this group has completed numerous studies involving animal models, including sheep, to evaluate implant design. Unlike the osseointegrated compressive design used in our study, their implant consists of a press-fit ribbed titanium stem with a porous coated subcutaneous collar. They have demonstrated good histologic and radiographic evidence of osseointegration as well as decreased infection risk from the outside environment [19–22]. They are currently working toward human trials.

Work underway overseas and at the previously stated US institution has been promising but compressive osseointegrative technology has the potential to achieve superior results. The Compress® system has been FDA approved since 2003 for use in limb-salvage procedures. It has several advantages making it an appealing design choice in the development of new osseointegrated transcutaneous prostheses. First, the technology is based upon Wolff's law in which a compressive force is applied to the bone-implant interface resulting in bone formation and osseointegration [23]. Not only does this design eliminate stress shielding from the implant, but also it seals the intramedullary canal to limit the spread of ascending medullary infection from the outside environment. Over the past few years, the longevity of these implants has been evaluated in orthopaedic literature. A recent study by Monument et al. evaluated 18 patients treated with compressive osseointegration of either the proximal or distal femur with a minimum of five years of follow-up. They demonstrated implant survivorship of 88% when evaluating for aseptic revision and 67% implant survivorship when including revision for oncologic failure, infection, arthrofibrosis, and mechanical failure [24]. A study by Healey et al. showed similar results; they retrospectively reviewed 82 patients treated with the Compress® Knee Arthroplasty for distal femoral replacements. They demonstrated an 85% implant survival rate at 5 years and 80% survival rate at 10 years. Further, of the failed implants, 62% (8/13) were the result of failures at the bone/implant interface [25]. In both studies, most implant failures were observed early in the postoperative period, with little change in outcome after the first two years. The other important advantage of these implants is the minimal amount of bone stock required for both implantation and removal. A study by Tyler et al. evaluated 11 patients who underwent removal of a compressive osseointegrated device from either the proximal or distal femur over an 11-year period. Intraoperative measurements revealed an average bone loss of 8 mm with removal of the implant [9]. Not only do these implants require minimal bone stock for implantation, but also they provide the surgeon with future options if revision surgery is required. The final advantage is the transcutaneous component of this device, which is more robust; in our small series, we had no implant failures. Some may consider the placement of a Compress® device in patients with poor bone quality, as often seen in transfemoral amputees, to be a risk factor for periprosthetic fracture; however, this has not been supported in the literature.[26, 27].

This study has several limitations. First, the number of animals included in the study is small (*N=4*). It is difficult to ascertain statistically significant conclusions based on these numbers; however, the ultimate goal of our study was to obtain data demonstrating the feasibility of this concept. Based on the data shown, this concept as a transdermal osseointegrated prosthesis is promising. Second, the follow-up for this study would be considered short-term at 16 weeks. However, these initial data allow us to feel positive about many of the short-term concerns such as acute infection or implant failure. Third, difficulty maintaining lack of weight bearing was another limitation not initially anticipated. All animals immediately ambulated after the initial amputation and implantation of the spindle. Although the cross pins through the anchor plug do provide some rotational control, the device is designed for limited weight bearing until bony apposition develops along the spindle. Further, this immediate weight bearing likely contributed to the fractures seen in two of the animals. This was successfully addressed with the developed splinting technique. Finally, the last limitation was the use of both long and short anchor plugs in a small study; however, there is not published data that compares one to the other. Although the shorter anchor plug has been commercially available for quite some time without any massive clinical failures, one possible advantage to the use of the shorter plug is in the setting of very little residual femur; this device can still be used with as little as approximately 5 cm of bone. This could potentially take someone who physically acts more like a hip disarticulation, since the residual limb cannot support a prosthesis, to a functional extremity. However, the longer plug may be seen as stronger, since the longer anchor plug creates less cantilevering leading to a more equally distributed force across the end of the bone. Future human trials would allow for more clinically relevant patient-specific outcomes with minimal risk to the patient and with potential profound advantages.

Osseointegrated transcutaneous prosthetic devices for human use are not widely available in the United States and the current implants being used in other countries have several features that could be improved. Taking these limitations into consideration, we felt that the best way to address these issues, such as osseointegration of the bone-implant interface, the amount of bone stock required for implantation/removal, and the sturdiness of the external prosthesis, could be addressed with an implant utilizing Compress® technology. Our proof-of-concept study, using a large animal model, demonstrated osseointegration is possible at the bone-implant interface and no occurrences of transcutaneous adapter implant failures in a worst-case scenario. Although our numbers were small and the results were based on a short time period, the goal of our pilot study was to obtain initial data as a feasibility study to demonstrate that this concept has merit.

Subsequent to this animal study being performed, a case series has been conducted on humans with this device, with substantial success [28]. These devices have been performed under the custom regulatory process. There were three complications in 13 patients: two fractures that were revised and maintained their revised prosthesis and one taper mismatch which was corrected. No infections were noted in this small study. Our group intends on collaborating with the FDA IDE study soon for further investigation.

Disclosure

An earlier version of this work was presented at "ISOLS/MSTS Annual Meeting," 2015.

Authors' Contributions

Brian T. Grisez was responsible for data analysis, drafting of the manuscript, and approval of the final version; Andrew E. Hanselman was responsible for data acquisition, drafting of the manuscript, and approval of final version; Karim W. Boukhemis was responsible for data acquisition and approval of final version; Trapper A. J. Lalli was responsible for data acquisition and approval of final version; Brock A. Lindsey was responsible for research design, data acquisition, critical revision of manuscript, and approval of final version. All authors have read and approved the final submitted manuscript.

Acknowledgments

The institution of the authors (Brian T. Grisez, Andrew E. Hanselman, Karim W. Boukhemis, Trapper A. J. Lalli, and Brock A. Lindsey) received funding from Zimmer Biomet, Inc., Warsaw, IN.

References

[1] N. L. Dudek, M. B. Marks, S. C. Marshall, and J. P. Chardon, "Dermatologic conditions associated with use of a lower-extremity prosthesis," *Archives of Physical Medicine and Rehabilitation*, vol. 86, no. 4, pp. 659–663, 2005.

[2] R. L. Waters and S. Mulroy, "The energy expenditure of normal and pathologic gait," *Gait & Posture*, vol. 9, no. 3, pp. 207–231, 1999.

[3] H. Van De Meent, M. T. Hopman, and J. P. Frölke, "Walking ability and quality of life in subjects with transfemoral amputation: A comparison of osseointegration with socket prostheses," *Archives of Physical Medicine and Rehabilitation*, vol. 94, no. 11, pp. 2174–2178, 2013.

[4] K. Hagberg and R. Brånemark, "One hundred patients treated with osseointegrated transfemoral amputation prostheses - Rehabilitation perspective," *Journal of Rehabilitation Research and Development*, vol. 46, no. 3, pp. 331–344, 2009.

[5] P.-I. Branemark, "Osseointegration and its experimental background," *The Journal of Prosthetic Dentistry*, vol. 50, no. 3, pp. 399–410, 1983.

[6] J. Sullivan, M. Uden, K. P. Robinson, and S. Sooriakumaran, "Rehabilitation of the trans-femoral amputee with an osseointegrated prosthesis: The United Kingdom experience," *Prosthetics and Orthotics International*, vol. 27, no. 2, pp. 114–120, 2003.

[7] A. Nebergall, C. Bragdon, A. Antonellis, J. Kärrholm, R. Brånemark, and H. Malchau, "Stable fixation of an osseointegated implant system for above-the-knee amputees: Titel RSA and radiographic evaluation of migration and bone remodeling in 55 cases," *Acta Orthopaedica*, vol. 83, no. 2, pp. 121–128, 2012.

[8] J. Tillander, K. Hagberg, L. Hagberg, and R. Brånemark, "Osseointegrated titanium implants for limb prostheses attachments: Infectious complications," *Clinical Orthopaedics and Related Research*, vol. 468, no. 10, pp. 2781–2788, 2010.

[9] W. K. Tyler, J. H. Healey, C. D. Morris, P. J. Boland, and R. J. O'Donnell, "Compress® periprosthetic fractures: Interface stability and ease of revision," *Clinical Orthopaedics and Related Research*, vol. 467, no. 11, pp. 2800–2806, 2009.

[10] H. H. Aschoff, A. Clausen, and T. Hoffmeister, "The endo-exo femur prosthesis–a new concept of bone-guided, prosthetic rehabilitation following above-knee amputation," *Zeitschrift für Orthopädie und Unfallchirurgie*, vol. 147, no. 5, pp. 610–615, 2009.

[11] H. H. Aschoff, R. E. Kennon, J. M. Keggi, and L. E. Rubin, "Transcutaneous, distal femoral, intramedullary attachment for above-the-knee prostheses: An endo-exo device," *The Journal of Bone & Joint Surgery*, vol. 92, no. 2, pp. 180–186, 2010.

[12] C. J. Pendegrass, A. E. Goodship, and G. W. Blunn, "Development of a soft tissue seal around bone-anchored transcutaneous amputation prostheses," *Biomaterials*, vol. 27, no. 23, pp. 4183–4191, 2006.

[13] C. J. Pendegrass, D. Gordon, C. A. Middleton, S. N. Sun, and G. W. Blunn, "Sealing the skin barrier around transcutaneous implants," *The Journal of Bone & Joint Surgery (British Volume)*, vol. 90-B, no. 1, pp. 114–121, 2008.

[14] B. J. Farrell, B. I. Prilutsky, R. S. Kistenberg, J. F. Dalton, and M. Pitkin, "An animal model to evaluate skin–implant–bone integration and gait with a prosthesis directly attached to the residual limb," *Clinical Biomechanics*, vol. 29, no. 3, pp. 336–349, 2014.

[15] K. A. Drygas, R. Taylor, C. G. Sidebotham, R. R. Hugate, and H. Mcalexander, "Transcutaneous tibial implants: A surgical procedure for restoring ambulation after amputation of the distal aspect of the tibia in a dog," *Veterinary Surgery*, vol. 37, no. 4, pp. 322–327, 2008.

[16] C. L. Peters, J. L. Hines, K. N. Bachus, M. A. Craig, and R. D. Bloebaum, "Biological effects of calcium sulfate as a bone graft substitute in ovine metaphyseal defects," *Journal of Biomedical Materials Research Part A*, vol. 76, no. 3, pp. 456–462, 2006.

[17] B. M. Willie, R. D. Bloebaum, W. R. Bireley, K. N. Bachus, and A. A. Hofmann, "Determining relevance of a weight-bearing ovine model for bone ingrowth assessment," *Journal of Biomedical Materials Research Part A*, vol. 69, no. 3, pp. 567–576, 2004.

[18] G. N. Duda, K. Eckert-Hübner, R. Sokiranski, A. Kreutner, R. Miller, and L. Claes, "Analysis of inter-fragmentary movement as a function of musculoskeletal loading conditions in sheep," *Journal of Biomechanics*, vol. 31, no. 3, pp. 201–210, 1997.

[19] T. G. R. Chou, C. A. Petti, J. Szakacs, and R. D. Bloebaum, "Evaluating antimicrobials and implant materials for infection prevention around transcutaneous osseointegrated implants in a rabbit model," *Journal of Biomedical Materials Research Part A*, vol. 92, no. 3, pp. 942–952, 2010.

[20] S. Jeyapalina, J. P. Beck, K. N. Bachus, O. Chalayon, and R. D. Bloebaum, "Radiographic evaluation of bone adaptation adjacent to percutaneous osseointegrated prostheses in a sheep model," *Clinical Orthopaedics and Related Research*, vol. 472, no. 10, pp. 2966–2977, 2014.

[21] S. Jeyapalina, J. P. Beck, R. D. Bloebaum, and K. N. Bachus, "Progression of bone ingrowth and attachment strength for stability of percutaneous osseointegrated prostheses," *Clinical Orthopaedics and Related Research*, vol. 472, no. 10, pp. 2957–2965, 2014.

[22] T. J. Shelton, J. Peter Beck, R. D. Bloebaum, and K. N. Bachus, "Percutaneous osseointegrated prostheses for amputees: Limb compensation in a 12-month ovine model," *Journal of Biomechanics*, vol. 44, no. 15, pp. 2601–2606, 2011.

[23] M. J. Kramer, B. J. Tanner, A. E. Horvai, and R. J. O'Donnell, "Compressive osseointegration promotes viable bone at the endoprosthetic interface: retrieval study of Compress implants," *International Orthopaedics*, vol. 32, no. 5, pp. 567–571, 2008.

[24] M. J. Monument, N. M. Bernthal, A. J. Bowles, K. B. Jones, and R. L. Randall, "What are the 5-year survivorship outcomes of compressive endoprosthetic osseointegration fixation of the femur?" *Clinical Orthopaedics and Related Research*, vol. 473, no. 3, pp. 883–890, 2014.

[25] J. H. Healey, C. D. Morris, E. A. Athanasian, and P. J. Boland, "Compress knee arthroplasty has 80% 10-year survivorship and novel forms of bone failure," *Clinical Orthopaedics and Related Research*, vol. 471, no. 3, pp. 774–783, 2013.

[26] A. C. Pedtke, R. L. Wustrack, A. S. Fang, R. J. Grimer, and R. J. O'Donnell, "Aseptic failure: how does the compress implant compare to cemented stems?" *Clinical Orthopaedics and Related Research*, vol. 470, no. 3, pp. 735–742, 2012.

[27] A. A. Bhangu, M. J. Kramer, R. J. Grimer, and R. J. O'Donnell, "Early distal femoral endoprosthetic survival: Cemented stems versus the Compress® implant," *International Orthopaedics*, vol. 30, no. 6, pp. 465–472, 2006.

[28] R. L. McGough, M. A. Goodman, R. L. Randall, J. A. Forsberg, B. K. Potter, and B. Lindsey, "The Compress® transcutaneous implant for rehabilitation following limb amputation," *Der Unfallchirurg*, vol. 120, no. 4, pp. 300–305, 2017.

14

PEEK versus Silicon Interspinous Spacer for Reduction of Supradjacent Segment Degeneration following Decompression and Short-Segment Instrumentation for Degenerative Lumbar Spinal Stenosis

Panagiotis Korovessis,[1] Vasileios Syrimpeis [1], Vasileios Tsekouras,[1] Konstantinos Vardakastanis,[1] and Peter Fennema[2]

[1] *Orthopaedics Department, General Hospital of Patras, Tsertidou Str 1, 26224, Greece*
[2] *AMR Advanced Medical Research GmbH, Hofenstrasse 89b, CH-8708 Männedorf, Switzerland*

Correspondence should be addressed to Vasileios Syrimpeis; siva@upatras.gr

Academic Editor: Hiroshi Hashizume

Purpose. A retrospective study that aims to report Adjacent Segment Degeneration (ASD) incidence and spinopelvic balance in short lumbosacral instrumentation for degenerative lumbar spinal stenosis. Although ASD is a common complication following lumbar fusion, the effect of an interspinous spacer (IS) in the supradjacent segment in short lumbosacral instrumented fusion and its interaction with spinopelvic balance has not been studied adequately. *Methods.* From 55 consecutive age-, diagnosis-, and gender-matched patients aged 60±11 years, 17 (Group R) received PEEK IS; 18 (Group S) received Silicon IS compared with 20 controls (Group C) without receiving any IS. The functional outcome was evaluated with VAS and ODI. Spinopelvic balance was evaluated using SVA, T_{12}-S_1 LL, SS, PT, PI, and supradjacent segment disc heights. All spines were preoperatively balanced (SVA<40 mm). *Results.* The follow-up averaged out to 56±11 months. VAS and ODI scores improved postoperatively in all 3 groups. SS and anterior disc height in the supradjacent free segment increased postoperatively compensatory to spinal alterations. Although 6, 4, and 5 patients from Groups R, S, and C, respectively, showed radiological progression of the preoperative degeneration grade in the supradjacent disc, only 2, 1, and 2 patients in Groups R, S, and C, respectively, developed symptomatic ASD in the 1st supradjacent segment solely. No additional surgery was required in any patient. *Conclusion.* ASD incidence in the supradjacent segment following short lumbar fusion did not statistically significantly differ between PEEK and Silicon IS. There was a trend towards lower ASD incidence in Silicon IS. IS reduced ASD in both 1st and 2nd supradjacent segments. The authors speculate that soft stabilization provided by IS may be more advantageous for preventing ASD. This trial is registered with *ClinicalTrials.gov*NCT03477955.

1. Introduction

Decompression and instrumented fusion is the most commonly performed procedure for the treatment of degenerative lumbar spinal stenosis (DLSS) [1, 2]. Instrumented spinal fusion increases significantly motion and forces acting mainly on the supradjacent segment of the instrumented lumbar area [3] resulting in ASD and less commonly in symptomatic adjacent segment disease [4].

ASD incidence ranges from 0 to 100% [5] while the reported risk for symptomatic ASD per year ranged from 0.6 to 3.9% [6]. ASD in DLSS occurs most frequently (89%) in the supradjacent segment of instrumented fusion, while it is rare (3.7%) in the subjacent segment [7]. Among the reported risk factors for ASD following spinal fusion, age, preexisting segment degeneration, and sagittal imbalance have been included [5, 6, 8].

Although sagittal balance restoration is important in patients undergoing deformity surgery [9], sagittal balance restoration is less emphasized in patients with DLSS. Old age, PI-LL mismatches, high PT, and high disability index scores were associated with sagittal imbalance [10, 11]. There

Table 1: Patients with circumferential fusion presented per group and level of PLIF insertion.

Group	Segments fused			
	L4/L5	*L5/S1*	*No PLIF*	Total
R	12	2	3	**17**
S	9	4	5	**18**
C	12	3	5	**20**
Total	**33**	**9**	**13**	**55**

exists an interaction between sagittal imbalance and ASD, while both are associated with poor health quality and pain [10, 12, 13].

Although there is no recommendation, there are clinical studies that reported successful use of IS to prevent ASD following lumbar spine fusion [8, 14–16].

Based on previous clinical studies [5, 14–16] the authors hypothesized that by adding an IS at the supradjacent segment, above a rigid short lumbosacral instrumentation, in a balanced spine, a decreased incidence of ASD may occur.

The *primary outcome measure* of this study was the ASD incidence in the spines that received PEEK IS versus those that received Silicon IS; and the *secondary outcome measure* was to correlate potential spinopelvic alignment changes postoperatively with ASD.

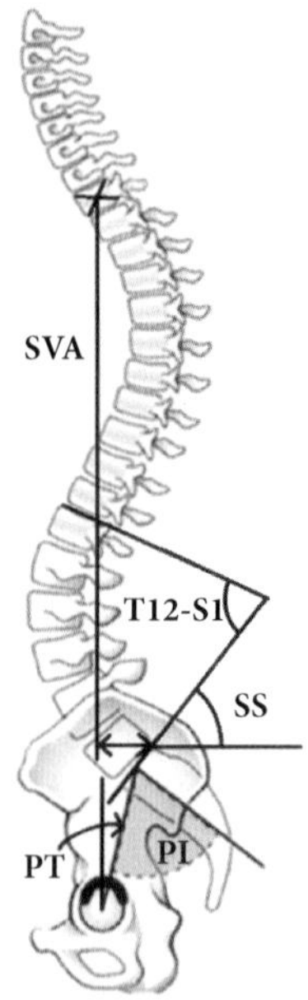

Figure 1: The radiological parameters PI, SS, PT, LL (T_{12}-S_1), SVA, and SL.

2. Patients and Methods

This study included initially two consecutive selected groups (R and S) of 20, gender-, age-, and diagnosis-matched adult patients each. The patients underwent a primary wide decompression plus 1- or 2 segment pedicle screw fixation with posterolateral instrumented fusion with the addition of PLIF in one segment or no PLIF (Table 1), between April 2006 and November 2009 for symptomatic DLSS. No concomitant decompression in the adjacent segment was performed in any patient of the three groups because the degeneration grades were low and there were no stenosis symptoms from the adjacent segment. The *inclusion criteria* were preoperative MRI with degeneration grades ≤III [17] at the 1st supradjacent lumbar segment. The patients were randomly selected to receive one of two IS: Wallis IS (Zimmer, Inc., San Clemente, CA, USA) (Group R) or the DIAM IS (Medtronic Inc., Sunnyvale, CA, USA) (Group S). Twenty individuals from our historical series (Group C), who had received by the first author the same surgery without the addition of IS and similar degeneration grade in the adjacent segments (two above and one below fusion), were selected to fit diagnosis, age, functional, and radiological parameters (Table 2). The insertion of IS was performed according to the manufactures' instructions, with meticulous preservation of the capsule and facet joints in the unfused segments to reduce iatrogenic ASD.

The *exclusion criteria* were body mass index ≥40kg/m^2, severe osteoporosis, lumbar fracture, preoperative SVA>4 cm, spondylolisthesis grades ≥II or spondylolytic lesion, and acquired spinous process insufficiency in the supradjacent segment cephalad to instrumentation. All patients had moderate to severe lower back pain and/or numbness in the lower extremity/-ies before surgery and had received for a minimum of 6 months conservative therapy without relief. Patients were assessed with the ODI score and the lower limb pain plus the back pain magnitude with the VAS (0–10 scale). This clinical trial was approved by the institutional ethical committee and informed consent was obtained from all individual participants.

The preoperative and postoperative roentgenographic work-up included the following: (a) standing whole spine anteroposterior digital roentgenogram, (b) lateral digital roentgenograms, (c) sitting lateral dynamic (flexion/extension), and (d) supine oblique views for spinal fusion estimation.

Pelvic Incidence (PI) (the angle between the line perpendicular to the sacral plate at its midpoint and the line connecting this point to the femoral heads axis), Sacral Slope (SS) (the angle between the horizontal and the sacral plate), Pelvic Tilt (PT) (the angle created by a line running from the sacral end plate midpoint to the center of the bifemoral heads and the vertical axis), T_{12}–S_1 Lordosis (LL) (the angle formed by the lines drawn at the upper endplate of T_{12}-vertebra and upper endplate of S_1), and SVA (the distance from the posterior S_1 endplate edge to the T_1-plumbline) were measured (Figure 1). In addition, Segmental Lordosis (SL) (the angle formed between the upper and lower endplates at the supradjacent unfused segment), anterior disc height (ADH), and posterior disc height (PDH) were measured (Figure 2). Sagittal imbalance according to Schwab et al. is defined when SVA≥40 mm [13]. Spinal fusion was radiologically evaluated 8-12 months postoperatively using the Christensen grading [18].

The modified Pfirrmann [17] MRI classification (Table 3 and Figure 3) was used both preoperatively and 3-5 years

Table 2: Baseline radiographic parameters comparison (P-values, unpaired t-test).

Group	T12-S1 (LL)	SVA	SS	PI	PT	SL	ADH	PDH
Wallis vs DIAM	0.74	0.55	0.6	0.73	0.37	0.21	0.0005	0.023
DIAM vs Control	0.16	0.14	0.16	0.06	0.09	0.008	0.008	0.024
Control vs Wallis	0.08	0.06	0.32	0.06	0.7	0.68	0.68	0.009

Table 3: The Modified Grading System for Lumbar Disc Degeneration∗. This material is used after author's permission [17].

Grade	Signal from Nucleus and Inner Fibers of Annulus	Distinction Between Inner and Outer Fibers of Annulus at Posterior Aspect of Disc	Height of Disc
1	Uniformly hyperintense, equal to CSF	Distinct	Normal
2	Hyperintense (>presacral fat and <CSF)±hypointense intranuclear cleft	Distinct	Normal
3	Hyperintense though < presacral fat	Distinct	Normal
4	Mildly hyperintense (slightly > outer fibers of annulus)	Indistinct	Normal
5	Hypointense (=outer fibers of annulus)	Indistinct	Normal
6	Hypointense	Indistinct	<30% reduction in disc height
7	Hypointense	Indistinct	30%-60% reduction in disc height
8	Hypointense	Indistinct	>60% reduction in disc height

∗Grades 1, 2, and 3 are based on the signal intensity of the nucleus and inner fibers of annulus. For grade 4, the margins between the inner and other fibers of the annulus at the posterior margin of the disc are indistinct. For grade 5, the disc is uniformly hypointense, although there is no loss of disc space height. For grades 6, 7, and 8, there is progressive loss of disc space height. These could be broadly classified as mild and moderate to severe loss of disc space height. Very occasionally, although obvious disc collapse is present, hyperintense signal from the nucleus and inner fibers of the annulus is preserved. This is referred to by a double entry, e.g., 4/7 with the former reporting the disc signal and the latter reporting the degree of collapse.

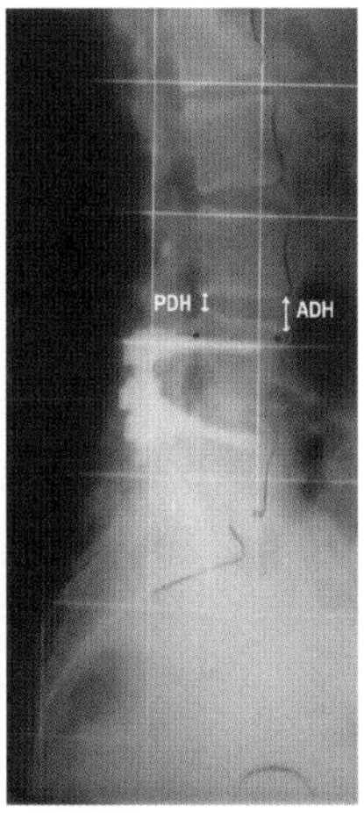

Figure 2: Anterior disc height ratio (ADHr) and posterior disc height ratio (PDHr).

postoperatively for disc degeneration grading in the 1st and 2nd supradjacent and subjacent segment (Tables 4 and 5). ASD with clinical significance was defined as the worsening of low back pain despite solid fusion and the absence of any surgery-related complication. Facet joint injection with local anesthetic under image intensifier was made for identification and localization of the pain source.

Sitting lateral dynamic X-rays (flexion/extension) and supine oblique views for spinal fusion determination were used in all 55 patients. CT scan was used for spinal

Table 4: Pfirrmann degeneration grade in MRI in the 1st supradjacent segment preoperatively till the final observation.

Group	**Preoperatively**		**Postoperatively (>3 years postop)**			
	II	**III**	**II**	**III**	**IV**	**V**
R (n=17)	*8*	*9*	8	7	0	**2∗**
S (n= 18)	*7*	*11*	7	9	1	**1∗**
C (n=20)	*8*	*12*	8	8	2	**2∗**

∗Cases with symptomatic ASD.

determination of the posterolateral and PLIF spinal fusion rate.

The reliability (intra- and interrater) of the disc degeneration grade and spinal fusion in each particular spine was tested by two independent unbiased observers: one senior orthopedic radiologist and one experienced spine surgeon using the kappa value. Difference in grading more than one degree was regulated by consensus.

Subjects of Groups R, S, and C were followed through discharge for 3 to 5 years. Functional and radiological examination results were recorded for this study 6 and 24 months and thereafter once every 2 years after index surgery and until the final observation (Tables 6 and 7).

2.1. Interspinous Spacers. Second-generation Wallis (Figure 4) is a floating system, consisting of a PEEK (polyetheretherketone) block that is considered in this study compared to

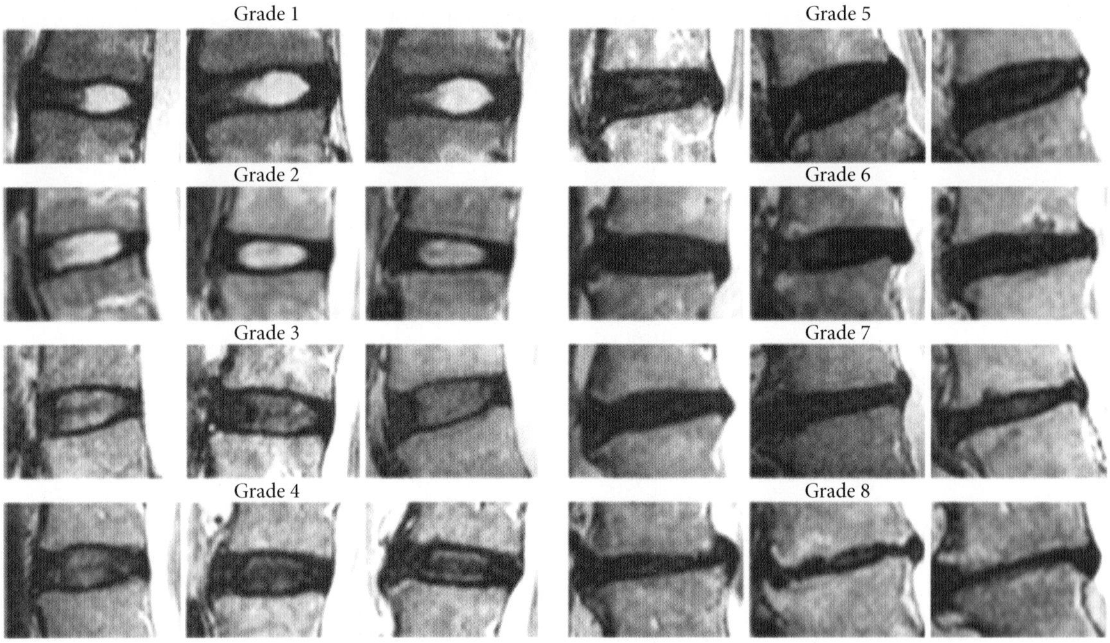

FIGURE 3: MRI images of the Modified Grading System for Lumbar Disc Degeneration. This material is used after author's permission [17].

TABLE 5: Pfirrmann classification in the 2nd supradjacent and subjacent segment preoperatively till the final follow-up.

2nd Supradjacent Group	**Preoperatively**		**Postoperatively**		
	II	III	I	II	III
R (n=17)	*16*	*1*	15	2	0
S (n= 18)	*17*	*1*	16	2	0
C (n=20)	*18*	*2*	17	3	0
Subjacent Group	I	II	I	II	III
R (n=14/17)**	11	3	10	4	0
S (n= 16/18)*	12	4	11	3	2
C (n=17/20)* * *	14	3	13	3	1

*,**,* * * The segments per group with L5-S1 fusion that were excluded from ASD evaluation.

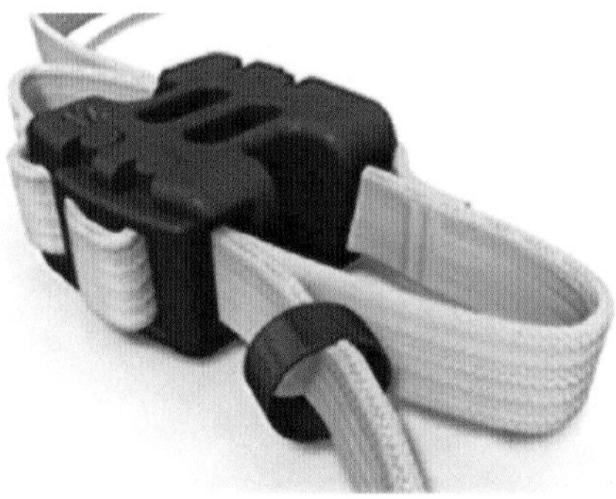

FIGURE 4: The second-generation Wallis interspinous spacer.

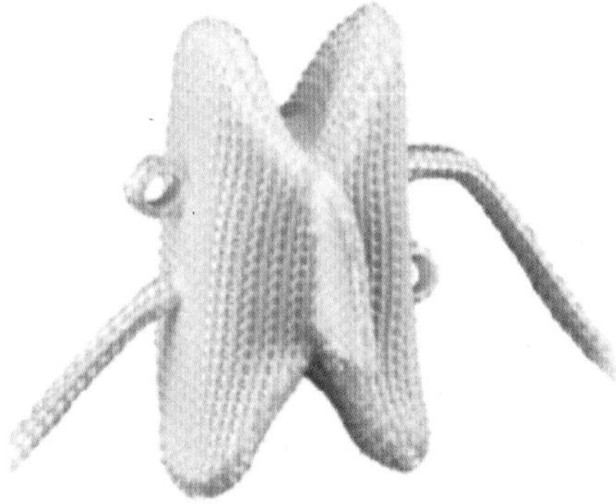

FIGURE 5: The DIAM interspinous spacer.

DIAM rigid. It is augmented by two woven Dacron ribbons, which are wrapped around the spinous processes and fixed under tension.

DIAM (Figure 5) is a silicon core covered by a polyester sleeve. It is held in position by three mesh bands, two around each spinous process and one around the supraspinous ligament.

DIAM's and Wallis' potential benefits are their alternative to spinal fusion, their fit between the interspinous processes,

TABLE 6: Functional outcomes of 55 patients who received short lumbosacral fusion.

Group	ODI						VAS-Leg						VAS-Back					
	Preop	Post Op	pre/post	Post Op-2	F-up	Post-2/F-up	Preop	Post Op	pre/post	Post Op-2	F-up	Post-2/F-up	Preop	Post Op	pre/post	Post Op-2	F-up	Post-2/F-up
	ODI	6 months	P-value	2 Years	max	P-value	VAS	6 months	P-value	2 Years	max	P-value	VAS	6 months	P-value	2 Years	max	P-value
R	37±12	18±16%	**0.001**	19±14%;	20±15%;	0.56	5.9 ± 1.1	2.3 ± 0.5	**0.001**	2.4 ± 0.4	2.6 ± 0.5	0.56	4.3 ± 0.4	1.5 ± 0.3	**0.001**	1.6 ± 0.4	1.6 ± 0.3	0.91
S	39±12%	20±16%	**0.001**	21±15%	20±12%	0.84	5.5 ± 0.5	2.1 ± 0.4	**0.001**	2.5 ± 0.6	2.7 ± 0.5	0.65	4.7 ± 1.1	2.0 ± 0.1	**0.001**	2.2 ± 021	2.3 ± 0.2	0.67
C	38±12%	19±14%.	**0.001**	20±13%.	21±13%.	0.91	5.7 ± 0.3	2.2 ± 0.2	**0.001**	2.6 ± 0.3	2.6 ± 0.5	0.82	4.7 ± 0.3	2.1 ± 0.2	**0.001**	2.1 ± 0.3	2.1 ± 0.23	0.56

TABLE 7: Changes of radiographic parameters preoperatively till the last follow-up in Groups R, S, and C (paired t-test).

Group	Preop	Postop 6 mon	Pre/Post P-value	Postop-2 2 years	F-up max	Postop-2/F-up P-value
			Lordosis T12-S1(Cobb degrees)			
R	48±11	43±8	0.15	43±7	44±8	**0.12**
S	47±13	49±11	0.49	48±11	48±13	0.64
C	39±16	41±13	0.58	40±12	42±12	0.32
			SL (Cobb degrees)			
R	18±8	23±6	**0.082**	22±6	23±6	0.78
S	22±12	23±10	0.67	23±9	23±10	0.49
C	22±16	26±8	0.27	27±6	26±9	0.65
			SS (Cobb degrees)			
R	31±8	34±7	**0.015**	33±8	34±6	0.30
S	33±10	31±7	0.46	30±6	31±7	0.82
C	27±10	31±10	**0.054**	30±12	31±10	0.63
			PDH (Cobb degrees)			
R	4±1	5±2	0.38	5±2	5±2	0.72
S	6±2	7±2	0.38	7±2	6±1	0.72
C	4±2	4±2	0.23	4±2	4±2	0.50
			SVA (mm)			
R	11±19	9±18	0.37	9±15	10±17	0.54
S	12±18	9±16	0.54	8±14	9±17	0.45
C	14±18	12±15	0.91	13±16	12±15	0.33
			ADH (Cobb degrees)			
R	6±2	7±2	0.34	7±3	6±2	**0.06**
S	10±2	12±1	0.34	11±3	11±2	0.15
C	7±3	7±2	0.71	6±3	6±2	**0.039**
			PT (Cobb degrees)			
R	33±2	25±10	0.52	24±11	26±9	**0.08**
S	23±7	22±9	0.17	23±9	24±8	0.17
C	28±7	29±6	0.18	28±7	30±6	0.73

and their function as a shock absorber that reduces loads from the surrounding vertebrae [3, 14, 19, 20].

2.2. Statistical Data Analysis. Data were analyzed using the SPSS Software (v.18, SPSS, Inc., Chicago, IL, USA). Continuous data were reported as mean±SD.

Global and individual group statistical analysis was performed using the Fisher exact test for categorical variables.

Simple linear regression analysis was used to compare different parameters.

Two-sided p-values<0.05 were considered statistically significant.

Clinical success was defined as a ≥20 percentage point improvement in pain VAS score and a ≥15 percentage point improvement in ODI.

The kappa value was used for inter- and intrarater agreement in the evaluation of spinal fusion and Pfirrmann degeneration grade.

The research that is reported in the manuscript has been performed with the approval of the GHP's Ethics Committee and was carried out in compliance with the Helsinki Declaration.

3. Results

From the 60 patients who were initially enrolled in this study, 55 patients were finally separated in three groups: 17 patients (Group R); 18 patients (Group S); and 20 patients (Group C); they were finally available for the latest evaluation after they have completed a minimum of 3 years of follow-up after index surgery.

The female/male ratio per group was as follows: Group R 10:7; Group S 12:6; and Group C 13:7. The age of the patients in Groups R, S, and C were 64±17, 59±13, and 61±12 years, respectively, (p=0.49) (Table 8).

The L5-S1 segment was included in the fusion in two, four, and three patients in each of the Groups R, S, and

TABLE 8: Demographic characteristics at baseline of 55 patients.

Characteristics	Group R	Group S	Group C	P-Value
Number	17	18	20	
Female/male ratio	(10:7)	(12:6)	(13:7)	0.72
Age	64±17	59±13	61±12	0.49

C, respectively (Table 1). Whenever the L5-S1 segment was included in the instrumentation, it was reinforced with a PLIF.

TLIF received 14/17 patients in Group R, 13/18 in Group S, and 15/20 in Group C (Table 1). A single TLIF was used in the patients who received circumferential fusion.

The inter- and intrarater kappa-values for Pfirrmann degeneration grading pre- to postoperatively at the1st and 2nd supradjacent and subjacent segments ranged from 0.82 to 0.91. The inter- and intrarater kappa-values for Christensen spinal fusion evaluation ranged from 0.93 to 0.97.

The mean follow-up was 56±11 months, range 37 to 70 months, and did not differ between Groups R, S, and C (Fisher, p=0.24).

For the 5 patients, who were not available for the final observation (>3 years) for different reasons (residence change, death due to unrelated reasons) and were excluded from the analysis, in the reviewed charts, no complications or other surgery-related events or revision surgery had been recorded until the latest observation.

3.1. Functional Results. All 3 groups showed statistically significant improvements in all clinical outcomes six months postoperatively, without further significant changes until the final observation. No significant differences between the groups in the changes of functional scores (VAS, ODI) were shown (Table 6).

3.2. Roentgenographic/MRI Results. Preoperatively, disc degeneration grade increases with age (P<0.01).

SS increased significantly (P=0.015) in the 6-month postoperative evaluation in Group R, while it increased marginally statistically significantly (P=0.054) in Group C.

ADH at the IS insertion segment increased significantly (P=0.039) in Group R and marginally significantly (P=0.06) in Group C, 2 years postoperatively until the final observation (Table 7).

3.3. Complications

3.3.1. Surgical. Accidental dural tears occurred and were sutured in the same session in two patients (one in each of the Groups S and C). Deep hematomas occurred in the first week postoperatively in one patient in Group C and in one patient in Group S and were evacuated successfully.

Urinary tract infection occurred in two patients (one in Group R and one in Group C).

Pneumonia turned up in one patient in Group S and was treated with antibiotics.

No intraoperative spinous processes fracture occurred during PEEK or Silicon IS implantation.

3.3.2. Radiological. In 6, 4, and 5 patients of Group R, Group S, and Group C, respectively, there was a progression of Pfirrmann degeneration grade at the 1st IS insertion segment (Table 4). In the 2nd supradjacent and subjacent segments, ASD grade remained postoperatively<III grades (Tables 4 and 5).

Adjacent Segment Disease. Only 2 patients (12%) in Group R, 1 patient (5%) in Group S, and 2 patients (10%) in Group C (P=0.43) developed adjacent segment disease with pain localized solely in the 1st supradjacent segment. There was no patient operated on for adjacent segment disease (Table 4).

4. Discussion

Regarding the first outcome measure, ASD incidence in the supradjacent segment was similar in Groups R and S. Regarding the second outcome measure, there were no significant changes in sagittal spinopelvic alignment in any group.

However, in this study there was a trend that, in the spines that received Silicon IS, the symptomatic ASD was lower (5%) compared to PEEK (12%) and controls (10%). This is in compliance with the previously reported results with transpedicular instrumentation (12.2–18.5%) [21]. Consistently, with previous papers, no patient developed symptomatic ASD in the subjacent and 2nd supradjacent segment [22, 23]. In a previous similar study [14], the incidence of ASD both in the 1st and 2nd cephalad supradjacent unfused segment, following transpedicular fixation without IS, was higher (28.6%), than in the PEEK (Wallis) group (4.1%). Previous studies [14, 21] showed that the addition of Wallis protected both supradjacent segments from ASD and this was shown in our study with PEEK and Silicon IS. Postoperatively there was an increase of degeneration grade in the supradjacent segment only in the spines with grade III disc degeneration, justifying a previous study [24].

Sagittal spinal imbalance with impact on ASD may occur following instrumented lumbar fusion, because spinal fusion alters the biomechanics of the spine. Subsequently, the loss of motion at the fused levels is at least theoretically compensated by changes of sagittal spinopelvic balance and increased motion in the unfused segments [25]. Among the different spinopelvic parameters that were studied in this paper, there was only a postoperative increase of SS that represented an essential compensatory mechanism to resist the reduction of the anteversion of the pelvis, even in preoperatively balanced spines [16]. Furthermore, the increase of anterior disc height in the spines of Groups R and C may indicate adaptation in order to maintain the preoperative sagittal balance.

Spinal fusion is considered the gold standard for treatment of spinal degenerative disease, although there are several complications associated with this technique, such as nonunion, instrumentation failure, infection, and pain in the donor area if an iliac bone graft is used. Moreover, an increased range of movement at adjacent segments after spinal fusion may increase the risk of ASD. To avoid some of these undesirable effects, dynamic stabilization systems and motion-preserving surgeries (disc replacement, Graff ligamentoplasty, and Dynesys) are increasingly gaining interest in order to avoid the adverse effects of spinal fusion [26].

Wallis and DIAM represent newer advents of dynamic stabilization for the unfused lumbar spine similarly with that provided by Graff ligaments and Dynesys elastic stabilization. A recent clinical study that compared Dynesys stabilization with PLIF fixation in the lumbar degenerative disease showed that Dynesys stabilization partially preserves the range of motion of the stabilized segments, limits hypermobility in the upper adjacent not-fixed segment, and may prevent the occurrence of ASD [27].

In the relative literature there are contradictory results regarding the usefulness of IS in reducing ASD in DLSS [14, 19, 20]. IS related complications such as recurrent lumbar disc herniation, bone resorption, spinous process fractures, and dural tear at the level of IS insertion have been reported [20]. In this series there were two cases of dural tear that were successfully sutured. The absence of spinous process fractures and osteolysis may be due to the lack of significant osteoporosis in our patients.

Few temporary neurologic complications were observed in this series mostly related to PLIF insertion and nerve root retraction as in other similar studies also reported with Dynesys dynamic stabilization and PLIF [27].

The *strengths of the study* are as follows: (a) an interesting hypothesis that the use of an IS in the most commonly degenerated segment, which is supradjacent to rigid lumbar fusion, may reduce symptomatic ASD; (b) while all three groups were selected consecutively, the patients were treated by the same one experienced surgeon; (c) there was a meticulous assessment of specified radiographic and functional parameters; and (d) prespecified inclusion and exclusion criteria were established.

The *limitations of this study* are as follows: (a) the small number of patients in each group; (b) the retrospective design of the study; and (c) the lack of power analysis preoperatively.

In conclusion, the present study found that short lumbosacral fixation in balanced spines does not significantly alter the preoperative spinopelvic alignment. No significant differences in symptomatic ASD incidence were found between PEEK, Silicon IS, and groups without IS, but there was a trend towards lower ASD in the Silicon Group. Further prospective studies with a greater number of patients and longer follow-up, focusing on clinical and radiographical outcomes, are warranted.

Ethical Approval

The research that is reported in the manuscript has been performed with the approval of the General Hospital of Patras (GHP) ethics committee. All procedures performed in studies involving human participants were in accordance with the ethical standards of the institutional and/or national research committee and with the 1964 Helsinki Declaration and its later amendments or comparable ethical standards.

References

[1] S. S. Rajaee, H. W. Bae, L. E. A. Kanim, and R. B. Delamarter, "Spinal fusion in the United States: analysis of trends from 1998 to 2008," *The Spine Journal*, vol. 37, no. 1, pp. 67–76, 2012.

[2] K. Hu and D. Feng, "Fusion Surgery for Lumbar Spinal Stenosis," *The New England Journal of Medicine*, vol. 375, no. 6, pp. 597–601, 2016.

[3] C.-H. Lee, S.-J. Hyun, K.-J. Kim, T.-A. Jahng, S. H. Yoon, and H.-J. Kim, "The efficacy of lumbar hybrid stabilization using the DIAM to delay adjacent segment degeneration: an intervention comparison study with a minimum 2-year follow-up," *Neurosurgery*, vol. 73, no. 2, pp. 224–232, 2013.

[4] C. Zhang, S. H. Berven, M. Fortin, and M. H. Weber, "Adjacent segment degeneration versus disease after lumbar spine fusion for degenerative pathology," *Journal of Spinal Disorders & Techniques*, vol. 29, no. 1, pp. 21–29, 2016.

[5] P. Gillet, "The fate of the adjacent motion segments after lumbar fusion," *Journal of Spinal Disorders & Techniques*, vol. 16, no. 4, pp. 338–345, 2003.

[6] K. E. Radcliff, C. K. Kepler, A. Jakoi et al., "Adjacent segment disease in the lumbar spine following different treatment interventions," *The Spine Journal*, vol. 13, no. 10, pp. 1339–1349, 2013.

[7] G. Cheh, K. H. Bridwell, L. G. Lenke et al., "Adjacent segment disease followinglumbar/thoracolumbar fusion with pedicle screw instrumentation: a minimum 5-year follow-up," *The Spine Journal*, vol. 32, no. 20, pp. 2253–2257, 2007.

[8] M. D. Helgeson, A. J. Bevevino, and A. S. Hilibrand, "Update on the evidence for adjacent segment degeneration and disease," *The Spine Journal*, vol. 13, no. 3, pp. 342–351, 2013.

[9] Y. J. Kim, K. H. Bridwell, L. G. Lenke, S. Rhim, and G. Cheh, "An analysis of sagittal spinal alignment following long adult lumbar instrumentation and fusion to l5 or S1: Can we predict ideal lumbar lordosis?" *The Spine Journal*, vol. 31, no. 20, pp. 2343–2352, 2006.

[10] S. D. Glassman, K. Bridwell, J. R. Dimar, W. Horton, S. Berven, and F. Schwab, "The impact of positive sagittal balance in adult spinal deformity," *The Spine Journal*, vol. 30, no. 18, pp. 2024–2029, 2005.

[11] N. Takeda, T. Kobayashi, Y. Atsuta, T. Matsuno, O. Shirado, and A. Minami, "Changes in the sagittal spinal alignment of the elderly without vertebral fractures: A minimum 10-year longitudinal study," *Journal of Orthopaedic Science*, vol. 14, no. 6, pp. 748–753, 2009.

[12] S. Dohzono, H. Toyoda, T. Matsumoto, A. Suzuki, H. Terai, and H. Nakamura, "The influence of preoperative spinal sagittal balance on clinical outcomes after microendoscopic laminotomy in patients with lumbar spinal canal stenosis," *Journal of Neurosurgery: Spine*, vol. 23, no. 1, pp. 49–54, 2015.

[13] V. Lafage, F. Schwab, A. Patel, N. Hawkinson, and J.-P. Farcy, "Pelvic tilt and truncal inclination: two key radiographic parameters in the setting of adults with spinal deformity," *The Spine Journal*, vol. 34, no. 17, pp. E599–E606, 2009.

[14] P. Korovessis, T. Repantis, S. Zacharatos, and A. Zafiropoulos, "Does Wallis implant reduce adjacent segment degeneration above lumbosacral instrumented fusion?" *European Spine Journal*, vol. 18, no. 6, pp. 830–840, 2009.

[15] R. J. Crawford, R. I. Price, and K. P. Singer, "The effect of interspinous implant surgery on back surface shape and radiographic lumbar curvature," *Clinical Biomechanics*, vol. 24, no. 6, pp. 467–472, 2009.

[16] J. C. Le Huec, S. Charosky, C. Barrey, J. Rigal, and S. Aunoble, "Sagittal imbalance cascade for simple degenerative spine and consequences: algorithm of decision for appropriate treatment.," *European spine journal : official publication of the European Spine Society, the European Spinal Deformity Society, and the European Section of the Cervical Spine Research Society*, vol. 20, pp. 699–703, 2011.

[17] J. F. Griffith, Y.-X. J. Wang, G. E. Antonio et al., "Modified Pfirrmann grading system for lumbar intervertebral disc degeneration," *The Spine Journal*, vol. 32, no. 24, pp. E708–E712, 2007.

[18] F. B. Christensen, M. Laursen, J. Gelineck, S. P. Eiskjær, K. Thomsen, and C. E. Bünger, "Interobserver and intraobserver agreement of radiograph interpretation with and without pedicle screw implants: the need for a detailed classification system in posterolateral spinal fusion," *The Spine Journal*, vol. 26, no. 5, pp. 538–544, 2001.

[19] J. Sénégas, J.-M. Vital, V. Pointillart, and P. Mangione, "Long-term actuarial survivorship analysis of an interspinous stabilization system," *European Spine Journal*, vol. 16, no. 8, pp. 1279–1287, 2007.

[20] Y. Floman, M. A. Millgram, Y. Smorgick, N. Rand, and E. Ashkenazi, "Failure of the Wallis interspinous implant to lower the incidence of recurrent lumbar disc herniations in patients undergoing primary disc excision," *Journal of Spinal Disorders & Techniques*, vol. 20, no. 5, pp. 337–341, 2007.

[21] T. L. Schulte, F. Leistra, V. Bullmann et al., "Disc height reduction in adjacent segments and clinical outcome 10 years after lumbar 360◦ fusion," *European Spine Journal*, vol. 16, no. 12, pp. 2152–2158, 2007.

[22] S. Imagama, N. Kawakami, Y. Matsubara et al., "Radiographic Adjacent Segment Degeneration at 5 Years after L4/5 Posterior Lumbar Interbody Fusion with Pedicle Screw Instrumentation: Evaluation by Computed Tomography and Annual Screening with Magnetic Resonance Imaging," *Clinical Spine Surgery*, vol. 29, no. 9, pp. E442–E451, 2016.

[23] J. Anandjiwala, J. Y. Seo, K. Y. Ha, and et al, "Adjacent segment degeneration after instrumented posterolateral lumbar fusion: a prospective cohort study with a minimum five-year follow-up," *The Spine Journal*, vol. 20, pp. 1951–1960, 2011.

[24] H. Wang, L. Ma, D. Yang et al., "Incidence and risk factors for the progression of proximal junctional kyphosis in degenerative lumbar scoliosis following long instrumented posterior spinal fusion," *Medicine (United States)*, vol. 95, no. 32, Article ID e4443, 2016.

[25] V. Lafage, N. Gangnet, J. Sénégas, F. Lavaste, and W. Skalli, "New interspinous implant evaluation using an in vitro biomechanical study combined with a finite-element analysis," *The Spine Journal*, vol. 32, no. 16, pp. 1706–1713, 2007.

[26] M. Kanayama, T. Hashimoto, K. Shigenobu, D. Togawa, and F. Oha, "A minimum 10-year follow-up of posterior dynamic stabilization using graf artificial ligament," *The Spine Journal*, vol. 32, no. 18, pp. 1992–1996, 2007.

[27] Y. Zhang, J.-L. Shan, X.-M. Liu, F. Li, K. Guan, and T.-S. Sun, "Comparison of the dynesys dynamic stabilization system and posterior lumbar interbody fusion for lumbar degenerative disease," *PLoS ONE*, vol. 11, no. 1, Article ID 0148071, 2016.

15

The Impact of Pinless Navigation in Conventionally Aligned Total Knee Arthroplasty

P. Koenen, M. M. Schneider, T. R. Pfeiffer, B. Bouillon, and H. Bäthis

Department of Orthopaedics, Trauma Surgery and Sports Medicine, Cologne-Merheim Medical Center, University of Witten/Herdecke, Cologne, Germany

Correspondence should be addressed to P. Koenen; paola.koenen@googlemail.com

Academic Editor: Allen L. Carl

Background. Restoration of the mechanical axis is a main objective in total knee replacement (TKR). Aim of this study was to analyse the verification tool of a pinless navigation system in conventional TKR (cTKR). *Methods.* In a prospective study, 147 TKR were performed by conventional technique. Using the "pinless verification" mode of a smartphone based navigation system, the cutting block position and final resection plane for distal femur and proximal tibial resection were measured. If necessary, the block position or resection level were optimized, corrections were protocolled. Postoperatively, standardized radiographs were performed. *Results.* In 65.3%, intraoperative measurements changed the surgical procedure (corrections: 20.4% femoral, 25.9% tibial, 19% both). The additional time for surgery compared to cTKR averaged 6 minutes (79 ± 15 versus 73 ± 17 minutes). Using navigation data, the final femoral and tibial axes were in 93% within a range of ±2°. A mean difference of 1.4° and 1.6° could be shown between the final measurement of the navigation system and the postoperative mLDFA and mMPTA. *Conclusion.* Intraoperative pinless navigation has impact on the surgical procedure in the majority of cTKR. It represents a less time-consuming tool to improve implant position while maintaining the routine of conventional technique.

1. Introduction

Total knee replacement (TKR) has been established as standard therapy for severe osteoarthritis. Restoration of the mechanical axis is a main objective in TKR, as it is attributed to good long-term results. Numerous radiological and clinical studies have proven that computer-assisted total knee replacements (CAS-TKR) are more precise regarding limb alignment reconstruction as well as implant position compared to the conventional technique [1–3]. Moreover registry data from the Australian joint registry have demonstrated a reduced revision rate of CAS-TKR compared to conventional technique for younger patients on a large patient data base [4]. In spite of its valuable advantages, the navigation technique is still not used as routine [5]. Main limitations are higher costs and additional time required for the surgical procedure [6, 7]. Further disadvantages are a prolonged training curve for new users [3, 8] and morbidity due to the placement of bony reference arrays such as fractures and infections [9, 10]. However, in conventional TKR, no standardized intraoperative technique is available to verify the result of surgery with respect to limb alignment. Only navigation technology offers the opportunity to improve the accuracy of the procedure. In order to bridge this gap and to address some of the aforementioned disadvantages of the navigation technique, recent developments have focused on the introduction of more user-friendly devices and workflows. Pinless navigation systems have been developed to offer an intraoperative verification tool for conventional arranged cutting guides without the need of reference arrays fixed to the bone of the patient [11].

The aim of the study was to analyse the verification tool of a pinless navigation system in conventional total knee arthroplasty. Furthermore, it was questioned whether verification data of a pinless navigation system had impact on the surgical procedure and therefore may affect alignment in conventional total knee arthroplasty. It was hypothesized that in the majority of conventional TKR intraoperative acquired pinless navigation data influence the surgical procedure as defined by a correction of the cutting block position or resection plane.

2. Materials and Methods

2.1. Study Design. In a prospective study, 147 consecutive TKR were included. Approval was given by the local ethics committee (113/2012). For all knee arthroplasties a cemented, cruciate-retaining implant design was used (PFC Sigma Total Knee System, DePuySynthes Orthopedics, Kirkel, Germany). Surgery was performed by one senior surgeon. The "pinless verification" module of the image-free, smartphone based navigation system DASH (BrainLAB, Munich, Germany) was used, which is also implemented within the "Knee3" software-module of the company.

Exclusion criteria were age < 18 years, the absence of a written consent, and the use of a semiconstrained or constrained implant design.

2.2. Navigation System. The DASH system works as an image-free navigation system. All joint information is digitized during surgery without the need for additional preoperative diagnostic. Within the "pinless verification" workflow no reference arrays have to be attached to the femoral or tibial bone. The essential hardware is provided by a sterile draped Apple iPod touch® that is included into a handheld cradle and serves as the operating and display unit. The iPod works remotely with the separated computer platform that is included into the infrared-camera stand using secured Wireless-LAN connection. The software can be used, as preferred by the surgeon, femur or tibia first.

2.3. Surgical Technique. All arthroplasties were performed in tibia first technique. The conventional alignment technique was applied (DePuy HP-Instruments-Set®) using extramedullary alignment at the proximal tibia and intramedullary alignment at the distal femur. The femoral alignment guide was set to 5–7° valgus dependent on the preoperatively determined anatomical-mechanical axis angle (AMA-angle). Within the "pinless verification" workflow of the DASH system the resection guide is placed to a preliminary resection position using the conventional instruments. Without any additional arrangement a limited number of anatomical landmarks (femur: Whiteside line, tibia: insertion of the anterior cruciate ligament, medial and lateral malleolus) have to be digitized using the handheld cradle to acquire an accurate 3D position of the cutting block. The surgeon gets instant and comprehensive information of the resection level, the flexion/extension position, and the varus/valgus alignment, which is displayed on the sterile draped iPod. If the position was satisfying the surgery proceeded. If a relevant displacement of the cutting jig of at least 1.5° varus/valgus was measured, correction was performed and the result was digitized again. A cut-off value of 1.5° varus/valgus was chosen, as a range of ±2° is considered as safe zone for individual axes of tibia and femur. A tibial slope of 5° was aimed; correction was performed if this value was missed by at least 2°. Verification of rotational orientation of the femoral component is not supported by the system and was determined ligament-balanced using conventional spacer blocks. For verification of the performed resection plane, a maximum of two landmarks (femur: centre of the femoral head by hip pivoting, tibia: medial and lateral malleolus) have to be digitized. Again, only in case of satisfying alignment data the surgery proceeded; otherwise correction was performed and again the result was measured.

These data were stored for the final patient report. It was recorded whether and to which degree the alignment data of the navigation system were used to optimize the cutting block position or the final resection plane by the surgeon. The surgical procedure is illustrated in Figure 1.

2.4. Operating Room Time. Time needed for the navigation process including all coronal bone resections and measurements of the navigation system was measured. Furthermore, the length of the surgical procedure (skin to skin) was documented for each patient. OR (operating room) time was compared to a control group including 125 conventional TKR performed in 2012 by the same senior surgeon.

2.5. Full-Length Weight-Bearing Radiographs. Axial limb alignment was evaluated on standardized full-length weight-bearing radiographs before and after the surgery. Radiographs were performed according to an internal standardized protocol based on the recommendations described by Cooke et al. [12]. Postoperative radiographs were delayed until full knee extension was achieved to minimize errors due to incorrect rotation or knee flexion. Alignment measurements were performed using the digital planning software mediCAD version 2.20 (Hectec, Niederviehbach, Germany).

2.6. Statistical Analysis. Statistical analysis was performed using GraphPad Prism 6 (La Jolla, California, USA). Means, standard deviations, and ranges were calculated. An unpaired, two-tailed t-test was performed to compare OR times of cTKR and DASH TKR. A paired, two-tailed t-test was performed to compare differences between the initial conventional alignment and the final resection plane as well as differences of the final measurement and postoperative mLDFA/mMPTA. Values of $p \leq 0.05$ were considered statistically significant.

3. Results

147 computer-assisted primary total knee replacements were included. 48 patients (32.7%) were male and 99 (67.3%) were female. Their mean age was 65 years ranging from 27 to 87 years. 73 (49.7%) patients had surgery on the right knee; 74 (50.3%) on the left knee. The preoperative mechanical axis measured by X-ray was between 24.5° varus and 22.9° valgus, respectively.

In 63.3% (93), the intraoperative measurements of the navigation system had impact on the surgical procedure. In 20.4% (30) only the femoral resection and in 25.9% (38) only the tibial resection were modified. In 19.0% (28) of TKR both the femoral and tibial resection were modified within the same surgical procedure while in 34.7% (51) the initial conventional cutting block position was maintained (Figure 2). The initial orientation of the tibial cutting block

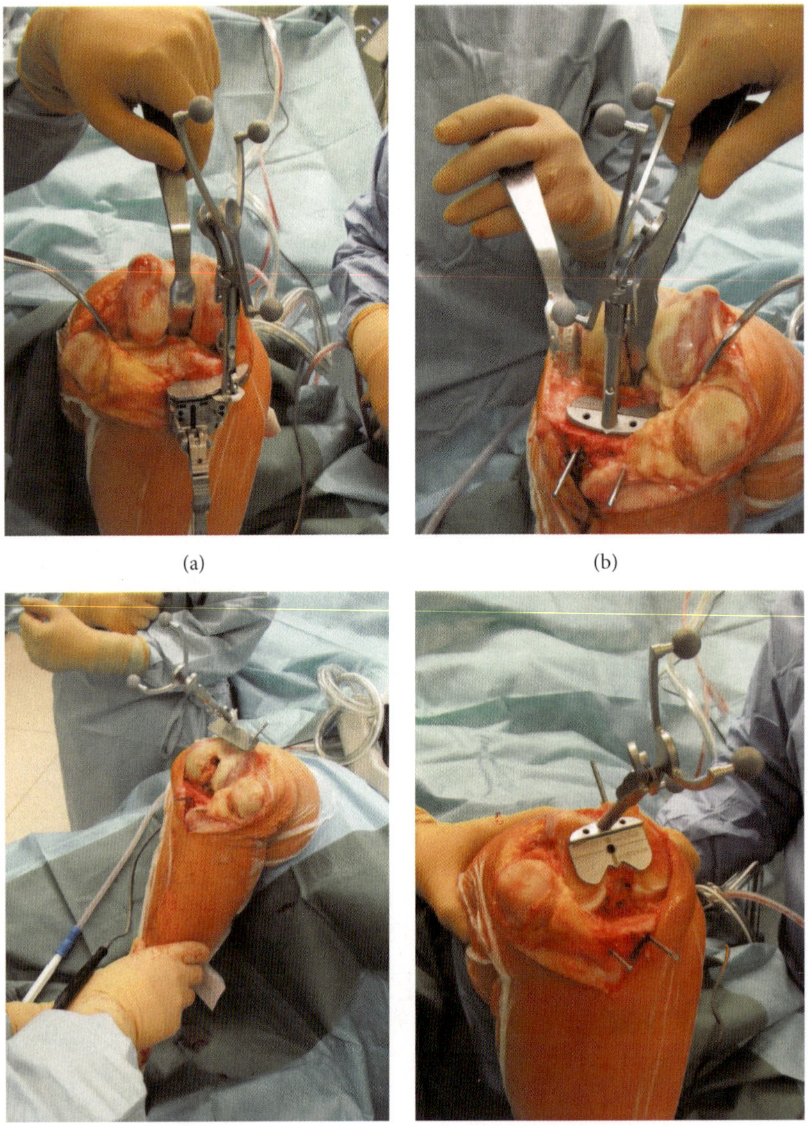

(a) (b) (c) (d)

FIGURE 1: Surgical procedure using the "pinless verification" workflow of the DASH system. (a) Cutting block verification at the proximal tibia, (b) cut verification at the proximal tibia, (c) cutting block verification at the distal femur, and (d) cut verification at the distal femur.

ranged from 5° varus to 3.5° valgus. The initial orientation of the femoral cutting block was between 6° varus and 4° valgus, demonstrating a substantial variability with a significant number of outliers of the conventional technique (Figure 3). Moreover, in 11.8% (18) both the initial femoral and tibial orientation of the cutting block were displaced to the same direction. Readjustment of the cutting block in the coronal plane or a correction of the final resection plane was carried out in equal parts in the direction of varus and valgus, respectively (femur 43.1% and 56.9%, tibia 53% and 47%; Figure 4). The mean degree of correction was 1.5 ± 1.4° (0–7.5°) at the femur and 1.2 ± 1.0° (0–6.5°) at the tibia. Differences between the initial conventional alignment and the final resection plane were shown to be statistically significant for femur ($p = 0.02$), but not for tibia ($p = 0.29$).

The mean duration of surgery was 79 ± 15 minutes in the navigation group compared to 73 ± 17 minutes in the conventional group, which was statistically significant ($p = 0.005$). The overall time for all coronal bone resections and measurements of the navigation system averaged 11.5 ± 4.5 minutes (Figure 5).

By navigation data the final femoral and tibial axis were in 93% within a range of ±2°. A mean difference of 1.4 ± 1.2° (0–5.4°) and 1.6 ± 1.2° (0–5.0°) could be shown between the final measurement of the navigation system and the mLDFA (mechanical Lateral Distal Femoral Angle) and mMPTA (mechanical Medial Proximal Tibial Angle) in the postoperative full-length weight-bearing radiograph, respectively. Differences were not statistically significant (mLDFA: $p = 0.39$, mMPTA: $p = 0.55$).

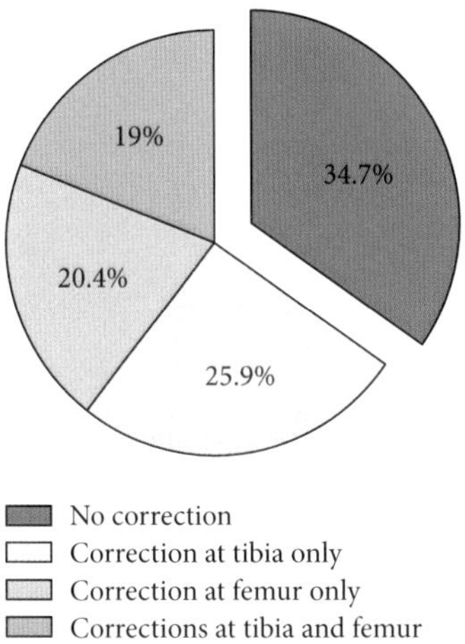

FIGURE 2: Change of surgical procedure due to the intraoperatively acquired data of the navigation system, presented as percentage of all arthroplasties.

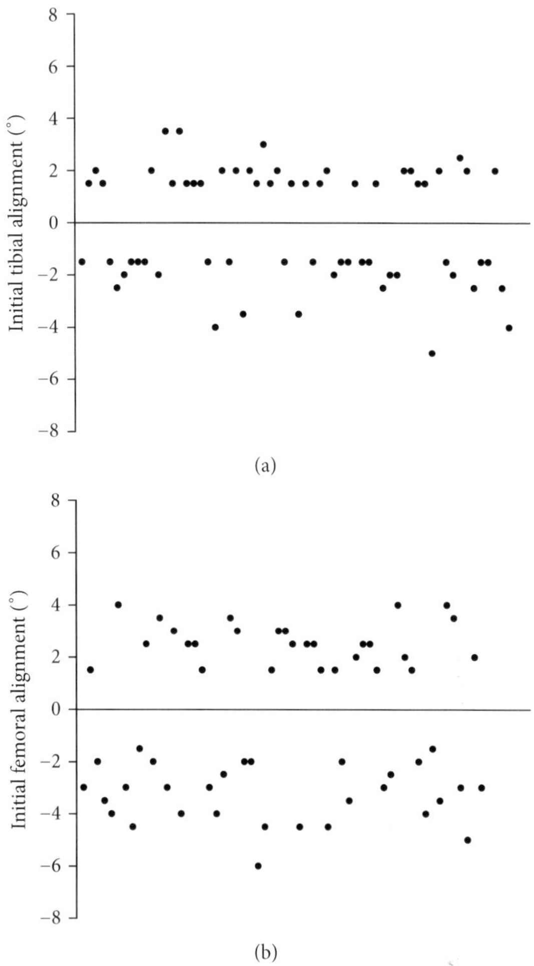

FIGURE 3: Initial tibial (a) and femoral (b) alignment by using the conventional extramedullary (tibia) and intramedullary (femur) alignment technique. Only cases, in which corrections were performed (− varus, + valgus), are shown.

4. Discussion

Restoration of the mechanical axis is one of the main objectives in TKR. Earlier studies have shown that an alignment in the coronal plane within the range of 3° varus/valgus is associated with a better survival of the prosthesis [1, 2, 8, 13, 14]. Considering various meta analyses from different groups, CAS in total knee arthroplasty has been proven to be more accurate regarding restoration of the mechanical axis compared to the conventional technique [1–3]. Despite this valuable advantage, CAS-TKR has not yet become routine due to disadvantages like additional costs and prolonged procedure time [6, 7]. However, besides navigation technology, no standardized technique is available to verify the implant position and leg alignment in TKR intraoperatively. This is in strict contrast to trauma surgery, where intraoperative X-ray technology is used as a matter of routine to verify the reposition of a fracture or implant position, when performing osteosynthesis.

This study shows that only in one-third of arthroplasties the initial conventional alignment was considered satisfying by the surgeon, accepting a maximum displacement of the resection plane of 1.5° or less from the neutral alignment position. In our study, the initial femoral and tibial alignment by the conventional technique showed a significant number of outliers. Moreover, in 11.8% of cases both the initial femoral and tibial alignment deviated in the same direction. As a consequence maintaining the initial alignment would have led to a substantial malalignment. Therefore, in the majority of arthroplasties the intraoperatively acquired data of the navigation system did have a significant influence on the surgical procedure. This is in accordance with various comparative studies, describing that implant alignment and a resulting leg alignment within a range of ±3° are only achieved at most 80% using the conventional technique [2, 13, 15]. In addition there is no learning curve in improving leg alignment with improved surgical experience [16].

By now, only navigation technology is able to improve the accuracy of the procedure. The described verification module of the DASH system using pinless technique offers the opportunity to bridge this gap. It may be used as intra-operative verification tool in conventional TKR to monitor implant position and to correct the resulting alignment during the surgical procedure. Pinless navigation systems have been developed to address some of the drawbacks of the navigation technique. While lacking disadvantages as the morbidity of Steinman pins or lengthening of OR time [11], pinless navigation systems have been shown to be comparable in accuracy to conventional computer-assisted surgery. The concept of the DASH system, presenting the information in line with the working field of the surgeon, leads to an instant visual feedback of the surgeon's movements within the surgical field. The simplified software algorithm and the intuitive handling have been shown to facilitate the computer-assisted surgical procedure even for navigation beginners [17]. Furthermore, this new technique represents a

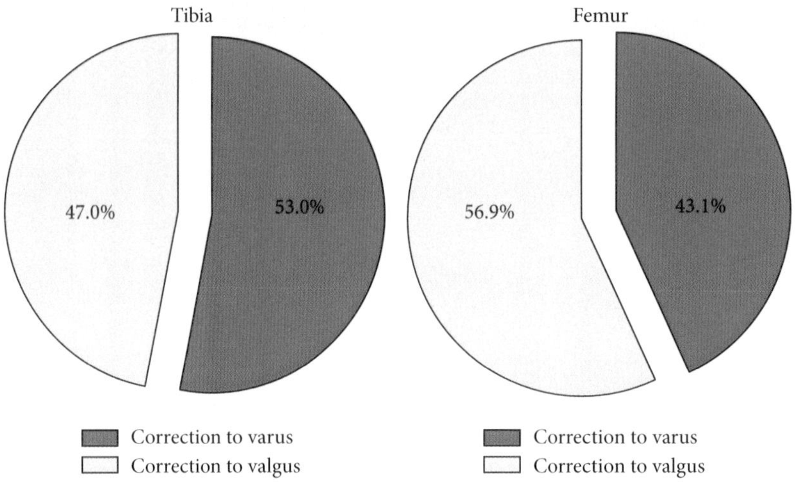

FIGURE 4: Change of surgical procedure, presented as percentage for the femoral and tibial bone resection, separately. The direction of the required correction is shown.

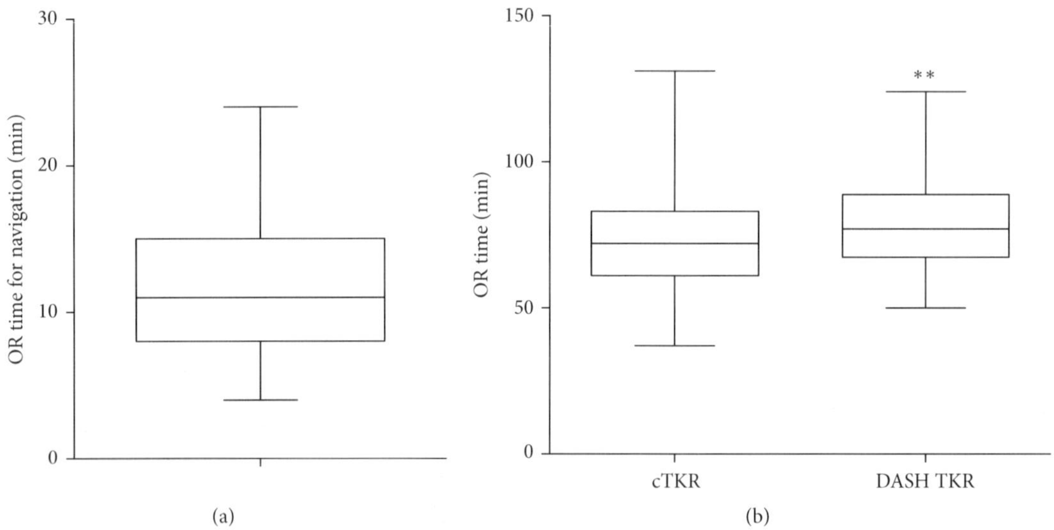

FIGURE 5: (a) Expenditure of time for all coronal bone resections and measurements of the navigation system, presented as boxplot. (b) OR time for DASH TKR ($n = 144$) and conventional TKR (cTKR; $n = 125$), shown as mean ± SD. $^{**}p < 0.01$.

great possibility for surgical trainees in the context of learning the conventional technique of TKR [18]. However, the DASH system does not provide all features of established navigation systems. Verification of rotational alignment of the femoral component is not supported by the system, as well as a ligament balancing support. An additional option for defining the rotational orientation of the femoral component is not implemented to the pinless verification workflow as freehand navigation techniques have not been able to demonstrate superior precision of rotational implant orientation due to the difficult digitization of landmarks for short axes, for example, epicondylar axis [19–21]. Therefore the rotational alignment within this study was performed in a conventional ligament-balanced technique using spacer blocks.

The precision of the DASH system could be shown to be comparable to established navigation systems with regard to reconstruction of the limb alignment. The final tibial and femoral axes were in 93% within a range of ±2°, which is considered as safe zone for individual axes of tibia and femur.

We measured a mean expenditure of time for the whole navigation process of 11.5 minutes. The surgical procedure was extended by only 6 minutes compared to the conventional technique. In contrast, Bauwens et al. found that the use of established navigation systems extended OR time by 15 minutes [7].

Limitations of the study are mainly due to a lacking control group. In spite of a prospective design we did not include a control group. Therefore, conclusions regarding radiological outcomes are restricted.

5. Conclusion

Pinless navigation using a verification workflow as an augmentation to the conventional technique of TKR is a helpful tool to verify cutting block position and resection plane while using the conventional alignment technique. Thereby an improved implant position might be achieved, whereas only a short additional OR time is required. Major disadvantages associated with established navigation systems like fixation of reference arrays or severely increased OR time are eliminated with this technique.

Ethical Approval

All procedures involving human participants were in accordance with the 1964 Helsinki Declaration and its later amendments.

References

[1] T. Cheng, S. Zhao, X. Peng, and X. Zhang, "Does computer-assisted surgery improve postoperative leg alignment and implant positioning following total knee arthroplasty? A meta-analysis of randomized controlled trials?" *Knee Surgery, Sports Traumatology, Arthroscopy*, vol. 20, no. 7, pp. 1307–1322, 2012.

[2] M. Tingart, C. Lüring, H. Bäthis, J. Beckmann, J. Grifka, and L. Perlick, "Computer-assisted total knee arthroplasty versus the conventional technique: how precise is navigation in clinical routine?" *Knee Surgery, Sports Traumatology, Arthroscopy*, vol. 16, no. 1, pp. 44–50, 2008.

[3] C. Lüring, H. Bäthis, M. Tingart, L. Perlick, and J. Grifka, "Computer assistance in total knee replacement—a critical assessment of current health care technology," *Computer Aided Surgery*, vol. 11, no. 2, pp. 77–80, 2006.

[4] R. N. de Steiger, Y.-L. Liu, and S. E. Graves, "Computer navigation for total knee arthroplasty reduces revision rate for patients less than sixty-five years of age," *The Journal of Bone & Joint Surgery—American Volume*, vol. 97, no. 8, pp. 635–642, 2015.

[5] B. Rath, H.-R. Springorum, J. Beckmann et al., "Importance of computer-assisted navigation in total knee arthroplasty - Results of a nationwide survey in Germany," *Zeitschrift für Orthopädie und Unfallchirurgie*, vol. 149, no. 2, pp. 173–177, 2011.

[6] C. Xie, K. Liu, L. Xiao, and R. Tang, "Clinical outcomes after computer-assisted versus conventional total knee arthroplasty," *Orthopedics*, vol. 35, no. 5, pp. e647–e653, 2012.

[7] K. Bauwens, G. Matthes, M. Wich et al., "Navigated total knee replacement: a meta-analysis," *The Journal of Bone & Joint Surgery—American Volum*, vol. 89, no. 2, pp. 261–269, 2007.

[8] P. M. Bonutti, D. Dethmers, S. D. Ulrich, T. M. Seyler, and M. A. Mont, "Computer navigation-assisted versus minimally invasive TKA: benefits and drawbacks," *Clinical Orthopaedics and Related Research*, vol. 466, no. 11, pp. 2756–2762, 2008.

[9] J. Beldame, P. Boisrenoult, and P. Beaufils, "Pin track induced fractures around computer-assisted TKA," *Orthopaedics & Traumatology: Surgery & Research*, vol. 96, no. 3, pp. 249–255, 2010.

[10] E. T. Berning and R. M. Fowler, "Thermal damage and tracker-pin track infection in computer-navigated total knee arthroplasty," *The Journal of Arthroplasty*, vol. 26, no. 977, pp. e21–e24, 2011.

[11] C. Baier, G. Maderbacher, H. R. Springorum et al., "No difference in accuracy between pinless and conventional computer-assisted surgery in total knee arthroplasty," *Knee Surgery, Sports Traumatology, Arthroscopy*, vol. 22, no. 8, pp. 1819–1826, 2014.

[12] T. D. V. Cooke, E. A. Sled, and R. A. Scudamore, "Frontal plane knee alignment: a call for standardized measurement," *The Journal of Rheumatology*, vol. 34, no. 9, pp. 1796–1801, 2007.

[13] A. Ensini, F. Catani, A. Leardini, M. Romagnoli, and S. Giannini, "Alignments and clinical results in conventional and navigated total knee arthroplasty," *Clinical Orthopaedics and Related Research*, no. 457, pp. 156–162, 2007.

[14] J. M. Sikorski, "Alignment in total knee replacement," *The Journal of Bone & Joint Surgery (British Volume)*, vol. 90, no. 9, pp. 1121–1127, 2008.

[15] H. Bäthis, S. Shafizadeh, T. Paffrath, C. Simanski, J. Grifka, and C. Lüring, "Are computer assisted total knee replacements more accurately placed? A meta-analysis of comparative studies," *Der Orthopäde*, vol. 35, no. 10, pp. 1056–1065, 2006.

[16] J. Mahaluxmivala, M. J. K. Bankes, P. Nicolai, C. H. Aldam, and P. W. Allen, "The effect of surgeon experience on component positioning in 673 press fit condylar posterior cruciate-sacrificing total knee arthroplasties," *The Journal of Arthroplasty*, vol. 16, no. 5, pp. 635–640, 2001.

[17] C. Schnurr, P. Eysel, and D. P. König, "Displays mounted on cutting blocks reduce the learning curve in navigated total knee arthroplasty," *Computer Aided Surgery*, vol. 16, no. 5, pp. 249–256, 2011.

[18] R. Iorio, D. Mazza, G. Bolle et al., "Computer-assisted surgery: A teacher of TKAs," *The Knee*, vol. 20, no. 4, pp. 232–235, 2013.

[19] M. A. Katz, T. D. Beck, J. S. Silber, R. M. Seldes, and P. A. Lotke, "Determining femoral rotational alignment in total knee arthroplasty: Reliability of techniques," *The Journal of Arthroplasty*, vol. 16, no. 3, pp. 301–305, 2001.

[20] J. Jerosch, E. Peuker, B. Philipps, and T. Filler, "Interindividual reproducibility in perioperative rotational alignment of femoral components in knee prosthetic surgery using the transepicondylar axis," *Knee Surgery, Sports Traumatology, Arthroscopy*, vol. 10, no. 3, pp. 194–197, 2002.

[21] W. P. Yau, A. Leung, K. Y. Chiu, W. M. Tang, and T. P. Ng, "Intraobserver errors in obtaining visually selected anatomic landmarks during registration process in nonimage-based navigation-assisted total knee arthroplasty: a cadaveric experiment," *The Journal of Arthroplasty*, vol. 20, no. 5, pp. 591–601, 2005.

Outcome after 52 Salto Ankle Prostheses Implanted by a Single Surgeon

Frank W. M. Faber,[1] Monique J. L. Mastboom,[2] Sabine T. van Vliet-Koppert,[2] Ilse C. E. Bouman,[3] and Paulien M. van Kampen[1]

[1]*Department of Orthopaedic Surgery, Bergman Clinics, Rijswijk, Netherlands*
[2]*Department of Orthopaedic Surgery, LUMC, Leiden, Netherlands*
[3]*Department of Orthopaedic Surgery, HAGA Hospital, The Hague, Netherlands*

Correspondence should be addressed to Frank W. M. Faber; f.faber@bergmanclinics.nl

Academic Editor: Panagiotis Korovessis

While ankle arthrodesis was traditionally the gold standard method of treatment for disabling end-stage ankle arthritis, total ankle replacement (TAR) has been an acceptable alternative. The satisfaction rate of patients with TAR however differs. The purpose of our study is to investigate whether implant survival and results with special emphasis on the satisfaction rate of patients treated with a TAR implanted by a single surgeon were comparable to the literature. This was a retrospective cohort study in a teaching hospital. Data was collected from 52 patients who received a total ankle replacement (TAR) between 05/2002 and 06/2014. The mean follow-up time was 4.2 years (95% CI 3.3 – 5.0). Results showed a high satisfaction rate of 94% and 94% survival of the TAR after 5 years. We conclude that TAR with the Salto prosthesis is, in our hands, a reliable solution for end-stage ankle arthritis, with results comparable to the literature.

1. Introduction

While ankle arthrodesis was traditionally the gold standard method of treatment for disabling end-stage ankle arthritis, total ankle replacement (TAR) has been an acceptable alternative [1–4]. Drawbacks of ankle fusion are nonunion, quite long postoperative immobilization, and in the long-term arthritis in the adjacent joints [5, 6]. Disadvantages of TAR are the technical difficulty of the procedure, causing a considerable learning curve [7–9] and uncertain long-term survival of the implant [3, 10, 11]. The satisfaction rate of patients with TAR also differs. Conflicting reports exist about the cause for this difference in satisfaction. Spirt et al. [12] and Henricson et al. [13] found a worse result in younger patients, focusing on implant survival, complication rates, and revision rates. Tenenbaum et al. [14] and Dematracopoulous et al. [15] reported equal results in different age groups, considering clinical outcomes, gait improvement, and patient reported outcome. Schenk et al. [16] reported 6.9% unsatisfied patients, mostly because of conversion of the prosthesis to an arthrodesis. Other factors influencing implant survival, and with that patient satisfaction, are preoperative alignment, body weight, and proper operative technique. Furthermore, management of the expectations of the patients and explicit information in the preoperative phase is of influence [17]. The purpose of our study is to investigate whether implant survival and results with special emphasis on the satisfaction rate of our patients treated with a TAR were comparable to the literature.

2. Patients and Methods

2.1. Study Design and Setting. This was a retrospective cohort study. Data was collected from patients who received a total ankle replacement (TAR) between 05/2002 and 06/2014 in the HAGA Hospital, the Hague, in the Netherlands. All surgeries were performed by the same Orthopedic Surgeon specialized in foot and ankle surgery (FF). The study was enlisted by the

Medical Ethical Committee Southwest Holland (15-103) and was declared not to subdue to Medical Research Involving Human Subjects Act. The board of directors of the hospital approved the study.

2.2. Participants. Patients who received a TAR in the previous mentioned time window were included in the study. Patients with the following criteria were included: symptomatic ankle osteoarthritis (Kellgren-lawrence score of 3+ or 4 despite conservative treatment), age≥ 65 years (except rheumatoid patients), BMI ≤ 30, American Society of Anesthesiologists (ASA) stage 1, 2, or 3, adequate bone-quality, ≤10° varus or valgus deformity, and no (extreme) sport wish. Exclusion criteria for a TAR were neurological disorders, bad peripheral circulation, osteonecrosis of talus or tibia, and infection present. The operation was performed under spinal or general anesthesia. Half an hour prior to surgery and 24 hours postoperatively intravenous antibiotics were administered. Standard anterior approach was used and an uncemented SALTO® prosthesis (Tornier SA, Saint Ismier, France) was placed (a third-generation ankle prosthesis, three components, and mobile bearing). Postoperative treatment consisted of a lower leg cast: first 2 weeks non-weight-bearing followed by 2 weeks full-weight-bearing. After cast removal, an intensive physical therapy program was followed for at least 6 weeks. The questionnaires were distributed with a minimum of 1 year follow-up and the postoperative X-rays were made the first day after surgery and 4 weeks postoperatively. The follow-up X-rays were performed with AP and lateral weight-bearing X-rays on a 2-yearly routine base.

2.3. Variables. Patients' satisfaction was measured by asking one question: "would you choose the TAR again in a similar situation?"

Revision of the TAR was defined as any secondary operation in which a prosthetic component was exchanged and/or conversion to an arthrodesis had to be performed, for any reason.

Functional outcome was measured by the Foot Function Index (FFI) [18]. We used the validated Dutch Version using verbal rating scales provided by Kuyvenhoven et al. [19]. The second outcome measure was the American Orthopaedic Foot and Ankle Society (AOFAS) questionnaire [20].

2.4. Measurement. Radiological outcome for the position of the prosthesis components is measured in degrees on first weight-bearing postoperative X-ray compared to last postoperative X-ray (Figure 1). Measurements, calculated as angular deviation according to the perfect position, are performed as described by Valderrabano et al. [21].

Radiographic analysis were performed by one independent senior orthopaedic surgeon (SvVK).

2.5. Statistical Methods. Continuous baseline characteristics were presented as mean with 95% confidence interval between square brackets. Nominal data was presented in counts and percentages. Statistical analyses were conducted in SPSS version 17 (IBM Co., Armonk, NY, USA). For all statistical analyses, a two-tailed p-value less than 0.05 was considered to be statistically significant.

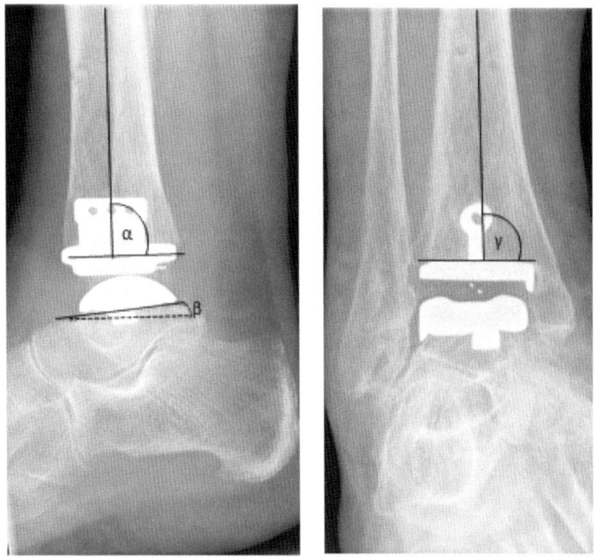

FIGURE 1: Radiological angles. Perfect tibial position is defined as γ angle 90 degrees and in the sagittal plane position of the tibial component with an inclination till 7 degrees (α = +7; according to the manufacturer of the Salto prosthesis). Perfect talar position is placement of this component parallel to the sole of the foot (β angle 0 degrees). An angle-difference over time of 5 degrees or more is considered significant and is classified as migration. Malposition is defined as an angulation of a component of more than 10 degrees from the perfect position as defined by Schimmel [7].

Patient satisfaction was presented in percentages. A Kaplan-Meier curve was presented for survival analysis with revision for any reason as endpoint. All functional outcomes were presented as mean with 95% confidence interval (CI) and the radiological outcomes as median and IQR.

3. Results

3.1. Participants. A total 52 patients were included in the study. The mean follow-up time was 4.2 years (95% CI 3.3 – 5.0, range 0.1 – 13.7).

All baseline characteristics are presented in Table 1.

3.2. Outcome. In total 48 of the 51 patients would choose the TAR again in a similar situation (94% satisfaction rate). One answer was missing, because we were unable to contact this patient. Two patients were dissatisfied with the TAR; one patient required a conversion to an arthrodesis for septic loosening and the other dissatisfied patient had persistent pain, but had good function and perfect radiological images. This TAR was converted to an ankle arthrodesis for suspicion of low grade infection, which was not confirmed. Pain persisted even after an uneventful solid ankle fusion with allograft.

Table 1: Baseline characteristics.

Age, mean	Years, range	70 [49 – 86]
Gender	Male	26 [50%]
	Female	26 [50%]
Side	Left	19 [64%]
	Right	33 [37%]
ASA	1	21 [40%]
	2	26 [50%]
	3	2 [4%]
	Missing	3 [6%]
Smoking	No	44 [85%]
	Yes	7 [14%]
	Missing	1 [2%]
Indication	Post-traumatic	29 [56%]
	Primary Osteoarthritis	18 [35%]
	Rheumatoid Arthritis	4 [8%]
	Rheumatoid Arthritis and Post-traumatic	1 [2%]

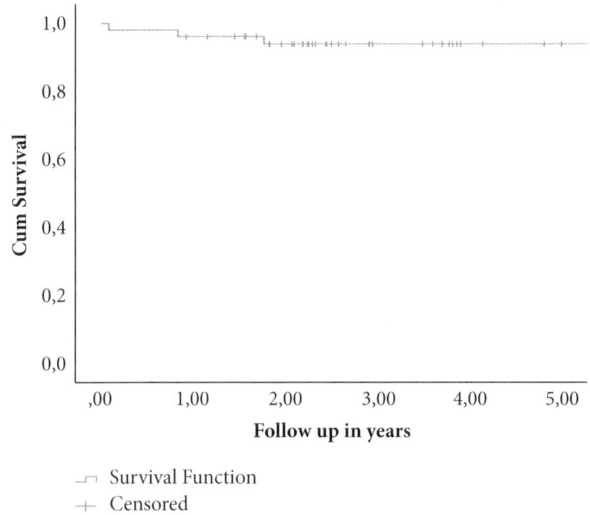

Figure 2: Survival of the TAR in years. At 2,5 years 29 were at risk and at 5 years 15 were at risk. The overall survival time is 11 with a 95% confidence interval of 10-13.

Three of all patients had an ankle arthrodesis on the contralateral side. These patients all preferred their TAR over their ankle arthrodesis.

In Figure 2 the Kaplan-Meier curve is presented. The survival of the TAR after 5 years is 94% with 15 patients at risk.

The functional and radiological results are presented in Table 2. The mean total AOFAS score was 85 out of a maximum of 100 points. The mean total FFI was 36 out of a maximum of 115 (with 23 as lowest and best score).

Not for all the 52 patients clinical and radiological data could be collected. The patients that were converted to an arthrodesis were excluded. In addition, we were unable to reach one patient (like mentioned above) and one patient was not willing to come to the hospital and only answered the satisfaction question on the phone. This explains the different numbers in the first column.

3.3. Complications. Five talar component malpositions were noted at postoperative weight-bearing X-rays. Four malpositions of the tibial part were discovered, of which one was treated with a reoperation within two weeks: repositioning of the tibial component leading to a satisfactory result afterwards. Preoperatively, 2 medial malleolus fractures and 1 lateral malleolus fracture occurred. All fractures were fixed during the ankle replacement procedure.

Three patients suffered from prolonged wound healing: more than 4 weeks postoperatively wound leakage was present: these all resolved with prolonged immobilization and antibiotics.

During the follow-up period in 4 cases, conversion to an arthrodesis was necessary. Two patients needed conversion because of aseptic loosening caused by multiple cysts; one patient suffered from severe wound problems and an acute deep infection. One conversion was performed because of persistent pain and suspicion of low grade infection, which was not confirmed during reoperation.

4. Discussion

TAR is known as a technically demanding procedure and a considerable learning curve is described by several authors [7–9]. Yet, equally functional results are described by Reuver et al. [22] in low volume centres: the AOFAS score of these authors had an average of 75 (SD ± 15). Our study, single surgeon and low volume, shows an even higher average AOFAS score of 85 (SD ± 17). This difference could be explained because the senior author of this series (FF) already had considerable experience in TAR with another type ankle prosthesis (STAR) before he started implanting the Salto prosthesis. The functional outcome of this study is comparable to other series that also described the FFI and/or the AOFAS score as an outcome parameter. The FFI found by Kerkhoff et al. [23] and Schimmel et al. [7] were 33 and 32, respectively. The AOFAS score varied from 73 to 85 [16, 24–27]. Bonnin, who is actually one of the inventers of the Salto prosthesis, described an AOFAS score of 79 points, with a follow-up of 7–11 years [28]. So, in our hands, the functional results are certainly not inferior.

In our study 48 of the 51 patients (94%) would have the TAR performed again in a similar situation, of whom some are even revised and converted to an arthrodesis. Yet, 2 of the 2 dissatisfied patients had a revision. So implant survival and satisfaction are definitely related. Implant survival can be improved by proper technique, for instance, component placement in proper alignment [3, 29]. Our survival rate is 94% after 5 years with 15 patients at risk. This is better than the results described by Henricsson et al. [13], that is, 78% survival at 5 years. One study found a 94% implant survival at 5 years, even 87% survival at 10 years, which dropped quite steep to 64% after 15 years [30]. One of our exclusion criteria for a TAR is age: we excluded patients younger than 65 years, in whom we prefer an arthrodesis, except for rheumatoid patients. These patients often have other joint impairments

Table 2

		N			Range
FFI	Activity	45	Mean [95% CI]	18 [16 -20]	[9-43]
	Pain	45	Mean [95% CI]	16 [14 – 18]	[9-39]
	Restriction	45	Mean [95% CI]	8 [7 -9]	[5-16]
	Total	45	Mean [95% CI]	42 [37 – 47]	[25-94]
AOFAS	Alignment	45	Mean [95% CI]	9 [8 – 10]	[0-10]
	Function	45	Mean [95% CI]	41 [38 – 45]	[5-50]
	Pain	45	Mean [95% CI]	34 [32 – 37]	[20-40]
	Total	45	Mean [95% CI]	85 [80 – 90]	[26-100]
Radiological outcome	First alpha	49	Median [IQR]	6 [4]	[-3 - 12]
	Last alpha	47	Median [IQR]	5 [4]	[-3-14]
	First beta	49	Median [IQR]	-4 [8]	[-15-9]
	Last beta	47	Median [IQR]	-4 [9]	[-15-8]
	First gamma	49	Median [IQR]	0 [2]	[-4-5]
	Last gamma	47	Median [IQR]	0 [4]	[-5-7]

(hindfoot, midfoot), which probably benefit when the ankle joint is kept mobile instead of fused. Gait analysis showed a more normal gait in TAR patients than in patients who had an arthrodesis [31]. Although the age selection criterion seems justifiable in terms of long-term implant survival, reports in the literature are conflicting. Kofoed and Lundberg-Jensen [32] and Skyttä et al. [33] described no influence of age; Tenenbaum et al. [14] reported equal functional improvement in patients over 70 years patients and aged 50-60 years. In contrast with this, Henricson et al. [13] and Raikin et al. [34] all reported worse results in younger patients. Because of our high patient satisfaction and the good survival rate compared with the literature, we consider performing TARs in younger patients. We realize we have to inform this younger group about the risk of a conversion to an arthrodesis later in life.

The strong points of this study were the independent investigators who performed the patient investigations at follow-up, the high follow-up percentage, and the use of one and the same prosthesis, with an unchanged design by the same surgeon. A weak point is its retrospective design, so no preoperative clinical scores were available.

5. Conclusion

We conclude that TAR with the Salto prosthesis is, in our hands, a reliable solution for end-stage ankle arthritis, with results comparable to the literature.

Disclosure

Level of clinical evidence is retrospective cohort study, Level 3.

References

[1] C. L. Saltzman, R. G. Kadoko, and J. S. Suh, "Treatment of isolated ankle osteoarthritis with arthrodesis or the total ankle replacement: a comparison of early outcomes," *Clinics in Orthopedic Surgery*, vol. 2, no. 1, pp. 1–7, 2010.

[2] J. Morash, D. M. Walton, and M. Glazebrook, "Ankle Arthrodesis Versus Total Ankle Arthroplasty," *Foot and Ankle Clinics*, vol. 22, no. 2, pp. 251–266, 2017.

[3] J. A. Mann, R. A. Mann, and E. Horton, "STAR™ ankle: Long-term results," *Foot & Ankle International*, vol. 32, no. 5, pp. 473–484, 2011.

[4] R. Zaidi, S. Cro, K. Gurusamy et al., "The outcome of total ankle replacement: A systematic review and meta-analysis," *The Bone & Joint Journal*, vol. 95, no. 11, pp. 1500–1507, 2013.

[5] L. M. Coester, C. L. Saltzman, J. Leupold, and W. Pontarelli, "Long-term results following ankle arthrodesis for post-traumatic arthritis," *The Journal of Bone & Joint Surgery*, vol. 83, no. 2, pp. 219–228, 2001.

[6] R. A. Mann and K. M. Rongstad, "Arthrodesis of the ankle: A critical analysis," *Foot & Ankle International*, vol. 19, no. 1, pp. 3–9, 1998.

[7] J. J. P. Schimmel, L. H. B. Walschot, and J. W. K. Louwerens, "Comparison of the short-term results of the first and last 50 scandinavian total ankle replacements: Assessment of the learning curve in a consecutive series," *Foot & Ankle International*, vol. 35, no. 4, pp. 326–333, 2014.

[8] A. Haskell and R. A. Mann, "Perioperative complication rate of total ankle replacement is reduced by surgeon experience," *Foot & Ankle International*, vol. 25, no. 5, pp. 283–289, 2004.

[9] F. G. Usuelli, C. Maccario, A. Pantalone, N. Serra, and E. W. Tan, "Identifying the learning curve for total ankle replacement using a mobile bearing prosthesis," *Journal of Foot and Ankle Surgery*, vol. 23, no. 2, pp. 76–83, 2017.

[10] A. Henricson, J.-Å. Nilsson, and Å. Carlsson, "10-year survival of total ankle arthroplasties: A report on 780 cases from the Swedish Ankle Register," *Acta Orthopaedica*, vol. 82, no. 6, pp. 655–659, 2011.

[11] G. Labek, H. Klaus, R. Schlichtherle, A. Williams, and M. Agreiter, "Revision rates after total ankle arthroplasty in sample-based clinical studies and national registries," *Foot & Ankle International*, vol. 32, no. 8, pp. 740–745, 2011.

[12] A. A. Spirt, M. Assal, and S. T. Hansen Jr., "Complications and failure after total ankle arthroplasty," *The Journal of Bone & Joint Surgery*, vol. 86, no. 6, pp. 1172–1178, 2004.

[13] A. Henricson, A. Skoog, and Å. Carlsson, "The Swedish Ankle Arthroplasty Register: An analysis of 531 arthroplasties between 1993 and 2005," *Acta Orthopaedica*, vol. 78, no. 5, pp. 569–574, 2007.

[14] S. Tenenbaum, J. Bariteau, S. Coleman, and J. Brodsky, "Functional and clinical outcomes of total ankle arthroplasty in elderly compared to younger patients," *Journal of Foot and Ankle Surgery*, vol. 23, no. 2, pp. 102–107, 2017.

[15] C. A. Demetracopoulos, S. B. Adams, R. M. Queen, J. K. Deorio, J. A. Nunley, and M. E. Easley, "Effect of Age on Outcomes in Total Ankle Arthroplasty," *Foot & Ankle International*, vol. 36, no. 8, pp. 871–880, 2015.

[16] K. Schenk, S. Lieske, M. John et al., "Prospective study of a cementless, mobile-bearing, third generation total ankle prosthesis," *Foot & Ankle International*, vol. 32, no. 8, pp. 755–763, 2011.

[17] E. Pinsker, T. Inrig, T. R. Daniels, K. Warmington, and D. E. Beaton, "Symptom Resolution and Patient-Perceived Recovery Following Ankle Arthroplasty and Arthrodesis," *Foot & Ankle International*, vol. 37, no. 12, pp. 1269–1276, 2016.

[18] E. Budiman-Mak, K. J. Conrad, and K. E. Roach, "The foot function index: A measure of foot pain and disability," *Journal of Clinical Epidemiology*, vol. 44, no. 6, pp. 561–570, 1991.

[19] M. M. Kuyvenhoven, K. J. Gorter, P. Zuithoff, E. Budiman-Mak, K. J. Conrad, and M. W. M. Post, "The Foot Function Index with verbal rating scales (FFI-5pt): A clinimetric evaluation and comparison with the original FFI," *The Journal of Rheumatology*, vol. 29, no. 5, pp. 1023–1028, 2002.

[20] H. B. Kitaoka, I. J. Alexander, R. S. Adelaar, J. A. Nunley, M. S. Myerson, and M. Sanders, "Clinical rating systems for the ankle-hindfoot, midfoot, hallux, and lesser toes," *Foot & Ankle International*, vol. 15, no. 7, pp. 349–353, 1994.

[21] V. Valderrabano, B. Hintermann, and W. Dick, "Scandinavian total ankle replacement: A 3.7-Year average followup of 65 patients," *Clinical Orthopaedics and Related Research*, no. 424, pp. 47–56, 2004.

[22] J. M. Reuver, N. Dayerizadeh, B. Burger, L. Elmans, M. Hoelen, and N. Tulp, "Total ankle replacement outcome in low volume centers: Short-term followup," *Foot & Ankle International*, vol. 31, no. 12, pp. 1064–1068, 2010.

[23] Y. R. A. Kerkhoff, N. M. Kosse, W. P. Metsaars, and J. W. K. Louwerens, "Long-term Functional and Radiographic Outcome of a Mobile Bearing Ankle Prosthesis," *Foot & Ankle International*, vol. 37, no. 12, pp. 1292–1302, 2016.

[24] A. Frigg, B. Nigg, L. Hinz, V. Valderrabano, and I. Russell, "Clinical relevance of hindfoot alignment view in total ankle replacement," *Foot & Ankle International*, vol. 31, no. 10, pp. 871–879, 2010.

[25] E. P. McConnell and R. M. Queen, "Correlation of Physical Performance and Patient-Reported Outcomes Following Total Ankle Arthroplasty," *Foot & Ankle International*, vol. 38, no. 2, pp. 115–123, 2017.

[26] J.-L. Besse, N. Brito, and C. Lienhart, "Clinical evaluation and radiographic assessment of bone lysis of the AES total ankle replacement," *Foot & Ankle International*, vol. 30, no. 10, pp. 964–975, 2009.

[27] T. Kraal, H. J. L. Van Der Heide, B. J. Van Poppel, M. Fiocco, R. G. H. H. Nelissen, and H. C. Doets, "Long-term follow-up of mobile-bearing total ankle replacement in patients with inflammatory joint disease," *The Bone & Joint Journal*, vol. 95, no. 12, pp. 1656–1661, 2013.

[28] M. Bonnin, F. Gaudot, J.-R. Laurent, S. Ellis, J.-A. Colombier, and T. Judet, "The salto total ankle arthroplasty: Survivorship and analysis of failures at 7 to 11 years," *Clinical Orthopaedics and Related Research*, vol. 469, no. 1, pp. 225–236, 2011.

[29] N. Espinosa, M. Walti, P. Favre, and J. G. Snedeker, "Misalignment of total ankle components can induce high joint contact pressures," *The Journal of Bone & Joint Surgery*, vol. 92, no. 5, pp. 1179–1187, 2010.

[30] H. Koivu, I. Kohonen, K. Mattila, E. Loyttyniemi, and H. Tiusanen, "Long-term Results of Scandinavian Total Ankle Replacement," *Foot & Ankle International*, vol. 38, no. 7, pp. 723–731, 2017.

[31] S. Singer, S. Klejman, E. Pinsker, J. Houck, and T. Daniels, "Ankle arthroplasty and ankle arthrodesis: gait analysis compared with normal controls," *The Journal of Bone & Joint Surgery*, vol. 95, no. 24, pp. 2195–2202, 2013.

[32] H. Kofoed and A. Lundberg-Jensen, "Ankle arthroplasty in patients younger and older than 50 years: A prospective series with long-term follow-up," *Foot & Ankle International*, vol. 20, no. 8, pp. 501–506, 1999.

[33] E. T. Skyttä, H. Koivu, A. Eskelinen, M. Ikävalko, P. Paavolainen, and V. Remes, "Total ankle replacement: A population-based study of 515 cases from the Finnish Arthroplasty Register," *Acta Orthopaedica*, vol. 81, no. 1, pp. 114–118, 2010.

[34] S. M. Raikin, K. Sandrowski, J. M. Kane, D. Beck, and B. S. Winters, "Midterm Outcome of the Agility Total Ankle Arthroplasty," *Foot & Ankle International*, vol. 38, no. 6, pp. 662–670, 2017.

17

The Effect of Season and Weather on Orthopaedic Trauma: Consult Volume Is Significantly Correlated with Daily Weather

J. M. Wilson,[1] C. A. Staley,[1] A. L. Boden,[2] A. R. Boissonneault,[1] A. M. Schwartz,[1] and M. L. Schenker[1]

[1]*Department of Orthopaedic Surgery, Emory University School of Medicine, Atlanta, Georgia, USA*
[2]*Emory University School of Medicine, Atlanta, Georgia, USA*

Correspondence should be addressed to J. M. Wilson; jacobmwilson12@gmail.com

Academic Editor: Hiroshi Hashizume

Introduction. On-call orthopedic clinicians have long speculated that daily consult volume is closely correlated with weather. While prior studies have demonstrated a relationship between weather and certain fracture types, the effect of weather on total orthopaedic consult volume has not yet been examined. The aim of this study was to investigate this relationship. *Methods.* We retrospectively reviewed orthopaedic consult data from 405 consecutive days at an urban, level one trauma center. The number, mechanism of injury, and type of consult were collected, along with daily weather data (temperature, wind, and precipitation). Statistical analysis was then performed to determine the relationship between weather and orthopaedic trauma consults. *Results.* A total of 4543 consults were received during the study period. There was a significant difference in total number of consults between months of the year ($p<0.001$). A post hoc analysis revealed that this was due to increased volume in the summer months relative to the winter months (i.e., August 13.7 consults/day; January 9.3 consults/day). Average daily temperature and consult volume were also positively correlated ($p<0.001$, $r= 0.30$). While there was no significant association between precipitation and total consult volume, when there was over 0.25 inches of rain, there were less penetrating trauma ($p=0.034$) and motorcycle collision consults ($p=0.013$). *Conclusion.* Weather parameters, specifically average temperature and precipitation, were found to be associated with daily orthopedic consult type and volume. Additionally, consult volume varies significantly between months of the year. Because trauma centers are often resource scarce, this is an important relationship to understand for proper resource allocation.

1. Introduction

Clinicians have long speculated that daily trauma volume is closely correlated with the weather, and to many familiar with the care of the traumatically injured this seems anecdotally obvious. Not surprisingly, this conjecture has been the subject of numerous studies, primarily examining the number of general surgery trauma admissions and emergent cases as it relates to daily weather conditions [1–13]. Orthopedic injuries have also received attention in this regard, as a number of studies have examined the relationship between weather and fracture-specific patterns—most notably hip, forearm, and distal radius fractures [14–24].

Given the medical morbidity and mortality associated with hip fractures in the geriatric population, [25] hip fractures have understandably been of particular interest. Because ground level falls are a common mechanism of injury, multiple studies have demonstrated a higher incidence of hip fractures in the winter months [16, 21, 24, 26]. A similar trend has been demonstrated in distal radius fractures [20, 23]. Pediatric orthopedic injuries, on the other hand, have been shown to increase with warm temperatures and decrease with significant precipitation [15]. Unfortunately, the current literature on adult orthopaedic trauma is limited to only a handful of specific fracture types. To our knowledge, only one study has examined the effect of weather metrics on orthopedic consult volume and this was in a pediatric population [15]; however, no similar study exists in adults.

At publicly-funded, urban, level I trauma centers, there are limited resources available, despite the inherently high demands of often severely injured patients. These centers treat a large number of patients and orthopedic trauma typically accounts for a significant portion of this volume. The strain of this large number of resource-intensive patients on the healthcare system becomes problematic, as constraints on operating room availability can increase time to surgery for urgent cases [27]. Examining only a few specific fracture types, while useful, does not fully elucidate the strain that increased volume places on a hospital's staffing and resources. Additionally, severity of injury has been something that prior studies have had difficulty capturing. This study examined severity in two ways: (1) for patients who required a trauma activation, Injury Severity Scores (ISS) were collected from the trauma registry and (2) the number of orthopaedic cases booked as urgent or emergent was examined.

The current study sought to delineate what effect various weather variables, in addition to day of the week, month, and season, have on the total orthopedic trauma volume seen at an American College of Surgeons (ACS)-verified urban, level I trauma center. We hypothesized that orthopedic trauma consult volume as well injury severity in these patients is significantly affected by these parameters. This study aims to provide useful information for optimal resource allocation—consult and operating room coverage, implant availability, and operating room block time. Proper resource allocation could conceivably optimize care of patients from the time they arrive to the trauma center, through definitive care.

2. Materials and Methods

This is an IRB approved, retrospective review of orthopedic consults at an ACS-verified urban, level one trauma center in the southeastern United States. Orthopaedic consults were queried for 405 consecutive days ranging from December 2015 to January 2017. Hand and spine call at our institution is shared with plastic surgery and neurosurgery, respectively, so these consults were excluded from analysis. Additionally, the on-call resident covers orthopedic consults for a local pediatric hospital and these were also excluded. Therefore, the patient population included patients over the age of 18 years who required an orthopedic trauma consult.

The following metrics were collected for each of the 405 days: total number of inpatient consults and outpatient consults, total number of combined consults, age, admitting service, injury or reason for consult, and number of urgent/emergent consults. Mechanism of injury [motor vehicle crash (MVC), motorcycle crash (MCC), ground level fall (GLF), gunshot wound (GSW), fall from height (FFH), pedestrian versus auto (PVA), and other blunt mechanism)], Injury Severity Score (ISS), and Glasgow Coma Score (GCS) were queried from the local trauma database for all inpatient consults. This information is available for all patients who required a trauma activation. Given the volume of patients included in this series, this information was collected for only the inpatient consults, because outpatient consults were less likely to require trauma activation and we assumed these patients were not severely injured.

For the purposes of this study, urgent or emergent consults were defined as one of the following: open fractures (ballistic injuries were not included in this cohort), compartment syndrome, septic joint, and traumatic arthrotomy.

Inpatient consults included those patients who arrived to the emergency department (ED) and were admitted, as well as those patients who are already admitted to the hospital with a subsequent orthopedic injury or concern prompting consultation. Outpatient consults were those patients who were evaluated in the emergency department, treated by the orthopedic service, and discharged home with follow-up. Fracture types were classified into the following broad categories: foot (talus, midfoot, metatarsal, and phalanx), calcaneus, femur (shaft and distal), hip (including all femoral neck and peritrochanteric fractures), acetabulum, pelvic ring, tibia (plateau and shaft), pilon, ankle, humerus, both bone forearm fractures, and distal radius fractures. Patients who were multiply injured were tabulated as one overall consult, but each injury was also tabulated independently for categorical analysis.

Weather metrics were gathered from the National Climatic Data Center (NCDC) online databases (https://www.ncdc.noaa.gov). Weather data was collected at a nearby weather station, located 9.3 miles from the institution where the consults were received and well within the catchment range of the hospital. The following weather metrics were collected: precipitation amount, snow amount, average, maximum, and minimum temperature, average wind speed, and fastest 5 seconds of wind speed (when available).

Statistical analysis was completed using Stata (StataCorp. 2015. Stata Statistical Software: Release 14. College Station, TX: StataCorp LP) software. Analysis of variance (ANOVA), independent samples t-tests, and Pearson correlation were then performed to determine the relationship between weather and orthopaedic trauma consults. Findings were considered significant when $p<0.05$. Where appropriate, correlation coefficients as well as odds ratios are reported.

3. Results

3.1. Consult Characteristics. During the 405-day study period, there were a total of 5,725 orthopedic consults. Once hand (715 consults) and spine (467 consults) were excluded, 4543 orthopedic trauma consults met inclusion criteria and were included in this study. This equates to an average of 0.46 consults per hour and 11.21 consults per day. Of these, 2874 (63%) were inpatient consults and 1669 (37%) were outpatient consults. Ultimately, 2055 (71.55%) of the inpatient consults required trauma activation and therefore were available for further evaluation. Specific injuries included foot fractures (693 consults), calcaneus fractures (126 consults), femur fractures (74 consults), hip fractures (269 consults), tibia fractures (530 consults), pilon fractures (79 consults), both bone forearm fractures (57 consults), humerus fractures (301 consults), distal radius fractures (291 consults), and ankle fractures (524 consults). The remaining consults did not fit into a specified injury category. There were 503 emergent or urgent consults—382 open fractures, 50 septic joints, 13 cases of compartments syndrome, and 58 traumatic arthrotomies (Table 1).

TABLE 1: Number and type of consults over study period.

Consults	Number of consults
Total	4543
Inpatient	2874
Outpatient	1669
Trauma Activation	2055
Urgent/Emergent	503
Foot Fractures	693
Calcaneus	126
Ankle	524
Both Bone Forearm	57
Femur	374
Hip	269
Acetabulum	193
Pelvic Ring	294
Tibia	530
Pilon	59
Humerus	301
Distal Radius	291
Total Urgent/Emergent Consults	503
Open Fractures	382
Traumatic Arthrotomy	58
Septic Joints	50
Compartment Syndrome	13

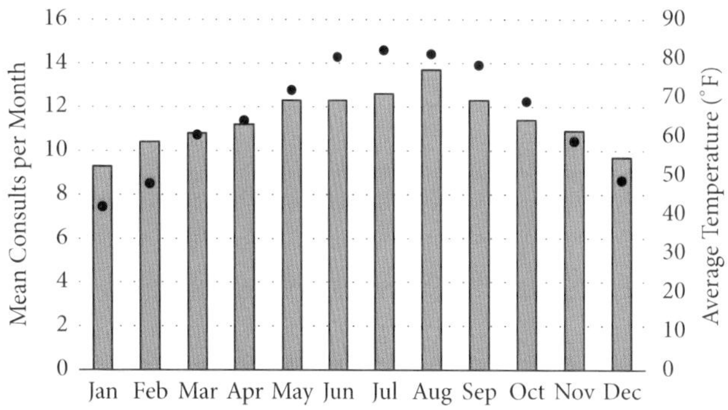

FIGURE 1: Average number of consults per month and average daily temperature per month (scatter plot). The average daily number of consults increases with increasing average monthly temperature.

3.2. Consult Variation with Month of Year. A one-way between-subjects ANOVA was conducted to compare the effects of the month of the year on the total number of orthopaedic consults. There was a significant increase in the number of consults in the summer months of the year, with August demonstrating peak consult volume (p<0.001; see Figure 1). A Bonferroni post hoc analysis of pairwise differences revealed that this was due to increased volume in summer months when compared to winter months. Specifically, the following were found to be significant: December versus July (p=0.046) and August (p<0.001); January versus May (p=0.009), June (p=0.009), July (p=0.001), August (p<0.001), and September (p=0.012); February versus August (p=0.020). No other pairwise differences were significant (Figure 1).

3.3. Consult Variation with Day of the Week. ANOVA analysis was also utilized to attempt to identify any variations in consult volume by day of the week (Monday, Tuesday, Wednesday, etc.). This analysis revealed no statistically significant variation between days of the week or between weekdays and weekends.

3.4. Consult Volume Variation with Temperature. Pearson correlation was utilized to compare total orthopaedic consult volume to daily temperature. There was a significant positive correlation between average daily temperature and total orthopaedic consult volume (r=0.30, p<0.001; see Figure 2). Furthermore, subgroup analysis with Pearson correlation revealed weak, but significant, correlation between average daily temperature and lower extremity trauma (foot, ankle, and pilon; r=0.15, p=0.002), motorcycle crash mechanism (r=0.19, p<0.001), and total blunt trauma (r=0.20, p<0.001). Temperature did not significantly correlate with any other mechanism of injury, nor with any other injury types (Figure 2).

3.5. Mechanism of Injury/Consult Volume with Total Precipitation. Independent sample t-tests were used to determine the influence of precipitation on consults. There was no significant association between daily precipitation and total consult volume (p = 0.407; Figure 2(c)). However, when there was over a quarter inch of rain in a single day, there were significantly less penetrating trauma consults (p=0.034) and significantly less motorcycle collisions (p=0.013). Pearson correlation was also utilized to further delineate the relationship between total daily precipitation and consult type and mechanism, and there was no correlation with total consult volume. There was a weak, but significant, negative correlation between precipitation and motorcycle collision consults (r = -0.12, p=0.013; see Table 2). There was also a trend toward a significant negative correlation between total daily precipitation and consults from gunshot wounds (r= -0.091; p= 0.067; Table 2).

3.6. Mechanism of Injury/Consult Volume and Wind Speed. Pearson correlation revealed no significant correlation between wind speed (maximum 5-second gust or average daily wind speed) and consult volume (p = 0.776). There were no significant correlations found between wind speed and types of consult or mechanism of consult. (Table 2, Figure 2)

3.7. Severity of Injury and Weather. Weather parameters did not significantly correlate with ISS scores or urgent/emergent consult volume. Consult Injury Severity Score was not correlated with average daily temperature (p=0.514), total precipitation (p=0.704), or wind speed (p=0.809). Similarly, open fracture consults were not associated with temperature (p=0.410), precipitation (p= 0.415), or wind (p=0.352).

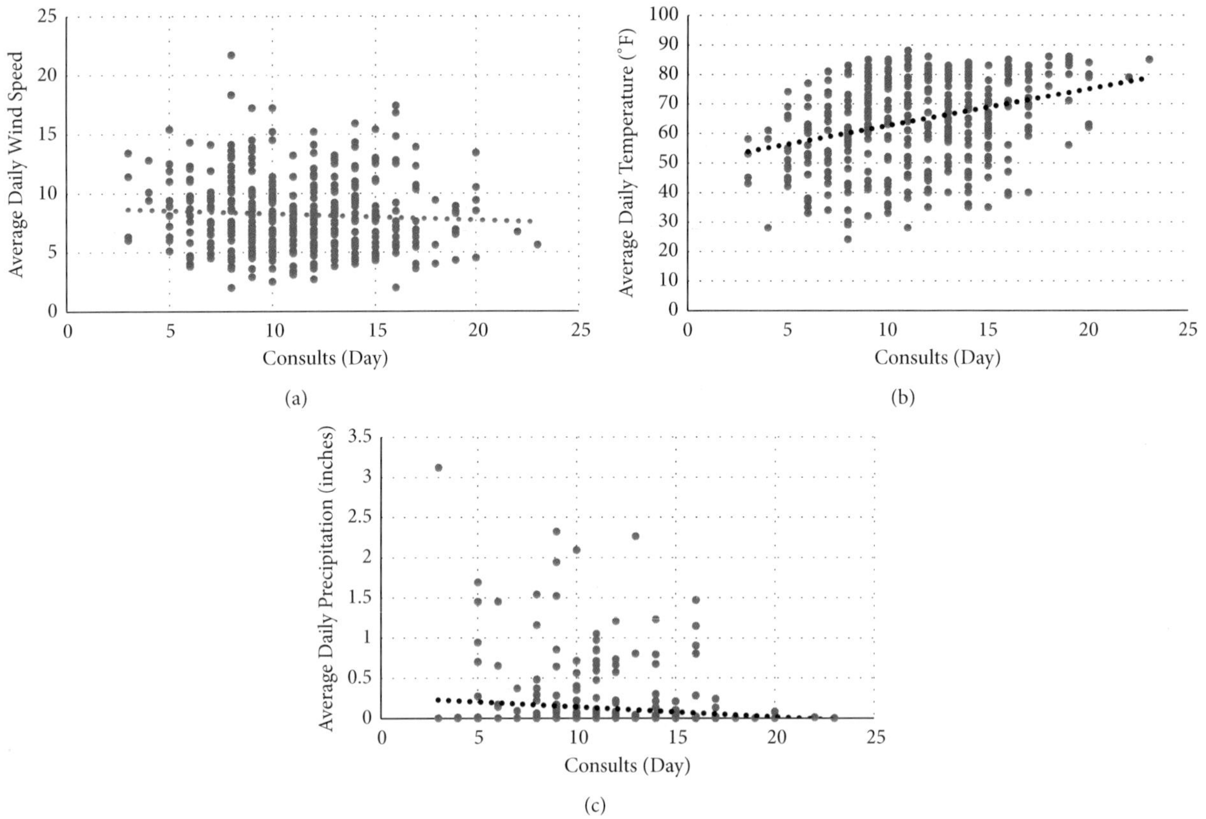

FIGURE 2: Relationship between total orthopedic consults and weather parameters: (a) average daily wind speed, (b) average daily temperature (r=0.30, p<0.001), and (c) average daily precipitation. Average daily wind speed and average daily precipitation were not significantly correlated to consult volume.

TABLE 2: Pearson Correlation analysis of weather parameters versus consult type and mechanism of injury. Statistically significant values are in bold.

Type of Consult	v. Temperature	v. Wind	v. Total Precipitation
Total Consults	**r=0.30, p<0.001**	r=-0.01, p=0.776	r=-0.04, p=0.407
Lower Extremity (Foot, ankle, pilon)	**r=0.15, p=0.002**	r=0.01, p=0.764	r=<-0.01, p=0.999
Long Bone (Tibia, Femur)	r=0.01, =0.922	r=-0.03, p=0.508	r=-0.05, p=0.373
Pelvis (hip, acetabulum, pelvic ring)	r=-0.002, p=0.967	r=<0.01, p=0.989	r=0.03, p=0.595
Upper Extremity (BBFFx, DR, Humerus)	r=0.03, p=0.584	r<-0.01, p=0.993	r=-0.03, p=0.565
Mechanism of Injury			
GSW	r=0.04, p=0.381	r=-0.03, p=0.514	r=-0.091, p=0.067
MVC	r=0.06, p=0.215	r=0.06, p=0.257	r=0.02, p=0.687
MCC	**r=0.19, p<0.001**	r=0.02, p=0.665	**r=-0.12, p=0.013**
Total Penetrating	r=0.04, p=0.385	r=-0.02, p=0.664	r=-0.09, p=0.063
Total Blunt	**r=0.20, p<0.001**	r=0.04, p=0.386	r=-0.072, p=0.146

There were also no significant correlations found with traumatic arthrotomies, septic joints, or compartment syndromes.

4. Discussion

Weather having an effect on human behavior and injury is not a novel concept [28]. In his 1842 "thermic law of delinquency," Adolphe Quetelet hypothesized that violent crimes were more prevalent in the summer months. While there have been multiple reports on the incidence of specific fracture types and total pediatric orthopaedic consult volume, [1–8, 17] with regards to weather, there has been, to our knowledge, no report examining total adult orthopedic trauma consult volume as it relates to various weather metrics. Most studies have concluded that, in the pediatric population, total trauma admissions and fracture incidences are increased in the spring and summer. The opposite has been found in geriatric populations where hip fracture rates are increased during winter months.

In the present study, we examined the effect of various weather parameters on all orthopedic trauma consult volume. Our data demonstrated that consult volume was positively correlated with temperature and, as such, there were significantly more daily consults in summer months when compared with winter months. Adverse weather (precipitation, wind, and snow) was not found to have a significant effect on total consult volume. However, when precipitation was greater than 0.25 inches there was significantly less penetrating and motorcycle crash consult volume. There was no difference in severity of injury or the number of urgent/emergent consults with variation in weather parameters. Our results also did not demonstrate a significant difference in consult volume by day of the week, a finding that was anecdotally surprising.

A strength of our study is that data was analyzed from over 400 consecutive days. The study was performed at a high volume, level one trauma center, with weather data available from the National Weather Service in close proximity to the treating hospital. Additionally, all data was from one center and daily consult data was compared directly to daily observed weather. We were also able to investigate the effect of weather on consult severity by comparing average consult ISS and daily number of urgent/emergent consults to weather variables.

The retrospective nature of our design limits the conclusions that can be drawn, and the generalizability of our results may be limited. Hospitals in areas with a similar climate to the southeastern United States are likely to experience similar patterns to those demonstrated in our study. However, more northern climates, with significantly lower temperatures and higher amounts of winter precipitation, may experience different seasonal variation in total consult volume, given the wider ranges of both temperature and precipitation between winter and summer months. Additionally, it must be noted that this study was conducted at a high-volume, level one trauma center in a major metropolitan area. Generalizing the results to smaller, nonlevel one centers outside of a metropolitan area is of unknown appropriateness. Lastly, our database only allows for identification of diagnosis at time of consult. Therefore, we likely underestimate the incidence of both septic joint and compartment syndrome as the workup may have been pending when reported or the condition may have yet to develop in the case of compartment syndrome.

Seasonal variation in consult volume and subsequently case volume is an important relationship to understand. The emergency department literature has examined volume variation and utilizes this information to appropriately allocate bed and staffing resources [29–31]. In orthopedics, this would be a novel concept but one that makes good sense. Implant availability, resident and faculty call coverage, and operating room block time availability should be properly allocated to match local seasonal variation needs. Orthopedic trauma surgeons would likely benefit from understanding their local variation and reserve more operating block time for trauma in the "busy season" and schedule elective cases intentionally at slower times of the year.

5. Conclusion

In conclusion, our study has demonstrated that total orthopedic trauma consult volume is positively correlated with temperature and this translates to higher orthopedic trauma volume in the summer months when compared to winter months. This variation should be anticipated by similar centers and efforts should be made to optimize patient care through proper resource appropriation.

References

[1] V. P. Ho, C. W. Towe, J. Chan, and P. S. Barie, "How's the weather? relationship between weather and trauma admissions at a level i trauma center," *World Journal of Surgery*, vol. 39, no. 4, pp. 934–939, 2015.

[2] L.-W. Lin, H.-Y. Lin, C.-Y. Hsu, H.-H. Rau, and P.-L. Chen, "Effect of weather and time on trauma events determined using emergency medical service registry data," *Injury*, vol. 46, no. 9, pp. 1814–1820, 2015.

[3] T. Bhattacharyya and F. H. Millham, "Relationship between weather and seasonal factors and trauma admission volume at a level I trauma center," *Journal of Trauma - Injury Infection and Critical Care*, vol. 51, no. 1, pp. 118–122, 2001.

[4] B. Zangbar, P. Rhee, V. Pandit et al., "Seasonal variation in emergency general surgery," *Annals of Surgery*, vol. 263, no. 1, pp. 76–81, 2016.

[5] B. Joseph, P. Rhee, and B. Zangbar, "Reply: Seasonal Variation in Emergency General Surgery: Why is February Underrepresented?" *Annals of Surgery*, vol. 266, no. 6, p. e75, 2017.

[6] S. T. Ward, R. J. Mithen, M. S. Mohamed, and G. R. Mufti, "Seasonal variation in emergency referrals to a Surgical Assessment Unit," *International Journal of Clinical Practice*, vol. 63, no. 1, pp. 121–125, 2009.

[7] A. M. Ali and K. Willett, "What is the effect of the weather on trauma workload? A systematic review of the literature," *Injury*, vol. 46, no. 6, pp. 945–953, 2015.

[8] W. R. Rising, J. A. O'Daniel, and C. S. Roberts, "Correlating weather and trauma admissions at a level I trauma center," *Journal of Trauma - Injury Infection and Critical Care*, vol. 60, no. 5, pp. 1096–1110, 2006.

[9] W. G. Atherton, W. M. Harper, and K. R. Abrams, "A year's trauma admissions and the effect of the weather," *Injury*, vol. 36, no. 1, pp. 40–46, 2005.

[10] W. K. M. Kieffer, D. V. Michalik, K. Gallagher, I. McFadyen, J. Bernard, and B. A. Rogers, "Temporal variation in major trauma admissions," *Annals of the Royal College of Surgeons of England*, vol. 98, no. 2, pp. 128–137, 2016.

[11] Z. J. O'Connor, S. D. Helmer, C. L. Yates, J. G. Ward, A. Khandelwal, and J. M. Haan, "An evaluation of the effect of wind speed on trauma admissions and injury severity at a Midwest Level I Trauma Center," *The American Surgeon*, vol. 78, no. 5, pp. 614–616, 2012.

[12] K. A. Friede, M. C. Osborne, and D. J. Erickson, "Predicting trauma admissions: the effect of weather, weekday, and other variables," *Minnesota Medicine*, vol. 92, pp. 47–49, 2009.

[13] R. M. Eisele and J. Schuld, "Seasonal Variation in Emergency General Surgery: Why Is February Underrepresented," *Annals of Surgery*, vol. 266, no. 6, pp. e74–e75, 2017.

[14] C. Jantzen, H. L. Jorgensen, and M. T. Thomsen, "Daily number of fractures is associated with road temperature in an urban area," *The Danish Medical Journal*, vol. 61, no. 3, p. A4794, 2014.

[15] K. S. Livingston, P. E. Miller, A. Lierhaus, T. H. Matheney, and S. T. Mahan, "Does Weather Matter? The Effect of Weather Patterns and Temporal Factors on Pediatric Orthopedic Trauma Volume," *The Open Orthopaedics Journal*, vol. 10, no. 1, pp. 550–558, 2016.

[16] A. Odeń, J. A. Kanis, E. V. McCloskey, and H. Johansson, "The effect of latitude on the risk and seasonal variation in hip fracture in Sweden," *Journal of Bone and Mineral Research*, vol. 29, no. 10, pp. 2217–2223, 2014.

[17] J. Weston-Simons, C. M. Jack, C. Doctor, K. Brogan, D. Reed, and D. Ricketts, "The impact of snow on orthopaedic trauma referrals," *Injury*, vol. 43, no. 7, pp. 1033–1036, 2012.

[18] J.-J. Sinikumpu, T. Pokka, K. Sirniö, R. Ruuhela, and W. Serlo, "Population-based research on the relationship between summer weather and paediatric forearm shaft fractures," *Injury*, vol. 44, no. 11, pp. 1569–1573, 2013.

[19] K. Matter-Walstra, M. Widmer, and A. Busato, "Seasonal variation in orthopedic health services utilization in Switzerland: The impact of winter sport tourism," *BMC Health Services Research*, vol. 6, p. 10, 2006.

[20] K. Wareham, A. Johansen, M. D. Stone, J. Saunders, S. Jones, and R. A. Lyons, "Seasonal variation in the incidence of wrist and forearm fractures, and its consequences," *Injury*, vol. 34, no. 3, pp. 219–222, 2003.

[21] S. Douglas, A. Bunyan, K. H. Chiu, B. Twaddle, and N. Maffulli, "Seasonal variation of hip fracture at three latitudes," *Injury*, vol. 31, no. 1, pp. 11–19, 2000.

[22] I. R. Murray, C. R. Howie, and L. C. Biant, "Severe weather warnings predict fracture epidemics," *Injury*, vol. 42, no. 7, pp. 687–690, 2011.

[23] A. M. Giladi, M. J. Shauver, A. Ho, L. Zhong, H. M. Kim, and K. C. Chung, "Variation in the incidence of distal radius fractures in the U.S. elderly as related to slippery weather conditions," *Plastic and Reconstructive Surgery*, vol. 133, no. 2, pp. 321–332, 2014.

[24] S. Mirchandani, G. B. Aharonoff, R. Hiebert, E. L. Capla, J. D. Zuckerman, and K. J. Koval, "The effects of weather and seasonality on hip fracture incidence in older adults," *Orthopedics*, vol. 28, no. 2, pp. 149–155, 2005.

[25] G. S. Keene, M. J. Parker, and G. A. Pryor, "Mortality and morbidity after hip fractures," *British Medical Journal*, vol. 307, no. 6914, pp. 1248–1250, 1993.

[26] O. C. Román, J. M. Tenías, M. Estarlich, and F. Ballester, "Systematic review of the association between climate and hip fractures," *International Journal of Biometerology*, vol. 59, no. 10, pp. 1511–1522, 2015.

[27] R. Runner, T. Moore, and W. Reisman, "Value of a dedicated saturday orthopaedic trauma operating room," *Journal of Orthopaedic Trauma*, vol. 30, no. 1, pp. e24–e29, 2016.

[28] L. A. Quetelet, "A treatise on man and the development of his faculties. 1842," *Obesity Research*, vol. 2, no. 1, pp. 72–85, 1994.

[29] K. A. Faryar, *The Effects of Weekday, Season, Federal Holidays, and Severe Weather Conditions on Emergency Department Volume in Montgomery County*, Wright State University, Dayton, Ohio, 2013.

[30] G. Joseph, "Fixing the Crowded Emergency Department, Part 3 — Implementing the Solution," *Common Sense*, vol. 21, no. 1, pp. 22–24, 2014.

[31] G. Joseph, "Fixing the Crowded Emergency Department, Part 2 — Creating the Analytic Model," *Common Sense*, vol. 20, no. 6, pp. 23–25, 2013.

18

Efficacy of Self-Directed Learning in the Supracondylar Fracture Performance Improvement Module at an Academic Pediatric Orthopedic Institution

Eric W. Edmonds,[1,2] John W. Kemppainen,[3] Joanna H. Roocroft,[1] John Munch,[1] and Tracey P. Bastrom[1]

[1] *Rady Children's Hospital, San Diego, CA, USA*
[2] *University of California, San Diego, CA, USA*
[3] *Helen DeVos Children's Hospital, Grand Rapids, MI, USA*

Correspondence should be addressed to Eric W. Edmonds; eedmonds@rchsd.org

Academic Editor: Panagiotis Korovessis

Maintenance of certification (MOC) within a medical society requires continuing medical education that demonstrates life-long learning, cognitive expertise, and practice-based self-assessment. This prospective study sought to evaluate whether a self-directed Practice Improvement Module (PIM) would improve pediatric orthopedic patient outcomes, thus demonstrating evidence of life-long learning (Part II MOC credit) in treating supracondylar humerus fractures. Six surgeons and 113 patients were included. There was no significant difference in actual fracture outcome before or after PIM at any level of surgeon experience regarding radiographic appearance or need for reoperation ($p > 0.10$). Junior staff demonstrated a statistically significant improvement in the percentage of time that marking the operative site was documented in the chart by the surgeon before (38%) and after (65%) PIM ($p = 0.02$). The self-directed education portion of the supracondylar fracture PIM led to modest improvement in documentation habits among junior staff, without impact on overall patient outcomes. Therefore, the PIM appears to be less useful in providing evidence for life-long learning as it relates to surgical outcomes (Part II MOC/CME), yet, it may directly benefit practice-based self-assessment (Part IV MOC), and the self-assessment and Personal Improvement Plan may be the most important portion of the PIM to improve outcomes.

1. Introduction

Maintenance of certification (MOC) within a medical society requires continuing medical education that demonstrates life-long learning, cognitive expertise, and practice-based self-assessment. These can be defined in four distinct parts [1]. Part I is "Evidence of Professional Standing" which can be defined as having state licensure to practice medicine. Part II is "Evidence of Life-Long Learning" which is defined as having Continuing Medical Education (CME) credits and Self-Assessment Examination (SAE). Part III is "Evidence of Cognitive Expertise" which is one's ability to secure and pass a recertification examination. Part IV is "Evidence of Practice-Based Self-Assessment" which is defined as clinical case review and performance improvement activity.

As part of the American Board of Orthopaedic Surgery (ABOS) MOC process, POSNA released a Practice Improvement Module (PIM) for supracondylar humerus fractures, which was initially intended to satisfy the MOC requirement for practice-based self-assessment (Part IV MOC), but at the time of this study it was approved by the ABOS for Part II MOC credit [2]. The POSNA PIM is comprised of three sections. Section 1 consists of 33 questions pertaining to the preoperative evaluation, treatment, and follow-up of operatively treated supracondylar humerus fractures. The process involves the surgeon collecting specified data on 10 consecutive cases of supracondylar fractures treated surgically via the ABOS Scribe database. The surgeon then receives a report from the ABOS, comparing their responses to others that have submitted the same data. From this information, the surgeon can then begin Section 2 of the PIM, which involves the development of a Personal Action Plan. This plan is centered on areas of improvement highlighted by comparing their entered data to other ABOS diplomats. They are then directed to complete a CME activity. There are currently two methods to obtain the CME required to move onto Section 3: Option #1, which requires the completion of 4 out of 6 items (see Supplementary Appendix A), or Option #2, attending a POSNA annual meeting breakout session. Once this has been completed, then the surgeon would implement their Personal Action Plan and collect data on 10 subsequent cases to assess how his or her practice has changed.

Since the PIM process is intended to provide MOC credit (whether it is Evidence of Life-Long Learning or Evidence of Practice-based Self-Assessment), it is reasonable to assess the process and to validate its purpose. The POSNA PIM is one of the first Practice Improvement Modules to be approved for utilization and future PIM development will likely be based on the success of this first attempt. This study assesses the ability of the self-directed standardized CME portion of the PIM system to affect clinical outcomes among junior and senior staff at a level-one pediatric trauma center, attempting to validate its ability to demonstrate either life-long learning or practice-based self-assessment. We asked the following question: Does the POSNA-developed supracondylar humerus fracture PIM self-directed standardized CME improve pediatric orthopedic patient outcomes with this condition, thus demonstrating evidence of life-long learning for the surgeon (evidence for Part II MOC credit)?

2. Materials and Methods

A prospective study of surgeons treating supracondylar fractures operatively at a single institution was carried out over an enrollment period of 14 months (October 2012 to December 2013). Fractures treated by both junior (less than 2 years in practice) and senior staff were enrolled, with each surgeon confirmed to have completed at least 10 supracondylar humerus fracture surgeries prior to the study, to negate discrepancies in experience level [3]. The methodology of the PIM was altered for the purposes of this study and the surgeons were blinded to the questions and measures being obtained. Therefore, they did not fully participate in the transition between Sections 1 and 2 of the PIM, meaning that no improvement opportunities were identified and therefore no Personal Action Plans were developed. Instead, in an attempt to keep the surgeons blind to the study outcomes, after they had performed the initial 10 surgeries included in the study, the surgeons then underwent a self-driven computer-based education by completing 4 of 6 CME activities established by the PIM (see Supplementary Appendix A), as the official instructions were that only 4 were required and the remaining two items are courses to attend and are difficult to coordinate for study purposes. As intended in the PIM, the CME activity was self-paced and standardized, and no posttest or verification was completed.

Section 3 of the PIM was then completed with data collection and enrollment continuing after the surgeon education sessions to reach a target of 10 post-PIM cases for each surgeon. Even though the surgeons were the subjects being studied, our Institutional Review Board asked that each patient being reviewed be consented prospectively for their data to be collected. Research staff members then audited the enrolled cases from Sections 1 and 3. The questionnaire included in the POSNA PIM (Supplementary Appendix B) was utilized as the data collection sheet. Additionally, since the study was conducted at an academic institution with multiple midlevel and resident providers, data on whether the treating surgeon dictated the note was also recorded. The two questions pertaining to alignment on X-ray were answered by one of the surgeon authors who was not participating in the enrollment of cases, so that none of the participating surgeons were unblinded to the PIM questionnaire or measures of outcome.

Descriptive statistics before to after PIM education data were calculated to determine completeness of the record according to the PIM. Clinical (ROM compared to contralateral, limb alignment compared to contralateral) and radiographic (anterior humeral line and AP alignment) outcomes that were part of the PIM questionnaire were also compared before and after PIM. Furthermore, documentation and outcomes were compared by level of experience (junior versus senior staff). Proportions were compared utilizing chi-square analysis and all analyses were performed utilizing SPSS v. 12 (SPSS Inc., Chicago, IL).

3. Results

Six surgeons (4 junior and 2 senior) treated adequate numbers of supracondylar fractures for data before and after PIM session and 113 patients were included. There were 22 patients (19%) treated by senior staff before PIM education and 22 patients (19%) treated by senior staff after PIM education. There were 34 patients (30%) treated by junior staff before PIM and 35 (31%) treated after PIM education. Thus, a total of 56 patients (50%) were treated prior to staff PIM education and 57 (50%) were treated after staff PIM education. There were no significant differences in the proportion of times where the treating surgeon was the originator of the clinic notes before and after PIM ($p > 0.05$).

Before PIM, 27/56 (48%) of patients had at least a 6-week minimum follow-up visit. This increased to 37/57 (65%) after PIM education, although this was not statistically significant ($p = 0.073$). Detailed information of chart audits based on the PIM questions is presented in Table 1.

There was no significant difference in actual fracture outcome before and after PIM at any level of surgeon experience regarding radiographic appearance or need for reoperation ($p > 0.10$). Outcomes based on level of training, regardless of PIM status, are demonstrated in Table 2. Posttreatment radiographs demonstrated that the anterior humeral line passed through the central 1/3 of the capitellum in 70% of the junior staff cases and in 53% of the senior staff cases ($p = 0.064$). Alignment on the AP radiograph was anatomic within 5 degrees in 80% of the junior staff cases and in 93% of the senior staff cases ($p = 0.051$). For patients with available data, range of motion was contralateral within 10 degrees in 85% of the junior staff cases and in 63% of the senior staff

TABLE 1: Detailed response rates for PIM questions before and after PIM education, based on level of experience as well as for the cohort as a whole. Significant differences are noted via bold values; differences at alpha < 0.10 are in italics.

	Junior	Senior	All
Preoperative assessment			
Limb perfusion documented			
Before PIM	94%	95%	95%
After PIM	97%	91%	95%
Neuro deficit/exam documented			
Before PIM	97%	100%	*98%*
After PIM	86%	95%	*90%*
AP/lateral X-rays obtained			
Before PIM	97%	100%	98%
After PIM	86%	95%	90%
Treatment assessment			
Time of injury available to determine length of time between injury and treatment			
Before PIM	9%	18%	13%
After PIM	6%	9%	7%
Informed consent obtained and documented in op. note			
Before PIM	100%	95%	98%
After PIM	100%	98%	98%
Site signed and documented in op. note			
Before PIM	**38%**	100%	63%
After PIM	**65%**	86%	74%
Surgical pause performed and documented in op. note			
Before PIM	97%	77%	89%
After PIM	97%	91%	95%
Preop. antibiotics given and charted in op. note			
Before PIM	76%	86%	80%
After PIM	86%	86%	86%
Limb perfusion documented after reduction and fixation			
Before PIM	24%	14%	20%
After PIM	37%	5%	25%
Lateral pins only?			
Before PIM	76%	73%	75%
After PIM	69%	72%	70%
Degree of flexion in cast documented			
Before PIM	18%	18%	18%
After PIM	29%	18%	26%
Neuro deficit/exam documented prior to discharge			
Before PIM	44%	64%	52%
After PIM	54%	64%	58%
Limb perfusion documented prior to discharge			
Before PIM	*35%*	68%	48%
After PIM	*66%*	55%	61%
Aftercare and outcome at final follow-up			
Pins removed at 3 weeks?			
Before PIM	*76%*	73%	75%
After PIM	*51%*	76%	61%
Cast d/c at 3 weeks?			
Before PIM	68%	64%	66%
After PIM	46%	62%	52%

Table 1: Continued.

	Junior	Senior	All
Limb perfusion documented at last f/u?			
Before PIM	85%	59%	75%
After PIM	89%	77%	84%
Neuro deficit/exam documented at last f/u?			
Before PIM	85%	82%	84%
After PIM	91%	95%	93%
On A/P X-ray, was alignment within 5 degrees anatomic?			
Before PIM	76%	95%	84%
After PIM	83%	91%	86%
On lateral, does anterior humeral line pass through central 1/3 of capitellum?			
Before PIM	74%	55%	66%
After PIM	66%	50%	59%
Patient has minimum 6-week f/u?			
Before PIM	41%	59%	48%
After PIM	57%	77%	65%
Physical exam documented elbow alignment at final visit?			
Before PIM	57%	31%	44%
After PIM	55%	35%	46%
Range of motion documented at final visit?			
Before PIM	76%	82%	79%
After PIM	83%	91%	76%
Time of return to unrestricted activity known?			
Before PIM	100%	92%	96%
After PIM	80%	94%	87%
Reoperation?			
Before PIM	0%	0%	0%
After PIM	5%*	0%	3%*

*1 patient had reoperation for septic elbow.

Table 2: Summary of clinical and radiographic outcomes based on experience.

	Junior	Senior	p value	Combined
Anatomic AP alignment within 5 degrees	55/69 (80%)	41/44 (93%)	0.051	96/113 (85%)
Anterior humeral line passing through central 1/3 of capitellum	48/69 (70%)	23/44 (53%)	0.064	71/113 (63%)
ROM within 10 degrees of other side*	17/20 (85%)	15/24 (63%)	0.095	32/44 (73%)
Clinical alignment within 5 degrees of contralateral upper extremity*	19/19 (100%)	9/10 (90%)	0.345	28/29 (97%)

*n is reduced for these variables, as those with <6-week follow-up or those where the outcome of interest was not recorded in visit note are excluded from the analysis.

cases ($p = 0.095$). Of the patients with available data, only one had documented clinical alignment that was not contralateral within five degrees.

Junior staff demonstrated a statistically significant improvement in the percentage of documented that the operative site was signed: from pre- (38%) to post- (65%) PIM ($p = 0.02$). They also demonstrated a nonsignificant increase in the documentation of limb perfusion prior to discharge (35%, before, and 66%, after; $p = 0.10$).

4. Discussion

At a level 1 academic children's hospital, the POSNA supracondylar fracture PIM self-directed education led to modest improvement in documentation habits among junior staff but did not affect overall clinical or radiographic outcomes. There are no comparative studies within orthopedics to help guide the utility of this particular PIM, but there is some evidence outside our field regarding the utility of Part II and Part IV MOC as well as PIMs.

Reflection regarding the ability of the PIM to affect patient outcomes requires a more basic level of assessing the MOC process, for which there has also been work looking into the utility of both MOC Part II and MOC Part IV [4]. Using a national database of physicians treating type 2 diabetes, Galliher and colleagues were able to demonstrate that both Part II and Part IV MOC correlated with greater improvements in care for patients treated by physicians participating in MOC in comparison to those treated by physicians not participating in MOC, suggesting that the PIM could affect patient outcomes. Yet, the authors note that they cannot make a direct association with the improvement in care and the participation in the Part II and Part IV exercises.

Previous study on the utility of a PIM has been performed, but the methods and conclusions are vague [5]. The American Board for Internal Medicine developed an osteoporosis PIM and then assessed the changes being seen by the participating physicians. Their methodology did not blind the participants from the outcome measures, which allowed them to review the results from all three sections of their PIM. Their conclusions were that the participating physicians could readily identify improvement opportunities within their practice and establish Personal Improvement Plans. Therefore, the authors concluded that the PIM assists the participant in evaluating their competency in practice-based learning and improvement (success regarding whether or not the PIM could change the quality improvement process for physicians).

Our study does not demonstrate an improvement in patient outcome based on the CME undertaken during the POSNA PIM but shows an improvement in documentation among young surgeons. It could be construed that improved "sign-your-site" documentation could be related to actually signing the extremity having surgery, which would then decrease the risk of wrong site surgery. However, our particular institution does not allow the patient to go back to the operating theater without the site being marked by the surgeon, so it truly is just an improvement in documentation by the surgeon concerning actions that they took. Moreover, the improved documentation of limb perfusion after PIM seen in our study could also represent an actual improvement in assessment of the patients prior to discharge, an improvement of care. A direct correlation remains difficult to state.

Although we had generally good clinical results and did not show a significant improvement in clinical outcomes after the self-directed learning portion of the PIM, this does not mean that there was not room for development. As a group, the surgeons did not achieve 100% compliance in any of the documentation or clinical measures outlined in the PIM. The authors of the PIM created its measured outcomes based on the best available evidence to maximize patient safety and clinical outcomes and, consequently, the goal of any orthopedic surgeon treating supracondylar humerus fractures should be to achieve 100% compliance in all measures. Based on this study, it appears that the self-directed standardized CME portion of the PIM alone does not achieve this goal. Perhaps the inclusion of the self-assessment and performance improvement plan would have allowed the self-reflection needed to see significant improvements in outcomes after the learning modules. Or perhaps the ability of a surgeon to seek specific CME related to their shortcomings in knowledge would improve patient outcomes rather than prescribing a standardized CME for all participants in the PIM process. Hence, the true value of this study may be that it demonstrates that standardized CME alone does not lead to measurable improvement in patient care.

One of the limitations of this study is the setting in which it was performed. Since it is an academic institution with frequent discussion of cases (both operative and nonoperative), as well as evaluation of surgical technique in a training environment, it may explain the lack of relationship between the PIM and clinical/radiographic outcomes in this study. A similar study, utilizing the same methods at a private practice without weekly conferences to assess the surgeons' radiographic outcomes, could have a completely different outcome from pre-PIM to post-PIM Section 2 CME. Future study on the efficacy of the PIM at impacting clinical outcomes at a nonacademic center may be valuable to confirm or refute this potential limitation.

Another limitation is the blinding of the surgeons to the transition from Section 1 to Section 2 of the PIM, eliminating the direct comparative feedback that would normally be available for identifying improvement opportunities, or the presence of a comparison group of surgeons that completed the Personal Improvement Plan. In order to prevent "gaming" of the results by the participating surgeons, it was imperative to keep the surgeons from knowing the measureable outcomes. This means that any changes seen from pre-PIM to post-PIM Section 2 self-study were purely the result of the CME undertaken and therefore accurately reflect changes related to the PIM (rather than changes related to an attempt to get a better score or demonstrating success in reaching the self-proclaimed goals of a Personal Improvement Plan). Admittedly, structured self-reflection of one's practice may more effectively drive clinical improvements than CME activities alone, and the omission of the Personal Improvement Plan may have tempered any potential benefits regarding clinical outcome. Perhaps the "gaming" of the results that we sought to prevent by blinding the surgeons is, in fact, the truly valuable component of the PIM that could lead to measurable improvements in patient care. However, after this study, we believe that the standardized CME portion (set in a general fashion by the PIM process and not related to a surgeons' Personal Improvement Plan) likely can be considered as ineffective in improving patient outcomes. A better methodology may be to allow surgeons to tailor their CME to meet their specific needs, based on their self-reflection.

Therefore, the next study will need to include the Personal Improvement Plan in order to determine whether the standardized CME can be useful in that setting. If it is not, then future PIMs will need to be modified to allow personal CME choices (rather than a standardized CME) that are based on the Personal Improvement Plan.

Another limitation is that the treating surgeons, as noted above, did not always perform the documentation themselves. Therefore, changes to documentation may not reflect changes in the practice of the treating surgeon. However, as with all academic centers, the attending surgeon is the owner of the chart and patient care. Therefore, from a medical-legal standpoint, the onus of documentation belongs to the attending surgeon, and with each note being cosigned, we believe that changes to the documentation do in fact represent changes to the treating surgeons' practice.

Currently, the ABOS intend to offer the supracondylar PIM for Part II MOC credit (Evidence of Life-Long

Learning). This study demonstrates that self-directed learning in the absence of self-reflection on one's practice does not significantly change clinical outcomes but may modestly change documentation patterns among young surgeons. However, the PIM system does appear to provide evidence for practice-based self-assessment, since it directly records surgeons' documentation habits in real time for outside MOC committee review. Improvements in practice habits may represent an improvement in patient care, which is the importance of Part IV MOC criteria. Therefore, reconsideration by the ABOS to utilize the POSNA supracondylar fracture PIM for Part IV MOC credit may be warranted. Future development of PIMs and MOC credits within medical societies should stress the importance of self-assessment of physician practice to affect patient outcomes, and the development of personalized CME may be warranted to utilize the PIMs for Part II MOC credit.

References

[1] J. K. Iglehart and R. B. Baron, "Ensuring physicians' competence - Is maintenance of certification the answer?" *The New England Journal of Medicine*, vol. 367, no. 26, pp. 2543–2549, 2012.

[2] A. A. Stans and G. A. Mencio, "Practice improvement modules: The pediatric supracondylar fracture PIM," *Journal of Pediatric Orthopaedics*, vol. 35, no. 5, pp. S37–S38, 2015.

[3] R. W. Liu, J. Roocroft, T. Bastrom, and B. Yaszay, "Surgeon learning curve for pediatric supracondylar humerus fractures," *Journal of Pediatric Orthopaedics*, vol. 31, no. 8, pp. 818–824, 2011.

[4] J. M. Galliher, B. K. Manning, S. M. Petterson et al., "Do professional development programs for maintenance of certification (MOC) affect quality of patient care?" *Journal of the American Board of Family Medicine*, vol. 27, no. 1, pp. 19–25, 2014.

[5] B. J. Hess, M. M. Johnston, W. F. Iobst, and R. S. Lipner, "Practice-based learning can improve osteoporosis care," *Journal of the American Geriatrics Society*, vol. 61, no. 10, pp. 1651–1660, 2013.

Epidemiology of C2 Fractures in the 21st Century: A National Registry Cohort Study of 6,370 Patients from 1997 to 2014

Anna-Lena Robinson,[1,2] Claes Olerud,[2] and Yohan Robinson[2]

[1]*Stockholm Spine Center, Upplands Väsby, Sweden*
[2]*Department of Surgical Sciences, Uppsala University Hospital, Uppsala, Sweden*

Correspondence should be addressed to Anna-Lena Robinson; anna-lena.robinson@spinecenter.se

Academic Editor: Allen L. Carl

Objective. C2 fractures are a common injury in the elderly population. Treatment is often complicated due to osteoporosis and patient comorbidity. This study aims to investigate the incidence and treatment trend of C2 fractures in Sweden. *Methods.* Patients with the principal and secondary diagnosis of fracture of the second vertebrae (ICD-10: S12.1) between 1997 and 2014 were identified in the Swedish National Patient Registry (NPR). *Results.* Between 1997 and 2014, 6,370 patients with a C2 fracture (51% male; age: 72 ± 18) were identified in the NPR. The incidence of C2 fractures increased from 3 to 6 per 100,000 ($r = 0.94$; $p < 0.01$), mainly due to an increase of incidence in the geriatric subgroup (≥70 years). The percentage of surgically treated patients decreased from 1997 to 2014 ($r = -0.80$; $p < 0.01$). Younger age, male gender, spinal cord injury, and earlier year of admission were associated with surgical treatment assignment. *Discussion.* This study documents a rising incidence of C2 fractures in the elderly during the last two decades in Sweden. Greater awareness of fractures, improved diagnostics, coding, and a higher activity level of the patients are plausible causes. The declining trend of surgical treatment warrants further study.

1. Introduction

Fractures of the second cervical vertebra (C2) are a common injury in both the elderly and the young and active population [1]. Previously published studies find 9–18% of cervical fractures to be C2 fractures, of which 35–78% are odontoid process fractures and 11–25% are traumatic C2 spondylolysis, Hangman's fractures [2–6].

In the elderly, the proportion of C2 fractures is greater than that in the younger population [7, 8]. The elderly population has grown during the last decades [9]; therefore it is likely that the incidence of C2 fractures has increased as well. About 89% of the C2 fractures in patients ≥ 70 years of age in two tertiary referral centres in Sweden are odontoid fractures [8]. On a regional level in Sweden, we report a growing incidence of elderly patients with C2 fractures, which has not been seen in the younger population [8].

Surgical treatment options vary depending on the type of C2 fracture. Odontoid fractures type 2 are commonly treated with anterior screw osteosynthesis or posterior C1-C2 fusion [10–13]. Hangman's fractures are treated surgically with anterior C2-C3 fusion, posterior direct osteosynthesis, or posterior C2-C3 fusion [14, 15].

Nonsurgical treatment of C2 fractures is commonly performed with a rigid cervical collar [16]. In cases of instability or dislocations a halo-vest treatment is possible [17, 18].

The availability of prospectively collected data in nationwide registries in Sweden allows tracking of epidemiology retrospectively without the necessity of repeated cross-sectional trials. This study aims to investigate the incidence and treatment trend of C2 fractures during the last two decades in the Swedish National Patient Registry.

2. Patients and Methods

2.1. Study Design. This national multiregistry cohort study used prospectively collected electronic healthcare data from the Swedish National Patient Registry (NPR) and Statistics Sweden between 1997 and 2014. The study protocol was approved by the Institutional Ethical Review Board (2010/131/1) and follows STROBE and RECORD statements [19].

2.2. Setting. The Swedish National Patient Registry is hosted by the Swedish National Board of Health and Welfare and contains all patient contacts within Sweden with a coverage of >90% for orthopaedic diagnoses [20]. Registered are main diagnosis and comorbidity using the International Classification of Diseases, Ninth Revision (ICD-9), until December 1996 and since then the ICD-10 code [21]. In the International Classification of Diseases, Tenth Revision (ICD-10), there is no subclassification for C2 fractures [21]. Treatment has been coded since 1997 using the Swedish classification of surgical procedures [22]. Furthermore, information on hospitalisation time is available from the registry. Statistics Sweden is an administrative agency, providing statistics to the government, different agencies, and researchers.

2.3. Participants. All patients registered with the main and secondary diagnosis of C2 fracture treated between 1 January 1997 and 31 December 2014 were extracted from the NPR. In this study, we wanted to calculate the incidence and treatment trend, and therefore both main and secondary diagnoses were included, so that most possible C2 fractures would be included for calculations. Prior to data transmission, the Swedish National Board of Health and Welfare anonymised the individual personal identification numbers using a key that remained with the agency. Patients younger than 20 years of age and older than 99 years at the date of fracture were excluded. Population registry data from January 1997 until December 2014 were abstracted from Statistics Sweden. An inclusion flow diagram was prepared according to CONSORT statements [23].

2.4. Variables. The ICD-10 code S12.1 (fracture of the second vertebrae) was used to identify patients with C2 fracture in the NPR. ICD-10 has been validated for all diagnosis with an accuracy from 89 to 95% [20] and also for orthopaedic diagnosis with an accuracy of 95% for principal and secondary diagnoses until the third position and 90% to the fourth position [24]. The specificity of the ICD-10 code S12.1 has been validated in a dataset of 172 patients with ICD-10 S12.1 from 2002 to 2014, where 0% false positive cases were found (specificity = 100%). Baseline data for the included individuals were collected from the NPR and presented in tabular form. Causes of injury codes were not extracted from the NPR, due to, for our purposes, unacceptably low accuracy of these codes [20, 24]. Patients receiving surgical treatment were identified, using Swedish surgical procedure codes for spinal fusion ("NAG") and spinal fracture treatment ("NAJ"). Nonsurgically treated cases with a change of treatment modality to surgery were registered as surgical patients. Subgroup analysis was performed for nongeriatric (20–69 years) and geriatric patients (70–99 years) and for nonsurgical and surgical treatment.

2.5. Statistical Methods. All statistical calculations were programmed in R version 3.3.0 (R Foundation for Statistical Computing, Vienna, Austria) [25]. Mean values were presented ± standard deviation if not indicated otherwise. Groups were compared with t-test for normally distributed variables; otherwise the Wilcoxon test was applied. Trends were analysed with linear regression and presented with correlation coefficient r. Group proportions were tested with χ^2 test. $p < 0.05$ was regarded as statistically significant. The age distribution differences of patients with C2 fractures treated with and without surgery were visualised with a density distribution plot. A logistic regression analysis identified covariates of surgical treatment assignment and was presented with 95% confidence intervals (CI) and statistical probability p [26]. As relevant covariates in a model for surgical treatment assignment, age [27], gender [28], CCI [29], and SCI [30] were determined by literature review. Before removing the cases below 20 years of age and older 100 from the dataset, a histogram of the age-related frequency of C2 fractures was prepared.

2.6. Data Access and Cleaning Methods. The authors did not have direct access to the national registry databases in this study but were provided with a predefined extract from the national registries by the Swedish National Board of Health and Welfare (specification number: 13062/2015).

Even though a clean patient registry dataset was provided, duplicates (recurrent admissions of the same patient or continued treatment in a secondary facility) had to be identified and removed from the extract. The secondary diagnoses of the duplicates were added to the original record prior to duplicate exclusion.

3. Results

3.1. Participants. The population of 20 to 99 years of age in Sweden 1997 was 6,689,671 (mean age: 39.9 years), and in 2014 it was 7,536,133 inhabitants (mean age: 41.2 years). Between 1997 and 2014, a total number of 11,077 cases were treated as inpatients due to a C2 fracture. The inclusion flow chart is shown in Figure 1.

3.2. Descriptive Data. 6,370 patients with the principal and secondary diagnosis of a C2 fracture (ICD-10: S12.1) were included. 51% were male. The mean age was 72 ± 18 years. The group was divided into nongeriatric patients < 70 years of age (n = 2,256) and geriatric patients ≥ 70 years of age (n = 4,114). 26% received surgical treatment: 34% in the nongeriatric group and 22% in the geriatric group (χ^2 test, $p < 0.01$). Stratified for gender (51% male, 49% female), 31% male and 22% female patients received surgical treatment (χ^2, $p < 0.01$).

Baseline data is shown in Table 1. The Charlson Comorbidity Index (CCI) was 4.9 ± 2.5, and spinal cord injury (SCI) was present in 2% (n = 140). 10% (n = 630) had a concomitant C1 fracture.

3.3. Outcome Data

3.3.1. Incidence of C2 Fractures. The incidence of C2 fractures doubled from 1997 to 2014 from 3 to 6 per 100,000 inhabitants

TABLE 1: Baseline values of patients according to treatment presented as count (n) or mean ± standard deviation.

	n	Age	Sex		CCI	SCI	C1	Spinal fracture			Surgical technique	
			Male	Female				Subaxial	T	L	Screw	Fusion
		Years	n	n		n	n	n	n	n	n	n
Surgical	1681	68 ± 17	1013	668	4.4 ± 2.3	77	236	194	90	30	168	1513
Nonsurgical	4689	73 ± 18	2277	2412	5.1 ± 2.6	63	394	272	186	122	0	0
All	6370	72 ± 18	3290	3080	4.9 ± 2.5	140	630	466	276	152	168	1513

n: number; SD: standard deviation; CCI: Charlson Comorbidity Index; SCI: spinal cord injury; T: thoracic; L: lumbar.

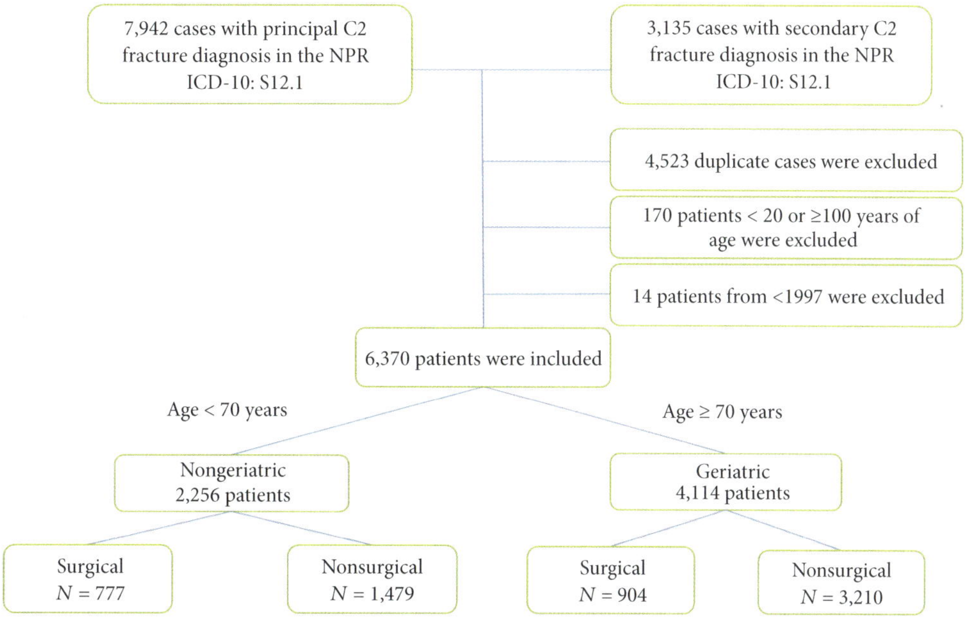

FIGURE 1: Inclusion flow diagram.

($r = 0.94$; $p < 0.01$). The incidence in the geriatric group increased linearly from 10.2 to 23.7 per 100,000 from 1997 to 2014, which was not found in the nongeriatric group (Figure 2) ($r = 0.89$; $p < 0.01$).

There was no significant difference of the C2 fracture incidence between the sexes in the subgroup of 80–89 and 90–99 years of age ($p = 0.43$ and $p = 0.46$). With regard to patients below the age of 80 years, C2 fractures were more common in men ($p < 0.01$) (Table 2). A bimodal distribution of age-related C2 fracture frequency was found with peaks at 20–25 years and at 80–85 years (Figure 3). From 1997 to 2014, the C2 fracture incidence quadrupled in the old geriatric patients (90–99 years), while it more than doubled in the age group of 80–89 years and it increased by 30% in the age group of 70–79 years (Figure 4).

3.3.2. C2 Fracture Treatment Trends in Sweden. Of the included patients, 26% were treated surgically. There was a higher density of nonsurgical treatment in the elderly (Figure 5). There has been linear trend from 1997 to 2014 towards nonsurgical treatment ($r = -0.8$; $p < 0.01$) (Figure 6). There was an even stronger trend towards nonsurgical treatment in the geriatric subgroup ($r = -0.95$; $p < 0.01$), compared to the younger age group. Treatment trends are shown in Figures 5, 6, and 7.

In a logistic regression model, the odds ratio of surgical treatment assignment was significantly greater for younger age, male gender, SCI, and earlier year of admission (Table 3).

4. Discussion

4.1. Key Results. This study documents a growing incidence and a declining surgical treatment trend of C2 fractures in the elderly during the last two decades in Sweden.

4.2. Interpretation

4.2.1. Incidence of C2 Fractures. Since 1997, the incidence of C2 fractures has risen from 3 to 6 per 100,000. As the elderly population has grown dramatically in Sweden, the number of hospital admissions due to elderly-specific C2 fractures increased during the last decade. Despite the 64% increase in the population of 90 to 99 years of age from 1997 to 2014,

Table 2: Incidence of C2 fractures per 100,000 within age subgroups according to gender (presented with p values of t-test for gender difference).

Age category Years	Female Per 100,000	Male Per 100,000	Both sexes Per 100,000	t-test p value
20–29	0.8	2.1	1.5	<0.01
30–39	0.5	1.4	1.0	<0.01
40–49	0.8	2.1	1.4	<0.01
50–59	1.7	3.0	2.4	<0.01
60–69	3.9	5.9	4.9	<0.01
70–79	9.2	13.6	11.2	<0.01
80–89	26.2	28.8	27.2	0.43
90–99	49.7	55.2	51.1	0.46

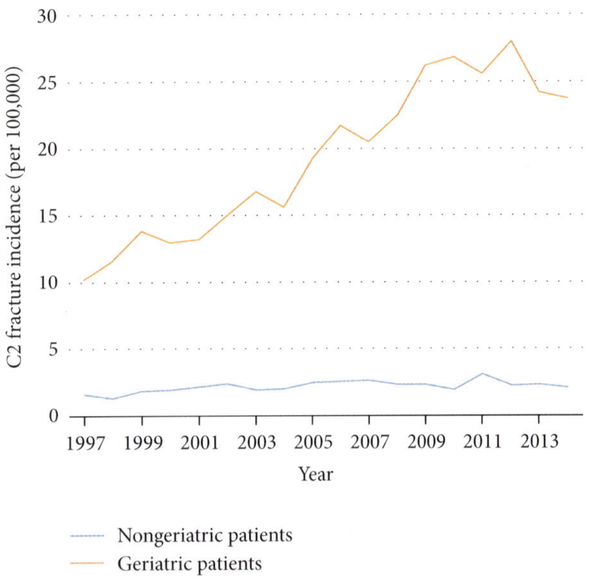

Figure 2: C2 fracture incidence per 100,000 of nongeriatric (blue) and geriatric (red) patients between 1997 and 2014.

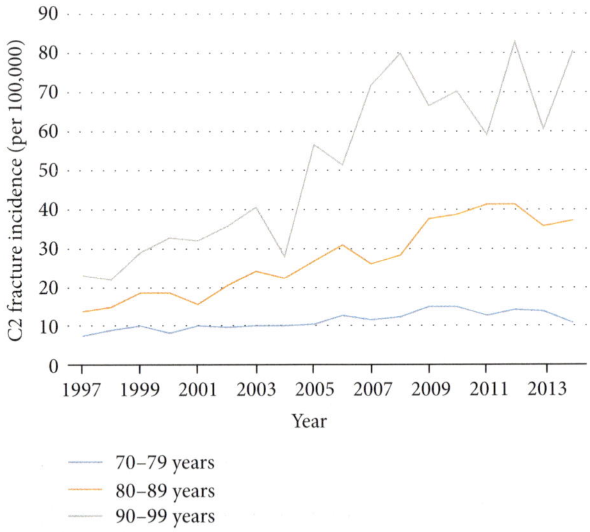

Figure 4: Incidence of C2 fractures between 1997 and 2014 per 100,000 in geriatric age categories: 70–79 years (blue), 80–89 years (orange), and 90–99 years (grey).

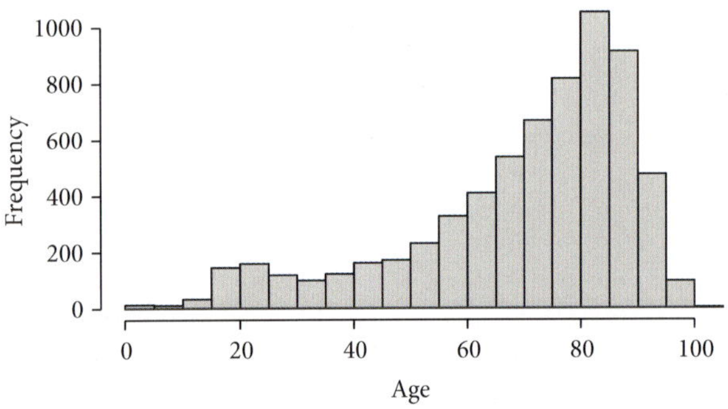

Figure 3: Age distribution of C2 fractures.

a 4-fold increase of the population-adjusted incidence of C2 fractures was found. This compares to the 70–79 years of age population which only increased by 13% but C2 fractures increased by 43%.

One explanation for the increased incidence of C2 fractures is a diagnostic bias, as we nowadays use a computed tomography instead of conventional radiographs as a first diagnostic instrument [31]. Beyond that, the number of falls in the elderly is substantial [32]. There is an increased rate of falls, 78%, for those with four or more risk factors [33, 34]. 5% of the falls cause a fracture [34]. The elderly receive better treatment for comorbidities compared to decades ago [35]. This leads to a higher activity level of the elderly, along with a higher risk of falling, but also the inactive persons stand a high risk of falls [32]. The orthostatic effect of medication like benzodiazepines and antihypertensive drugs may also lead to falls. Furthermore, the fact that the healthcare system in Sweden encourages geriatric patients to live in their own homes instead of nursing homes affects possibilities of supervision and accessibility, a plausible cause of domestic falls [35, 36]. Otherwise, patients at nursing homes stand a higher risk of falls [32, 34]. The combination of falls, a

TABLE 3: The assignment to surgical treatment was dependent on younger age, male gender, spinal cord injury, and earlier year of admission. Odds ratios are presented with 95% CI and p value.

	OR	95% CI 2.5%	95% CI 97.5%	p
Age	0.99	0.99	1.00	0.012
Male gender	1.42	1.26	1.59	<0.001
Spinal cord injury	2.94	2.08	4.16	<0.001
Charlson Comorbidity Index	0.96	0.92	1.00	0.072
Year of admission	0.96	0.94	0.97	<0.001

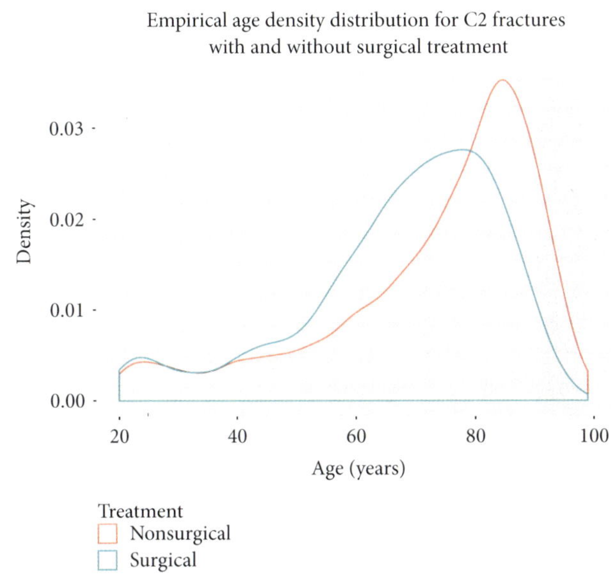

FIGURE 5: Empirical age distribution for C2 fractures with and without surgical treatment.

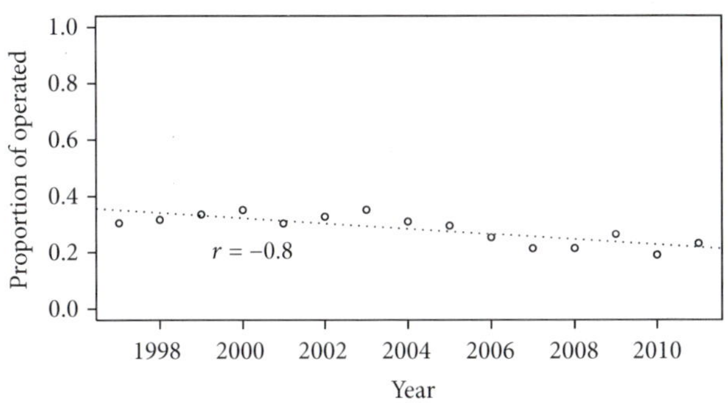

FIGURE 6: Annual proportion of surgically treated patients with C2 fractures.

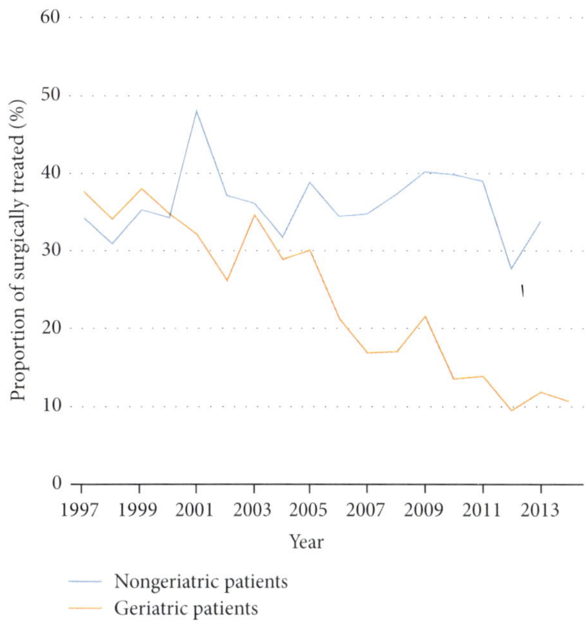

FIGURE 7: Proportion of surgically treated nongeriatric (blue) and geriatric (orange) patients with C2 fractures between 1997 and 2014.

stiff lower cervical spine, and osteoporosis could explain the increased incidence of C2 fractures in the elderly [37, 38].

4.2.2. C2 Fracture Treatment Trends in Sweden. There was a national trend towards nonsurgical treatment of C2 fractures in Sweden, foremost in the elderly, which does not confirm previously published results from other countries [37, 39, 40]. Fear of overtreatment could be a factor contributing to the trend of nonsurgical treatment of cervical fractures. The elderly patients' comorbidity could explain the physicians' tendency to use a cervical collar in the belief of avoiding harm. In contrast, recently published results suggest that surgical C2 fracture stabilisation reduces morbidity and mortality of elderly patients with greater comorbidity [37, 41]. In this registry study, we could not perform a subgroup analysis of C2 fracture subtypes, level of dislocation, or treatment allocation. Several authors recommend a treatment based on level of fracture dislocation besides comorbidity and age; this could not be investigated in our cohort [2, 6, 42].

4.2.3. Gender Differences in Treatment Assignment. This study pinpointed that men and women were treated differently. The proportion of women treated surgically was much lower than men. Thus, female patients received a probably inferior treatment with regard to survival [43]. Multiple studies have documented an implicit, unintended discrimination of female patients by their physicians [44, 45]. As treating surgeons, we should accept and acknowledge the fact that our treatment decisions are unintentionally affected by stereotypes as gender [40]. This will allow us to minimise implicit gender discrimination.

4.3. Strengths and Limitations. Due to the unmatched coverage and the high internal validity of the Swedish patient registry, the presented data is reliable. The national population-based cohort design of this study minimises the selection bias of tertiary referral centres. These often attract odd and unusual case referrals and distort the disease panorama. This national registry study has therefore advantages over many previously published cohort studies. Furthermore, registry studies have the strength of including the whole population instead of creating a sample of the population (as you would do in randomised controlled trials) [37]. This allows identification of even rare diseases or complications of treatments.

As the ICD-10 does not allow the differentiation of odontoid fractures from other C2 fractures, the NPR could not answer the question of proportion of C2 fracture subtypes. In a previous study from two regions in Sweden, we have revealed that about 63% of the C2 fractures are odontoid type 2 fractures in the elderly population ≥ 70 years, and 26% are odontoid type 3 fractures [8]; this means that a total 89% of the odontoid fractures in the elderly are either type 2 or type 3. We described an increase in the proportion of odontoid C2 fractures in the elderly from 2002 to 2014. Therefore, one can assume that the increase of C2 fractures in the geriatric subgroup from 1997 to 2014 found in the present study was largely due to an increase of odontoid type 2 and type 3 fractures. In the younger age group, our previous study from Sweden revealed a more differentiated panorama of C2 fractures, including 24% Hangman's fractures, 21% atypical fractures, 17% odontoid type 3 fractures, and 34% odontoid type 2 fractures [8]. In the present nationwide study, C2 fractures of the nongeriatric patients did not increase (Figure 2); thus, any conclusions regarding the C2 fracture subtype distribution would be speculative.

The availability of computed tomography for diagnostics of cervical injuries in the last two decades could have led to a diagnostic bias, where a greater number of C2 fractures would be detected during the recent years of this study [46, 47].

As the validity of the 4th digit of the fracture ICD-10 code (90%) is lower than the third digit (95%) [24], approximately 5% of C2 fractures were likely to be misdiagnosed as other cervical spine fractures (S12.0, S12.2, S12.7, S12.8, and S12.9). In contrast, the risk that fractures that are not C2 fractures were misdiagnosed as S12.1 is low, since the specificity of S12.1 was 100% (unpublished data).

A confounder not controlled for in this study is the comorbidity of osteoporosis. If the population's osteoporosis improved (i.e., due to better preventive healthcare measures), this would affect the risk of cervical spinal fractures [35].

As most other countries, Sweden has a geographically, health-economically, and ethnically unique population. The results presented in this study might not be generalizable to the rest of the world. Studies from national patient registries in other countries will have to validate our results in their specific settings.

5. Conclusion

This study identified an increased incidence of C2 fractures during the last decade along with a decreased proportion of surgically treated elderly patients. Results from ongoing randomised controlled trials, as the U-SOFT trial (ClinicalTrials.gov # NCT02789774), will facilitate an evidence-based treatment rationale for C2 fractures.

References

[1] L. D. Anderson and R. T. D'Alonzo, "Fractures of the odontoid process of the axis," *The Journal of Bone & Joint Surgery—American Volume*, vol. 56, no. 8, pp. 1663–1674, 1974.

[2] K. A. Greene, C. A. Dickman, F. F. Marciano, J. B. Drabier, M. N. Hadley, and V. K. H. Sonntag, "Acute axis fractures. Analysis of management and outcome in 340 consecutive cases," *The Spine Journal*, vol. 22, no. 16, pp. 1843–1852, 1997.

[3] M. D. Ryan and T. K. F. Taylor, "Odontoid fractures in the elderly," *Journal of Spinal Disorders & Techniques*, vol. 6, no. 5, pp. 397–401, 1993.

[4] U. Vieweg, B. Meyer, and J. Schramm, "Differential treatment in acute upper cervical spine injuries: A critical review of a single-institution series," *World Neurosurgery*, vol. 54, no. 3, pp. 203–211, 2000.

[5] E. C. Benzel, B. L. Hart, P. A. Ball, N. G. Baldwin, W. W. Orrison, and M. Espinosa, "Fractures of the C-2 vertebral body," *Journal of Neurosurgery*, vol. 81, no. 2, pp. 206–212, 1994.

[6] M. N. Hadley, C. A. Dickman, C. M. Browner, and V. K. H. Sonntag, "Acute axis fractures: A review of 229 cases," *Journal of Neurosurgery*, vol. 71, no. 5 I, pp. 642–647, 1989.

[7] H. Wang, M. Coppola, R. D. Robinson et al., "Geriatric trauma patients with cervical spine fractures due to ground level fall: Five years experience in a level one trauma center," *Journal of Clinical Medicine Research*, vol. 5, no. 2, Article ID 23519239, pp. 75–83, 2013.

[8] A.-L. Robinson, A. Möller, Y. Robinson, and C. Olerud, "C2 Fracture Subtypes, Incidence, and Treatment Allocation Change with Age: A Retrospective Cohort Study of 233 Consecutive Cases," *BioMed Research International*, vol. 2017, Article ID 8321680, 7 pages, 2017.

[9] United_Nations, "World Population Ageing 2013," United Nations, Department of Economic and Social Affairs, Population Division, 2013.

[10] C. Eap, L. Barresi, X. Ohl et al., "Odontoid fractures anterior screw fixation: A continuous series of 36 cases," *Orthopaedics & Traumatology: Surgery & Research*, vol. 96, no. 7, pp. 748–752, 2010.

[11] T. M. Frangen, C. Zilkens, G. Muhr, and C. Schinkel, "Odontoid fractures in the elderly: Dorsal C1/C2 fusion is superior to halo-vest immobilization," *Journal of Trauma - Injury Infection and Critical Care*, vol. 63, no. 1, pp. 83–89, 2007.

[12] P. L. Hénaux, F. Cueff, S. Diabira et al., "Anterior screw fixation of type IIB odontoid fractures in octogenarians," *European Spine Journal*, vol. 21, no. 2, pp. 335–339, 2012.

[13] A. F. Joaquim and A. A. Patel, "Surgical treatment of type II odontoid fractures: anterior odontoid screw fixation or posterior cervical instrumented fusion?" *Neurosurgical Focus*, vol. 38, no. 4, article E11, 2015.

[14] F. P. Ferro, G. D. Borgo, O. B. Letaif, A. F. Cristante, R. M. Marcon, and A. S. Lutaka, "Traumatic spondylolisthesis of the axis: epidemiology, management and outcome," *Acta Ortopédica Brasileira*, vol. 20, no. 2, pp. 84–87, 2012.

[15] R. Al-Mahfoudh, C. Beagrie, E. Woolley et al., "Management of typical and atypical Hangman's fractures," *Global Spine Journal*, vol. 6, no. 3, pp. 248–256, 2016.

[16] A. Patel, R. Zakaria, R. Al-Mahfoudh et al., "Conservative management of type II and III odontoid fractures in the elderly at a regional spine centre: a prospective and retrospective cohort study," *British Journal of Neurosurgery*, vol. 29, no. 2, pp. 249–253, 2015.

[17] C. E. U. Ekong, M. L. Schwartz, C. H. Tator, D. W. Rowed, and V. E. Edmonds, "Odontoid fracture: Management with early mobilization using the halo device," *Neurosurgery*, vol. 9, no. 6, pp. 631–637, 1981.

[18] R. J. Bransford, D. W. Stevens, S. Uyeji, C. Bellabarba, and J. R. Chapman, "Halo vest treatment of cervical spine injuries: A success and survivorship analysis," *The Spine Journal*, vol. 34, no. 15, pp. 1561–1566, 2009.

[19] E. I. Benchimol, L. Smeeth, A. Guttmann et al., "The REporting of studies Conducted using Observational Routinely-collected health Data (RECORD) Statement," *PLoS Medicine*, vol. 12, no. 10, Article ID e1001885, 2015.

[20] J. F. Ludvigsson, E. Andersson, A. Ekbom et al., "External review and validation of the Swedish national inpatient register," *BMC Public Health*, vol. 11, article 450, 2011.

[21] WHO, "Statistical Classification of Diseases and Related Health Problems," 2006, http://www3.who.int/icd/currentversion/fr-icd.htm.

[22] Socialstyrelsen, "Swedish Classification of Operations and Major Procedures," 2004, http://www.socialstyrelsen.se/Publicerat/2004/8608/2004-4-1.htm.

[23] D. Moher, S. Hopewell, K. F. Schulz et al., "CONSORT 2010 explanation and elaboration: updated guidelines for reporting parallel group randomised trials," *British Medical Journal*, vol. 340, article c869, 2010.

[24] M. F. Bergström, L. Byberg, H. Melhus, K. Michaelsson, and R. Gedeborg, "Extent and consequences of misclassified injury diagnoses in a national hospital discharge registry," *Injury Prevention*, vol. 17, no. 2, pp. 108–113, 2011.

[25] R.C.T.R.A.f., A language and environment for statistical, https://www.r-project.org/.

[26] S. C. Bagley, H. White, and B. A. Golomb, "Logistic regression in the medical literature: standards for use and reporting, with particular attention to one medical domain," *Journal of Clinical Epidemiology*, vol. 54, no. 10, pp. 979–985, 2001.

[27] B. I. Woods, J. B. Hohl, B. Braly, W. Donaldson III, J. Kang, and J. Y. Lee, "Mortality in elderly patients following operative and nonoperative management of odontoid fractures," *Journal of Spinal Disorders & Techniques*, vol. 27, no. 6, pp. 321–326, 2014.

[28] M. G. Fehlings, R. Arun, A. R. Vaccaro, P. M. Arnold, J. R. Chapman, and B. Kopjar, "Predictors of treatment outcomes in geriatric patients with odontoid fractures: AOSpine North America multi-centre prospective GOF study," *The Spine Journal*, vol. 38, no. 11, pp. 881–886, 2013.

[29] Y.-M. Ryang, E. Török, I. Janssen et al., "Early Morbidity and Mortality in 50 Very Elderly Patients after Posterior Atlantoaxial Fusion for Traumatic Odontoid Fractures," *World Neurosurgery* vol. 87, pp. 381–391, 2016.

[30] M. R. Konieczny, A. Gstrein, and E. J. Müller, "Treatment algorithm for dens fractures: non-halo immobilization, anterior screw fixation, or posterior transarticular C1-C2 fixation," *The Journal of Bone & Joint Surgery Series A*, vol. 94, no. 19, 2012.

[31] L. Barker, J. Anderson, R. Chesnut, G. Nesbit, T. Tjauw, and R. Hart, "Reliability and reproducibility of dens fracture classification with use of plain radiography and reformatted computer-aided tomography," *The Journal of Bone & Joint Surgery—American Volume*, vol. 88, no. 1, pp. 106–112, 2006.

[32] Y. Dionyssiotis, "Analyzing the problem of falls among older people," *Journal of General Internal Medicine*, vol. 5, pp. 805–813, 2012.

[33] M. E. Tinetti, M. Speechley, and S. F. Ginter, "Risk factors for falls among elderly persons living in the community," *The New England Journal of Medicine*, vol. 319, no. 26, pp. 1701–1707, 1988.

[34] L. Z. Rubenstein, "Falls in older people: epidemiology, risk factors and strategies for prevention," *Age and Ageing*, vol. 35, supplement 2, pp. ii37–ii41, 2006.

[35] O. Health Quality, "Prevention of falls and fall-related injuries in community-dwelling seniors: an evidence-based analysis," *Ontario Health Technology Assessment Series*, vol. 8, no. 2, pp. 1–78, 2008.

[36] M. E. Bravell, S. Berg, B. Malmberg, and G. Sundström, "Sooner or later? A study of institutionalization in late life," *Aging Clinical and Experimental Research*, vol. 21, no. 4-5, pp. 329–337, 2009.

[37] Y. Robinson, A.-L. Robinson, and C. Olerud, "Systematic review on surgical and nonsurgical treatment of type II odontoid fractures in the elderly," *BioMed Research International*, vol. 2014, Article ID 231948, 7 pages, 2014.

[38] J. Kaesmacher, C. Schweizer, A. Valentinitsch et al., "Osteoporosis Is the Most Important Risk Factor for Odontoid Fractures in the Elderly," *Journal of Bone and Mineral Research*, 2017.

[39] T. J. Choma, G. R. Rechtine, R. A. McGuire, and D. S. Brodke, "Treating the aging spine," *Journal of the American Academy of OrthopaedicSurgeons* , vol. 23, no. 12, pp. e91–e100, 2015.

[40] J. Chapman, J. S. Smith, B. Kopjar et al., "The AOSpine North America geriatric odontoid fracture mortality study: A retrospective review of mortality outcomes for operative versus nonoperative treatment of 322 patients with long-term follow-up," *The Spine Journal*, vol. 38, no. 13, pp. 1098–1104, 2013.

[41] S. Majercik, R. Z. Tashjian, W. L. Biffl et al., "Halo vest immobilization in the elderly: A death sentence?" *Journal of Trauma - Injury Infection and Critical Care*, vol. 59, no. 2, pp. 350–357, 2005.

[42] M. L. J. Apuzzo, J. S. Heiden, M. H. Weiss, T. T. Ackerson, J. P. Harvey, and T. Kurze, "Acute fractures of the odontoid process. An analysis of 45 cases," *Journal of Neurosurgery*, vol. 48, no. 1, pp. 85–91, 1978.

[43] D. R. Barlow, B. T. Higgins, E. M. Ozanne, A. N. A. Tosteson, and A. M. Pearson, "Cost effectiveness of operative versus non-operative treatment of geriatric type-II odontoid fracture," *The Spine Journal*, vol. 41, no. 7, pp. 610–617, 2016.

[11] T. M. Frangen, C. Zilkens, G. Muhr, and C. Schinkel, "Odontoid fractures in the elderly: Dorsal C1/C2 fusion is superior to halo-vest immobilization," *Journal of Trauma - Injury Infection and Critical Care*, vol. 63, no. 1, pp. 83–89, 2007.

[12] P. L. Hénaux, F. Cueff, S. Diabira et al., "Anterior screw fixation of type IIB odontoid fractures in octogenarians," *European Spine Journal*, vol. 21, no. 2, pp. 335–339, 2012.

[13] A. F. Joaquim and A. A. Patel, "Surgical treatment of type II odontoid fractures: anterior odontoid screw fixation or posterior cervical instrumented fusion?" *Neurosurgical Focus*, vol. 38, no. 4, article E11, 2015.

[44] P. M. Jonsson, I. Schmidt, V. Sparring, and G. Tomson, "Gender equity in health care in Sweden-Minor improvements since the 1990s," *Health Policy*, vol. 77, no. 1, pp. 24–36, 2006.

[45] K. Pukk, J. Lundberg, R. V. Penaloza-Pesantes, M. Brommels, and F. A. Gaffney, "Do women simply complain more? National patient injury claims data show gender and age differences.," *Quality Management in Healthcare*, vol. 12, no. 4, pp. 225–231, 2003.

[46] S. C. Gale, V. H. Gracias, P. M. Reilly, and C. W. Schwab, "The inefficiency of plain radiography to evaluate the cervical spine after blunt trauma," *The Journal of Trauma and Acute Care Surgery*, vol. 59, no. 5, pp. 1121–1125, 2005.

[47] J. F. Holmes and R. Akkinepalli, "Computed tomography versus plain radiography to screen for cervical spine injury: A meta-analysis," *Journal of Trauma - Injury Infection and Critical Care* vol. 58, no. 5, pp. 902–905, 2005.

Cut-Off Value of Medial Meniscal Extrusion for Knee Pain

Hiroaki Kijima,[1,2] Naohisa Miyakoshi,[1] Yuji Kasukawa,[1] Yoshinori Ishikawa,[1] Hayato Kinoshita,[1] Kentaro Ohuchi,[2] Masazumi Suzuki,[1] Nozomi Kaga,[1] Chie Sato,[2] Shuichi Chida,[1] and Yoichi Shimada[1,2]

[1] *Department of Orthopedic Surgery, Akita University Graduate School of Medicine, 1-1-1 Hondo, Akita 010-8543, Japan*
[2] *Akita Sports, Arthroscopy, and Knee Group (ASAKG), 1-1-1 Hondo, Akita 010-8543, Japan*

Correspondence should be addressed to Hiroaki Kijima; h-kijima@gd5.so-net.ne.jp

Academic Editor: Allen L. Carl

Purpose. Medial meniscal extrusion (MME) has attracted attention as an index of knee pain in conjunction with clinical symptoms that could be more useful than the diagnosis of knee osteoarthritis on X-ray. However, the size of MME that would cause knee pain has not been clarified. The aim of the present study was to investigate the cut-off value of MME for knee pain. *Methods.* A total of 318 knees were evaluated. The presence of current or past knee pain was confirmed by interview. Next, MME was measured using vertical sonographic images of the medial joint spaces during weightbearing. *Results.* Overall, 71 knees were painful (P-group), and 247 knees were not (N-group). MME was 5.9 ± 1.8 mm in the P-group and 2.9 ± 1.5 mm in the N-group ($P < 0.0001$). Analysis of the receiver operating characteristic curve showed that the cut-off value of MME for knee pain was 4.3 mm, with sensitivity of 0.8451 and specificity of 0.8502. In addition, 64% of knees without pain cases at the time of examination whose MME exceeded this cut-off value had past knee pain. *Conclusions.* The sensitivity and specificity of MME for knee pain were very high with a cut-off value of 4.3 mm.

1. Introduction

Knees diagnosed as having osteoarthritis on X-ray or magnetic resonance imaging (MRI) may not have pain. Thus, there is asymptomatic knee osteoarthritis. In addition, there are knees with severe pain and knees with only slight pain, even though they have similar imaging findings. Furthermore, even if imaging indicates knee osteoarthritis, knees without pain are rarely treated.

In recent years, many large-scale epidemiological investigations of knee osteoarthritis have been performed to develop guidelines for the diagnosis and treatment of knee osteoarthritis in order to prevent locomotive syndrome and extend healthy life expectancy, as well as standardize treatment policy [1–4]. Most diagnoses are made based on joint space narrowing or osteophyte formation on X-ray or cartilage evaluation on MRI [5], but, as noted above, these findings on X-ray images or MRI do not correlate with the degree of pain, which is the target of the treatment. Therefore, the results provided by this approach differ from epidemiological investigations of symptomatic knee osteoarthritis targeted for treatment, because imaging investigations include a considerable number of asymptomatic knee osteoarthritis cases.

It is necessary to perform epidemiological investigations of symptomatic knee osteoarthritis to standardize the treatment of knee osteoarthritis and to develop a treatment guideline for knee osteoarthritis. To that end, an index related to the degree of pain of knee osteoarthritis is necessary.

In recent years, two papers have reported that medial meniscal extrusion (MME), which can be measured on ultrasonography, is related to the degree of knee pain [6, 7]. Furthermore, MME has attracted attention as an index related to the clinical symptoms of knee osteoarthritis, unlike the X-ray diagnosis of knee osteoarthritis, which does not relate to the degree of knee pain.

MME is defined as deviation of the medial meniscus medially from the joint. Kenny reported for the first time in 1997 that MME represented decreased meniscal function [8]. Many reports demonstrated that MME participated in the progress of knee osteoarthritis, and it was shown that MME reflected cartilage damage more subtly than X-ray findings [9].

On the other hand, pain in the medial joint space during weightbearing is a representative symptom of knee osteoarthritis, but the cause of the pain has not been clarified. It has been confirmed that MME is greater during weightbearing than during nonweightbearing [10]. The soft tissues around the medial joint space may be stretched by this phenomenon, which may cause the pain of knee osteoarthritis through the affected mechanical receptors. However, the amount of displacement needed to cause pain has not been investigated. If this were to be clarified, epidemiological investigations of knee osteoarthritis that could become symptomatic could be easily performed by ultrasonography.

Therefore, the purpose of this study was to determine the cut-off value of MME for knee pain.

2. Materials and Methods

The bilateral knees (318 knees) of 159 members of the general population who underwent medical examinations in an area where the birthrate is falling and the population is aging were examined. The subjects' average age was 70 years (30–87 years); there were 154 males and 164 females. The subjects lived in a snowy agricultural area of the northeast district of Japan. In this area, medical examinations of the subjects are performed annually.

First, a questionnaire was used to check whether the participants had knee pain at the time of the examination or in the past. In this study, where the pain was located in the knee was not checked. Then, on ultrasonographic vertical images of the medial joint space in extended knees during weightbearing, the displacement length from the medial tibial condyle to the deep layer of the medial collateral ligament of the medial meniscus was measured by ultrasound examination (ACUSON S1000, Siemens Medical Solutions USA, Inc., Ultrasound Division, Mountain View, CA) to evaluate MME. This method of measurement for MME is the same as that of Kawaguchi et al. [10] and of many reports [6, 7]. Since the intraclass correlation coefficients of this method are 0.990 for intraobserver correlation and 0.989 for interobserver correlation [11], it is not necessary to check the intraclass correlation coefficients for MME evaluation with ultrasonography in our institution.

A receiver operating characteristic (ROC) curve for the relationship between pain and the amount of MME was created, and the cut-off value of MME for knee pain was determined as the point of maximal sensitivity and specificity.

Furthermore, the rate of knees with past knee pain without current pain that had MME beyond the cut-off value was compared with that of knees without current pain that had MME less than the cut-off value. The rates of knees with pain in the past were compared between the 2 groups with and without MME beyond the cut-off value using the chi-squared test. Significance was set at $P < 0.05$.

The approval for this study was given by the institutional review board, and an informed consent was obtained from each participant.

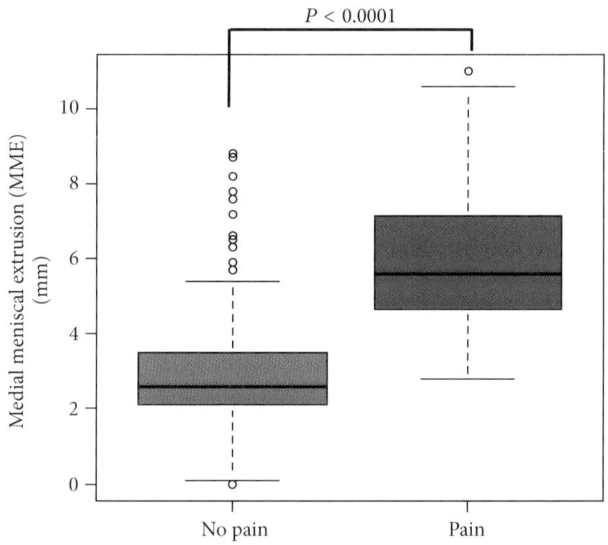

Figure 1: The relationship between medial meniscal extrusion (MME) and knee pain. MME is significantly greater in the P-group (5.9 ± 1.8 mm) than in the N-group (2.9 ± 1.5 mm; Student's t-test, $P < 0.0001$).

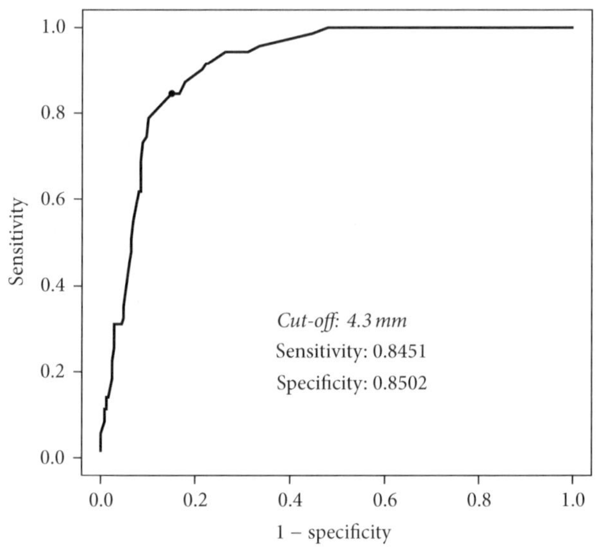

Figure 2: Receiver operating characteristic (ROC) curve of the amount of medial meniscal extrusion (MME) for knee pain. The cut-off value of MME for knee pain is 4.3 mm, with sensitivity of 0.8451 and specificity of 0.8502.

3. Results

The P-group had 26 male knees and 45 female knees, and the N-group had 129 male knees and 118 female knees. A total of 71 knees were painful (P-group) and 247 were not (N-group). MME was significantly greater in the P-group (5.9 ± 1.8 mm) than in the N-group (2.9 ± 1.5 mm; Student's t-test, $P < 0.0001$) (Figure 1).

The MME cut-off value for knee pain was 4.3 mm on ROC curve analysis, with sensitivity of 0.8451 and specificity of 0.8502 (Figure 2). Among the knees without current pain but

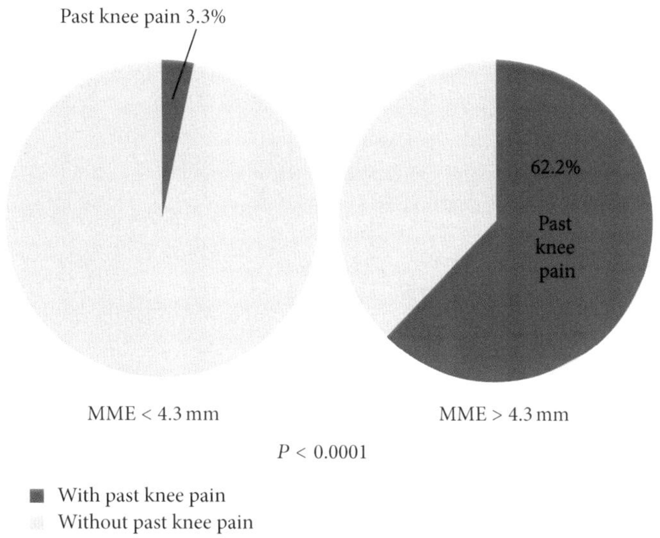

FIGURE 3: Rate of past knee pain in the N-group. In the N-group, the rate of knees with pain in the past among the knees with MME greater than 4.3 mm is significantly larger than that of knees with MME less than 4.3 mm.

with an MME beyond the cut-off value, 62% had a past history of knee pain.

In the N-group, the rate of knees with past knee pain was significantly higher among the knees with MME greater than 4.3 mm than that among the knees with MME less than 4.3 mm (chi-square test, $P < 0.0001$) (Figure 3).

4. Discussion

In this study, the presence of knee pain in the general population and the amount of MME were investigated using ultrasonography. When the MME cut-off value for knee pain was 4.3 mm based on the ROC curve analysis, the sensitivity and specificity were very high.

In the current diagnosis of early osteoarthritis of the knee, MME > 3 mm is one of the standard indices [12, 13]. In the present study, the MME cut-off value for pain was 4.3 mm, which is not very different from the 3.0 mm used for diagnosis.

In recent years, there have been many reports of the evaluation of MME by ultrasonography, and it has been found that MME on ultrasonography can show the progress of knee osteoarthritis, similar to MME evaluation by MRI [7, 10].

Though the evaluation of MME has been done previously by MRI, in the present study, MME was evaluated by ultrasonography, which provides an easy, noninvasive, and inexpensive approach. Furthermore, the evaluation with ultrasonography enables the measurement of MME during weightbearing. Other reports have shown that this method was used for medical examinations of the general population [14]. In addition, the reliability of this method has been demonstrated [11].

The first limitation of this study is that information about the knees other than MME and pain was not investigated, because the subjects were taken from the general population. In other words, knee pain due to injury or knee pain due to inflammatory diseases could not be excluded. Because the evaluation of MME was performed at a specific time point, a longitudinal study is necessary. In the future, it will be necessary to investigate the detailed causes of knee pain in the general population by adding more interview items and by evaluating the synovium with ultrasonography. In addition, by conducting such investigations, we can identify those who have knee pain or who are more likely to have knee pain at an early stage. This study demonstrated that this approach will contribute more efficiently to a longer healthy life expectancy for more persons by facilitating early intervention for their osteoarthritis.

The second limitation of this study is that the height, weight, and body mass index of the subjects were not assessed, though obesity is related to knee osteoarthritis. However, it is expected that MME increases if the subject is heavy because MME was checked during weightbearing in this study. In other words, the MME measurement may be suitable as an index of the pain of knee osteoarthritis, because the factor of weight is already included in the measured MME value.

The third limitation is that the number of subjects was relatively small. Using the results of this study, a larger-scale investigation of the relationships between MME and knee pain should be performed. By doing so, it will be possible to investigate in greater detail the relationship between past knee pain and MME, which became clear in this study. It may also help elucidate the natural relief mechanism of knee pain in osteoarthritis, and it may lead to the development of new therapies for knee osteoarthritis.

The final limitation of this study is that the reason for knee pain with large MME is not known. MME is greater with weightbearing than with nonweightbearing [10]. Therefore, during weightbearing, MME causes stretching of soft tissues around the medial joint space. This may cause the knee pain around the medial joint space during weightbearing, which is the key symptom of knee osteoarthritis. However, a tear (posterior horn in particular) of the medial meniscus, considered to be a cause of MME [15], may in itself be the cause of the knee pain.

However, from the results of the present study, it became clear that the amount of MME, which could be noninvasively investigated in several seconds with ultrasonography, was related to knee pain. Thus, it is now easy to conduct a large-scale epidemiological investigation to identify symptomatic knee osteoarthritis that should receive treatment with this method, instead of epidemiological investigations of knee osteoarthritis using only conventional imaging. In addition, the results of the current study help us better understand the mechanism of knee pain in osteoarthritis.

5. Conclusions

The MME cut-off value for knee pain was 4.3 mm based on ROC curve analysis, with sensitivity of 0.8451 and specificity of 0.8502.

Disclosure

The funding source did not have any role in the study design, collection, analysis, and interpretation of data; in the writing of the manuscript; and in the decision to submit the manuscript for publication. This research was presented in the 11th Biennial ISAKOS (International Society of Arthroscopy, Knee Surgery and Orthopaedic Sports Medicine) Congress in Shanghai, China.

Acknowledgments

This research was supported by Japan Orthopaedics and Traumatology Research Foundation, Inc., Grant no. 278.

References

[1] N. Yoshimura, S. Muraki, H. Oka, H. Kawaguchi, K. Nakamura, and T. Akune, "Association of knee osteoarthritis with the accumulation of metabolic risk factors such as overweight, hypertension, dyslipidemia, and impaired glucose tolerance in Japanese men and women: The ROAD study," *Journal of Rheumatology*, vol. 38, no. 5, pp. 921–930, 2011.

[2] N. Yoshimura, S. Muraki, H. Oka, H. Kawaguchi, K. Nakamura, and T. Akune, "Cohort profile: Research on osteoarthritis/osteoporosis against disability study," *International Journal of Epidemiology*, vol. 39, no. 4, Article ID dyp276, pp. 988–995, 2009.

[3] S. Muraki, H. Oka, T. Akune et al., "Prevalence of radiographic knee osteoarthritis and its association with knee pain in the elderly of Japanese population-based cohorts: The ROAD study," *Osteoarthritis and Cartilage*, vol. 17, no. 9, pp. 1137–1143, 2009.

[4] H. Oka, S. Muraki, T. Akune et al., "Fully automatic quantification of knee osteoarthritis severity on plain radiographs," *Osteoarthritis and Cartilage*, vol. 16, no. 11, pp. 1300–1306, 2008.

[5] S. Muraki, T. Akune, Y. En-yo et al., "Joint space narrowing, body mass index, and knee pain: The ROAD study (OAC1839R1)," *Osteoarthritis and Cartilage*, vol. 23, no. 6, pp. 874–881, 2015.

[6] H. Kijima, S. Yamada, K. Nozaka, H. Saito, and Y. Shimada, "Relationship between Pain and Medial Meniscal Extrusion in Knee Osteoarthritis," *Advances in Orthopedics*, vol. 2015, Article ID 210972, 2015.

[7] S. Yanagisawa, T. Ohsawa, K. Saito et al., "Population-based study of the relationship between medial meniscus radial displacement, determined by use of ultrasound screening, and knee pain," *Journal of Orthopaedic Science*, vol. 19, no. 6, pp. 954–958, 2014.

[8] C. Kenny, "Radial displacement of the medial meniscus and Fairbank's signs," *Clinical Orthopaedics and Related Research*, no. 339, pp. 163–173, 1997.

[9] G. Ohi, M. Kimura, H. Asagumo, S. Kanbayashi, A. Kobayashi, and M. Taki, "The relation between radial displacement of medial meniscus and grade of chondral lesion in early osteoarthritis of the knee," *East Japan Journal of Orthopaedic and Traumatology*, vol. 18, pp. 155–159, 2006.

[10] K. Kawaguchi, M. Enokida, R. Otsuki, and R. Teshima, "Ultrasonographic evaluation of medial radial displacement of the medial meniscus in knee osteoarthritis," *Arthritis and Rheumatism*, vol. 64, no. 1, pp. 173–180, 2012.

[11] T. Aki, A. Takahashi, M. Kashiwaba, N. Yamamoto, M. Kamimura, and E. Itoi, "Quantitative evaluation for the medial meniscal extrusion using ultrasonography," *Tohoku J Orthop Traumatol*, vol. 56, pp. 55–59, 2013.

[12] T. Magee, M. Shapiro, and D. Williams, "Prevalence of Meniscal Radial Tears of the Knee Revealed by MRI after Surgery," *American Journal of Roentgenology*, vol. 182, no. 4, pp. 931–936, 2004.

[13] S.-I. Bin, T.-W. Jeong, S.-J. Kim, and D.-H. Lee, "A new arthroscopic classification of degenerative medial meniscus root tear that correlates with meniscus extrusion on magnetic resonance imaging," *Knee*, vol. 23, no. 2, pp. 246–250, 2016.

[14] S. Yanagisawa, T. Ohsawa, K. Saito, T. Kobayashi, A. Yamamoto, and K. Takagishi, "Morphological evaluation and diagnosis of medial type osteoarthritis of the knee using ultrasound," *Journal of Orthopaedic Science*, vol. 19, no. 2, pp. 270–274, 2014.

[15] N. Gomi, K. Chikami, H. Nakamizo, T. Mashiba, S. Mori, and T. Yamamoto, "Relationship between a torn posterior horn of a medial meniscus and OA progression," *Arthroscopy Society Magazine Guidance & Contribution Rules*, vol. 31, pp. 23–28, 2006.

21

Intraoperative Disinfection by Pulse Irrigation with Povidone-Iodine Solution in Spine Surgery

Vincenzo De Luna, Federico Mancini, Fernando De Maio, Gabriele Bernardi, Ernesto Ippolito, and Roberto Caterini

Department of Orthopaedic Surgery, University of Rome Tor Vergata, Viale Oxford 81, 00133 Rome, Italy

Correspondence should be addressed to Gabriele Bernardi; bernardi.gab@gmail.com

Academic Editor: Allen L. Carl

Background. Deep wound infection in spine surgery is a debilitating complication for patients and increases costs. The objective of this prospective study was to evaluate the efficacy of wound pulse irrigation with a dilute povidone-iodine solution in the prevention of surgical site infection. *Methods.* 50 patients undergoing spinal surgery were randomly divided into two groups (A and B) of 25 patients each. In group A, wounds were irrigated with dilute (3%) povidone-iodine solution through a low-pressure pulsatile device. In group B, wounds were irrigated with saline solution through a bulb syringe. In both groups, specimens for bacterial culture were harvested from surgical site before and after irrigation. *Results.* In group A, no surgical site infection occurred; in group B, deep wound infection was observed in 3 patients. In both groups, before irrigation some cultures have been found positive for bacterial contamination. *Conclusion.* Our study seems to support the idea that low-pressure pulsating lavage of surgical wounds with povidone-iodine diluted to a nontoxic concentration of 3% is an effective therapeutic adjunct measure to prevent surgical site infection in spine surgery. However, the number of the enrolled patients is small and a significant statistical analysis is not practicable. This trial is registered with NCT03249363.

1. Introduction

Surgical site infection (SSI) in spine surgery is a serious complication in terms of healthy status of the patient, clinical outcome, and cost for the community. SSI in spine surgery usually requires prolonged antibiotic therapy and one or more surgical debridement operations that can aggravate patient morbidity. The causes of SSI are multifactorial, and they comprise patient and procedure specific risks. According to the best evidenced studies, well summarized by Schuster et al. [1], age (>60 years), diabetes, malnutrition, obesity, ASA score ≥ 3, higher glucose level, transfusions, posterior approach, and duration of surgery are the preoperative and intraoperative risk factors in spine surgery for which a statistically significant association with SSI has been reported. In 1991, the National Nosocomial Infections Surveillance System (NNIS) introduced Infection Risk Index (IRI) to monitor trends in infections and risk factors [2]. It permitted comparing the infection rates, considering the confounding factors secondary to the different types of surgery, to the risk of endogenous contamination and to the general clinical aspect of the patient. It was developed to predict a surgical patient's risk of acquiring a surgical wound infection with an index score ranging from 0 to 3 (Table 1).

Use of perioperative antibiotic treatment has been well supported by retrospective studies and randomized trials, and it should be utilized in any patients undergoing spine surgery [3–6]. However, despite antibiotic prophylaxis, studies on adult and on children report an overall infection rate ranging from 0.4% to 20% after spinal surgery [7–11]. In addition to antibiotic prophylaxis, many perioperative adjuncts have been used to reduce infection rates in spine surgery but few studies, with a low level of evidence, have been published on these measures [12–20]. The most utilized adjunct measures for preventing postoperative SSI are wound irrigation with povidone-iodine (PVP-I) or hydrogen peroxide and saline solution, silver impregnated dressing, closed wound suction drainage, and use of an ultraclean

Table 1: IRI score.

National Nosocomial Infections Surveillance
ASA Score
1-2: 0 points
3-4: 1 point
Duration of surgery
<75%: 0 points
>75%*: 1 point
Wound class
I-II**: 0 points
III-IV***: 1 point

*Above the threshold value of duration for that category of surgery (239 minutes); **clean, clean/contaminated; ***contaminated, dirty/infected; IRI: Infection Risk Index; ASA score + duration of surgery + wound class = IRI score.

air technology in the operating room. With regard to these measures in spinal surgery, the literature has shown a "moderate," "low," or "very low" level of evidence to support their efficacy in reducing the infection rate [13, 14]. PVP-I is often used as a surgical scrub and for antiseptic prophylaxis in open wounds and treatment of superficial and deep infections. The antiseptic function of PVP-I is characterized by a complex of polyvinylpyrrilidine and triiodine ions that acts against cell walls and inhibits the release of pathogenic factors, even of highly resistant microbiological organism [15, 16]. In a dilution of 1:25 to 1:200 (0.5–4% Poviderm), it has been considered, compared to other irrigating fluids such as soap, antibiotics, and chlorhexidine, the one with the greatest bactericidal efficacy and the lowest cell toxicity [21–23]. Often in orthopaedic surgery, PVP-I solution is utilized through a pulsatile irrigation device which combines irrigation lavage or pulsatile debridement technique with rapid suction removal of effluent. Many authors consider pulsed lavage more effective than bulb syringe in wound irrigation [24–26].

The purpose of this study was to evaluate the efficacy, in preventing SSI, of intraoperative pulsatile irrigation with a 2000 ml saline solution of PVP-iodine in a group of patients undergoing complex spine surgery with a posterior approach. To confirm and better assess the efficacy of intraoperative irrigation, specimens for bacterial culture were harvested by swabs from muscular tissue before and after irrigation of the wounds.

2. Materials and Methods

This is a single-center prospective cohort study of a total of 50 consecutive patients (20 males, 30 females; mean age of 41.7 years), operated from 2010 to 2012 for scoliosis. None of the patients showed clinical signs of infection before surgery, and for all of them it was the primary spinal surgery procedure. Operative treatments included 50 instrumented arthrodeses for scoliosis (21 degenerative, 27 idiopathic, and 2 congenital). All the surgeries were performed through posterior central surgical access with a length of skin incision ranged from 37 to 52 cm. Hardware and autologous bone graft (local bone and iliac crest bone) was added in all the patients to stabilize the vertebral segments. Before surgery, we assigned an Infection Risk Index (IRI score) to each patient (Table 1). Every patient received antibiotic prophylaxis (1000 mg of cefazolin i.v.) 1 hour before surgery which was repeated every 3 hours during surgery, and the same dose 2 times/die for at least 48 hours was received until suction drainage removal. Before surgical incision, the skin was disinfected and prepared as usual, utilizing Poviderm solution, sterile drapes, sterile clothes, and gloves. Before surgery we randomly divided this group of 50 patients into two groups of 25 patients each: group A (11 males, 14 females; mean age 41.4 years) and group B (9 males, 16 females; mean age 42.1 years). In group A, before applying the bone graft, low-pressure irrigation (Bio Pulse, Leader Medica) with PVP-I diluted to a 3% concentration (30 g/l) in 2 litres of saline for between 5 and 10 minutes was performed and then washed out by 1 litre of sodium chloride solution through a pulse irrigation device. In group B, low-pressure irrigation with 2 litres of saline solution for between 5 and 10 minutes was performed before applying bone graft. Before and after pulsatile irrigation with diluted PVP-I in group A and before and after pulsatile irrigation with saline solution in group B, we obtained samples for bacterial cultures from muscular tissue in order to better evaluate the antimicrobial action of the solutions utilized in the 2 groups. The culture was made on blood agar plates for a sufficient number of days to allow for bacterial growth. Using the 2009 Centers for Disease Control and Prevention National Health Safety Network criteria [27], we clinically defined the presence of infected cases, and both superficial and deep SSIs were included. According to these criteria, superficial SSI occurred within 30 days after surgery and involves only the skin and the subcutaneous tissue of the incision, while deep SSI occurred within 30 days after surgery if no hardware is implanted or within 1 year if hardware is present and the infection seems to be related to operative procedure and involves deep soft tissue of the incision. SSI was detected if positive cultures and clinical signs of infection were found [27, 28].

The statistical analysis was not significant (p value = 0.235 by Fisher exact test).

3. Results

Groups A and B were homogenous regarding sex, age, and Infection Risk Index score. The duration of surgery above the 75th percentile (> of 239 minutes) (Table 2) was common to all patients. In group A, 19 had risk index score grade I and 6, grade II; in group B, 18 had risk index score grade I and 7, grade II. In group A, no infections were diagnosed despite the fact that the first samples obtained by swabs from muscular tissue, before performing intraoperative pulse irrigation, were found positive for wound contamination in 4 of the 25 patients (*Staphylococcus epidermidis* in 1, *Enterococcus faecalis* in 2, and *Escherichia coli* in 1). However, the microbiological cultures on the second samples obtained after the PVP-I and saline pulse irrigation did not confirm the contamination and did not show any bacterial growth (Table 3). In group B, we diagnosed 3 deep wound infections (6% of the entire cohort) ($p < 0.05$). In the infected wounds,

Table 2: List of two-subgroup patients' age, sex, spine pathology, kind of treatment, IRI score, ASA, duration of surgery, wound class, and wound infection.

(a)

Group A (PVP-I pulse irrigation)	Sex	Age	Spine pathology	ASA score	Wound class	Duration of surgery	IRI score	Wound infection
(1)	M	19	AIS	0	0	1	I	No
(2)	M	59	DS	0	0	1	I	No
(3)	F	40	AIS	0	0	1	I	No
(4)	M	30	AIS	0	0	1	I	No
(5)	F	68	DS	0	0	1	I	No
(6)	M	70	DS	0	0	1	I	No
(7)	F	39	AIS	0	0	1	I	No
(8)	F	50	AIS	0	0	1	I	No
(9)	F	70	DS	1	0	1	II	No
(10)	M	44	AIS	0	0	1	I	No
(11)	M	75	DS	1	0	1	II	No
(12)	F	61	AIS	0	0	1	I	No
(13)	F	20	AIS	0	0	1	I	No
(14)	F	66	DS	1	0	1	II	No
(15)	F	59	DS	1	0	1	II	No
(16)	M	14	IS	0	0	1	I	No
(17)	M	62	DS	1	0	1	II	No
(18)	F	14	IS	0	0	1	I	No
(19)	M	38	AIS	0	0	1	I	No
(20)	F	13	IS	0	0	1	I	No
(21)	F	13	CS	0	0	1	I	No
(22)	F	15	IS	0	0	1	I	No
(23)	M	27	AIS	0	0	1	I	No
(24)	F	16	IS	0	0	1	I	No
(25)	M	54	DS	0	0	1	II	No

(b)

Group B (saline pulse irrigation)	Sex	Age	Spine pathology	ASA score	Wound class	Duration of surgery	IRI score	Wound infection
(1)	M	62	DS	0	0	1	I	No
(2)	F	51	AIS	0	0	1	I	No
(3)	M	46	DS	0	0	1	I	No
(4)	M	29	AIS	0	0	1	I	No
(5)	F	63	DS	1	0	1	II	Yes *E. coli*
(6)	F	20	AIS	0	0	1	I	Yes *E. coli*
(7)	F	21	AIS	0	0	1	I	No
(8)	F	71	DS	1	0	1	II	Yes *S. aureus*
(9)	M	60	DS	0	0	1	I	No
(10)	F	42	AIS	0	0	1	I	No
(11)	F	40	AIS	0	0	1	I	No
(12)	M	65	DS	0	0	1	I	No
(13)	F	73	DS	1	0	1	II	No
(14)	F	48	DS	1	0	1	II	No
(15)	F	50	DS	1	0	1	II	No

(b) Continued.

Group B (saline pulse irrigation)	Sex	Age	Spine pathology	ASA score	Wound class	Duration of surgery	IRI score	Wound infection
(16)	F	15	CS	0	0	1	I	No
(17)	M	27	AIS	0	0	1	I	No
(18)	M	41	AIS	0	0	1	I	No
(19)	F	66	DS	1	0	1	II	No
(20)	M	59	DS	1	0	1	II	No
(21)	F	17	IS	0	0	1	I	No
(22)	F	18	AIS	0	0	1	I	No
(23)	M	28	AIS	0	0	1	I	No
(24)	F	27	AIS	0	0	1	I	No
(25)	F	13	IS	0	0	1	I	No

AIS: adult idiopathic scoliosis, DS: degenerative scoliosis, IS: idiopathic scoliosis, and CS: congenital scoliosis.

we isolated *Escherichia coli* in 2 cases and *Staphylococcus aureus* in 1 case (Table 2). However in group B the samples before and after saline irrigation were positive in 4 cases *(2 Escherichia coli, 1 Staphylococcus aureus, and 1 Staphylococcus epidermidis)* (Table 3) but three of them (cases number 5, 6, and 8) developed SSI, while the case contaminated by *Staphylococcus epidermidis* (patient no. 1) did not develop clinical signs of wound infection in spite of previous wound contamination. At clinical presentation and after laboratory tests, all the infected patients were treated with surgical debridement, PVP-I and saline pulse irrigation, and at least 3 months of antibiotic therapy. The hardware was removed only in 1 of the infected patients, after the failure of the first surgical debridement (patient no. 6 in group B). At 2 years of follow-up after SSI treatment, we registered no signs of wound infection in any of these patients.

4. Discussion

Nowadays, postsurgical infections are becoming a serious problem also in developed countries as well for two main reasons: bacterium resistance to antibiotics and an increase in the number of surgical procedures. In the last 20 years, the number of spinal surgery procedures has increased and, although some of them are performed through minimally invasive technics, the risk of wound contamination and infection is still elevated and represents a very debilitating complication for the patient, with an increase of costs [29–33].

In a systematic review on the influence of perioperative risk factors and therapeutic interventions on infection rates after spine surgery, Schuster et al. [1] concluded that the causes of SSI are multifactorial and related to a complex interplay of patient and procedural influences.

As we found in our series of spinal operations, the risk was higher in patients with an IRI score > 0 (duration of surgery > 75% and ASA score > 2). In our patients, the ASA score was never more than 1, demonstrating a cohort in relative good general condition, while the index influencing infection risk was mostly the duration of surgery, always more than 4 hours (>75%). This correlation in increasing the risk of SSI was already underlined by Shiono et al. [34] with a study where they found that the probability of contamination by skin bacteria increases with the duration of surgery.

Povidone-iodine is an antiseptic agent with bactericidal activity against most pathogens including methicillin-resistant *Staphylococcus aureus* (MRSA) [35–38]. Cheng et al. [14] prospectively investigated 414 spinal surgery patients and compared wounds irrigated with PVP-I solution (3.5% concentration) to wounds irrigated with saline solution. They reported 0% infection rate in the PVP-I group and 3.4% of infection rate in the saline irrigated wounds (0.5% superficial infections and 2.9% deep infections).

Regarding cytotoxic effects of PVP-I, Kaysinger et al. [39] reported that the inhibitory effect of PVP-I on tibia and osteoblast cells isolated from embryonic chicks is significant only after exposure to concentrations of 5% betadine or higher. Recently Van Meurs et al. [40] in an in vitro study on antiseptic solutions for intraoperative irrigation reported that only diluted povidone-iodine was bactericidal at a concentration where some cell viability remained. They concluded that PVP-I diluted to a concentration of 1.3 g/l could be the optimal antiseptic for intraoperative irrigation.

In our study surgical wounds have been irrigated with PVP-I diluted to a 3% concentration (30 g/l) in normal saline solution, utilizing a pulsatile device. Experimental studies suggest that irrigation with high-pressure or low-pressure lavage may be effective for removing bacteria from contaminated wounds, but some studies have reported that high-pressure lavage can damage the bone and the surrounding soft tissues [26, 41–43]. In our patients, to reduce the risk of tissue damage, we opted for a low-pressure lavage in accordance with the result reported by Petrisor et al. [43], who examined "surgeons preferences in the initial management of open fracture wounds."

The aim of our study was to prospectively evaluate the effect of wound irrigation with PVP-I and saline solution through a pulsatile device for the prevention of SSI after long-duration instrumented spinal surgery.

In group A samples obtained before pulse irrigation with Poviderm, we observed 4 cases of wound contamination, but

Table 3: List of two-group patients' IRI score and wound contamination.

(a)

Group A (PVP-I pulse irrigation)	Infection index risk	Wound contamination (before pulse irrigation)	Wound contamination (after pulse irrigation)
(1)	I	Yes *(Staphylococcus epidermidis)*	No
(2)	I		
(3)	I		
(4)	I		
(5)	I		
(6)	I	Yes *(Enterococcus faecalis)*	No
(7)	I		
(8)	I	Yes *(Escherichia coli)*	No
(9)	II		
(10)	I		
(11)	II		
(12)	I		
(13)	I		
(14)	II	Yes *(Escherichia coli)*	No
(15)	II		
(16)	I		
(17)	II		
(18)	I		
(19)	I		
(20)	I		
(21)	I		
(22)	I		
(23)	I		
(24)	I		
(25)	II		

(b)

Group B (saline irrigation)	Infection index risk	Wound contamination (before pulse irrigation)	Wound contamination (after pulse irrigation)
(1)	I	Yes *(Staphylococcus epidermidis)*	Yes *(Staphylococcus epidermidis)*
(2)	I		
(3)	I		
(4)	I		
(5)	II	Yes *(Escherichia coli)*	Yes *(Escherichia coli)*
(6)	I	Yes *(Escherichia coli)*	Yes *(Escherichia coli)*
(7)	I		
(8)	II	Yes *(Staphylococcus aureus)*	Yes *(Staphylococcus aureus)*
(9)	I		
(10)	I		
(11)	I		
(12)	I		
(13)	II		
(14)	II		
(15)	II		
(16)	I		

(b) Continued.

Group B (saline irrigation)	Infection index risk	Wound contamination (before pulse irrigation)	Wound contamination (after pulse irrigation)
(17)	I		
(18)	I		
(19)	II		
(20)	II		
(21)	I		
(22)	I		
(23)	I		
(24)	I		
(25)	I		

no patient developed clinical signs of infection. On the other hand, when irrigation without PVP-I has been performed, wound contamination was present in 4 group B cases as well, but 3 (12%) of them developed SSI ($p = 0.235$).

However, contaminated surgical wounds do not always develop clinical signs of infection and patients with negative intraoperative cultures can develop postoperative infection [33, 34, 44]; in our series 3 wound infections have been diagnosed when PVP-I was not used and zero wound infections have been diagnosed when pulse irrigation with povidone-iodine has been performed.

5. Conclusions

In conclusion, it is clear that the causes of perioperative SSI are multifactorial, and they include specific patients and procedure risks. Because some of the risk factors are not modifiable, it is essential to maintain sterility during surgical procedure. Carefulness in wound sterility can be accomplished by the administration of pre- and intraoperative antibiotics and by the application of adjunct measures, such as PVP-I pulse irrigation. Although our cohort was homogeneous regarding general condition, mean age, surgical approach and technics, and duration of surgery, 8 cases were contaminated before wound closure; however, only 3 patients, not treated by PVP-I, developed SSI.

To the best of our knowledge, this is the first study that also uses bacterial cultures of samples obtained from the surgical site in order to show the efficacy of this adjunct method in preventing the risk of SSI.

This study can contribute to increasing the evidence of other available studies, by asserting that in order to reduce the risk of postoperative wound infection, pulse irrigation with dilute PVP-I and saline solution can be useful. However the number of the enrolled patients is small and a significant statistical analysis is not practicable; an additional study with a new group of patients is necessary to confirm these tantalizing preliminary results.

Ethical Approval

All procedures performed in studies involving human participants were in accordance with the ethical standards of the institutional and/or national research committee and with the 1964 Helsinki Declaration and its later amendments or comparable ethical standards.

References

[1] J. M. Schuster, G. Rechtine, D. C. Norvell, and J. R. Dettori, "The influence of perioperative risk factors and therapeutic interventions on infection rates after spine surgery: A systematic review," *Spine*, vol. 35, pp. S125–S137, 2010.

[2] National Nosocomial Infections Surveillance System, "National Nosocomial Infections Surveillance (NNIS) System Report, data summary from January 1992 through June 2004, issued October 2004," *American Journal of Infection Control*, vol. 32, no. 8, pp. 470–485, 2004.

[3] W. C. Watters III, J. Baisden, C. M. Bono et al., "Antibiotic prophylaxis in spine surgery: an evidence-based clinical guideline for the use of prophylactic antibiotics in spine surgery," *Spine Journal*, vol. 9, no. 2, pp. 142–146, 2009.

[4] F. G. Barker II, "Efficacy of prophylactic antibiotic therapy in spinal surgery: a meta-analysis," *Neurosurgery*, vol. 51, no. 2, pp. 391–401, 2002.

[5] R. F. Young and P. M. Lawner, "Perioperative antibiotic prophylaxis for prevention of postoperative neurosurgical infections. A randomized clinical trial," *Journal of Neurosurgery*, vol. 66, no. 5, pp. 701–705, 1987.

[6] D. W. Bratzler, E. P. Dellinger, K. M. Olsen et al., "Clinical practice guidelines for antimicrobial prophylaxis in surgery," *The American Journal of Health-System Pharmacy*, vol. 70, no. 3, pp. 195–283, 2013.

[7] C. A. Sansur, J. S. Smith, J. D. Coe et al., "Scoliosis research society morbidity and mortality of adult scoliosis surgery," *Spine*, vol. 36, no. 9, pp. E593–E597, 2011.

[8] C. Ho, D. J. Sucato, and B. S. Richards, "Risk factors for the development of delayed infections following posterior spinal fusion and instrumentation in adolescent idiopathic scoliosis patients," *Spine*, vol. 32, no. 20, pp. 2272–2277, 2007.

[9] A. I. Tsirikos, G. Lipton, W.-N. Chang, K. W. Dabney, and F. Miller, "Surgical correction of scoliosis in pediatric patients with cerebral palsy using the unit rod instrumentation," *Spine*, vol. 33, no. 10, pp. 1133–1140, 2008.

[10] P. D. Sponseller, "Pediatric revision spinal deformity surgery: Issues and complications," *Spine*, vol. 35, no. 25, pp. 2205–2210, 2010.

[11] P. D. Sponseller, D. M. LaPorte, M. W. Hungerford, K. Eck, K. H. Bridwell, and L. G. Lenke, "Deep wound infections after neuromuscular scoliosis surgery: a multicenter study of risk factors and treatment outcomes," *Spine*, vol. 25, no. 19, pp. 2461–2466, 2000.

[12] N. E. Epstein, "Do silver-impregnated dressings limit infections after lumbar laminectomy with instrumented fusion?" *Surgical Neurology*, vol. 68, no. 5, pp. 483–485, 2007.

[13] F.-Y. Chang, M.-C. Chang, S.-T. Wang, W.-K. Yu, C.-L. Liu, and T.-H. Chen, "Can povidone-iodine solution be used safely in a spinal surgery?" *European Spine Journal*, vol. 15, no. 6, pp. 1005–1014, 2006.

[14] M.-T. Cheng, M.-C. Chang, S.-T. Wang, W.-K. Yu, C.-L. Liu, and T.-H. Chen, "Efficacy of dilute betadine solution irrigation in the prevention of postoperative infection of spinal surgery," *Spine*, vol. 30, no. 15, pp. 1689–1693, 2005.

[15] M. F. Gruenberg, G. L. Campaner, C. A. Sola, and E. G. Ortolan, "Ultraclean air for prevention of postoperative infection after posterior spinal fusion with instrumentation: A comparison between surgeries performed with and without a vertical exponential filtered air-flow system," *Spine*, vol. 29, no. 20, pp. 2330–2334, 2004.

[16] S. E. Çelik and A. Kara, "Does Shaving the Incision Site Increase the Infection Rate After Spinal Surgery?" *Spine*, vol. 32, no. 15, pp. 1575–1577, 2007.

[17] D. M. Rogers, G. S. Blouin, and J. P. O'Leary, "Povidone-iodine wound irrigation and wound sepsis," *Surg Gynecol Obstet*, vol. 157, pp. 426–430, 1983.

[18] T. Ahl, N. Dalen, H. Jörbeck, and J. Hobom, "Air contamination during hip and knee arthroplasties: Horizontal laminar flow randomized vs. Conventional ventilation," *Acta Orthopaedica*, vol. 66, no. 1, pp. 17–20, 1995.

[19] C. Brandt, U. Hott, D. Sohr, F. Daschner, P. Gastmeier, and H. Rüden, "Operating room ventilation with laminar airflow shows no protective effect on the surgical site infection rate in orthopedic and abdominal surgery," *Annals of Surgery*, vol. 248, no. 5, pp. 695–700, 2008.

[20] A. G. Christodoulou, P. Givissis, P. D. Symeonidis, D. Karataglis, and J. Pournaras, "Reduction of postoperative spinal infections based on an etiologic protocol," *Clinical Orthopaedics and Related Research*, no. 444, pp. 107–113, 2006.

[21] J. Viljanto, "Disinfection of Surgical Wounds Without Inhibition of Normal Wound Healing," *Archives of Surgery*, vol. 115, no. 3, pp. 253–256, 1980.

[22] W. Lineaweaver, S. McMorris, D. Soucy, and R. Howard, "Cellular and bacterial toxicities of topical antimicrobials," *Plastic and Reconstructive Surgery*, vol. 75, no. 3, pp. 394–396, 1985.

[23] D. J. Crowley, N. K. Kanakaris, and P. V. Giannoudis, "Irrigation of the wounds in open fractures," *Journal of Bone and Joint Surgery - Series B*, vol. 89, no. 5, pp. 580–585, 2007.

[24] J. O. Anglen, "Wound Irrigation in Musculoskeletal Injury," *Journal of the American Academy of Orthopaedic Surgeons*, vol. 9, no. 4, pp. 219–226, 2001.

[25] S. N. Bhhaskar, D. E. Cutright, E. E. Runsuck, and A. Gross, "Pulsating water jet devices in debridement of combat wounds.," *Military Medicine*, vol. 136, no. 3, pp. 264–266, 1971.

[26] L. L. Brown, H. T. Shelton, G. H. Bornside, and I. Cohn Jr., "Evaluation of wound irrigation by pulsatile jet and conventional methods," *Annals of Surgery*, vol. 187, no. 2, pp. 170–173, 1978.

[27] D. H. Culver, T. C. Horan, R. P. Gaynes et al., "Surgical wound infection rates by wound class, operative procedure, and patient risk index. National Nosocomial Infections Surveillance System," *The American Journal of Medicine*, vol. 91, no. 3, pp. S152–S157, 1991.

[28] W. R. Jarvis, J. R. Edwards, and D. H. Culver, "Nosocomial infection rates in adult and pediatric intensive care units in the United States," *The American Journal of Medicine*, vol. 91, no. 3, supplement 2, pp. S185–S191, 1991.

[29] K. S. Kaye, D. J. Anderson, R. Sloane et al., "The effect of surgical site infection on older operative patients," *Journal of the American Geriatrics Society*, vol. 57, no. 1, pp. 46–54, 2009.

[30] M. J. Mcgirt, S. L. Parker, J. Lerner, L. Engelhart, T. Knight, and M. Y. Wang, "Comparative analysis of perioperative surgical site infection after minimally invasive versus open posterior/transforaminal lumbar interbody fusion: analysis of hospital billing and discharge data from 5170 patients—clinical article," *Journal of Neurosurgery: Spine*, vol. 14, no. 6, pp. 771–778, 2011.

[31] W. P. Weber, M. Zwahlen, S. Reck et al., "Economic burden of surgical site infections at a European university hospital," *Infection Control and Hospital Epidemiology*, vol. 29, no. 7, pp. 623–629, 2008.

[32] R. R. Calderone, D. E. Garland, D. A. Capen, and H. Oster, "Cost of medical care for postoperative spinal infections," *The Orthopedic Clinics of North America*, pp. 27–171, 1996.

[33] E. N. Perencevich, K. E. Sands, S. E. Cosgrove, E. Guadagnoli, E. Meara, and R. Platt, "Health and economic impact of surgical site infections diagnosed after hospital discharge," *Emerging Infectious Diseases*, vol. 9, no. 2, pp. 196–203, 2003.

[34] Y. Shiono, K. Watanabe, N. Hosogane et al., "Sterility of posterior elements of the spine in posterior correction surgery," *Spine*, vol. 37, no. 6, pp. 523–526, 2012.

[35] P. D. Goldenheim, "In vitro efficacy of povidone-iodine solution and cream against methicillin-resistant Staphylococcus aureus," *Postgraduate Medical Journal*, vol. 69, no. 3, pp. S62–S65, 1993.

[36] R. L. R. Hill and M. W. Casewell, "The in-vitro activity of povidone-iodinecream against Staphylococcus aureus and its bioavailability in nasal secretions," *Journal of Hospital Infection*, vol. 45, no. 3, pp. 198–205, 2000.

[37] A. R. McLure and J. Gordon, "In-vitro evaluation of povidone-iodine and chlorhexidine against methicillin-resistant Staphylococcus aureus," *Journal of Hospital Infection*, vol. 21, no. 4, pp. 291–299, 1992.

[38] C. Block, E. Robenshtok, A. Simhon, and M. Shapiro, "Evaluation of chlorhexidine and povidone iodine activity against methicillin-resistant Staphylococcus aureus and vancomycin-resistant Enterococcus faecalis using a surface test," *Journal of Hospital Infection*, vol. 46, no. 2, pp. 147–152, 2000.

[39] K. K. Kaysinger, N. C. Nicholson, W. K. Ramp, and J. F. Kellam, "Toxic effects of wound irrigation solutions on cultured tibiae and osteoblasts," *Journal of Orthopaedic Trauma*, vol. 9, no. 4, pp. 303–311, 1995.

[40] S. J. Van Meurs, D. Gawlitta, K. A. Heemstra, R. W. Poolman, H. C. Vogely, and M. C. Kruyt, "Selection of an optimal antiseptic solution for intraoperative irrigation: An in vitro study," *Journal of Bone and Joint Surgery - Series A*, vol. 96, no. 4, pp. 285–291, 2014.

[41] M. Bhandari, E. H. Schemitsch, A. Adili, R. J. Lachowski, and S. G. Shaughnessy, "High and low pressure pulsatile lavage of contaminated tibial fractures: An in vitro study of bacterial

adherence and bone damage," *Journal of Orthopaedic Trauma*, vol. 13, no. 8, pp. 526–533, 1999.

[42] D. R. Dirschl, G. P. Duff, L. E. Dahners, M. Edin, B. A. Rahn, and T. Miclau, "High Pressure Pulsatile Lavage Irrigation of Intraarticular Fractures: Effects on Fracture Healing," *Journal of Orthopaedic Trauma*, vol. 12, no. 7, pp. 460–463, 1998.

[43] B. Petrisor, K. Jeray, E. Schemitsch et al., "Fluid lavage in patients with open fracture wounds (FLOW): An international survey of 984 surgeons," *BMC Musculoskeletal Disorders*, vol. 9, article no. 7, 2008.

[44] A. Abdul-Jabbar, S. H. Berven, S. S. Hu et al., "Surgical site infections in spine surgery: identification of microbiologic and surgical characteristics in 239 cases," *Spine*, vol. 38, no. 22, pp. E1425–E1431, 2013.

22

Closed Reduction in a "Hyperextended Supine Position" with Percutaneous Transsacral-Transiliac and Iliosacral Screw Fixation for Denis Zone III Sacral Fractures

Hideto Irifune,[1,2] **Suguru Hirayama**,[1] **Nobuyuki Takahashi**,[2] **Mitsumasa Chiba**,[2] **and Toshihiko Yamashita**[2]

[1]*Department of Emergency Medicine Advanced Critical Care and Emergency Center, Sapporo Medical University School of Medicine, Sapporo, Japan*
[2]*Department of Orthopedic Surgery, Sapporo Medical University School of Medicine, Sapporo, Japan*

Correspondence should be addressed to Hideto Irifune; irifuneh@sapmed.ac.jp

Academic Editor: Andrew O'Brien

Background. Herein, we demonstrate the clinical results of closed reduction in a hyperextended supine position with transsacral-transiliac (TSTI) and iliosacral (IS) screw fixations for Denis zone III sacral fractures. *Patients and Methods.* Sixteen consecutive patients with Denis zone III sacral fractures who were treated between January 2009 and September 2016 were evaluated. All patients were treated using percutaneous TSTI/IS screw fixation during closed reduction performed with patients placed in a hyperextended supine position with body manipulation. The clinical and radiological results were evaluated, and the neurological outcomes were retrospectively assessed using Gibbon's classification system. The clinical outcomes were evaluated using the German Multicenter Study Group Pelvic Outcome Scale (POS). *Results.* The sacral kyphotic angle was reduced by $18.06^\circ \pm 15.26^\circ$ (mean kyphotic angle: pre-OP, $39.44^\circ \pm 20.56^\circ$; post-OP, $21.38^\circ \pm 7.39^\circ$), and fracture translation was reduced by 5.93 ± 4.95 mm (mean fracture translation: pre-OP, 8.69 ± 8.03 mm; post-OP 2.75 ± 3.97 mm). The mean initial Gibbon's score was 3.00 ± 1.32. Among 15 patients with a follow-up duration of over 12 months, the mean reduction loss in the sacral kyphotic angle was $5.87^\circ \pm 10.40^\circ$ and was 1.00 ± 3.00 mm for the fracture translation. The final Gibbon's score was 1.80 ± 1.21, and 73.3% of patients had good results based on the POS score. *Conclusions.* Although closed reduction in a hyperextended supine position with percutaneous posterior screw fixation is associated with some surgical limitations and technical difficulties, the procedure is minimally invasive and highly effective for stabilizing Denis zone III sacral fractures.

1. Introduction

Denis zone III sacral fractures are generally due to high-energy traumas such as falls from heights, traffic accidents, and crush injuries, with most of these fractures occurring in patients with polytrauma [1]. Zone III sacral fractures are relatively rare injuries, reportedly accounting for only 3–5% of all sacral fractures [2–4]. Importantly, these fractures are associated with a high rate of neurologic injury, including sensory and motor deficits in the lower legs; saddle anesthesia; and bowel, bladder, and sexual dysfunctions [2].

Historically, the standard treatment for Denis zone III sacral fractures did not involve surgery or was limited to sacral laminectomy [1, 5]. However, given the advances in internal fixation techniques, cases with minimal kyphosis and no neurological deficits can be treated using several commonly performed surgical procedures such as spinopelvic fixation [6], posterior plate fixation [7], and iliosacral screw fixation [8]. However, no clear guidelines currently exist regarding appropriate treatment strategies and indications for Denis zone III sacral fractures. Spinopelvic and posterior plate fixation have shown good reduction and neurological recovery but are associated with long operating times. Moreover, the surgery is performed in the prone position, which may be particularly disadvantageous for polytrauma patients.

In addition, the use of posterior plates and other spinal instrumentations may cause soft tissue damage and lead to wound complications. To minimize the risk of such complications, minimally invasive approaches have been increasingly used for these fractures. In recent reports, minimally invasive posterior screw fixations for pelvic ring fractures, including transsacral-transiliac (TSTI) and iliosacral (IS) screw fixations, have been reported to have a number of clinical and biomechanical advantages [9–13].

The purpose of the present study was to review our experiences and demonstrate the clinical results of closed reduction in a hyperextended supine position with percutaneous TSTI/IS screw fixation methods for Denis zone III sacral fractures.

2. Patients and Methods

Patients with Denis zone III sacral fractures classified as AO/OTA type C pelvic injuries, treated between January 2009 and September 2016, were selected from our trauma database. Patients who had undergone surgical treatment and had been followed up for a minimum of 12 months were selected for analysis. The patients' medical records were reviewed retrospectively, and the fractures were classified by the sacral level according to the method of Roy-Camille (as modified by Strange-Vognsen and Lebech) and the fracture morphology [1, 14, 15].

The following injury data were collected: demographics, mechanism of injury, associated injury, and the ISS. An initial clinical neurological examination was performed if the patient's condition permitted and was graded according to the classification system described by Gibbons et al [5, 16]. Preoperative imaging consisted of pelvic anterior-posterior radiographs and multislice CT scans. Collected postoperative data included the results from clinical and radiological assessments. Radiographic assessments of the sacral kyphotic angle, fracture translation, implant position, and decompression were performed using standard radiography of the pelvis and multislice CT [17, 18]. Additionally, multidisciplinary follow-up examinations were performed by an orthopedic surgeon (H.I.).

2.1. Reduction and Operative Techniques. During the 8-year study period, a standardized operative technique using closed reduction and posterior pelvic ring fixations (TSTI and/or IS screw fixation) was performed. In patients with combined sacral fractures and anterior pelvic ring injuries, staged and/or one-stage reconstruction was performed. Injuries of the anterior part of the pelvic ring were treated using an anterior extraperitoneal or percutaneous approach. Posterior pelvic ring fixation was performed through the percutaneous approach.

2.2. Operative Procedure. For posterior screw fixation, the patients were positioned supine on a radiolucent table and in hyperextension with handmade pillows placed vertical to the sacral fracture line (Figure 1(a)). Under fluoroscopic guidance, closed fracture reduction was performed. When the fracture reduction quality was insufficient, additional pillows were placed and/or manipulation of the patient's body was performed (Figure 1(b)). The manipulation maneuver involved putting a tow in the longitudinal direction while pushing the trunk and lower limbs to the table (Figure 1(c)). After closed reduction, percutaneous screw insertion was performed under fluoroscopic guidance (Figure 1(d)). In principle, two or more TSTI screws were inserted; when this was not possible, the TITS screws were set in combination with an IS screw. Screws utilized at our institute included 6.5 mm (diameter) cannulated cancellous screws provided by Depuy-Synthes, Inc. (partial thread; maximum length: 120 mm) and Meira, Inc. (partial and full thread; maximum length: 150 mm). Direct sacral decompression was not initially performed.

2.3. Postoperative Care. The patient was allowed to sit with the torso upright starting on postoperative day 1. Nonweight bearing activities were allowed 4 weeks after definitive surgery. Weight-bearing activities began 5 weeks after definitive surgery.

After definitive pelvic ring fixation, a follow-up CT was performed within 1 week to indirectly evaluate the decompression quality. If a remnant fracture fragment in the sacral canal and/or poor indirect decompression quality was found, a secondary direct sacral decompression was considered. One orthopedic trauma surgeon (H.I.) performed all operative procedures. Early and late complications associated with the surgical treatment were recorded.

2.4. Radiological Evaluation. The sacral kyphotic angulation of the Denis zone III sacral fracture was measured from sagittal CT reformations by measuring the angle between the posterior sacral cortices, superior and inferior to the level of the transverse fracture. Fracture translation was also measured from the sagittal CT reformations by measuring the displacement of the anterior cortex of the sacrum above and below the transverse fracture (Figure 2). All measurements involving the preoperative, postoperative, and final radiographs, as well as the CT images, were performed by the first author.

2.5. Outcome Evaluation. Lower extremity sensory and motor function and rectal examinations were performed pre- and postoperatively to identify injuries to the lower lumbosacral plexus. Neurological deficits from cauda equina injuries were classified according to the method of Gibbons et al [5]. Improvements in neurological function at the final follow-up were similarly assessed.

The clinical outcomes were evaluated at the final follow-up using the clinical criteria of the German Multicenter Study Group Pelvis Outcome Scale (POS) [19]. These clinical criteria (pain, functional impairment, persistent neurological and urological impairments, and bowel dysfunction) are based on the clinical results and range from 1 to 4 points; a POS score of 3–4 points is considered to be a good outcome, whereas a score of 1–2 points indicates a poor outcome.

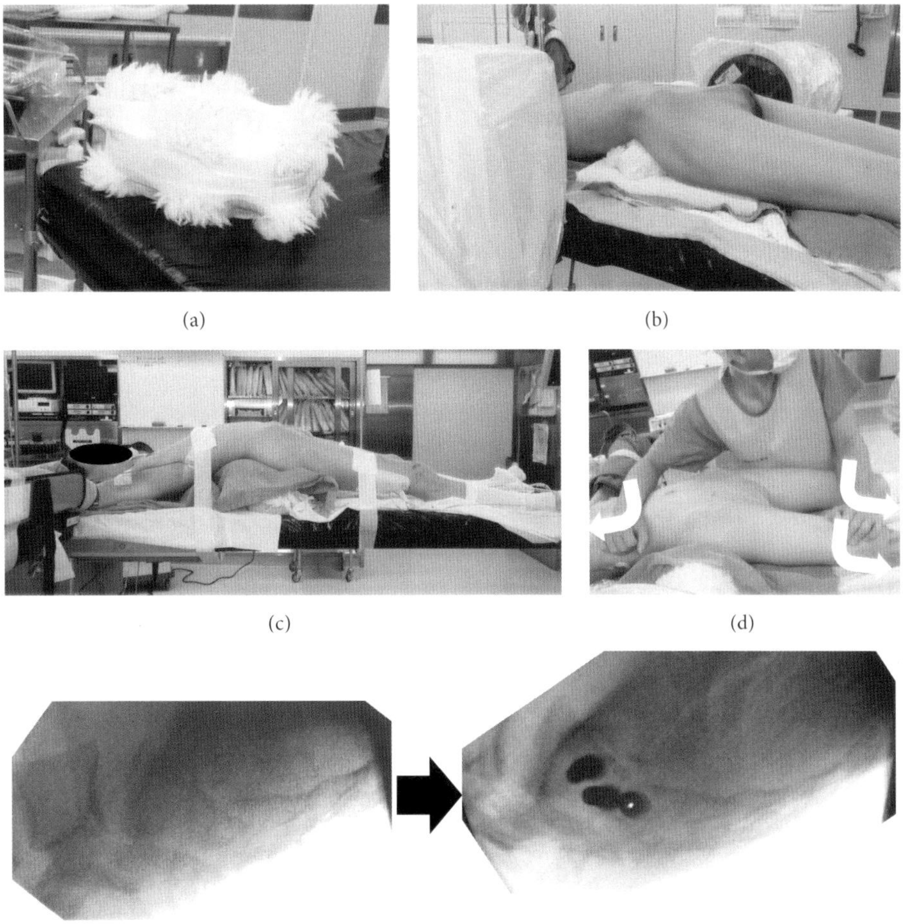

(a) (b) (c) (d) (e)

Figure 1: Closed reduction procedure in "hyperextended" supine position with manipulation. (a) A hand-made reduction pillow is shown.(b) The intraoperative position and "hyperextended" supine position is shown. (c) The manipulation maneuver is shown. (d) Intraoperative images are shown. The left image was taken before reduction maneuver and the right image was taken after the maneuvers. If good reduction was obtained, screw insertion was done in the same position. (e) Intraoperative fluoroscopic images pre- and postreduction maneuver. In this case, good reduction was obtained.

2.6. Statically Analysis. Data was enrolled through Microsoft Excel 2016 (Microsoft, Redmond, WA), followed by a statistical analysis using IBM SPSS Statistics, version 19 (SPSS, Chicago, IL). Data are given in terms of arithmetic mean and standard deviation. The initial, postoperative, and final follow-up data were analyzed using paired t-test. Data differences were considered significant for values of $p < 0.05$.

3. Results

3.1. Patient Demographics (Table 1). Sixteen patients (6 men, 10 women) with Denis zone III sacral fractures classified as AO/OTA type C pelvic injuries were identified. Table 1 presents the patient demographics, mechanism of injury, ISS, fracture patterns, initial Gibbons' grade, and operative procedures. At the time of injury, the mean age of the patients was 29.50 ± 11.12 years (range: 16–50 years). All patients sustained high-energy traumas. The mechanisms of injury included falls from a height (n = 12; 11 suicidal and 1 accidental), traffic accidents (n = 3), and crush injuries (n = 1).

The mean ISS was 25.94 ± 13.88 (range: 9–50). Thirteen of the 16 patients showed associated injuries, including 9 cases of associated injuries of the head and trunk with an Abbreviated Injury Scale Score ≥3. Other injuries of the spine and extremities were present in 10 patients, while two patients experienced pelvic fracture and urinary tract injuries. At the time of initial examination, neurological deficits were observed in 12 out of 16 patients, with a mean Gibbons' grade of 3.13 ± 1.25 (range: 1–4).

3.2. Fracture Types. The transverse fractures involved the following levels of the sacrum: S1 (n=1), S2 (n=7), S2-3 (n=2), S3 (n=3), S3-4 (n=1), S2 + S3-4 (n=1), and S2 + S3 (n=1). The fracture patterns were classified using the Roy-Camille classification system and the fracture morphology. Roy-Camille type 2 fractures occurred in 12 patients and type 3 fractures occurred in 4 patients. Further, H-shaped (n=3),

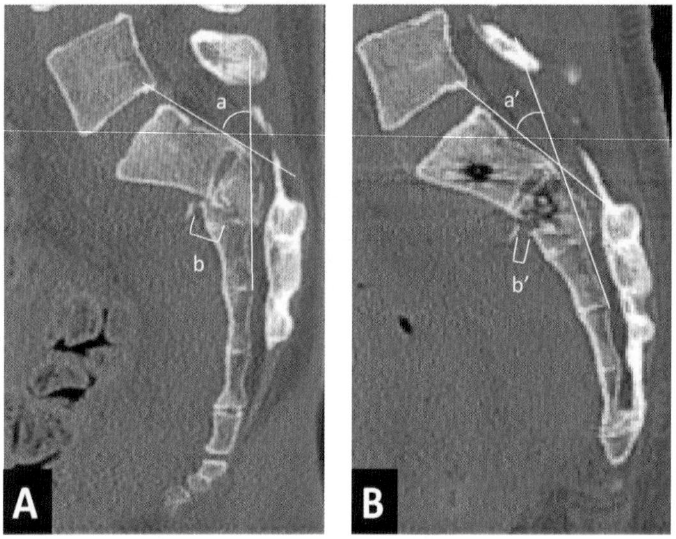

(a) (b)

FIGURE 2: Radiological measurement methods. (a) A preoperative CT scan of the sacrum in the sagittal plane is shown. (b) A postoperative CT scan of the sacrum in the sagittal plane is shown. a and a': sacral kyphotic angle; b and b': sacral fracture translation.

T-shaped (n=4), U-shaped (n=7), and Y-shaped fractures (n=2) were found. A Morel-Lavallée lesion was observed in 1 case, while no cases of open fracture were found.

3.3. Operative Treatment (Table 2). Posterior percutaneous internal fixation was performed between 0 and 8 days after the injury (median: 1.31 ± 2.73 days). The operative methods for posterior pelvic ring stabilization included 12 cases of 2- or 3-TSTI screw fixation only (Figures 3 and 4), 1 bilateral S1 IS and S2 TSTI screws fixation, 1 unilateral S1 and S2 IS screw fixations, and 2 bilateral S1 and S2 IS screw fixations (Figure 5). Additional primary fixation was performed in 9 patients, including pubic rami screw fixation (n=4), pubic rami plate fixation (n=1), pubic rami screw/plate and anterior sacroiliac plate fixation (n=1), symphysis plate fixation (n=2), and plate fixations for acetabular fractures (n=2) (Figure 5). The mean operative time for posterior definitive fixation was 64.69 ± 98.65 minutes (range: 10–420 minutes).

Additional operations due to remnant bone fragments and neurological deficits were performed in 5 patients, including delayed direct sacral decompression (n=5). Posterior implant removal was routinely performed in 14 patients after the fractures had healed.

3.4. Pre- and Postoperative Radiological Results (Table 2). The mean preoperative and postoperative sacral kyphotic angles were 39.44°± 20.57° (range: 13–89°) and 21.38°± 7.39° (range, 11–36°), respectively. The mean postoperative reduction angle of the sacral kyphosis was 18.06°± 15.26° (range: 2–57°). The kyphotic angle was improved with a significant difference (p<0.05, 95% confidence interval (CI) 9.93 to 26.19) The mean preoperative and postoperative translations were 8.69 ± 8.03 mm (range: 0–35 mm), 2.75 ± 3.97 mm (range: 0–16 mm), respectively. The mean postoperative translation reduction was 5.93 ± 4.95 mm (range: 0–19 mm). The fracture translation was also improved with a significant difference (p<0.05, 95%CI 3.30 to 8.57).

3.5. Radiological, Neurological, and Clinical Outcomes at Final Follow-Up (Table 2). Fifteen patients were followed for more than 12 months. At the final follow-up (mean: 27.53 ± 19.64 months; range: 12–71 months), the mean sacral kyphotic angle and reduction loss were 27.93°± 13.01° (range: 13–60°) and 5.87°± 10.40° (range: -1-32°), respectively. The kyphotic angle was decreased with a significant difference between post-OP and final follow-up (p<0.05, 95%CI -11.62 to -0.11). The mean sacral translation and reduction loss were 3.80 ± 6.71 mm (range: 0-24 mm) and 1.00 ± 3.00 mm (range: -2-8 mm), respectively. The translation was maintained with a no difference (p=0.22, 95%CI -2.66 to 0.66). The mean Gibbons' grade was 1.80 ± 1.21 (range: 1–4) and 8 out of 12 patients (66.71%) with neurological symptoms showed improvement in neurological status. The Gibbons grade was improved with a significant difference (p<0.05, 95%CI 0.65 to 2.02). The mean POS score was 2.93 ± 1.28 (range: 1-4). The clinical results as indicated by the POS score were good and poor in 73.3% (11/15) and 26.7% (4/15) of the patients, respectively (Table 2).

3.6. Complications. All patients showed bone union. No case of deep and/or superficial wound infection was noted. Screw loosening was observed in 3 patients; one patient had greater reduction loss (case 3; bilateral S1 and S2 IS screws, see Figure 5). Further, screw malposition was observed in 4 patients; however, in these cases, no new neurological deficits were observed postoperatively.

Table 1: Preoperative clinical data and operative procedures.

Patients No.	Age/Sex	Mechanism of Injury	Level of transverse fracture	Classifications		ISS	Day of OP	OP procedure	
				R-C	Description			Anterior	Posterior
1	25/M	FOH	S2	2	U	34	0		S1; TSTI(P), S2; TSTI(P)
2	20/M	FOH	S2	2	H	22	0	PR screw	S1; IS×2(P) S2; IS×2(P)
3	25/F	FOH	S2	2	H	29	0	acetabulum plate	S1; IS×2(P) S2; IS×2(P)
4	40/F	FOH	S2/3	2	T	43	0		S1; TSTI(P) S2; TSTI(P)
5	16/F	WTA	S3	2	Y	17	7	PR screw×2	S1; TSTI(P) S2; TSTI(P)
6	21/M	FOH	S2	2	T	13	1		S1; TSTI(F) S2; TSTI(F)
7	29/F	FOH	S2	2	U	10	0		S1; TSTI×2(F) S2; TSTI(F)
8	20/M	CR	S3/4	2	Y	35	8	PR screw, PR plate	S1; TSTI(F) S2; TSTI(F)
9	18/F	FOH	S3	2	U	50	0		S1; TSTI(F) S2; TSTI(F)
10	25/F	FOH	S3	2	H	34	0	acetabulum plate	S1; TSTI(F) S2; TSTI(F)
11	29/M	FOH	S2	3	U	9	0		S1; IS×2(P) S2; TSTI(F)
12	23/F	FOH	S2, S3/4	2	U	16	0		S1; TSTI×2(F) S2; TSTI(F)
13	50/M	FOH	S2/3	3	T	25	5	symphysis plate	S1; IS(P) S2; TSTI(F)
14	39/F	WTA	S2, S3	2	T	10	0	PR screw×2	S1; TSTI(F) S2; TSTI(F)
15	49/F	FOH	S1	3	U	50	0	symphysis plate	S1; TSTI×2(F)
16	43/F	CTA	S2	3	U	18	0	PR screw×2	S1; TSTI(F) S2; TSTI(F)

ISS: Injury Severity Score; R-C: Roy-Camille; OP: operative; TSTI: transsacral-transiliac screw; IS: iliosacral screw; U: U-shaped; H: H-shaped; T: T-shaped; FOH: fall from height; CR: crush injury; TA: traffic accident; F: female; M: male; P: partial threads screw; F: full thread screw.

TABLE 2: Radiological and clinical findings.

Patient No.	Kyphotic angle			Fracture translation			Gibbons		POS clinical	FU month
	Initial	post-OP	Final	Initial	Post-OP	Final	Initial	Final		
1	33	17	20	10	2	3	1	1	4	12
2	50	36	35	12	0	0	4	1	4	24
3	63	28	60	11	6	14	4	4	1	71
4	24	16	16	0	0	0	4	4	1	64
5	31	22	22	9	4	4	4	1	4	14
6	46	31	30	5	2	0	4	2	3	18
7	65	25	36	12	0	0	4	2	3	12
8	21	13	13	3	0	0	3	1	4	48
9	89	32	32	8	3	1	4	2	3	32
10	27	15	15	11	3	3	3	1	4	19
11	32	21	24	5	0	0	1	1	4	15
12	58	23	40	35	16	24	4	4	1	40
13	13	11	-	4	2	-	1	-	-	2
14	31	21	21	0	0	0	2	1	3	12
15	28	17	41	8	4	6	4	4	1	20
16	20	14	14	6	2	2	1	1	4	17

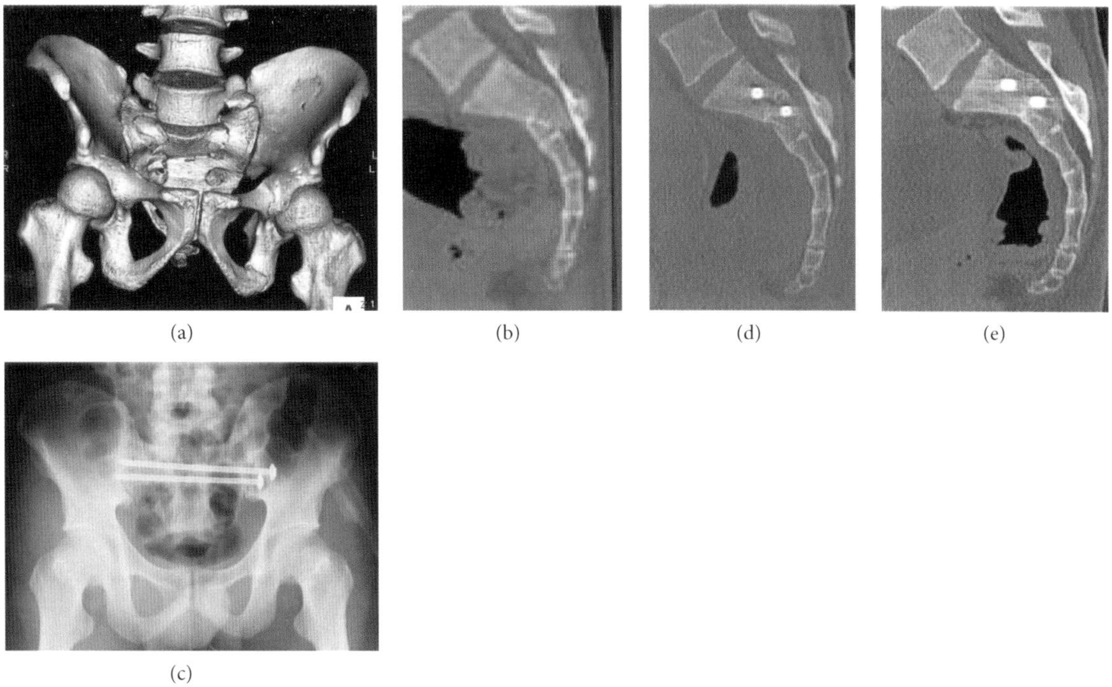

Figure 3: Case 1. A 25-year-old man who was injured from a fall from a height underwent S1 and S2 TSTI partial threaded screw fixation for a Roy-Camille type 2 U-shaped transverse sacral fracture. (a) Preoperative 3-dimensional CT reconstruction of the pelvis is shown. (b) Preoperative CT scan of the sacrum in the sagittal plane is shown (preoperative sacral kyphotic angle: 33°; fracture translation: 10 mm). (c) Postoperative anteroposterior radiograph of the pelvis is shown. (d) Postoperative CT scan of the sacrum in the sagittal plane is shown (postoperative sacral kyphotic angle: 17°; fracture translation: 2 mm). (e) Final follow-up CT scan of the sacrum in the sagittal plane is shown. Slight reduction loss was observed.

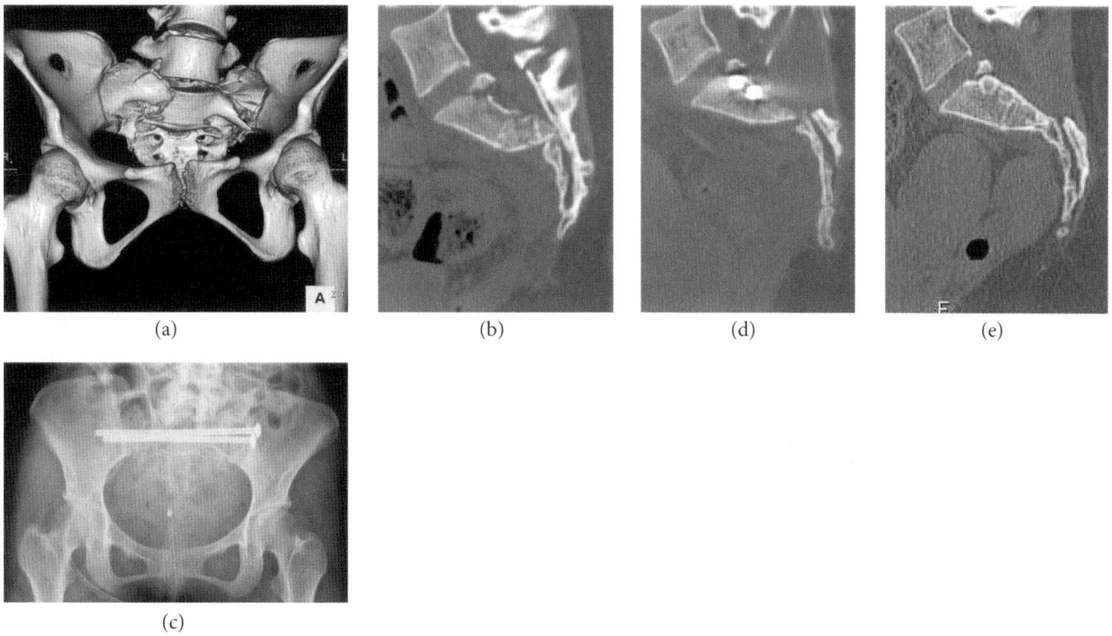

Figure 4: Case 9. An 18-year-old man who was injured from a fall from a height underwent S1 and S2 TSTI full threaded screw fixation for a Roy-Camille type 2 U-shaped transverse sacral fracture. (a) Preoperative 3-dimensional CT reconstruction of the pelvis is shown. (b) Preoperative CT scan of the sacrum in the sagittal plane is shown (preoperative sacral kyphotic angle: 89°; fracture translation: 8 mm). (c) Postoperative anteroposterior radiograph of the pelvis is shown. (d) Postoperative CT scan of the sacrum in the sagittal plane is shown (preoperative sacral kyphotic angle: 32°; fracture translation: 3 mm). (e) Final follow-up CT scan of the sacrum in the sagittal plane is shown. Good reduction quality was maintained.

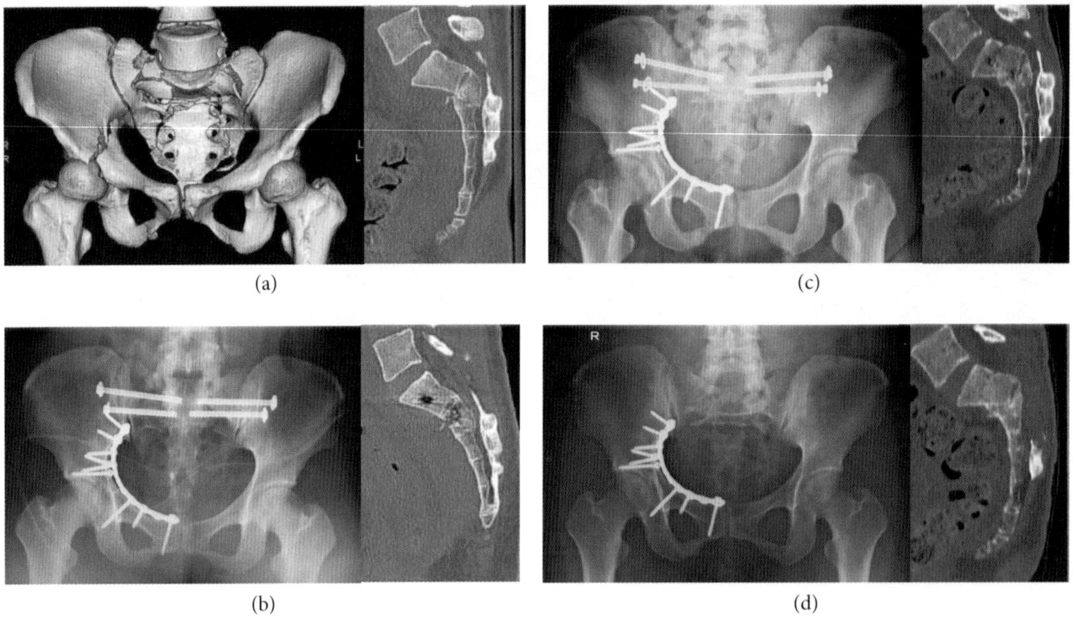

FIGURE 5: Case 3. This case had the greatest loss of reduction. A 25-year-old woman who was injured from a fall from a height underwent unilateral S1 and S2 bilateral iliosacral partial threaded screw fixation for a Roy-Camille type 2 H-shaped transverse sacral fracture. (a) Preoperative 3-dimensional and sagittal plane CT reconstruction of the pelvis is shown (preoperative sacral kyphotic angle: 63°; fracture translation: 11 mm). (b) Postoperative anteroposterior radiograph and CT scan of the sacrum in the sagittal plane is shown (postoperative sacral kyphotic angle: 28°; fracture translation: 6 mm). (c) The anteroposterior radiograph and CT scan of the sacrum in the sagittal plane taken one month after the initial operative treatment is shown (sacral kyphotic angle: 60°; fracture translation: 14 mm). IS screw loosening was observed. Secondary sacral decompression was performed. (d) Final follow-up anteroposterior radiograph and CT scan of the sacrum in the sagittal plane is shown. Bone healing was achieved, but reduction loss and bladder/bowel dysfunction remained.

4. Discussion

The present study aimed to show that closed reduction in a hyperextended supine position with manipulations and percutaneous TSTI/IS screw fixation is useful for treating Denis zone III sacral fractures. Currently, the present study is the largest case series regarding closed reduction and percutaneous screw fixation for these fractures [8, 10, 11, 13]. Furthermore, the present study includes the greatest number of cases involving the supine position maneuver.

Denis zone III sacral fractures may be H-, U-, T-, or Y-shaped [20], and sacral dislocations may be anterior or posterior [1]. When treating these fractures, it is important to reduce the sacral kyphotic angle fracture translation and to maintain this reduced position. Previously, the outcomes of several treatments for these fractures have been reported. Siebler et al. reported the results of conservative treatment [21], and found that the sacral kyphotic angle increased by 4.1° (from 36.4° to 40.5°) posttreatment. In terms of operative treatment, Schildhauer et al., Tan et al., and Lindahl et al. reported that using spinopelvic fixation, the initial kyphotic angles of 43°, 32°, and 38° were improved to the final angles of 21°, 19°, and 22°, respectively [6, 20, 22]. Nork et al. reported that, after using IS screw fixation, the kyphotic angle was reduced from 29.2° to 28.2° [8], whereas König et al. reported that, after using TSTI screw fixation in 3 patients, the sacrococcygeal and pelvic incidence angles were reduced from 84° and 75° preoperatively to 58° and 56° postoperatively, respectively (reduction losses of 14° and 15°, respectively) [10]. Ruatti et al. reported that, in a supine position, hyperlordosis, skeletal traction, and percutaneous IS screw fixation had good reduction results in 3 cases [13]. In the present study, the pre- and postoperative kyphotic angles were 40° and 22°, respectively, indicating a reduction loss of 4.9°. In terms of translation, Lindahl et al. reported that the mean pre- and postoperative translations with spinopelvic fixation were 15.5 and 5.8 mm, respectively [22], whereas in the present study, the corresponding values were 8.9 and 2.8 mm. In the present study, one patient with IS fixation only (Case 3) was observed to have a high reduction loss and screw loosening. Taken together, these clinical data suggest that TSTI screw fixation is equal to spinopelvic fixation. Furthermore, Min et al. reported that 2-TSTI screw fixation was superior to spinopelvic fixation in a zone 2 sacral fracture model from a biomechanical viewpoint [23]. Therefore, we believe that TSTI screw fixation in the supine position is an effective, rigid, and minimally invasive procedure for Denis zone III sacral fracture fixation.

Denis zone III sacral fractures have been reported to result in neurological injury of varying severity in up to 100% of patients [6–8, 20–22, 24]. Accordingly, in the present study, neurological deficits were seen in 12 of 16 patients (75%). However, neurological recovery has been shown to occur in 50–100% of patients with these fractures [6–8, 10, 20, 21]. Early surgical treatment of the sacrum, including restoration of spinopelvic stability and decompression of the nerve roots, indirectly or directly, is thought to provide the best possible environment for neurological recovery. Schildhauer et al. reported that neurological recovery depends on the extent of nerve damage at the time of injury [6]. However, Siebler et al., in their study of nonoperative treatment, reported that the recovery rate was still as high as 85.7%. [21] Thus, the best treatment method, in terms of neurological outcomes, remains unclear. In the present study, the overall neurological recovery rate was 66.7% (8/12). A lack of neurological recovery was observed in four cases (cases 3, 4, 12, and 15). Of these, one case (case 4) involved a spinal cord injury merger. In an additional case (cases 12), decompression of the postoperative sacral canal was deemed sufficient; however, no neurological recovery was observed. In cases 3 and 15, because of a suspected reduction loss in the kyphotic angle and translation, additional nerve decompression surgery was performed (case 3); however, nerve recovery could not be obtained. In addition, four cases (cases 6, 7, 8, and 9; see Figure 4) underwent additional decompression because of remnant fragment and/or insufficient neurological recovery and were finally considered to have sufficient neurological recovery. Based on our experience and the report by Schildhauer et al. [6], the likelihood of neurological recovery appears to be dependent on the degree of nerve damage at the time of injury. However, for maximum neurological recovery, we consider indirect or direct nerve decompression to be necessary. Hence, in our treatment strategy, indirect reduction and decompression are performed in the acute phase and if the postoperative CT shows incomplete decompression and/or remnant fracture fragments in the sacral canal, secondary direct sacral decompression is consequently performed.

We consider TSTI/IS screw fixation to be a less invasive method, associated with a relatively low complication rate. In our series, the mean operative time was approximately 65 minutes. In cases involving TSTI or IS screw insertion only, the screw insertion time was approximately 10 minutes per screw. In addition, the time required for our preoperative closed reduction procedure is about 20 to 30 minutes. Hence, in cases requiring only closed reduction and screw fixation, patients can be treated in the acute phase. Furthermore, in cases involving screw fixation only, the patient is positioned supine, which is often the most comfortable position for polytrauma patients. In addition, TSTI/IS screw fixation is associated with a very low profile and few surgical site complications. In fact, in our study, no surgical site complications were observed. In past reports using different approaches, the surgical site complication rate was as high as 38% [6, 7, 20]. Spinopelvic fixation is associated with a particularly high complication rate in pelvic ring fracture treatment [6, 20], and posterior soft tissue complications are associated with poorer outcomes.

There are several limitations to the present study. First, the study population was relatively small and did not allow for a highly powered statistical analysis; therefore, our conclusions should be interpreted with caution. Second, there are operative limitations for TSTI/IS screw fixation. In TSTI/IS screw fixation for zone III sacral fractures, at least two screw insertions (2 TSTI screws, or 1 TSTI screw and 1 IS screw) are required, as the screws need to provide resistance against the vertical load shear force and the rotational force of the sacral vertebral body. However, it has been reported that ilio-sacro-iliacal corridors for intraosseous implants were not inserted in 18–25% and 10–12% of S1 and S2 cases, respectively; moreover, a high frequency of this issue has been reported for female patients [25–27]. Thus, owing to anatomical variance and different fracture types, this method is not always useful.

In conclusion, the current study showed that closed reduction in a hyperextended supine position with TSTI/IS screw fixation is effective for treating Denis zone III sacral fractures in terms of the fracture reduction, loss of reduction, neurological recovery, and clinical outcomes. Thus, despite some limitations, we believe that our procedure is an effective and appropriate method for treating Denis zone III sacral fractures.

References

[1] R. Roy-Camille, G. Saillant, G. Gagna, and C. Mazel, "Transverse fracture of the upper sacrum: Suicidal jumper's fracture," *The Spine Journal*, vol. 10, no. 9, pp. 838–845, 1985.

[2] F. Denis, S. Davis, and T. Comfort, "Sacral fractures: An important problem: Retrospective analysis of 236 cases," *Clinical Orthopaedics and Related Research*, no. 227, pp. 67–81, 1988.

[3] T. J. Albert, M. J. Levine, H. S. An, J. M. Cotler, and R. A. Balderston, "Concomitant noncontiguous thoracolumbar and sacral fractures," *The Spine Journal*, vol. 18, no. 10, pp. 1285–1291, 1993.

[4] M. Hessmann, J. Degreif, A. Mayer, S. Atahi, and P. M. Rommens, "Transverse sacral fracture with intrapelvic intrusion of the lumbosacral spine: Case report and review of the literature," *Journal of Trauma - Injury Infection and Critical Care*, vol. 49, no. 4, pp. 754–757, 2000.

[5] K. J. Gibbons, D. S. Soloniuk, and N. Razack, "Neurological injury and patterns of sacral fractures," *Journal of Neurosurgery*, vol. 72, no. 6, pp. 889–893, 1990.

[6] T. A. Schildhauer, C. Bellabarba, S. E. Nork, D. P. Barei, M. L. Chip Routt Jr., and J. R. Chapman, "Decompression and lumbopelvic fixation for sacral fracture-dislocations with spino-pelvic dissociation," *Journal of Orthopaedic Trauma*, vol. 20, no. 7, pp. 447–457, 2006.

[7] A. J. G. Gribnau, P. B. V. Hensbroek, R. Haverlag, K. J. Ponsen, H. D. Been, and J. C. Goslings, "U-shaped sacral fractures: Surgical treatment and quality of life," *Injury*, vol. 40, no. 10, pp. 1040–1048, 2009.

[8] S. E. Nork, C. B. Jones, S. P. Harding, S. K. Mirza, and M. L. C. Routt Jr., "Percutaneous stabilization of U-shaped sacral fractures using iliosacral screws: Technique and early results," *Journal of Orthopaedic Trauma*, vol. 15, no. 4, pp. 238–246, 2001.

[9] S. A. Tabaie, J. G. Bledsoe, and B. R. Moed, "Biomechanical comparison of standard iliosacral screw fixation to transsacral locked screw fixation in a type C zone II pelvic fracture model," *Journal of Orthopaedic Trauma*, vol. 27, no. 9, pp. 521–526, 2013.

[10] M. A. König, U. Seidel, P. Heini et al., "Minimal-invasive percutaneous reduction and transsacral screw fixation for u-shaped fractures," *Journal of Spinal Disorders & Techniques*, vol. 26, no. 1, pp. 48–54, 2013.

[11] M. J. Gardner and M. L. C. Routt Jr., "Transiliac-transsacral screws for posterior pelvic stabilization," *Journal of Orthopaedic Trauma*, vol. 25, no. 6, pp. 378–384, 2011.

[12] S. S. Bederman, J. M. Hassan, K. N. Shah, P. D. Kiester, N. N. Bhatia, and D. P. Zamorano, "Fixation techniques for complex traumatic transverse sacral fractures: A systematic review," *The Spine Journal*, vol. 38, no. 16, pp. E1028–E1040, 2013.

[13] S. Ruatti, G. Kerschbaumer, E. Gay, M. Milaire, P. Merloz, and J. Tonetti, "Technique for reduction and percutaneous fixation of U- and H-shaped sacral fractures," *Orthopaedics & Traumatology: Surgery & Research*, vol. 99, no. 5, pp. 625–629, 2013.

[14] S. Mehta, J. D. Auerbach, C. T. Born, and K. R. Chin, "Sacral fractures," *Journal of the American Academy of Orthopaedic Surgeons*, vol. 14, no. 12, pp. 656–665, 2006.

[15] H. H. Strange-Vognsen and A. Lebech, "An unusual type of fracture in the upper sacrum," *Journal of Orthopaedic Trauma*, vol. 5, no. 2, pp. 200–203, 1991.

[16] A. Tötterman, T. Glott, J. E. Madsen, and O. Røise, "Unstable sacral fractures: Associated injuries and morbidity at 1 year," *The Spine Journal*, vol. 31, no. 18, pp. E628–E635, 2006.

[17] P. M. Rommens, P. M. Vanderschot, and P. L. Broos, "Conventional radiography and CT examination of pelvic ring fractures. A comparative study of 90 patients," *Der Unfallchirurg*, vol. 95, no. 8, pp. 387–392, 1992.

[18] A. R. Vaccaro, D. H. Kim, D. S. Brodke et al., "Diagnosis and management of sacral spine fractures," *Instructional Course Lectures*, vol. 53, pp. 375–385, 2004.

[19] T. Pohlemann, A. Gänsslen, O. Schellwald, U. Culemann, and H. Tscherne, "Outcome after pelvic ring injuries," *Injury*, vol. 27, no. 2, pp. 31–38, 1996.

[20] G.-Q. Tan, J.-L. He, B.-S. Fu, L.-X. Li, B.-M. Wang, and D.-S. Zhou, "Lumbopelvic fixation for multiplanar sacral fractures with spinopelvic instability," *Injury*, vol. 43, no. 8, pp. 1318–1325, 2012.

[21] J. C. Siebler, B. P. Hasley, and M. A. Mormino, "Functional outcomes of Denis Zone III sacral fractures treated nonoperatively," *Journal of Orthopaedic Trauma*, vol. 24, no. 5, pp. 297–302, 2010.

[22] J. Lindahl, T. J. Mäkinen, S. K. Koskinen, and T. Söderlund, "Factors associated with outcome of spinopelvic dissociation treated with lumbopelvic fixation," *Injury*, vol. 45, no. 12, pp. 1914–1920, 2014.

[23] K. S. Min, D. P. Zamorano, G. M. Wahba, I. Garcia, N. Bhatia, and T. Q. Lee, "Comparison of two-transsacral-screw fixation versus triangular osteosynthesis for transforaminal sacral fractures," *Orthopedics*, vol. 37, no. 9, pp. e754–e760, 2014.

[24] M. A. Ayoub, "Displaced spinopelvic dissociation with sacral cauda equina syndrome: Outcome of surgical decompression with a preliminary management algorithm," *European Spine Journal*, vol. 21, no. 9, pp. 1815–1825, 2012.

[25] P. Vanderschot, C. Meuleman, A. Lefèvre, and P. Broos, "Trans iliac-sacral-iliac bar stabilisation to treat bilateral lesions of the sacro-iliac joint or sacrum: Anatomical considerations and clinical experience," *Injury*, vol. 32, no. 7, pp. 587–592, 2001.

[26] T. Mendel, H. Noser, J. Kuervers, F. Goehre, G. O. Hofmann, and F. Radetzki, "The influence of sacral morphology on the existence of secure S1 and S2 transverse bone corridors for iliosacroiliac screw fixation," *Injury*, vol. 44, no. 12, pp. 1773–1779, 2013.

[27] F. Gras, S. Hillmann, S. Rausch, K. Klos, G. O. Hofmann, and I. Marintschev, "Biomorphometric analysis of ilio-sacro-iliacal corridors for an intra-osseous implant to fix posterior pelvic ring fractures," *Journal of Orthopaedic Research*, vol. 33, no. 2, pp. 254–260, 2015.

23

Sustained Results in Long-Term Follow-Up of Autologous Chondrocyte Implantation (ACI) for Distal Femur Juvenile Osteochondritis Dissecans (JOCD)

Jennifer J. Beck, [1] **Dai Sugimoto**, [2,3,4] **and Lyle Micheli** [2,3,4]

[1] *Orthopedic Institute for Children/UCLA, Los Angeles, CA, USA*
[2] *The Micheli Center for Sports Injury Prevention, Waltham, MA, USA*
[3] *Boston Children's Hospital Orthopaedics and Sports Medicine, Boston, MA, USA*
[4] *Department of Orthopaedic Surgery, Harvard Medical School, Boston, MA, USA*

Correspondence should be addressed to Jennifer J. Beck; jennbeck1982@gmail.com

Academic Editor: Allen L. Carl

Introduction. Concern regarding ability of autologous chondrocyte implantation (ACI) to correct for the bone and cartilage pathology of knee juvenile osteochondritis dissecans (JOCD) exists. The purpose of this study was to determine long-term, patient-based outcomes of ACI treatment of JOCD in young patients. Authors hypothesized long-term outcomes are comparable to reported mid-term outcomes. *Methods.* A single institution, longitudinal cohort study design combining medical record review and outcome surveys was used. Inclusion criteria included isolated JOCD diagnosis, failed primary healing of operatively treated JOCD, ACI surgery > 5 years ago, and ≤20 years of age at time of ACI. *Results.* 10/26 eligible patients (38.5%) participated (M: F = 5:5, age at ACI: 18.3 ± 2.5 y, current age: 30.8 ± 5.1 y, and current BMI: 24.6 ± 2.1). Follow-up was 12.0 ± 4.5 y. Lesion size at ACI was 9.1 ± 1.9 cm^2. Femoral condyle location was medial = 6 and lateral = 4. All required treatment at some point for knee symptoms after ACI. During the past one year, four patients required treatment. Patient reported outcome scores at 12 years following ACI were IKDC score: 73.0 ± 3.6, KOOS scores including pain [88.7 ± 2.3], symptoms [78.2 ± 4.6], activity of daily living [94.7 ± 1.9], function, sports, and recreational activities [73.0 ± 5.3], and quality of life [57.5 ± 5.8], and Modified Cincinnati Knee Rating score was 77.9 ± 4.1. A moderate to good relationship was found between KOOS symptoms and BMI and lesion size. Function, sports, and recreational activities of the KOOS were greater in participants who had ≤1 lesion prior to ACI procedures ($p = 0.044$). *Conclusion.* This study of ACI treatment of knee JOCD patients confirms sustained, long-term results. Number of lesions prior to ACI procedure influenced status of function, sports, and recreational activities.

1. Introduction

Osteochondritis dissecans (OCD) is a focal alteration in subchondral bone risking disruption of overlying articular cartilage and possibly leading to premature osteoarthritis [1]. This condition is thought of as a primarily bone pathology with secondary effects on the overlying cartilage. The patients' symptoms, skeletal maturity, and radiographic staging guide treatment. Commonly found in the knee, plain radiographs are used reliably for diagnosis, staging [2], and management. Advanced imaging, such as MRI, is often used in conjunction with radiographs and physical exam for staging and surgical planning though inconsistencies in protocols and findings limit its clinical utility [3–5].

Increasingly being diagnosed in skeletally immature athletes, juvenile osteochondritis dissecans (JOCD) can be problematic to manage in young, skeletally immature, highly active patients. Histologic cartilage studies have determined age of 20 years as a transition period between adult and juvenile cartilage [6] defining JOCD as patients less than 20 years of age at time of presentation. Male patients have up to 4 times the risk of JOCD compared to female while patients aged 12-19 years have 3 times the risk in comparison with 6-11-year-old patients [7]. Approximately 30% of patients have bilateral lesions [8]. Primary surgical intervention of the knee JOCD is indicated for failure of nonoperative management, advanced stage, or advanced age [9] and consists of microfracture, drilling, or fixation depending on the stage [10].

Salvage options after failure of knee JOCD primary surgical intervention are controversial and include autograft and allograft options. Autologous Chondrocyte Implantation (ACI) is one surgical option for failed JOCD healing. Concern regarding ability of ACI to correct for the bone and cartilage pathology of knee JOCD exists. Reports of bone edema after matrix-assisted autologous chondrocyte transplantation (MACT) did not correlate with a poorer outcome [11]. Favorable factors for ACI success are patients who are younger, have higher preoperative symptom scores, have a single lesion on the trochlea or lateral femoral condyle, and had less than 2 previous procedures on the knee [12].

A trend towards improvement in JOCD treatment results of ACI over osteochondral autologous transplantation, synthetic scaffolds, and other autologous or allograft reconstruction techniques exists [13]. Outcomes of adult OCD lesions treated by ACI are impacted by size of the OCD lesion with success rates lower than JOCD patients [14, 15]. Mid-term results for JOCD have been promising with improved outcome scores reported [14, 16, 17] with earlier age at implantation improving surgical success. Mid-term result failure in adult OCD is estimated around 20% [18] versus 3% in JOCD [16].

Ten-year follow-up of adult OCD lesions treated with ACI found 7% failure with another 9% requiring a graft related procedure within the first year of implantation, no patient reached their preinjury activity level, and nearly half of patients had radiographic evidence of osteoarthritis [19]. Long-term outcomes have not been reported for ACI in knee JOCD, especially in a physically active, youth population. Therefore, the purpose of this study is to examine long-term outcomes of ACI on young patients who failed primary surgical treatment of knee JOCD. Authors hypothesize long-term outcomes of ACI are comparable to previously reported mid-term outcomes [16].

2. Materials and Methods

2.1. Study Methodology. A single institution, retrospective, longitudinal cohort study design combining medical record review and outcome surveys was developed. Prior to study initiation, IRB approval was obtained.

Patients were included if they had isolated distal femur JOCD diagnosis, failed primary healing of operatively treated JOCD, ACI surgery > 5 years ago, and < 20 years of age at time of ACI. Twenty-six patients were identified by record review. Ten patients were able to be contacted and consented for study participation. All patients were > 18 years of age and able to provide institution approved, informed consent. One patient was contacted and refused participation in this study. Fifteen patients were unable to be contacted despite multiple attempts via mail, phone calls, and email methods. Therefore, a total of 10 out of 26 eligible patients (38%) participated.

International Knee Documentation Committee (IKDC), Knee injury and Osteoarthritis Outcome Score (KOOS), and Modified Cincinnati Knee Rating outcome scores were collected. A uniquely created survey consisting of questions regarding a history of treatments after ACI surgery was also completed by study participants (Appendix).

Scores from the IKDC, KOOS, Modified Cincinnati Rating outcome, and the survey created for this investigation were entered into a database for data analysis. Medical records were thoroughly reviewed for the ten patients enrolled in the study. During medical record review, diagnosis, history of procedures prior to ACI, lesion location, lesion size, age at implantation, concomitant procedure performed during ACI, ACI procedure details, postoperative complications, and contralateral knee surgeries were extracted and documented to confirm JOCD history and status following ACI.

2.2. Statistical Analysis. Baseline characteristics of patients including current age, height, weight, and body mass index (BMI) along with history of JOCD and detailed information of orthopedic procedures prior to ACI were examined. Also, patients' outcome surveys including IKDC, KOOS, and Modified Cincinnati Knee Rating Scale scores were analyzed by a descriptive statistics using mean, standard deviation, median, and ranges. Frequency of treatment history since ACI surgery and within the last year was examined by count and percentages (%). Correlation coefficient analysis was used to find an association between the three patients' outcome scales and lesion size, BMI, and age at ACI implantation. Correlation coefficient values (r) were selected to determine strength of the association, and the following criteria were used: little or no relationship ($r = 0.00 - 0.25$), fair ($r = 0.26$-0.50), moderate to good ($r = 0.51$-0.75), good to excellent ($r = 0.76$-1.00) [20]. The patients' outcome surveys were compared based on sex (male versus females), ACI location (medial versus lateral), and number of lesions before ACI (≤1 versus >1). Because of the small sample size, nonparametric t-test, Mann–Whitney U test, was employed to investigate whether there is a significant difference in the IKDC, KOOS, and Modified Cincinnati Knee Rating Scales. Cohen's d was also used to express effect size along with the Mann–Whitney U test. The following Cohen's d was used to express effect sizes: 0.2-0.3 was small, 0.5 was medium, and ≥0.8 was large. Statistical significance of 0.05 was used. Statistical Package for the Social Sciences (version 21, SPSS Inc., Armonk, NY, USA) was used for all analyses.

3. Results

3.1. Baseline Characteristics. Baseline information of physical characteristic, JOCD history, and orthopedic procedures for JOCD prior to ACI were determined for the ten patients enrolled in this study (Table 1). Equal numbers of male and female patients were included (M: F = 5:5). Patients were on average 18 years old (range 15-22 years) at the time of ACI (Table 1(a)). Mean follow-up duration after ACI was 12.0 ± 4.5 years. The JOCD lesions included six medial femoral condyle and four lateral femoral condyle locations. Eight patients had a periosteal covering, one a porcine mucosa covering, and

TABLE 1

(a) Study participant information (N = 10)

	Mean ± SD	Median	Range
Physical characteristics			
Current Age (years)	30.8 ± 1.6	31.3	23.0-37.7
Height (cm)	1.80 ± 0.04	1.78	1.60-1.90
Weight (kg)	77.9 ± 4.6	78.9	55.8-105.0
Body Mass Index	24.6 ± 0.67	24.7	21.1-28.9
JOCD history			
Age at Time of ACI	18.3 ± 0.19	18.0	15.0-22.0
Lesion Size at Time of ACI	9.1 ± 1.9	7.4	2.3-24.0
Number of Lesions	1.2 ± 0.4	1.0	1.0-2.0
Number of Surgeries before ACI	2.5 ± 1.3	2.0	1.0-5.0
Number of Surgeries after ACI	0.6 ± 0.7	0.5	0.0-2.0

(b) Surgical history prior to ACI

Orthopaedic Procedure Prior to ACI	(N)
Isolated Marrow Stimulation	8
Fragment Fixation	4
Bone Graft/Removal of Hardware	1
Excision of fragment/loose bodies	4
Removal of Hardware	2
Other/Unknown	6
Total Procedures	25

one synthetic patch covering. These lesions were isolated knee pathology except one case of lateral femoral condyle OCD associated with unstable lateral discoid meniscus.

Prior to ACI, surgical treatment included an average of 2.5 surgical procedures (range 1-5, Table 1(a)) with average of 4.4 years (range, 1-11) from initial surgical treatment of OCD to ACI. Only one patient had one surgery prior to ACI implantation with the rest of the patients having 2+ procedures (Table 1(b)). All patients underwent marrow stimulation and lesion debridement at some points prior to ACI, typically at the time of ACI biopsy. There was less than one year between ACI biopsy and implantation in every patient.

3.2. Patient Outcomes. IKDC, KOOS, and Modified Cincinnati Knee Rating Scales scores at final follow-up were calculated (Table 2). All patients required treatment at some point for knee symptoms after ACI. Patient reported treatments in the last year and since ACI were described (Table 3).

The effects of gender, lesion size, BMI, and lesion location were compared with outcome scores (Table 4). Moderate to good correlation was found between BMI and lesion size with KOOS symptoms, though these did not reach statistical significance. Fair or little correlation was found between the other outcome scores and lesion size, BMI, and age at ACI implantation. There were no significant differences between the three outcome scales and sex (female versus male, Table 5) or lesion location (medial versus lateral, Table 6). However, statistical significance was detected by a comparison of number of lesions prior to ACI (≤1 versus >1, Table 7). The function, sports, and recreational activities of the KOOS score in ACI patients ≤1 lesion were significantly greater than those of ACI patients with > 1 ($p = 0.044$, Table 7). Also, nearly large effect size was found in the function, sports, and recreational activities of the KOOS score in ACI patients with >1 lesion compared to ACI patients with ≤1 (Cohen's d = 0.716, Table 7). Also, greater than moderate effect sizes were recorded in symptoms in KOOS (Cohen's d = 0.637, Table 7) and Modified Cincinnati Knee Rating Scales (Cohen's d = 0.525, Table 7) among ACI patients with ≤ 1 lesion relative to ACI patients with >1.

3.3. Subsequent Operations. Retrospective chart review found four patients underwent surgery after ACI during the follow-up period. Three patients were treated by the same senior, primary surgeon at the same institution where they initially received treatment. Two of these three patients underwent arthroscopic loose body excision with specific documentation of an intact ACI graft at six and thirteen years after ACI. The other patient required two arthroscopies for loose body excision, microfracture of the lesion happening four and seven years after implantation. Prior to ACI, this patient had associated symptomatic lateral discoid menisci bilaterally, requiring surgical treatment. Additionally, this patient required tibial bone graft to augment the open reduction, internal fixation of the OCD fragment before going on to ACI for failure of this treatment. The fourth surgical patient was treated at another institution

TABLE 2: Outcome of IKDC, KOOS, and Modified Cincinnati Knee Rating Scores.

	Mean ± SD	Median	Range
IKDC			
Total Score	73.0 ± 3.6	70	66.0-97.0
Symptoms			
Highest level of activity without pain	2.6 ± 0.3	2.5	2.0-4.0
Pain in the past 4 weeks	7.1 ± 0.7	7.5	4.0-10.0
Severity of pain	6.5 ± 1.1	8.0	2.0-10.0
Stiffness or swelling in the past 4 weeks	3.4 ± 0.2	3.0	3.0-4.0
Highest level of activity without swelling	2.9 ± 0.4	3.0	1.0-4.0
Locking or catching in the past 4 weeks	0.5 ± 0.2	0.5	0.0-1.0
Highest level of activity without giving way	2.9 ± 0.4	3.0	1.0-4.0
Sports Activity			
Highest level of activity on a regular basis	2.4 ± 0.3	2.0	1.0-4.0
Ability to perform			
Go up stairs	3.6 ± 0.2	4.0	3.0-4.0
Go down stairs	3.5 ± 0.3	4.0	2.0-4.0
Kneel on the front your knee	2.4 ± 0.3	2.0	1.0-4.0
Squat	2.6 ± 0.4	2.5	1.0-4.0
Sit with your knee bent	3.6 ± 0.3	4.0	2.0-4.0
Rise from a chair	3.7 ± 0.2	4.0	3.0-4.0
Run straight ahead	3.4 ± 0.3	4.0	2.0-4.0
Jump and land on your involved leg	2.9 ± 0.2	3.0	2.0-4.0
Stop and start quickly	3.3 ± 0.3	3.0	2.0-4.0
Function			
0-10 scale prior to knee injury	7.5 ± 1.3	10.0	1.0-10.0
0-10 scale based on current function	8.3 ± 0.4	8.0	7.0-10.0
KOOS			
Symptoms	78.2 ± 4.6	73.2	60.7-100.0
Pain	88.7 ± 2.3	91.7	77.8- 97.2
Function, activity of daily living	94.7 ± 1.9	97.8	83.8-100.0
Function, sports and recreational activities	73.0 ± 5.3	72.5	45.0-100.0
Quality of life	57.5 ± 5.8	59.4	25.0- 81.3
Modified Cincinnati Knee Rating Scales			
Total Score	77.9 ± 4.1	77.0	60.0-100.0
Sign/Symptoms Questions			
Pain Intensities	13.3 ± 1.2	12.0	8.0-20.0
Swelling	8.2 ± 0.52	8.0	6.0-10.0
Giving way	16.4 ± 1.4	20.0	8.0-20.0
Overall Activity Level	15.1 ± 1.1	16.0	12.0-20.0
Walking	9.6± 0.3	10.0	8.0-10.0
Stairs	8.9 ± 0.4	8.0	8.0-10.0
Running Activities	3.1 ± 0.5	3.0	0.0-5.0
Jumping and Twisting	3.2 ± 0.5	4.0	0.0-5.0

undergoing repeat arthroscopy and ACI resection with reports of ACI "failure" and loose bodies five years after initial ACI implantation. These last two cases can be defined as ACI failure, which was a rate of 20% at an average of twelve years.

In addition to ipsilateral reoperation, chart review showed two patients had contralateral knee surgery for OCD lesions, both requiring a second surgery for excision and microfracture.

4. Discussion

To our knowledge, this is the first long-term study of ACI treatment of knee JOCD patients using patients' reported

Table 3: Description of treatment history.

Have you had any treatments on your knee since ACI surgery?	**Frequency (%)**
Yes	10/10 (100%)
No	0/10 (0.0%)
If yes, what type of treatments have you had?	
Physical Therapy	8/10 (80.0%)
Brace	5/10 (50.0%)
Steroid Injection	0/10 (0.0%)
Visco Injection	1/10 (10.0%)
Activity Modification	6/10 (60.0%)
Work Restrictions	1/10 (10.0%)
Oral Medications	1/10 (10.0%)
Surgical Intervention	4/10 (40.0%)
Have you had any treatments on your knee during last year?	
Yes	4/10 (40.0%)
No	6/10 (60.0%)
If yes, what type of treatments have you had in last year?	
Physical Therapy	0/4 (0.0%)
Brace	2/4 (50.0%)
Steroid Injection	3/4 (75.0%)
Visco Injection	2/4 (50.0%)
Activity Modification	0/4 (75.0%)
Work Restrictions	3/4 (75.0%)
Oral Medications	1/4 (25.0%)
Surgical Intervention	1/4 (25.0%)

Table 4: Correlation coefficient analysis of the patients' outcome scores, lesion size, BMI, and age at ACI implantation.

	Lesion Size	**BMI**	**Age at ACI Implantation**
IKDC Total Score	- 0.29	- 0.28	- 0.08
KOOS Symptoms	- 0.51*	- 0.51*	0.32
KOOS Pain	0.04	- 0.49	- 0.03
KOOS Function, activity of daily living	- 0.02	0.01	- 0.09
KOOS Function, sports and recreational activities	- 0.30	- 0.18	0.23
KOOS Quality of life	- 0.12	- 0.06	0.22
Modified Cincinnati Knee Rating Total Scores	- 0.01	0.40	- 0.36

Values were expressed by correlation coefficient value r. *Two variables: moderate to good relationships were found between KOOS symptoms and lesion size ($p = .135$) and KOOS symptoms and BMI ($p = .133$), but were nonsignificant.

Table 5: Comparison of the patients' reported outcome scores by sex.

	Females (N = 5)	**Males (N = 5)**	**P-values**	**Effect Size**
IKDC				
Total Score	69.4 ± 5.5	74.2 ± 13.0	0.841	0.234
KOOS				
Symptoms	82.9 ± 13.0	73.6 ± 15.7	0.222	0.307
Pain	89.0 ± 6.3	88.3 ± 8.7	0.840	0.046
Function, activity of daily living	96.8 ± 4.9	92.7 ± 6.8	0.421	0.327
Function, sports and recreational activities	80.0 ± 10.0	66.0 ± 20.4	0.151	0.399
Quality of life	61.3 ± 16.8	53.8 ± 21.0	0.690	0.193
Modified Cincinnati Knee Rating Scales				
Total Score	77.4 ± 12.6	80.0 ± 12.5	0.972	0.103

Table 6: Comparison of the patients' reported outcome scores by OCD location.

	Medial (N = 6)	Lateral (N = 4)	P-values	Effect Size
IKDC				
Total Score	69.5 ± 4.8	75.3 ± 14.8	0.914	0.255
KOOS				
Symptoms	75.0 ± 13.6	83.0 ± 16.3	0.476	0.257
Pain	87.6 ± 6.6	90.3 ± 8.6	0.610	0.173
Function, activity of daily living	95.3 ± 5.6	93.8 ± 7.3	0.762	0.115
Function, sports and recreational activities	68.3 ± 14.0	80.0 ± 20.4	0.476	0.292
Quality of life	62.5 ± 13.1	50.0 ± 24.5	0.476	0.303
Modified Cincinnati Knee Rating Scales				
Total Score	77.8 ± 9.4	80.0 ± 16.5	0.998	0.082

Table 7: Comparison of the patients' reported outcome scores by number of OCD lesions before ACI.

	≤ 1 OCD Lesion (N = 8)	> 1 OCD Lesion (N = 2)	P-values	Effect Size
IKDC				
Total Score	72.8 ± 10.8	68.0 ± 1.4	0.711	0.298
KOOS				
Symptoms	81.7 ± 14.0	64.3 ± 5.1	0.089	0.637†
Pain	89.0 ± 7.2	87.5 ± 9.8	0.889	0.087
Function, activity of daily living	95.0 ± 6.2	93.4 ± 7.3	0.711	0.117
Function, sports and recreational activities	78.1 ± 14.1	52.5 ± 10.6	0.044*	0.716†
Quality of life	58.6 ± 20.0	53.1 ± 13.3	0.711	0.160
Modified Cincinnati Knee Rating Scales				
Total Score	80.9 ± 12.4	70.0 ± 1.4	0.400	0.525†

*Statistically significant differences were noted with $p < 0.05$. †Moderate effect size was found.

outcome measures: KOOS, IKDC, Modified Cincinnati Knee Rating scores, and treatment history survey. Compared to previously reported literature [16], outcome scores observed in this study showed sustained improvement through twelve years. Thus our hypothesis was confirmed that ACI is a valid long-term treatment option for JOCD. Lesion size and BMI had only moderately correlated with KOOS symptom score and had poor correlation with other patient-based outcomes. Sex and lesion location also did not show any statistical differences with long-term outcome measures. However, number of lesions prior to ACI procedures demonstrated interesting findings. ACI patients with ≤1 lesion showed greater than moderate effect sizes on KOOS symptoms, KOOS-function, sports, and recreational activities, and Modified Cincinnati Knee Rating Scales compared to ACI patients with >1 lesion. Although statistical significance value was observed in only one variable (KOOS-function, sports, and recreational activities), all components of the three outcome surveys were more favorable for ≤1 lesion. Thus, number of lesions before ACI procedures may potentially influence a long-term outcome of ACI.

Microfracture results, as the original treatment technique for OCD, are the baseline to which other techniques are compared. Several studies have compared osteochondral autologous transplantation to microfracture with results showing improved outcomes for a sustained period of time of osteochondral autologous transplantation over microfracture [21, 22]. Athletic patients had a higher return to activities and results were improved when patients were treated at a younger age [19]. In the only comparison study involving pediatric patients with an average age of 14 years (12 to 18), 91% had good to excellent outcomes with osteochondral autologous transplantation and only 56% with microfracture [23].

Histological studies that examined developmental changes of focal cartilage lesions over four years after ACI reported characteristics of articular cartilage over hyaline cartilage [24, 25]. Additionally, histologic studies comparing ACI to other cartilage restoration techniques showed ACI had similar articular cartilage architecture to osteochondral autografts and improved articular cartilage architecture to microfracture [26]. Given increasing life expectancy and increased activity levels, adolescents with articular cartilage lesions require the cartilage restoration procedure that most closely resembles native articular cartilage.

However, the majority of cartilage restoration studies focused on adult patients. ACI outcomes for isolated full-thickness chondral lesions have been reported up to twenty years after index surgery. Improvement in outcome scores has been sustained through this time period [12, 15, 18, 19, 24, 27–31]. Nearly half of adults who underwent ACI procedures reduced their sports intensity and only 40% maintained "similar" training on average five years after surgery [32]. Although the results did not exactly match with clinical outcomes, magnetic resonance imaging (MRI) between 9 and 18 years after implantation indicated the tissue quality of the repair was similar to surrounding articular cartilage with restoration of the defect area in the majority of patients [33]. These outcomes are considered to defer from ACI outcomes in JOCD due to the lack of underlying bone pathology and involvement.

Recent systematic review of ACI in the adolescent knee followed for 52 months (12 to 74 months) showed an average improvement of outcome scores near 40% with graft hypertrophy being the most common complication [34]. Adolescent patients undergoing ACI for OCD have 96% good to excellent outcomes at the mid-term [17]. Similarly, 96% of patients also returned to high impact sports and 60% returned to a level equal to or higher than prior to their knee injury [17]. Improved results were seen in patients with shorter duration of symptoms (<12 months) and fewer surgeries [17, 34]. Looking at soccer specifically, younger patients, isolated lesions, shorter duration of symptoms, and lower number of surgeries correlated with improved rate of returning to soccer [35]. Our study was underpowered to be able to compare previous surgery numbers with outcomes. However, these previous studies demonstrated prompt treatment of JOCDs is paramount given their improved results.

Compared to the results of this study, a shorter follow-up study employed a similar cohort of JOCD patients with several years of follow-up duration (minimum of two years and mean follow-up time of four years) [16]. The study reported Modified Cincinnati Knee Rating score of 72 with an overall failure rate of 3% while the current study had a score of 78 and a failure rate of 20%. Nineteen percent of patients had undergone a subsequent surgical procedure by four-year follow-up in the previous study while the current study showed an increased surgical rate to 40% by twelve-year follow-up. Graft hypertrophy and graft failure were the common causes of need for subsequent surgery. The same senior author was involved in both studies and there is a high likelihood that patients enrolled in our study were also involved in the earlier study. However, previous databases were not available to confirm this suspicion.

Rosa et al. [36] published a similar study to the current study and concluded that ACI is an effective, durable solution for full-thickness cartilage and osteochondral lesions of the knee in young patients. With similar 12-year follow-up, 15 patients with average age of 21 years (range 13-45 years, standard deviation of 8.9 years) were treated with ACI for full-thickness cartilage and osteochondral lesions. Only seven patients were OCD patients and none of their patients had prior surgeries to treat their lesions. Average lesion size was slightly smaller than the current study (5.08 ± 2.01 versus 9.1 ± 1.9 cm^2). Similarly, a two-step ACI technique was performed in both studies.

The majority of our results were comparable in these two similar studies. Failure of ACI has been previously defined [16] as subsequent operation that either (1) necessitated removal of the graft, (2) confirmed a loss of defect fill, or (3) violated the subchondral bone (e.g., abrasion chondroplasty, microfracture, drilling, unicompartmental arthroplasty, or total knee arthroplasty). Both studies recorded two failures resulting in graft resection, though Rosa et al. did not define which patients, isolated cartilage or osteochondral lesions, failed. Outcome scores were similar between Rosa et al. and the current study with IKDC (76.3 versus 73.0), KOOS Pain (79.6 versus 88.7), symptoms (76.4 versus 78.2), activities of daily living (85.1 versus 94.7), and sports (70.3 versus 73.0). Despite these similar scores, Rosa et al. had a higher knee quality of life KOOS score of 74.2 compared to 57.5 documented in this study. Despite high scores on the rest of the outcome measures, speculation as to the lower knee quality of life in the current study is likely related to activity expectations of a younger population and their frustration with any hindrance in activity.

In addition to clinical outcomes, Rosa et al. were able to obtain MRI images around 12 years after surgery on a majority of their patients. Using the Magnetic Resonance Observation of Cartilage Repair Tissue (MOCART) system, the authors detected a significant decrease in MOCART score from short- to long-term follow-up with significant correlation with degree of defect repair and pain KOOS scores [36].

In 2012, the AAOS announced Clinical Practice Guidelines of the diagnosis and treatment of OCD [37]. Statements 8 and 12 stated that the work group is unable to recommend for or against a specific cartilage repair technique in symptomatic cases among skeletally immature or mature patients. The strength of recommendation of these particular statements was "inconclusive". This work group, however, had "consensus" level recommendation for offering surgery to skeletally mature or immature patients with symptomatic OCDs despite limited literature. This current study may help providing scientifically quality evidence and clinically valuable knowledge into long-term outcomes of JOCD treatment with ACI.

In 2016, the German Society of Orthopedics and Trauma (DGOU) work group on "Clinical Tissue Regeneration" provided guidelines on the use of ACI for knee cartilage defects [38]. Specified indications for ACI in the knee joint to include full-thickness, symptomatic cartilage defects of OCD stages 3 and 4 per ICRS-OCD, possibly in combination with subchondral reconstruction with use in children and adolescents. The group agreed that effect of subchondral edema is largely unknown due to limited available research as only one paper published on the topic concluded they were unable to find correlation between edema and outcomes [11]. Successful subchondral reconstruction has been described with subchondral defects greater than 3 mm undergoing one- or two-stage subchondral reconstruction [30]. Though the current study was not designed to comment on subchondral edema or subchondral reconstruction, our long-term results showed that knee JOCD patients can be successfully treated with ACI.

While ACI is a viable option for cartilage defects of the knee, excision/debridement, bone marrow stimulation, and allograft or autograft osteocartilaginous reconstructions are also available options for surgeons. Mundi et al. [39] published a meta-analysis with systematic review of Level 1 studies of cartilage restoration techniques of the knee. Synthesizing 12 studies completed in Europe on adult patients with variable pathology underwent, meta-analysis indicated no difference between outcomes of ACI and microfracture at 2 years despite majority of individual studies stating improvement of ACI outcomes over microfracture. Also, another limitation of this meta-analysis was not able to analyze comparison of ACI versus osteochondral autograft transplantation due to poor study methodologies and data collections. Therefore, their findings concluded an inability to determine a single best technique for cartilage restoration.

Only two studies have compared ACI versus other surgical treatment options for OCD. A 3-year observational, adult cohort showed ACI had improved knee function scores and greater relief from pain and swelling than debridement [40]. A prospective, randomized study comparing ACI versus mosaicplasty in adults demonstrated superiority of ACI over mosaicplasty with limited 19-month outcome being a main weakness of the study [41]. The relatively short duration of follow-up duration and small sample size of these studies are common limitations. With poor long-term clinical outcomes [42, 43] and evidence of early osteoarthritic changes on radiographs [44], JOCD fragment excision and debridement are less than desirable surgical techniques. Long-term results of osteochondral allografts [45, 46] and autografts [47, 48] indicated promise, but must be used with care in skeletally immature patients and near open physes of the distal femur. In short, surgeons who are planning to conduct future studies need to consider improving study methodologies and outcomes in order to determine the best treatment option for the individual patients, especially skeletally immature patients.

The senior author of this study has noted that most OCD lesions that fail to heal and have undergone fragment removal have necrotic bone at the base of the lesion. Ideally, vascularity must be restored to this base before ACI is attempted. This is usually best done by patterned drilling of the lesion with a .045 smooth pin at least six months prior to implant. MRI can be used to determine the depth required to bypass the necrotic bone. Using microfracture awls are not advised due to the risk of insufficient depth of penetration.

4.1. Limitation. Weaknesses of our study include small sample size, which limits generalizability of the current data. Nonsignificant findings by sex and lesion size analysis may be due to the small sample sizes. In addition, clinical or radiographic follow-up at final outcome point would have assisted understanding current status of ACI on patients' perception. At the time of ACI in our patient cohort, this surgical technique was still being developed and validated and therefore was not widely completed accounting for our small sample size. This small sample likely represents some of the first patients undergoing ACI for failed surgical treatment of JOCD. These patients had transitioned from teenage to adult life often moving away from the institution where their ACI was completed and therefore were unable to be examined and evaluated at final outcome.

5. Conclusion

The current study aimed to define long-term follow-up of JOCD patients undergoing ACI. The outcome data from patients' records and surveys indicated the ACI can be a viable treatment through twelve years despite the high need for continued treatment. The analysis showed a moderate to good relationship was found between KOOS symptoms and both BMI and lesion size while sex and lesion location had no effect on outcome scores. Additionally, number of lesions before ACI procedures may be an important factor for a long-term effect. In order to confirm the study outcome of this study, future study needs to have a bigger data sample size.

Appendix

Uniquely Created Survey of Treatments Rendered since Time of ACI Procedure

Thank you for agreeing to participate in our study. We would like to ask you some additional follow up questions about how you are doing. Please answer them as best you can.

Name: —

Biological Sex: —

Height: —

Weight: —

Current Occupation: —

(1) Have you required any treatment for your knee since your ACI surgery? □ Yes □ No

If Yes,

Please mark all non-operative treatments required since your ACI:

□ PT

□ Brace

□ Steroid Injection

□ Visco injection

□ Activity modification

□ Work restrictions

□ Oral medications

□ Other: —

Please mark all non-operative treatments required in the **last year**:

□ PT

□ Brace

□ Steroid Injection

□ Visco injection

□ Activity modification

□ Work restrictions

□ Oral medications

□ Other: —

(2) Please mark all imaging studies of your knee you've had in the past five years:

□ Xray

□ MRI

Table 8

	What was the name of the procedure?	What date was the surgery (month/year)?	Who was the surgeon?
1.			
2.			
3.			
4.			
5.			

□ CT

□ Bone scan

(4) Where were they completed?—

(5) Please list any additional surgeries to your knee after having ACI performed by Dr. Micheli? See Table 8

(6) Can we contact you if we have further questions regarding your treatment history? □ Yes □ No

Disclosure

This study was independently, internally funded without external support.

References

[1] E. W. Edmonds and K. G. Shea, "Osteochondritis dissecans: editorial comment," *Clinical Orthopaedics and Related Research*, vol. 471, no. 4, pp. 1105-1106, 2013.

[2] E. J. Wall, J. D. Polousky, K. G. Shea et al., "Novel radiographic feature classification of knee osteochondritis dissecans: A multicenter reliability study," *The American Journal of Sports Medicine*, vol. 43, no. 2, pp. 303–309, 2015.

[3] J. M. Ellermann, B. Donald, S. Rohr et al., "Magnetic Resonance Imaging of Osteochondritis Dissecans: Validation Study for the ICRS Classification System," *Academic Radiology*, vol. 23, no. 6, pp. 724–729, 2016.

[4] C. E. Quatman, C. C. Quatman-Yates, L. C. Schmitt, and M. V. Paterno, "The clinical utility and diagnostic performance of MRI for identification and classification of knee osteochondritis dissecans," *The Journal of Bone & Joint Surgery*, vol. 94, no. 11, pp. 1036–1044, 2012.

[5] B. P. Robbach, A. C. Paulus, T. R. Niethammer et al., "Discrepancy between morphological findings in juvenile osteochondritis dissecans (OCD): a comparison of magnetic resonance imaging (MRI) and arthroscopy," *Knee Surgery, Sports Traumatology, Arthroscopy*, vol. 24, no. 4, pp. 1259–1264, 2016.

[6] H. Schmal, J. M. Pestka, G. Salzmann, P. C. Strohm, N. P. Südkamp, and P. Niemeyer, "Autologous chondrocyte implantation in children and adolescents," *Knee Surgery, Sports Traumatology, Arthroscopy*, vol. 21, no. 3, pp. 671–677, 2013.

[7] J. I. Kessler, H. Nikizad, K. G. Shea, J. C. Jacobs, J. D. Bebchuk, and J. M. Weiss, "The demographics and epidemiology of osteochondritis dissecans of the knee in children and adolescents," *The American Journal of Sports Medicine*, vol. 42, no. 2, pp. 320–326, 2014.

[8] T. Cooper, A. Boyles, W. P. Samora, and K. E. Klingele, "Prevalence of bilateral JOCD of the knee and associated risk factors," *Journal of Pediatric Orthopaedics*, vol. 35, no. 5, pp. 507–510, 2014.

[9] L. Salci, O. Ayeni, M. Abouassaly et al., "Indications for surgical management of osteochondritis dissecans of the knee in the pediatric population: a systematic review.," *The Journal of Knee Surgery*, vol. 27, no. 2, pp. 147–155, 2014.

[10] J. L. Yellin, I. Gans, J. L. Carey, K. G. Shea, and T. J. Ganley, "The surgical management of osteochondritis dissecans of the knee in the skeletally immature: A survey of the Pediatric Orthopaedic Society of North America (POSNA) membership," *Journal of Pediatric Orthopaedics*, vol. 37, no. 7, pp. 491–499, 2017.

[11] G. Filardo, E. Kon, A. Di Martino et al., "Is the clinical outcome after cartilage treatment affected by subchondral bone edema?" *Knee Surgery, Sports Traumatology, Arthroscopy*, vol. 22, no. 6, pp. 1337–1344, 2014.

[12] E. Kon, F. Vannini, R. Buda et al., "How to Treat Osteochondritis Dissecans of the Knee: Surgical Techniques and New Trends," *The Journal of Bone and Joint Surgery-American Volume*, vol. 94, no. 1, pp. e1-1-8, 2012.

[13] S. P. Krishnan, J. A. Skinner, W. Bartlett et al., "Who is the ideal candidate for autologous chondrocyte implantation?" *The Journal of Bone & Joint Surgery (British Volume)*, vol. 88-B, no. 1, pp. 61–64, 2006.

[14] S. P. Krishnan, J. A. Skinner, R. W. J. Carrington, A. M. Flanagan, T. W. R. Briggs, and G. Bentley, "Collagen-covered autologous chondrocyte implantation for osteochondritis dissecans of the knee. Two- to seven-year results," *The Journal of Bone & Joint Surgery (British Volume)*, vol. 88, no. 2, pp. 203–205, 2006.

[15] C. Pascual-Garrido, N. A. Friel, S. S. Kirk et al., "Midterm Results of Surgical Treatment for Adult Osteochondritis Dissecans of the Knee," *The American Journal of Sports Medicine*, vol. 37, no. 1_suppl, pp. 125–130, 2017.

[16] L. J. Micheli, J. B. Moseley, A. F. Anderson et al., "Articular cartilage defects of the distal femur in children and adolescents: Treatment with autologous chondrocyte implantation," *Journal of Pediatric Orthopaedics*, vol. 26, no. 4, pp. 455–460, 2006.

[17] K. Mithöfer, T. Minas, L. Peterson, H. Yeon, and L. J. Micheli, "Functional outcome of knee articular cartilage repair in adolescent athletes," *The American Journal of Sports Medicine*, vol. 33, no. 8, pp. 1147–1153, 2005.

[18] B. J. Cole, T. DeBerardino, R. Brewster et al., "Outcomes of Autologous Chondrocyte Implantation in Study of the Treatment of Articular Repair (STAR) Patients With Osteochondritis Dissecans," *The American Journal of Sports Medicine*, vol. 40, no. 9, pp. 2015–2022, 2012.

[19] D. Martinčič, D. Radosavljevič, and M. Drobnič, "Ten-year clinical and radiographic outcomes after autologous chondrocyte implantation of femoral condyles," *Knee Surgery, Sports Traumatology, Arthroscopy*, vol. 22, no. 6, pp. 1277–1283, 2014.

[20] L. G. Portney and M. P. Watkins, *Foundations of clinical research: applications to practice*, NJ, Prentice Hall Upper Saddle, 2000.

[21] R. Gudas, A. Gudaite, A. Pocius et al., "Ten-year follow-up of a prospective, randomized clinical study of mosaic osteochondral autologous transplantation versus microfracture for the treatment of osteochondral defects in the knee joint of athletes," *The American Journal of Sports Medicine*, vol. 40, no. 11, pp. 2499–2508, 2012.

[22] R. Gudas, E. Stankevičius, E. Monastyreckiene, D. Pranys, and R. J. Kalesinskas, "Osteochondral autologous transplantation versus microfracture for the treatment of articular cartilage defects in the knee joint in athletes," *Knee Surgery, Sports Traumatology, Arthroscopy*, vol. 14, no. 9, pp. 834–842, 2006.

[23] R. Gudas, R. Simonaityte, E. Čekanauskas, and R. Tamošiunas, "A prospective, randomized clinical study of osteochondral autologous transplantation versus microfracture for the treatment of osteochondritis dissecans in the knee joint in children," *Journal of Pediatric Orthopaedics*, vol. 29, no. 7, pp. 741–748, 2009.

[24] L. Peterson, M. Brittberg, I. Kiviranta, E. L. Åkerlund, and A. Lindahl, "Autologous chondrocyte transplantation: biomechanics and long-term durability," *The American Journal of Sports Medicine*, vol. 30, no. 1, pp. 2–12, 2002.

[25] L. Peterson, T. Minas, M. Brittberg, A. Nilsson, E. Sjögren-Jansson, and A. Lindahl, "Two-to 9-year outcome after autologous chondrocyte transplantation of the knee," *Clinical Orthopaedics and Related Research*, no. 374, pp. 212–234, 2000.

[26] A. C. DiBartola, J. S. Everhart, R. A. Magnussen et al., "Correlation between histological outcome and surgical cartilage repair technique in the knee: A meta-analysis," *The Knee*, vol. 23, no. 3, pp. 344–349, 2016.

[27] A. E. Beris, M. G. Lykissas, I. Kostas-Agnantis, and G. N. Manoudis, "Treatment of full-thickness chondral defects of the knee with autologous chondrocyte implantation: A functional evaluation with long-term follow-up," *The American Journal of Sports Medicine*, vol. 40, no. 3, pp. 562–567, 2012.

[28] A. M. Bhosale, J. H. Kuiper, W. E. Johnson, P. E. Harrison, and J. B. Richardson, "Midterm to Long-Term Longitudinal Outcome of Autologous Chondrocyte Implantation in the Knee Joint," *The American Journal of Sports Medicine*, vol. 37, no. 1_suppl, pp. 131–138, 2017.

[29] T. Minas, A. Von Keudell, T. Bryant, and A. H. Gomoll, "The John Insall Award: A Minimum 10-year Outcome Study of Autologous Chondrocyte Implantation," *Clinical Orthopaedics and Related Research*, vol. 472, no. 1, pp. 41–51, 2014.

[30] P. Niemeyer, S. Porichis, M. Steinwachs et al., "Long-term outcomes after first-generation autologous chondrocyte implantation for cartilage defects of the knee," *The American Journal of Sports Medicine*, vol. 42, no. 1, pp. 150–157, 2014.

[31] L. Peterson, H. S. Vasiliadis, M. Brittberg, and A. Lindahl, "Autologous chondrocyte implantation: a long-term follow-up," *The American Journal of Sports Medicine*, vol. 38, no. 6, pp. 1117–1124, 2010.

[32] J. M. Pestka, M. J. Feucht, S. Porichis, G. Bode, N. P. Südkamp, and P. Niemeyer, "Return to Sports Activity and Work after Autologous Chondrocyte Implantation of the Knee: Which Factors Influence Outcomes?" *The American Journal of Sports Medicine*, vol. 44, no. 2, pp. 370–377, 2016.

[33] H. S. Vasiliadis, B. Danielson, and M. Ljunberg, "Autologous chondrocyte implantation in cartilage lesions of the knee: long-term evaluation with magnetic resonance imaging and delayed gadolinium-enhanced magnetic resonance imaging technique," *The American Journal of Sports Medicine*, vol. 38, no. 5, pp. 943–949, 2010.

[34] A. C. DiBartola, B. M. Wright, R. A. Magnussen, and D. C. Flanigan, "Clinical Outcomes After Autologous Chondrocyte Implantation in Adolescents' Knees: A Systematic Review," *Arthroscopy - Journal of Arthroscopic and Related Surgery*, vol. 32, no. 9, pp. 1905–1916, 2016.

[35] K. Mithöfer, L. Peterson, B. R. Mandelbaum, and T. Minas, "Articular cartilage repair in soccer players with autologous chondrocyte transplantation: Functional outcome and return to competition," *The American Journal of Sports Medicine*, vol. 33, no. 11, pp. 1639–1646, 2005.

[36] D. Rosa, G. Balato, G. Ciaramella, E. Soscia, G. Improta, and M. Triassi, "Long-term clinical results and MRI changes after autologous chondrocyte implantation in the knee of young and active middle aged patients," *Journal of Orthopaedics and Traumatology*, vol. 17, no. 1, pp. 55–62, 2016.

[37] H. G. Chambers, K. G. Shea, and J. L. Carey, "AAOS Clinical Practice Guideline: Diagnosis and Treatment of Osteochondritis Dissecans," *American Academy of Orthopaedic Surgeon*, vol. 19, no. 5, pp. 307–309, 2011.

[38] P. Niemeyer, D. Albrecht, S. Andereya et al., "Autologous chondrocyte implantation (ACI) for cartilage defects of the knee: a guideline by the working group 'Clinical Tissue Regeneration' of the German Society of Orthopaedics and Trauma (DGOU)," *The Knee*, vol. 23, no. 3, pp. 426–435, 2016.

[39] R. Mundi, A. Bedi, L. Chow et al., "Cartilage Restoration of the Knee," *The American Journal of Sports Medicine*, vol. 44, no. 7, pp. 1888–1895, 2016.

[40] F. H. Fu, D. Zurakowski, J. E. Browne et al., "Autologous chondrocyte implantation versus debridement for treatment of full-thickness chondral defects of the knee: An observational cohort study with 3-year follow-up," *The American Journal of Sports Medicine*, vol. 33, no. 11, pp. 1658–1666, 2005.

[41] G. Bentley, L. C. Biant, R. W. J. Carrington et al., "A prospective, randomised comparison of autologous chondrocyte implantation versus mosaicplasty for osteochondral defects in the knee," *The Journal of Bone & Joint Surgery (British Volume)*, vol. 85, no. 2, pp. 223–230, 2003.

[42] J. W. Michael, A. Wurth, P. Eysel, and D. P. König, "Long-term results after operative treatment of osteochondritis dissecans of the knee joint—30 year results," *International Orthopaedics*, vol. 32, no. 2, pp. 217–221, 2008.

[43] R. W. Wright, M. McLean, M. J. Matava, and R. A. Shively, "Osteochondritis dissecans of the knee: Long-term results of excision of the fragment," *Clinical Orthopaedics and Related Research*, no. 424, pp. 239–243, 2004.

[44] J. R. D. Murray, J. Chitnavis, P. Dixon et al., "Osteochondritis dissecans of the knee; long-term clinical outcome following arthroscopic debridement," *The Knee*, vol. 14, no. 2, pp. 94–98, 2007.

[45] R. Lyon, C. Nissen, X. C. Liu, and B. Curtin, "Can fresh osteochondral allografts restore function in juveniles with osteochondritis dissecans of the knee? Knee," *Clinical Orthopaedics and Related Research*, vol. 471, no. 4, pp. 1166–1173, 2013.

[46] G. Raz, O. A. Safir, D. J. Backstein, P. T. H. Lee, and A. E. Gross, "Distal femoral fresh osteochondral allografts: Follow-up at a mean of twenty-two years," *Journal of Bone and Joint Surgery - American Volume*, vol. 96, no. 13, pp. 1101–1107, 2014.

[47] K. Sasaki, T. Matsumoto, T. Matsushita et al., "Osteochondral autograft transplantation for juvenile osteochondritis dissecans of the knee: A series of twelve cases," *International Orthopaedics*, vol. 36, no. 11, pp. 2243–2248, 2012.

24

Posttraumatic Spinal Cord Injury without Radiographic Abnormality

Kivanc Atesok,[1] Nobuhiro Tanaka,[2] Andrew O'Brien,[3] Yohan Robinson,[4] Dachling Pang,[5,6,7] Donald Deinlein,[1] Sakthivel Rajaram Manoharan,[1] Jason Pittman,[1] and Steven Theiss[1]

[1]*Department of Orthopaedic Surgery, University of Alabama at Birmingham, Birmingham, AL, USA*
[2]*Department of Orthopaedic Surgery, Hiroshima University, Hiroshima, Japan*
[3]*Royal Victoria Hospital and Royal Belfast Hospital for Sick Children, Belfast, UK*
[4]*Department of Surgical Sciences, Uppsala University Hospital, Uppsala, Sweden*
[5]*Department of Pediatric Neurosurgery, University of California, Davis, CA, USA*
[6]*Regional Centre for Paediatric Neurosurgery, Kaiser Permanente Hospitals, Oakland, CA, USA*
[7]*Great Ormond Street Hospital For Children, NHS Trust, London, UK*

Correspondence should be addressed to Kivanc Atesok; Katesok@uabmc.edu

Academic Editor: John P. Kostuik

"Spinal Cord Injury without Radiographic Abnormality" (SCIWORA) is a term that denotes objective clinical signs of posttraumatic spinal cord injury without evidence of fracture or malalignment on plain radiographs and computed tomography (CT) of the spine. SCIWORA is most commonly seen in children with a predilection for the cervical spinal cord due to the increased mobility of the cervical spine, the inherent ligamentous laxity, and the large head-to-body ratio during childhood. However, SCIWORA can also be seen in adults and, in rare cases, the thoracolumbar spinal cord can be affected too. Magnetic resonance imaging (MRI) has become a valuable diagnostic tool in patients with SCIWORA because of its superior ability to identify soft tissue lesions such as cord edema, hematomas and transections, and discoligamentous injuries that may not be visualized in plain radiographs and CT. The mainstay of treatment in patients with SCIWORA is nonoperative management including steroid therapy, immobilization, and avoidance of activities that may increase the risk of exacerbation or recurrent injury. Although the role of operative treatment in SCIWORA can be controversial, surgical alternatives such as decompression and fusion should be considered in selected patients with clinical and MRI evidence of persistent spinal cord compression and instability.

1. Introduction

The acronym SCIWORA (Spinal Cord Injury without Radiographic Abnormality) was first defined in 1982 by Pang and Wilberger Jr. in a series of 24 children who suffered traumatic myelopathy with no radiographic evidence of fractures, dislocations, or malalignment of the spine [1]. Pang and Pollack described SCIWORA as a syndrome in which there are clinical signs of traumatic spinal cord injury (SCI) without overt traumatic vertebral column disruption as displayed by spine X-rays, computed tomographic (CT) scans, myelograms, and dynamic flexion/extension X-rays [2]. The first human magnetic resonance imaging (MRI) scan was done in 1977, and distinctive MRI signal patterns of acute SCI were first described in 1987 [3, 4]. Hence, the original report from Pang and Wilberger Jr. that introduced SCIWORA into medical literature did not include MRI in the definition of this syndrome; Pang acknowledged the diagnostic potential of MRI in patients with SCIWORA two decades later [5]. It might be sensible to ask, "Would SCIWORA still exist if MRI was readily available for use in acute SCI only a few years earlier?" The answer would probably be "Yes," since MRI is never the first-line imaging modality in the setting of acute spinal trauma. Plain X-rays and CT are almost invariably performed before MRI, since MRI scans require more time, space, and patient transfer that might not be practical in emergency management of trauma patients.

SCIWORA is more commonly seen in the pediatric age group than in adults and involves the cervical spine more frequently than the thoracolumbar spine. The incidences have been reported between 13 to 19% and 10 to 12% of spinal injuries in children and adults, respectively [6–9]. SCIWORA is far more common in males than females [6, 8–10]. In a systematic review, Carroll et al. [10] documented that, of 368 pediatric patients with SCIWORA, approximately 68.5% were male, and 31.5% were female. Cervical spine was involved in 87% of the patients; thoracic spine was involved in 9.5%; lumbar spine was involved in 1.5%; and in 2%, the SCI spanned the cervical and thoracic levels. Evidence from the adult population indicating that thoracolumbar spine can also be involved with SCIWORA is limited to occasional case reports [11, 12]. The reasons for increased frequency of SCIWORA in the pediatric age group with a predilection for the cervical spinal cord include the large head-to-body ratio, increased mobility of the cervical spine, inherent ligamentous laxity, immaturity of neck musculature, incomplete ossification of the vertebrae, and shallow angulation of facet joints during childhood [2, 5, 12]. Interestingly, several studies showed that the upper cervical spine was more susceptible to SCIWORA in younger children than in older children, where the lower cervical spine is more commonly affected [2, 10, 13]. This finding is supported by the fact that the fulcrum of movement is at the upper levels of the cervical spine (between C2 and C4) in younger children and shifts to lower levels (C5-C6) in adolescents and adults [14, 15]. It is conceivable that SCIWORA is seen less frequently in adults as a result of age-related changes in bone morphology and a decrease in ligamentous laxity. Furthermore, the thoracic spine has a more stable and stiff structure compared to the cervical spine due to the surrounding rib cage and costovertebral articulations. Similarly, both the thoracic and lumbar spine have larger bony surfaces that increase axial loading capacity and stability [12].

2. Pathophysiology

Several mechanisms have been proposed to cause SCIWORA including spinal cord traction injury due to hyperflexion, extrinsic cord damage from hyperextension, and parenchymal cord damage resulting from edema or vascular injury [12]. The two-hit hypothesis is one of the possible pathophysiological explanations for delayed cord damage in patients with SCIWORA. After the primary injury from direct impact, a subsequent secondary insult to spinal cord parenchyma from complex cellular-level reactions to the primary injury can worsen the clinical picture [18]. Traumatic SCI may cause increased Na^+ influx into the cells through voltage-gated channels, which may lead to increased H^+ influx and intracellular acidosis through the activation of the Na^+/H^+ exchanger in an attempt by the cell to pump out accumulating intracellular Na^+ [19]. Likewise, increased Na^+ influx after SCI may cause reversal of Na^+/Ca^{++} exchanger that results in an increase in Na^+ extrusion and intracellular Ca^{++} accumulation with apoptosis of the neurons [18, 19]. These changes trigger intracellular events such as free radical-mediated cell damage, lipid peroxidation, and activation of membrane lipases. Consequently, a cascade of secondary inflammatory reactions, edema, and ischemia resulting in further spinal cord parenchymal insult can occur [18, 19].

3. Mechanism of Injury

The most common causes of injury in patients with SCIWORA are sports injuries, motor vehicle collisions, falls, and abuse [2, 10, 13]. In a series of 297 children who suffered from SCIWORA, Knox [13] demonstrated age-related variations in the mechanism of injury. Between 0 to 10 years, the most common cause of injury was found to be motor vehicle collisions (38–40%). However, sports injuries were the most common injury mechanism in children between 11 and 17 years of age (57%). In adult patients with SCIWORA, falls appear to be the most common mechanism of injury. Como et al. [20] reported that, of the 24 adult patients with SCIWORA, 67% had a mechanism of fall. In another study from Sharma et al. [9] of 12 adult SCIWORA patients, five (42%) were injured in motor vehicle accidents, and four (33%) fell from height. The difference between the two studies in terms of the most common mechanism of injury can be attributed to the difference in the number of patients included in each study (24 versus 12 patients, resp.). The literature includes sporadic publications reporting on thoracic SCIWORA cases in adults following motor vehicle accidents [11, 12]. Despite insufficient evidence, this may indicate the severity of the injury mechanism required to cause SCIWORA in the biomechanically more stable thoracic spine.

4. Diagnostic Evaluation

After the initial management in the field, diagnostic evaluation of patients with presumed SCI should start with a detailed history which can be possibly taken from eyewitnesses to determine the mechanism of injury [5]. More often than not, there are associated injuries of the head, thorax, abdomen, face, vasculature, pelvis, and the extremities. In a study of nationwide pediatric admissions, Knox [13] reported that 87% of patients with SCIWORA had associated injuries, and head trauma was the most common injury (between 28 to 64%), followed by orthopaedic injuries (10%), facial injuries (9%), thoracic injuries (9%), and gastrointestinal injuries (4%). It is imperative to detect and address these injuries, which can also provide clues to the mechanism of injury [5].

4.1. Clinical Findings. Clinical examination focusing on neurological findings may reveal a broad range of neurological deficits. Although clinical signs and symptoms can be observed from the moment of injury, neurological deficits may only become apparent several days after the injury due to second-hit phenomenon, edema, or a developing hematoma around the cord [21].

Table 1: Summarized descriptions of ASIA Impairment Scale (AIS) Grades A, B, C, D, and E. Please note that only patients with an initial SCI and neurological findings receive an AIS grade. *(Source: with permission from American Spinal Injury Association: International Standards for Neurological Classification of Spinal Cord Injury.)*

American Spinal Injury Association (ASIA) Impairment Scale (AIS)		
Grade		Description
A	Complete	No sensory or motor function is preserved in the sacral segments S4-5
B	Sensory incomplete	Sensory but not motor function is preserved below the neurological level and includes the sacral segments S4-5 AND no motor function is preserved more than three levels below the motor level on either side of the body
C	Motor incomplete	Motor function is preserved at the most caudal sacral segments for voluntary anal contraction OR the patient meets the criteria for sensory incomplete status
D	Motor incomplete	Motor incomplete status as defined above, with at least half (half or more) of key muscle functions below the single NLI having a muscle grade ≥ 3
E	Normal	If sensation and motor function are graded as normal in all segments and the patient had prior deficits, then the AIS grade is E

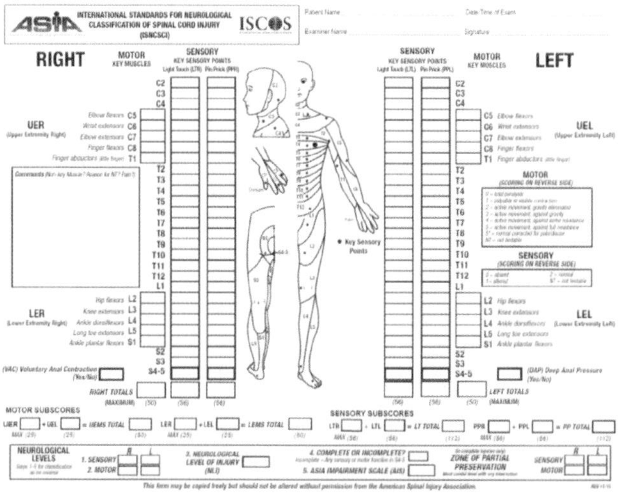

Figure 1: American Spinal Injury Association (ASIA) Injury Scale. *(Source: with permission from American Spinal Injury Association: International Standards for Neurological Classification of Spinal Cord Injury.)*

A thorough neurological examination immediately after the injury may indicate the level of SCI and help to monitor the progress of patients at later stages of their management. It is advisable to use one of the SCI scales, such as the American Spinal Cord Injury Association (ASIA) scale (Figure 1), and report the neurological examination findings as ASIA Impairment Scale (AIS) grades (Table 1) [22]. Published reports indicate that patients with SCIWORA may present with a wide range of neurological findings, including para/hemiparesis/plegia, paresthesia, changes in tendon reflexes, loss of bladder and bowel function, signs of anterior/central/posterior cord or Brown-Séquard syndrome in addition to local pain, sensitivity, abrasions, and bruising around the vertebral column [2, 11, 12, 17, 23].

In a retrospective case series from Martinez-Perez et al. [8] that included 48 adult patients diagnosed with SCIWORA, two patients had complete SCI with AIS grade A; five patients were documented as AIS grade B; 15 patients had AIS grade C; and 26 patients had AIS grade D SCI at admission. Neurological assessment of the patients at one-year follow-up revealed that neither of the two patients with complete SCI showed improvement after admission. All but eight patients (two grade B, two grade C, and 6 grade D) with incomplete SCI had improvement of at least one grade on AIS at one-year follow-up [8].

It should be kept in mind that neurological findings in SCIWORA patients may not always be prominent, and there may be fluctuations in severity.

4.2. Plain Radiographs and CT. In all patients with traumatic SCI, anteroposterior (AP), lateral (LAT), and odontoid views of the cervical spine are obtained. Depending on the level of injury, AP and LAT views of the thoracic and lumbar spine are added. If plain films do not reveal any abnormalities, then thin-section CT scans with coronal and sagittal three-dimensional (3D) reconstructions are performed. By definition, neither plain X-rays nor CT will reveal any signs of vertebral column fractures, dislocations, or malalignment in patients with SCIWORA syndrome despite the neurological findings of traumatic SCI in clinical assessment. In a postmortem study with 30 cases whose autopsy findings indicated gross or microscopic injuries to the spinal column or cord, Makino et al. [16] found that six patients (SCIWORA group) had no postmortem multidetector CT (MDCT) scan findings suggestive of direct or indirect trauma to the cervical spine. Although 58% (14/24) of non-SCIWORA cases had MDCT-detectable perivertebral hemorrhage, none of the SCIWORA subjects had hemorrhages detectable in postmortem MDCT images (Figure 2). The results of this study point out that even using a more advanced CT imaging technique such as MDCT may not provide conclusive evidence of spinal cord injury in SCIWORA patients [16].

4.3. Dynamic Imaging. If standard AP and LAT plain X-ray and CT images do not reveal any fracture or dislocation, the stability of the spine can be assessed by dynamic flexion and extension radiographs. Although conceptually dynamic imaging might be seen as an alternative modality in the

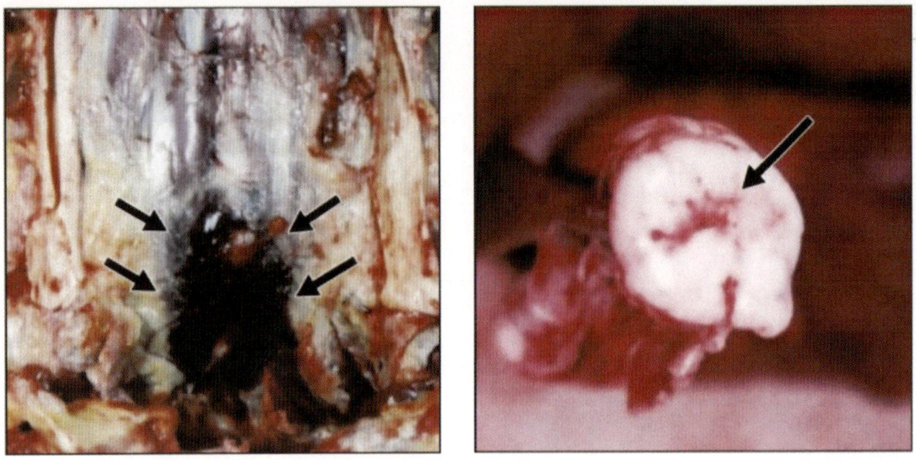

(a) (b)

Figure 2: Autopsy photographs of a 44-year-old man found dead near his bicycle. Cause of dead was not explainable based on external examination and investigation. MDCT scan did not reveal any fractures, dislocations, or other signs of trauma. (a) Autopsy revealed perivertebral hemorrhage (arrows) anterior to C6 and C7. (b) Macroscopic axial autopsy photographs show hemorrhage (arrow) in cervical spinal cord at C5. *(Source: with permission from [16].)*

diagnostic algorithm of SCIWORA patients, current evidence does not provide enough support for its routine use. Pang and Pollack [2] obtained dynamic cervical films during the first week after injury in 55 children with SCIWORA and noted that, in most, severe paraspinous muscle spasm prevented adequate flexion. The authors repeated the dynamic films after spasm had subsided and showed late stability in only one patient who had anterior subluxation of C4 on C5 that was masked on previous studies due to spasm [2].

Several investigators have studied the role of dynamic imaging in spinal clearance of obtunded trauma patients and their findings revealed that flexion and extension views do not provide any advantage over CT and are not cost effective as a diagnostic modality in cervical spine clearance [24–26]. Considering that the patients in these studies were unconscious and in a relatively relaxed state [24–26], performing adequate dynamic imaging with meaningful results in conscious SCIWORA patients with paraspinous muscle spasm would be highly unlikely. Hence, we do not recommend using dynamic imaging in SCIWORA patients who already had negative plain X-rays and CT images.

4.4. MRI. The advent of MRI provided superior visualization of the soft tissue structures and enabled better recognition of the pathologies involving intervertebral disks, ligaments, and neural tissues including the spinal cord and nerve roots. As a result, MRI has become the gold standard diagnostic imaging modality in patients with presumed SCI [27]. There are characteristic pathomorphological soft tissue changes in SCIWORA patients that could only be detected using MRI but not in plain films or CT images including spinal cord hematomas, transections, discoligamentous injuries, spinal cord edema, and compression [28–31].

Machino et al. [32] studied MRI examinations from 100 SCIWORA patients. The authors detected changes in signal intensity that could be due to spinal cord hemorrhage, contusion, or edema in 92% of the patients. Furthermore, the authors measured the range of signal changes based on the height of the C3 vertebral body from the patients' own sagittal MRI images and found that larger signal changes were predictive of more severe symptoms and poorer outcomes. Boese and Lechler [33] suggested grouping SCIWORA patients based on MRI findings. Patients with no detectable abnormalities in MRI were defined as Type I, and all the patients with detectable MRI abnormalities were included in Type II. The Type II patients were further divided into three groups: extraneural, intraneural, and coexistence of both intra- and extraneural abnormalities. The latter authors identified 36 studies, including 605 adult SCIWORA patients with reported MRI findings [33]. In 43 patients (7.1%), no MRI abnormalities were detected (Type I), while 562 (92.9%) had abnormal MRI scan results (Type II). Of these, 71 patients (11.7%) had extraneural; 223 patients (36.9%) had intraneural; and 268 patients (44.3%) had combined extra- and intraneural MRI abnormalities. Intraneural abnormalities included edema, hemorrhage, contusion, and partial or complete transection. Extraneural findings were disc herniation, ligamentum flavum bulging, prevertebral soft tissue swelling, or ligamentous abnormalities [33]. There is evidence in the literature suggesting that SCIWORA patients with no detectable MRI abnormalities usually have a better prognosis and recovery rate than the patients with MRI abnormalities [34, 35].

In some cases, repeating the MRI scan may reveal abnormalities which were not evident in the initial examination, or changes in the extent of the previously identified MRI abnormalities [23, 28, 36]. Liu et al. [28] performed MRI in 59 SCIWORA patients with neurological deficiencies at the cervical or thoracic level. Two patients with neurologic deficits were classified as normal on initial MRI. These

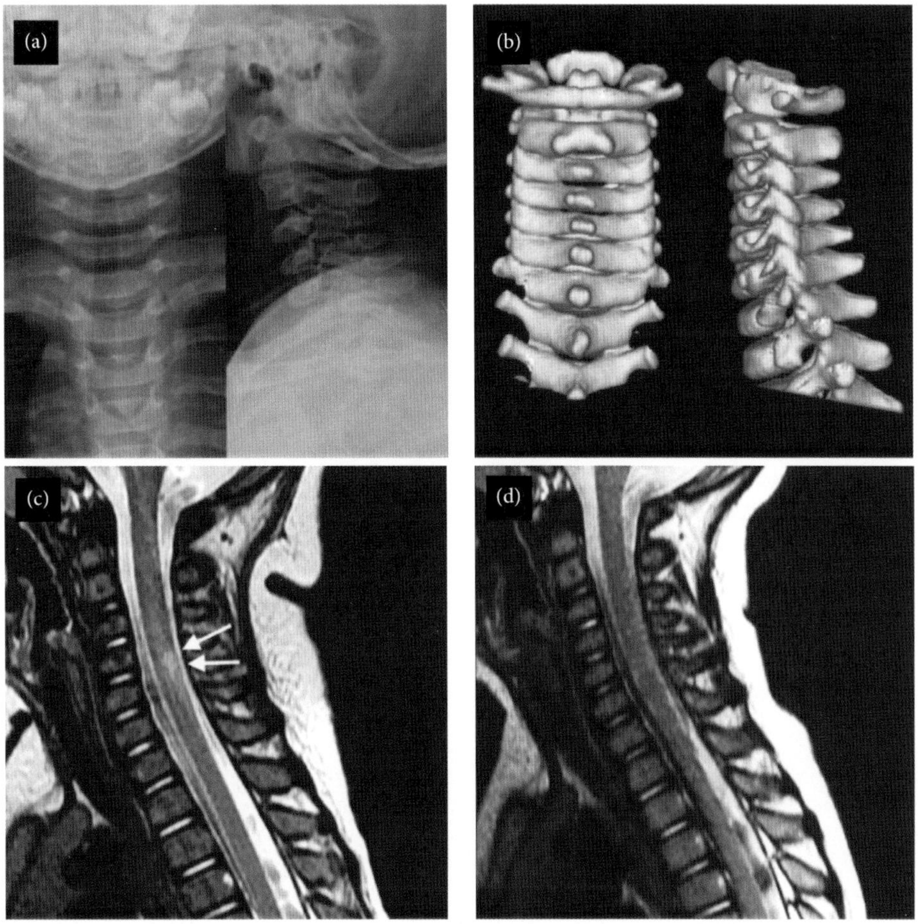

Figure 3: A 12-month-old female infant presented with nausea, vomiting, and drowsiness to emergency room after falling from a height of less than 30 cm. She had no neurological deficit at presentation, and cervical spine plain radiographs (a) and CT with 3D reconstruction (b) showed no abnormal findings. (c) Seven days after the injury the patient developed right sided hemiparesis and cervical MRI revealed increased intensity (arrows) in the T2-weighted images at the level of C6. (d) Repeat cervical MRI one month later shows that increased signal intensity has disappeared. The patient continued to improve neurologically until 24 months after the injury and returned to near-normal. *(Source: with permission from [17].)*

patients had repeat MRI scans 72 hours after the initial trauma, which revealed positive MRI abnormalities, and they underwent surgical interventions. Schellenberg et al. [23] reported on an 18-year-old male who was involved in a car accident as the seat-belted driver. Although the patient presented with paraplegia, his initial plain X-rays, CT, and MRI of the spine were normal. A repeat MRI scan five days after the collision revealed a new abnormal signal (10 mm in size) at the level of T3-T4, representing spinal cord edema. Ouchida et al. [36] performed MRI scan of 68 SCIWORA patients within 48 hours after the injury and repeated the MRIs two weeks after the injury to measure the changes in signal intensity and range. Repeat MRI scans revealed higher-grade signal intensity in 24 patients and attenuation in range of signal intensity as measured based on C3 vertebral height. Moreover, there was a significant negative correlation between the signal intensity grade and range and clinical symptom severity at two weeks. This negative correlation was absent in the acute MRI. The authors suggested that "delayed MRI can provide useful information about the state of the spinal cord after the acute phase..." [36].

Regardless of the timing or number of scans, MRI appears as the sole diagnostic modality that may aid orthopaedic surgeons in understanding the mystery of SCIWORA syndrome, which does not reveal any findings in plain X-rays and CT (Figure 3).

4.5. Somato Sensory Evoked Potentials (SSEPs). SSEPs are signals generated by the nervous system in response to electrical stimulation of a peripheral nerve. Since the SSEP signals are series of waves that reflect sequential activation of neural structures along the somatosensory pathways, monitoring these signals by electrodes positioned along these pathways can aid in detecting any dysfunction from the level of the peripheral nerve, through the spinal root, spinal cord, brain stem, and thalamocortical projections, up to the primary somatosensory cortex. Moreover, recording signal changes both at the craniovertebral junction and at the cortex can help distinguish between a spinal cord injury and thalamic or cortical dysfunction. Although SSEPs are routinely used for intraoperative neuromonitoring during surgery of the spine, literature support for their use in patients with SCIWORA is quite limited [5, 37, 38]. Moreover, evidence shows that SSEP changes are highly specific but not equally sensitive indicators of postoperative/postinjury neurological deficits [39]. Pang [5] used SSEPs as an adjunct in the initial evaluation of children with presumed SCIWORA. In the study of 95 children with SCIWORA, 50 had both MRI and SSEP data. SSEP recordings obtained within 24 hours after injury were found to be slightly more sensitive than MRI in patients with persistent (88% versus 64%, resp.) or transient (39% versus 27%, resp.) neurological deficits. The author suggested "Normal SSEPs should not be counted against an abnormal neurological examination in deciding whether myelopathy is present. Thus, SSEP recording should be regarded as a special rather than a routine test within the diagnostic algorithm of SCIWORA."

5. Treatment

Although Advanced Trauma Life Support (ATLS) protocols and the initial steps of resuscitation after traumatic SCI are universally accepted, the method utilized to approach patients diagnosed with SCIWORA may vary between institutions; no definitive treatment protocol has been established yet.

5.1. Nonsurgical Treatment. Since overt signs of spinal trauma, such as fractures and dislocations, are absent in SCIWORA, nonsurgical strategies, including immobilization and corticosteroid therapy, are the mainstay of treatment. Immobilization immediately after the injury and at the early stages is performed using hard collars for cervical SCIWORA, or restriction of patients' movements with bedrest and log-rolling for thoracolumbar SCIWORA [5]. After the general condition of the patient has improved and other systemic injuries have been addressed, based on the level of SCI, a cervical or cervical-thoracic brace or thoracolumbar orthosis is applied, and the patient is allowed to get out of the bed and walk. Braces or orthosis are used for a minimum of three months until the reassessment of the neurological condition. At three-month follow-up, a decision as to whether the patient should have another MRI is made on an individual basis. Although the latter is the most widely accepted immobilization protocol, some authors suggest using halter traction with a minimal weight for the first three weeks and immobilization in an extended cervical collar until three months after the injury [35]. Interestingly, Bosch et al. [40] reported 21 patients with recurrent SCIWORA; 14 of them sustained their repeat episode while still wearing a rigid type of cervical brace. The remaining seven patients had their second injury either in a soft brace or beyond the time of immobilization. The authors suggested, "Bracing and immobilization do not prevent recurrent SCIWORA or improve outcomes in minor or severe SCIWORA once instability had been properly ruled out." They also stated that "...bracing is not uniformly indicated."

It is imperative to note that evidence to date does not include any randomized controlled trials to prove the superiority of one practice or suggestion over another. However, immobilization of the spine until the spine tenderness clears, the neurologic examination has normalized, and MRI is negative for instability is the universally accepted initial nonsurgical treatment approach [5, 10, 21, 35, 36, 40]. Regardless of the immobilization type, all SCIWORA patients are advised to refrain from any physical activities that may increase the risk of reinjury for approximately six months [21].

Posttraumatic spinal cord damage results from both primary (impact of trauma itself) and secondary mechanisms (subsequent cellular events and inflammatory response) that start at the moment of the injury and go on for days and even weeks [18]. The rationale for the use of steroid therapy in patients with SCIWORA is to prevent or minimize the secondary mechanisms that may cause damage to spinal cord after a traumatic injury. Although there is not enough evidence supporting routine use of high-dose intravenous (IV) methylprednisolone in SCIWORA patients, some studies suggest potential efficacy after SCI if it is started within the first eight hours of trauma with additional benefit by extending the maintenance dose from 24 to 48 hours [41]. Hence, IV methylprednisolone bolus of 30 mg/kg within eight hours of injury, followed by infusion at 5.4 mg/kg/hr for the next 48 hours can be beneficial in improving outcomes. In most SCIWORA cases, IV steroid therapy is started before an MRI scan can be completed and any detailed information with regard to pathological findings is available. Martinez-Perez et al. [8] reported that none of their 48 SCIWORA patients received corticosteroids during their hospitalization. In a prospective study including 45 consecutive SCIWORA patients, Mohanty et al. [35] routinely gave IV methylprednisolone to all the patients for 48 hours. Sharma et al. [9] administered methylprednisolone to seven of their 12 SCIWORA patients and stated "...the number of patients is too small to comment on the efficacy." The effect of high-dose IV methylprednisolone therapy on clinical outcomes in SCIWORA patients requires further investigation.

5.2. Surgical Treatment. There is controversy in the literature regarding surgical treatment of patients diagnosed with SCIWORA. Although the majority of published reports suggest significant improvement in neurological status without operative treatment [17, 28, 31, 35], surgical intervention can become necessary in selected cases if there are clear signs of instability with ligamentous injury and/or cord compression which does not improve [8, 9, 36]. In a series that included 48 adult SCIWORA patients, Martinez-Perez et al. [8] treated 14 patients operatively. Of those 14 patients, six were treated by an anterior approach, and eight underwent decompressive laminoplasty or laminectomy. There was an improvement of at least one point on the ASIA Impairment Scale in 86% of the patients who received operative treatment compared with 76% of the patients who were treated conservatively. In a systematic review, Carroll et al. [10] identified 433 pediatric SCIWORA patients, and there were records of treatment in

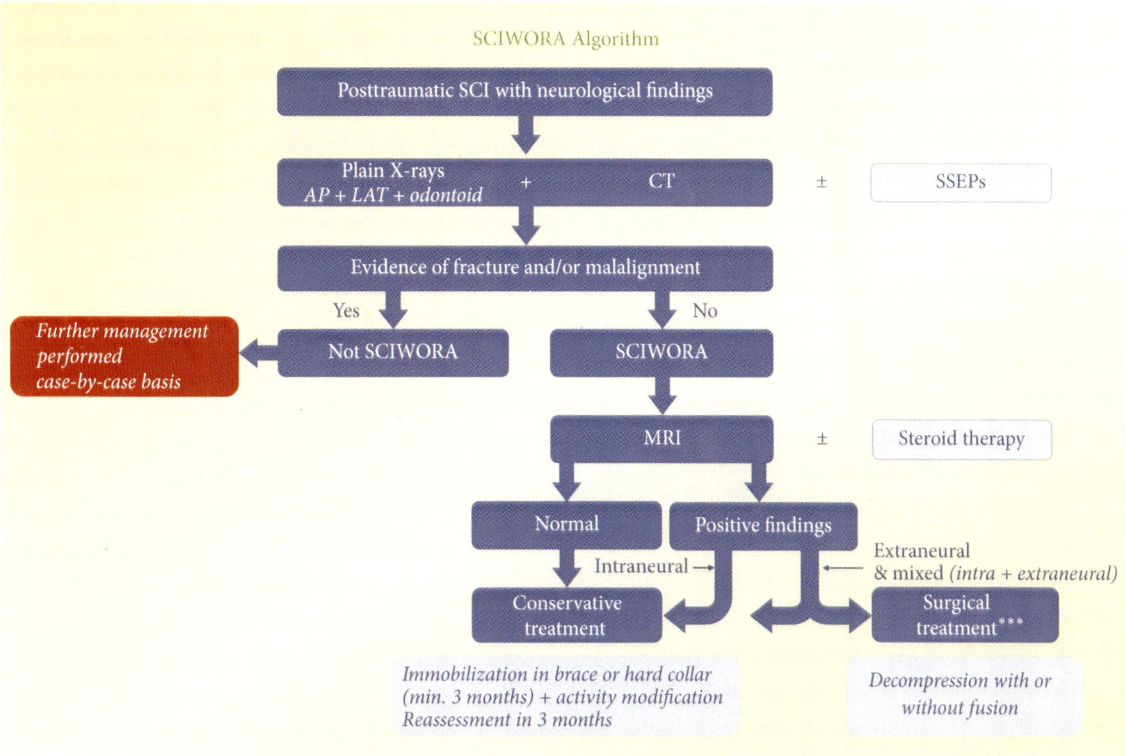

Figure 4: SCIWORA Algorithm. Pure intraneural MRI findings including edema or hemorrhage within the cord parenchyma is not an indication for surgery. Pure extraneural injury including severely injured ligaments or compression even without findings within the cord may be an indication for surgery. Patients with mixed extraintraneural MRI findings have the highest chance to require surgical treatment. Please note that there could be variations in diagnostic work up and treatment based on institutional or surgeons' preferences. ***Main indications for surgical treatment are cord compression and ligamentous instability along with worsening or not-improving neurological findings. *(Courtesy of University of Alabama at Birmingham, Department of Orthopaedic Surgery, Birmingham, AL, USA.)*

183 cases. Of those, only six were treated operatively without notable details in terms of operative indications, technique, or outcomes.

Based on current evidence and our previous experience, surgical treatment is not recommended in SCIWORA patients with normal or pure intraneural MRI findings (i.e., cord edema or contusion without compression) regardless of patient's neurological status. Although clear MRI evidence of ligamentous injury, instability, spinal cord compression along with worsening, or not-improving neurological findings should be indications for surgical decompression with or without fusion, no controlled study to date has compared the outcomes of surgical treatment in SCIWORA patients with outcomes of nonsurgical treatment (Figure 4).

6. Prognosis

In general, most SCIWORA patients show remarkable improvement in neurological status after the injury, and surgical treatment is rarely justifiable. However, the main reason for the priority of conservative treatment in the management of SCIWORA patients is not the mild nature of the injury, but the absence of bony involvement and malalignment. Hence, the injury itself should be recognized as dreadful, and the prognosis can be dismal with devastating complications such as permanent neurological impairments and death [2, 16].

The two main predictors of prognosis after SCIWORA are the initial neurological status and MRI findings [2, 5, 32, 34]. Pang [5] suggests that neurological status at admission is the only predictor of long-term outcome in children with SCIWORA. Children with complete SCI rarely improve. Those with severe but incomplete SCI often improve but seldom regain normal function. In Pang's experience and based on several other reports, patients with mild to moderate initial neurological deficits may have more chance to attain full recovery [5, 8, 28].

Martinez-Perez et al. [8] reported that, at one-year postinjury follow-up, complete recovery in neurological status (AIS grade E) was achieved only in patients with incomplete neurological injury (AIS grades C and D) at admission. Although this study could not demonstrate a significant association between the neurologic impairment at admission with recovery, their results indicate a tendency for the less-severe SCIs to recover completely, while the patients with complete SCIs failed to show any progress. The lack of statistical significance can be explained by limited patient numbers and unequal distribution of the patients to groups with different AIS grades due to retrospective nature of the study.

Correlation between the MRI findings and prognosis has been the focus of several investigators [9, 28, 32, 34–36]. Mohanty et al. [35] showed significant negative correlations ($P < 0.05$) between the length of MRI changes in the spinal cord and the recovery rate (−0.026) as well as the final motor score (−0.042). There was a significant negative correlation between the length of prevertebral hyperintensity in MRI and AIS at the time of presentation ($P < 0.001$), final follow-up ($P < 0.001$), and the rate of recovery ($P < 0.001$). Authors reported that SCIWORA cases with normal MRI findings and spinal cord edema showed a higher mean recovery rate at two years after the injury (95.56 ± 12.54 and 87.70 ± 21.67, resp.). The rates of recovery in patients with MRI findings of cord contusion and cord swelling were the lowest among the groups (48.72 ± 42.08 and 39.42 ± 1.68, resp.), and the differences in recovery rates between different spinal cord changes were statistically significant ($P < 0.05$). Supporting these results, Boese et al. [34] showed that the mean improvement of AIS grade in SCIWORA patients with no MRI abnormalities was higher compared to those with detectable MRI abnormalities (1.5 versus 0.9, resp.). These authors also noted that all the patients who required surgical decompression were presented with simultaneous extra- and intraneural MRI findings.

Although long-term prognosis (over two years) of SCIWORA patients has not been studied extensively in large patient groups, expecting further improvement in neurological status after the first two years may not be realistic. However, worsening in the long-term due to recurrent injuries and/or development of deformities has been reported by several authors [40, 42]. Bosch et al. [40] had 21 patients with recurrent SCIWORA; of those, 20 were older than eight years of age at the time of initial injury. Furthermore, recurrences occurred up to three years after the initial event. The majority of recurrences happened during sports activities, and this may explain the higher recurrence rate among children over eight years of age. Yalcin et al. [42] reported four patients who developed progressive neuromuscular scoliosis due to SCIWORA. Spinal deformities were first noticed at a mean of 17 months after the initial injury that led to surgical interventions at a mean of 6.5 years.

7. Summary

SCIWORA is a syndrome that defines posttraumatic SCI in patients with neurological findings without any evidence of fractures or malalignment in plain X-rays and CT. This condition is more commonly seen in the pediatric age group, with a predilection for the cervical spine. Proposed mechanisms of injury include hyperflexion, hyperextension, and parenchymal cord damage resulting from edema or vascular injury that can occur as a result of sports injuries, falls, and motor vehicle collisions. Diagnostic evaluation starts with a detailed history and physical examination, followed by plain X-rays and CT. SSEPs can be done selectively; dynamic imaging does not provide any additional information and has been dropped from the diagnostic algorithm in SCIWORA. With its superior ability to reveal soft tissue pathologies and prognostic value, MRI is accepted as the imaging modality of choice in patients diagnosed with SCIWORA. Nonsurgical treatment with cervical brace or collar for a minimum of three months and restriction of high-risk activities for six months is the mainstay of treatment. Steroid therapy has not proven to be effective in SCIWORA patients. Based on evidence from studies in patients with SCI in general, it can improve the outcomes if started within eight hours of injury and continued for 48 hours. Surgical treatment should be reserved for patients with clear MRI evidence of extraneural findings including spinal cord compression, ligamentous injury, and instability, along with worsening or not-improving neurological findings. Prognosis of SCIWORA depends on the initial neurological deficit and extent of spinal cord injury as evidenced by MRI. Although neurological improvement in patients with complete neurological deficit at initial presentation is highly unlikely, most patients with incomplete neurological injury show improvement. Even so, permanent disabilities and deformities in the long-term are among the complications encountered by SCIWORA patients.

References

[1] D. Pang and J. E. Wilberger Jr., "Spinal cord injury without radiographic abnormalities in children," *Journal of Neurosurgery*, vol. 57, no. 1, pp. 114–129, 1982.

[2] D. Pang and I. F. Pollack, "Spinal cord injury without radiographic abnormality in children-the sciwora syndrome," *Journal of Trauma - Injury Infection and Critical Care*, vol. 29, no. 5, pp. 654–664, 1989.

[3] A Short History of the Magnetic Resonance Imaging (MRI). http://www.teslasociety.com/mri.htm.

[4] M. V. Kulkarni, C. B. McArdle, D. Kopanicky et al., "Acute spinal cord injury: MR imaging at 1.5 T," *Radiology*, vol. 164, no. 3, pp. 837–843, 1987.

[5] D. Pang, "Spinal cord injury without radiographic abnormality in children, 2 decades later," *Neurosurgery*, vol. 55, no. 6, pp. 1325–1342, 2004.

[6] M. G. Hamilton and S. T. Myles, "Pediatric spinal injury: Review of 174 hospital admissions," *Journal of Neurosurgery*, vol. 77, no. 5, pp. 700–704, 1992.

[7] R. K. Osenbach and A. H. Menezes, "Pediatric spinal cord and vertebral column injury," *Neurosurgery*, vol. 30, no. 3, pp. 385–390, 1992.

[8] R. Martinez-Perez, P. M. Munarriz, I. Paredes, J. Cotrina, and A. Lagares, "Cervical spinal cord injury without computed tomography evidence of trauma in adults: magnetic resonance imaging prognostic factors," *World Neurosurgery*, vol. 99, pp. 192–199, 2017.

[9] S. Sharma, M. Singh, I. H. Wani et al., "Adult Spinal Cord Injury without Radiographic Abnormalities (SCIWORA): Clinical and Radiological Correlations," *Journal of Clinical Medicine Research*, vol. 1, no. 3, pp. 165–172, 2009.

[10] T. Carroll, C. D. Smith, X. Liu et al., "Spinal cord injuries without radiologic abnormality in children: A systematic review," *Spinal Cord*, vol. 53, no. 12, pp. 842–848, 2015.

[11] K. Khatri, K. Farooque, A. Gupta, and V. Sharma, "Spinal Cord Injury Without Radiological Abnormality Following Trauma to Thoracic Spine in an Adult Patient: A Case Report and Literature Review," *Archives of Trauma Research*, vol. 3, no. 3, 2014.

[12] G. Van Buul and F. C. Öner, "Thoracic spinal cord injury without radiographic abnormality in an adult patient," *The Spine Journal*, vol. 9, no. 3, pp. e5–e8, 2009.

[13] J. Knox, "Epidemiology of spinal cord injury without radiographic abnormality in children: a nationwide perspective," *Journal of Children's Orthopaedics*, vol. 10, no. 3, pp. 255–260, 2016.

[14] T. McCall, D. Fassett, and D. Brockmeyer, "Cervical spine trauma in children: a review," *Neurosurgical Focus*, vol. 20, no. 2, article E5, 2006.

[15] D. J. Nuckley, D. R. Linders, and R. P. Ching, "Developmental biomechanics of the human cervical spine," *Journal of Biomechanics*, vol. 46, no. 6, pp. 1147–1154, 2013.

[16] Y. Makino, H. Yokota, M. Hayakawa et al., "Spinal cord injuries with normal postmortem CT findings: A pitfall of virtual autopsy for detecting traumatic death," *American Journal of Roentgenology*, vol. 203, no. 2, pp. 240–244, 2014.

[17] S. H. Kim, S. H. Yoon, K. H. Cho, and S. H. Kim, "Spinal cord injury without radiological abnormality in an infant with delayed presentation of symptoms after a minor injury," *The Spine Journal*, vol. 33, no. 21, pp. E792–E794, 2008.

[18] J. N. Pettiford, J. Bikhchandani, D. J. Ostlie, S. D. St. Peter, R. J. Sharp, and D. Juang, "A review: The role of high dose methylprednisolone in spinal cord trauma in children," *Pediatric Surgery International*, vol. 28, no. 3, pp. 287–294, 2012.

[19] S. K. Agrawal and M. G. Fehlings, "Mechanisms of secondary injury to spinal cord axons in vitro: Role of Na+, Na+-K+-ATPase, the Na+-H+ exchanger, and the Na+-Ca2+ exchanger," *The Journal of Neuroscience*, vol. 16, no. 2, pp. 545–552, 1996.

[20] J. J. Como, H. Samia, G. A. Nemunaitis et al., "The misapplication of the term spinal cord injury without radiographic abnormality (SCIWORA) in adults," *Journal of Trauma and Acute Care Surgery*, vol. 73, no. 5, pp. 1261–1266, 2012.

[21] D. Szwedowski and J. Walecki, "Spinal cord injury without radiographic abnormality (SCIWORA) – Clinical and radiological aspects," *Polish Journal of Radiology*, vol. 79, no. 1, pp. 461–464, 2014.

[22] S. C. Kirshblum, S. P. Burns, F. Biering-Sorensen et al., "International standards for neurological classification of spinal cord injury (revised 2011)," *The Journal of Spinal Cord Medicine*, vol. 34, no. 6, pp. 535–546, 2011.

[23] M. Schellenberg, O. Islam, and R. Pokrupa, "Traumatic spinal cord injury without initial MRI abnormality: SCIWORA revisited," *Canadian Journal of Neurological Sciences*, vol. 38, no. 2, pp. 364–366, 2011.

[24] V. Spiteri, R. Kotnis, P. Singh et al., "Cervical dynamic screening in spinal clearance: Now redundant," *Journal of Trauma - Injury Infection and Critical Care*, vol. 61, no. 5, pp. 1171–1177, 2006.

[25] J. Anglen, M. Metzler, P. Bunn, and H. Griffiths, "Flexion and extension views are not cost-effective in a cervical spine clearance protocol for obtunded trauma patients," *Journal of Trauma - Injury Infection and Critical Care*, vol. 52, no. 1, pp. 54–59, 2002.

[26] L. Padayachee, D. J. Cooper, S. Irons et al., "Cervical spine clearance in unconscious traumatic brain injury patients: Dynamic flexion-extension fluoroscopy versus computed tomography with three-dimensional reconstruction," *Journal of Trauma - Injury Infection and Critical Care*, vol. 60, no. 2, pp. 341–345, 2006.

[27] D. Lammertse, D. Dungan, J. Dreisbach et al., "Neuroimaging in traumatic spinal cord injury: An evidence-based review for clinical practice and research," *The Journal of Spinal Cord Medicine*, vol. 30, no. 3, pp. 205–214, 2007.

[28] Q. Liu, Q. Liu, J. Zhao, H. Yu, X. Ma, and L. Wang, "Early MRI finding in adult spinal cord injury without radiologic abnormalities does not correlate with the neurological outcome: a retrospective study," *Spinal Cord*, vol. 53, no. 10, pp. 750–753, 2015.

[29] P. Mahajan, D. M. Jaffe, C. S. Olsen et al., "Spinal cord injury without radiologic abnormality in children imaged with magnetic resonance imaging," *Journal of Trauma and Acute Care Surgery*, vol. 75, no. 5, pp. 843–847, 2013.

[30] G. B. Kasimatis, E. Panagiotopoulos, P. Megas et al., "The adult spinal cord injury without radiographic abnormalities syndrome: Magnetic resonance imaging and clinical findings in adults with spinal cord injuries having normal radiographs and computed tomography studies," *Journal of Trauma - Injury Infection and Critical Care*, vol. 65, no. 1, pp. 86–93, 2008.

[31] C. K. Boese, M. Nerlich, S. M. Klein, A. Wirries, S. Ruchholtz, and P. Lechler, "Early magnetic resonance imaging in spinal cord injury without radiological abnormality in adults: A retrospective study," *Journal of Trauma and Acute Care Surgery*, vol. 74, no. 3, pp. 845–848, 2013.

[32] M. Machino, Y. Yukawa, K. Ito et al., "Can magnetic resonance imaging reflect the prognosis in patients of cervical spinal cord injury without radiographic abnormality?" *The Spine Journal*, vol. 36, no. 24, pp. E1568–E1572, 2011.

[33] C. K. Boese and P. Lechler, "Spinal cord injury without radiologic abnormalities in adults: A systematic review," *Journal of Trauma and Acute Care Surgery*, vol. 75, no. 2, pp. 320–330, 2013.

[34] C. K. Boese, D. Müller, R. Bröer et al., "Spinal cord injury without radiographic abnormality (SCIWORA) in adults: MRI type predicts early neurologic outcome," *Spinal Cord*, vol. 54, no. 10, pp. 878–883, 2016.

[35] S. P. Mohanty, N. S. Bhat, K. A. Singh, and M. Bhushan, "Cervical spinal cord injuries without radiographic evidence of trauma: A prospective study," *Spinal Cord*, vol. 51, no. 11, pp. 815–818, 2013.

[36] J. Ouchida, Y. Yukawa, K. Ito et al., "Delayed magnetic resonance imaging in patients with cervical spinal cord injury without radiographic abnormality," *The Spine Journal*, vol. 41, no. 16, pp. E981–E986, 2016.

[37] P. D. Thirumala, L. Bodily, D. Tint et al., "Somatosensory-evoked potential monitoring during instrumented scoliosis corrective procedures: Validity revisited," *The Spine Journal*, vol. 14, no. 8, pp. 1572–1580, 2014.

[38] J. S. Cheng, M. E. Ivan, C. J. Stapleton, A. Quinones-Hinojosa, N. Gupta, and K. I. Auguste, "Intraoperative changes in transcranial motor evoked potentials and somatosensory evoked potentials predicting outcome in children with intramedullary spinal cord tumors: Clinical article," *Journal of Neurosurgery: Pediatrics*, vol. 13, no. 6, pp. 591–599, 2014.

[39] P. D. Thirumala, S. R. Melachuri, J. Kaur et al., "Diagnostic accuracy of somatosensory evoked potentials in evaluating new neurological deficits after posterior cervical fusions," *The Spine Journal*, vol. 42, no. 7, pp. 490–496, 2017.

[40] P. P. Bosch, M. T. Vogt, and W. T. Ward, "Pediatric spinal cord injury without radiographic abnormality (SCIWORA): The absence of occult instability and lack of indication for bracing," *The Spine Journal*, vol. 27, no. 24, pp. 2788–2800, 2002.

[41] M. B. Bracken, "Steroids for acute spinal cord injury," *Cochrane Database of Systematic Reviews*, vol. 1, article CD001046, 2012.

25

Minimizing Stress Shielding and Cement Damage in Cemented Femoral Component of a Hip Prosthesis through Computational Design Optimization

Abdellah Ait Moussa, Justin Fischer, Rohan Yadav, and Morshed Khandaker

Department of Engineering and Physics, University of Central Oklahoma, Edmond, OK, USA

Correspondence should be addressed to Abdellah Ait Moussa; aaitmoussa@uco.edu

Academic Editor: Allen L. Carl

The average life expectancy of many people undergoing total hip replacement (THR) exceeds twenty-five years and the demand for implants that increase the load-bearing capability of the bone without affecting the short- or long-term stability of the prosthesis is high. Mechanical failure owing to cement damage and stress shielding of the bone are the main factors affecting the long-term survival of cemented hip prostheses and implant design must realistically adjust to balance between these two conflicting effects. In the following analysis we introduce a novel methodology to achieve this objective, the numerical technique combines automatic and realistic modeling of the implant and embedding medium, and finite element analysis to assess the levels of stress shielding and cement damage and, finally, global optimization, using orthogonal arrays and probabilistic restarts, were used. Applications to implants, fabricated using a homogeneous material and a functionally graded material, were presented.

1. Introduction

Between the two alternatives of total hip replacements, the cemented fixation method was mostly adopted owing to offering the immediate stability from cement-stem and cement-bone bonding interfaces after implant surgery [1, 2]. Clinical studies however reported that cemented hip prostheses fail to function properly due to the loosening of the fixations after long-term use [3, 4]; debonding of the cement-stem and cement-bone interfaces and the local fractures in the cement mantle were perceived as the primary mechanisms of cemented hip implant loosening [4]. Improved cementing techniques had then been developed to reduce the prevalence of loosening and to guarantee long-term fixation of the prosthesis [5–9]. Stress shielding of the bone received increased attention over the years [10]; whether cemented or uncemented implants were used, mechanical loosening owing to the physiological dynamic response of the bone is one of the main factors affecting the implants long-term durability. The presence of the femoral implant in the intramedullary canal reduces the loads normally applied to the bone of the proximal femur, resulting in periprosthetic bone resorption, bone loss, cortical bone thinning, and joint prosthesis failure [11–15]. Revision surgery to address such failure involves increased risks, complications, and costs. Given that the average life expectancy of many patients undergoing total hip arthroplasty (THA) exceeds 25 years, ongoing stress shielding is clinically important and the demand for implants which maximize the load-bearing capabilities of the bone is high [16, 17].

Implant design and material properties have great effects on the total hip joint stability and long-term performance. For instance, if the stem design and material lead to high stresses in the fixation area of the prosthesis, local fractures or fatigue failure of the cement is quite likely to occur. Observations from fatigue experiments and clinical studies had attributed the loosening of the cement-stem fixation to the local fractures initiated in the cement mantle adjacent to the stem that gradually propagated and produced separation of the stem-cement interfaces [4, 18, 19]. Concurrent with cement damage and stress shielding other studies revealed that stiffer implants induce high levels of stress shielding over the proximal femur and low levels of interface stress among the femur-implant constituents [20, 21], while in contrast less stress shielding and high levels of cement damage were observed with low stiffness implants [22].

The long-term survival of the cemented prosthesis is contingent on achieving a balance between stress shielding and cement damage; to this end a number of studies investigated several prospective modifications. In some of these investigations less stress shielding and improved implant stability were observed in fully cemented fixations [23] and with poly-methyl methacrylate (PMMA) instead of other bioactive bone cements [24]. It was also revealed that shorter stems had improved the overall stability of the cemented fixation and provided the femur with more proximal load [25]. Implant shape modification techniques were also investigated in cemented and cementless fixations; common design optimizations in the former fixation targeted the cement layer or cement-prosthesis interface with the objective of minimizing stress concentration in these areas [26–28]; however stress shielding of the bone was not quantified for use in the design analysis. Several shape optimization models were developed for cementless prostheses where one [27, 29–32] or more [33–35] performance criteria were used in the search method. In the most relevant of these studies [35], a three-dimensional model of the implant based on the commercial Tri-Lock (Depuy, Inc., Warsaw, IN, USA) was constructed using suitable interpolation between a fixed number of key cross sections and a simulation based structural optimization was used to identify new and improved designs. The major drawbacks of this form of optimization are the computing cost which is usually expensive; additionally they are prone to a risk of being trapped in local optima and the CAD interpretation of the shape optimization result is not trivial [36].

In the current study, we introduce a novel evolutionary technique to optimizing stem designs in a cemented hip prosthesis with the objective of minimizing stress shielding and cement damage. The self-regulated technique combines realistic and solid modeling of the implant and embedding medium, finite element to assess the levels of stress shielding, and cement damage in addition to a fast global optimization using orthogonal arrays and probabilistic restarts.

This paper is structured as follows; in Section 2 we introduce the computational technique used to realistically optimize the geometry of the stem of a cemented hip prosthesis. In Section 3, we apply the methodology thus introduced to identify the optimal stem design given two types of materials, Titanium alloy and a longitudinally inhomogeneous functionally graded material. In the final section, we conclude with a summary and discussion of future work.

2. The Computational Technique

In this section, we shall describe the general structure of the computational technique used to model and optimize the shape of a cemented hip implant with the objective of minimizing bone stress shielding and cement damage.

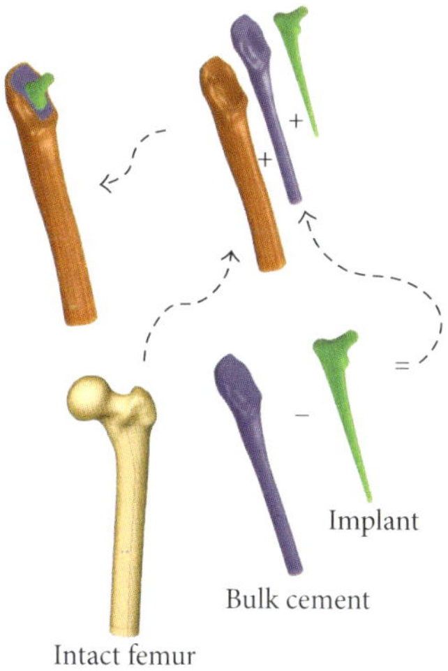

FIGURE 1: The intact femur bone was cut at its proximal part to allow for insertion of the implant. The geometry of the implant was deducted from the bulk cement represented and fixed length of the void inside the cortical bone. The implant and updated cement geometry were then aligned with the axis of the cortical bone and a femur-cement-implant construct was formed.

2.1. The Modeling of the Prosthesis. Our femur-prosthesis model is depicted in Figure 1, it consisted of a cortical bone representing the femur, the bone was cut at its proximal part to allow for insertion of the implant, and the cancellous bone was excluded for simplification. The implant was centered with the bone at its distal end and aligned with the axis of the femur; the cement filled the space between the implant and the bone and extended over the length of the stem. The cortical bone model was acquired from Sawbone Inc.

To accurately reproduce the geometry of the implant, we used a combination of mathematical and solid modeling. We flushed the sharp transition from the neck to the prosthesis axis with a four-point Bezier spline as depicted in Figure 2; we then selected 6 key cross sections with the centers and normal unit vectors, respectively, tangential to the prosthesis axis (cross sections 1, 2, and 3), the Bezier spline (cross section 4), and the neck axis (cross sections 5 and 6) as depicted on the same figure. The cross section on the distal end was circular with a fixed radius, the rest of the cross sections had variable shapes and sizes, and the characteristics equations of the cross-sectional profiles were modeled using (1) [35] where (a, b) are the lengths of the semiminor and semimajor axes in a local system of coordinates described by the x- and y-axes as depicted on the scaled up view of one of the cross sections; the exponent (p) is an integer number.

$$\left(\frac{x}{a}\right)^p + \left(\frac{y}{b}\right)^p = 1. \quad (1)$$

For more control over the shape and size of a cross section, the frontal and lateral sides were modeled according to (1), the sides shared the same exponent (p) and had identical lengths of the common semiaxis, and they may however have different lengths assigned to the opposite semiaxes as depicted in Figure 2. A total of four design variables $(a_1,$

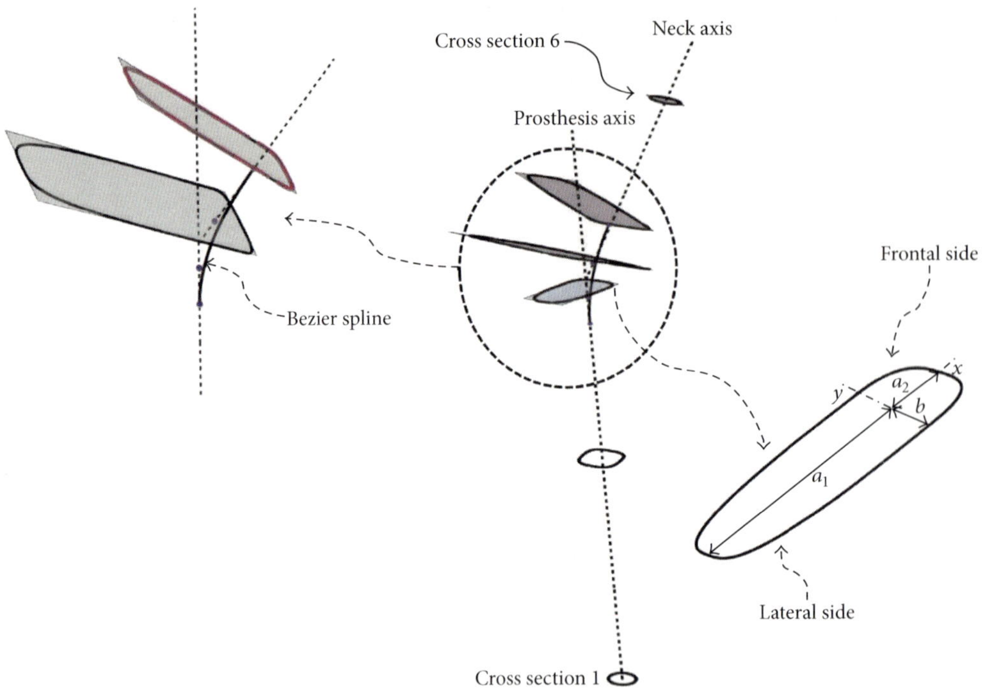

FIGURE 2: Skeleton of the hip implant. Each cross section is characterized by three geometrical parameters (a_1, a_2, b) in addition to the exponent (p) in (1). A four-point Bezier spline interpolated the sharp transition between the neck and prosthesis axes.

a_2, b, p) characterized the shape of each of the five cross sections, and together twenty parameters characterized the skeleton of the stem. A series of third-order Nonuniform Rational Basis Splines (NURBS) was interpolated between the different cross sections to produce the mathematical model depicted in Figure 3. The mathematical modeling of the stem was completed in Mathematica and different geometries are produced upon changes in the parameters of the cross sections.

To produce the accompanying solid model, we developed a program that imported the coordinates of a fixed but sufficient number of points on the surface of the implant model thus constructed to the graphical interface of SolidWorks; the flexibility of the structural programming in this software allowed for automatic interpolation among selected points along with surface mapping, solid modeling, and the optional lengthwise slicing of the implant as described in Figure 4. Using the same software, we successfully subtracted the material of the implant from the bulk cement and aligned the femur model together with the updated cement and implant geometries to produce the cemented femur-prosthesis model depicted in Figure 1. The procedure was automated to work with different prostheses models upon changes in the geometrical design parameters.

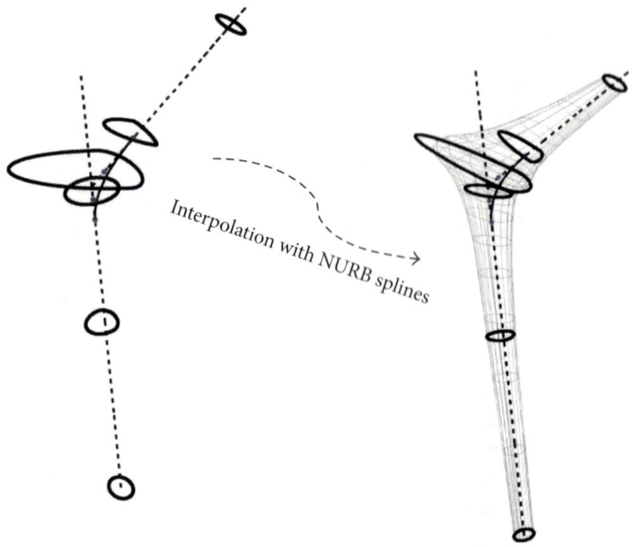

FIGURE 3: A series of NURB splines interpolated between the skeleton cross sections (left) to produce the hip model shown on the right.

2.2. The Finite Element Analysis. Previous studies [37] on the ability of computational methods to predict fatigue cracking in experimental models of a simplified femur structure showed that continuum damage mechanics can reliably predict cement fatigue locations in a timescale comparable with experimentation. Further studies [38] showed that a loading configuration including the hip joint contact force and the abductor force can adequately reproduce in vivo loading of cemented total reconstructions. Hereupon, a stress life fatigue analysis with constant amplitude (body load) and proportional loading, simulating average human walking condition, was conducted on the hip assembly thus constructed. The simulation setup in Figure 5(a) is similar

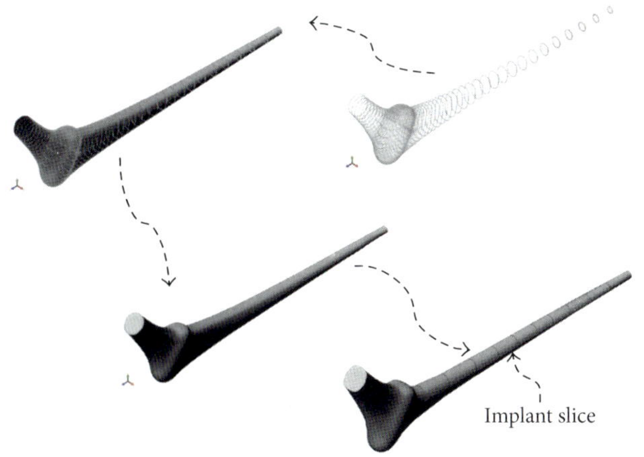

FIGURE 4: A fixed number of points were imported to the graphical interface of SolidWorks and interpolated with splines (top right), a closed surface envelope was mapped over the splines including the caps on both ends (top left), the enclosure was then filled, and a solid model of the implant was formed. The lengthwise slicing on the bottom right is optional.

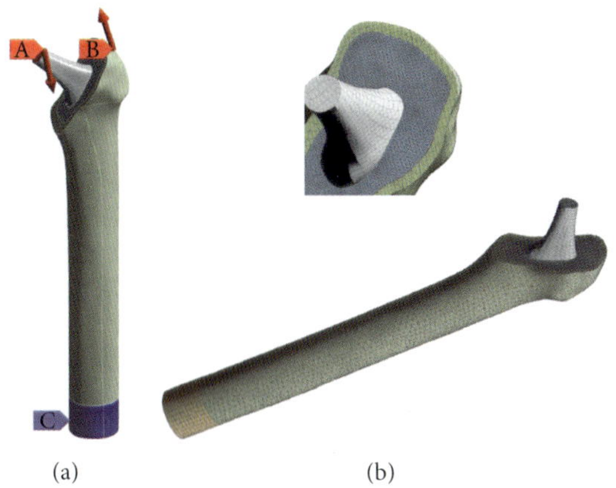

FIGURE 5: (a): (A) body force, (B) abductor muscle force, and (C) fixed support. (b): unstructured mesh with a combination of Tetrahedron, Patch Conforming, and Sweep Method was used for the assembly.

to that of Jeffers et al. [37]; it allowed a joint force of 2.5 kN to be applied at 10° angle from the axis of the femur and an abductor force of 1.5 kN at an angle of 15° together equivalent to 3.5 times bodyweight loading (assuming bodyweight of 700 N). Bonded and rough (no sliding) fixations were used at the bone/cement and cement/implant interfaces, respectively.

An unstructured mesh with a combination of Tetrahedron, Patch Conforming, and Sweep Method was used for the volumes of the implant, cement, and bone, the mesh was refined around the implant and on the boundary between the cement and bone, and a sample representation of this mesh is shown in Figure 5(b). We maintained the same global and local mesh controls in ANSYS Workbench 16.0 to ensure consistency of mesh element size among all models upon changes in geometry and/or material stiffness. The bone and PMMA cement were assumed homogeneous, isotropic, and linear elastic with modulus of elasticity of 18.6 GPa and 2.28 GPa, respectively; the Poisson's ratio was assumed constant among all materials and equal to 0.3 [39].

To estimate stress shielding of the bone, we used (2), where (σ_i, σ_i') are the calculated equivalent alternating (Von Mises) stresses, respectively, on a point of index (i) on the external surface of the intact femur in Figure 1 and a femur with implant. The index (i) runs from $(i = 1)$ to $(i = N = 3040)$ preselected locations along the length and around the femur model. σ_{av} is the average equivalent alternating stress over the external surface of the intact femur; the smaller the index, the less effective the stress shielding of the implanted bone.

$$\text{Stress Shielding Coefficient} = \frac{1}{\sigma_{av}} \left[\sum_{i=1}^{N} \left(\sigma_i - \sigma_i' \right)^2 \right]. \quad (2)$$

The total damage accumulation in the cement was evaluated by summing the local damage over the points in the cement nodes following (3), where (d_i) is the local fatigue damage at node (i) and $(i\max)$ is the total number of cement nodes. In calculating (d_i), we first used the Goodman criterion to correct for mean stress effects; the Von Mises stress was then used to convert the multiaxial stress to a single valued stress and the S-N curve of Davies et al. [40] was used to estimate the number of cycles to life (N_i) at mesh node (i). d_i was then assigned a value of 1 if the number of cycles to life is less than the design life and 0 otherwise. The term critical cement damage accumulation parameter was used as the failure index representing the percentage of the cement damaged at the design life of 2 million cycles [41–43].

$$\text{Critical Cement Damage Accumulation Parameter} = \sum_{i=1}^{i\max} d_i. \quad (3)$$

Stress distribution over the external surface of the bone for the intact femur in Figure 1 and a femur with Titanium implant (Titanium alloy Ti-6Al-4V with modulus of elasticity of 110 GPa and a Poisson's ratio of 0.3 [39]) were plotted in Figure 6, the abscissa refers to the length from the distal end of the implant, the ordinate pertains to the normalized stress at that location, and the normalization constant was taken as the average stress on the intact femur. Stress shielding of the bone with implant is clearly noticeable owing to the difference in stress distribution averaging between 40% and 50%; these percentages are consistent with experimental measurements [44]. The accumulated cement damage was plotted in Figure 7 as a function of the number of cycles. The growth rate of the fatigue damage is rapid and significant at early loading cycles as expected, gradually decreasing in subsequent stages of the loading. Inspection also indicated that the most likely sites for failure initiation were in the proximal anterior region and at the distal tip of the prosthesis; such fatigue scenario is generally consistent with experimentation [41–43].

The setup of the finite element analysis (FEA), including the application of the body and abductor force, interface

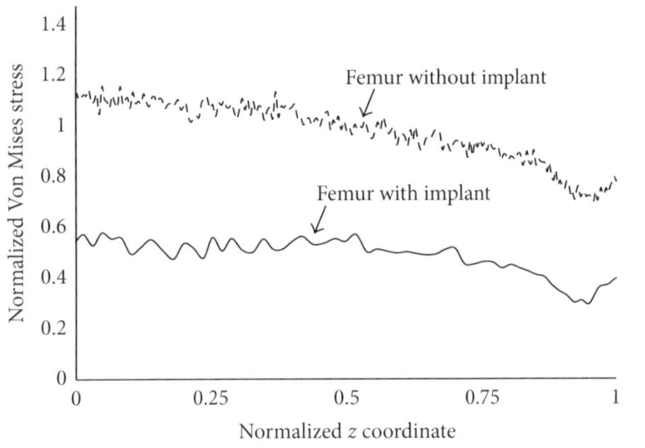

FIGURE 6: Stress distribution (moving average) over the surface of the cortical bone.

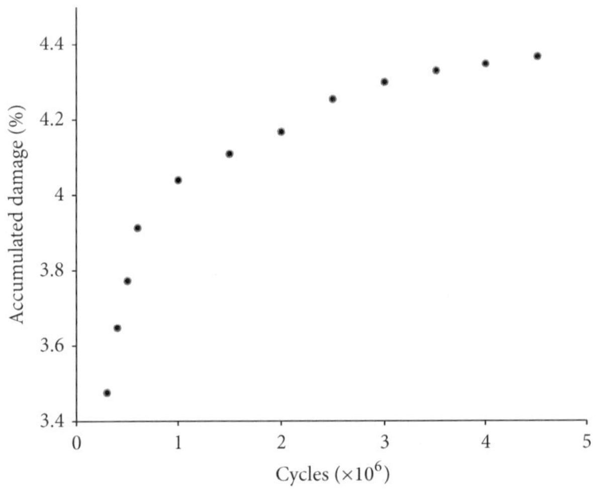

FIGURE 7: Accumulated damage within the cement as a function of the number of loading cycles (design life of 10^9 cycles). The growth rate of fatigue damage is rapid and significant at early loading cycles gradually decreasing in subsequent stages of the loading.

boundary conditions, material properties, assembly meshing, the setup, and solution of the fatigue analysis, was automated using a self-developed script for the ANSYS Workbench-Mechanical; the script is called every time the geometry and/or the material stiffness distribution were updated. Following geometrical updates of the implant, the ANSYS software exports data files with the calculated Von Mises stress over the bone surface and the calculated damage in the cement nodal points; these results are used to estimate the stress shielding coefficient and the critical cement damage accumulation parameter used in the optimization described in Section 2.3.

2.3. Optimization Setup and Procedure. Up to this point of the study, we successfully completed the mathematical modeling and programing of a model hip implant, the automatic reconstruction of a solid model that matches the geometry of the prosthesis; last but not least, we performed a fatigue analysis under average human walking condition in a self-regulated manner and were able to assess stress shielding through the stress shielding coefficient in (2) and the cement damage from the critical cement damage accumulation parameter in (3). Each element in this scenario can be rerun and different results may be achieved depending on the stem geometry and material properties. We initiated a self-regulated optimization process that reconfigured the geometry of the implant in a cemented prosthesis with the objective of minimizing a cost function defined as the sum of the squares of the normalized stress shielding coefficient and critical cement damage accumulation parameter; the normalization constants in (4) were, respectively, the maximum stress shielding coefficient and maximum critical cement damage accumulation parameter among all the design of experiments used throughout the optimization. The rationale of this technique is explained next.

$$\text{Objective function} = \left(\frac{\text{accu damage rate}}{\text{max accu damage rate}}\right)^2 + \left(\frac{\text{stress shielding coef}}{\text{max stress shielding coef}}\right)^2. \quad (4)$$

We identified twenty geometrical parameters among five cross sections (2 through 6 in Figure 2) that together control the geometry of the stem and cement mantle; fifteen of these parameters including the size of the principal axes in each cross section (a_1, a_2, and b in Figure 2) were set to take on any real value within their respective search intervals; the exponent (p) in (1) on the other hand was set to take on integer values alone. The design boundaries of the semimajor and semiminor axes were set so the cement thickness around the implant is maintained between 2.0 and 3.0 mm; additional constraints were added so the produced stem designs were clinically admissible.

Given the multiplicity of the design variables a fractional factorial based-design optimization following the Taguchi algorithm [45] was used; the methodology schematics is diagrammatically explained in Figure 8. We began with a fixed number of random vertices, where each vertex represented a possible geometrical configuration of the implant equivalent to twenty random values within the constrained boundaries of the design variables. We identified the vertex that is the farthest from the rest of the vertices using the variable variance probability (VVP) density defined in the appendix. For each parameter (x_i) in the vertex, we introduced two design values (x_i^1, x_i^2); we used (5) for the nonintegers, where Δx_i refers to the size of the domain of analysis of variable (x_i), and (6) was used for the integer exponents (p_i). With the design variables thus introduced, we initiated a two-level orthogonal array optimization following the Taguchi algorithm [45] to identify the combination of design variable (optimum vertex) that locally minimize the cost function in (4). The optimum vertex thus found was then added to the initial random vertices so to avoid selecting the same

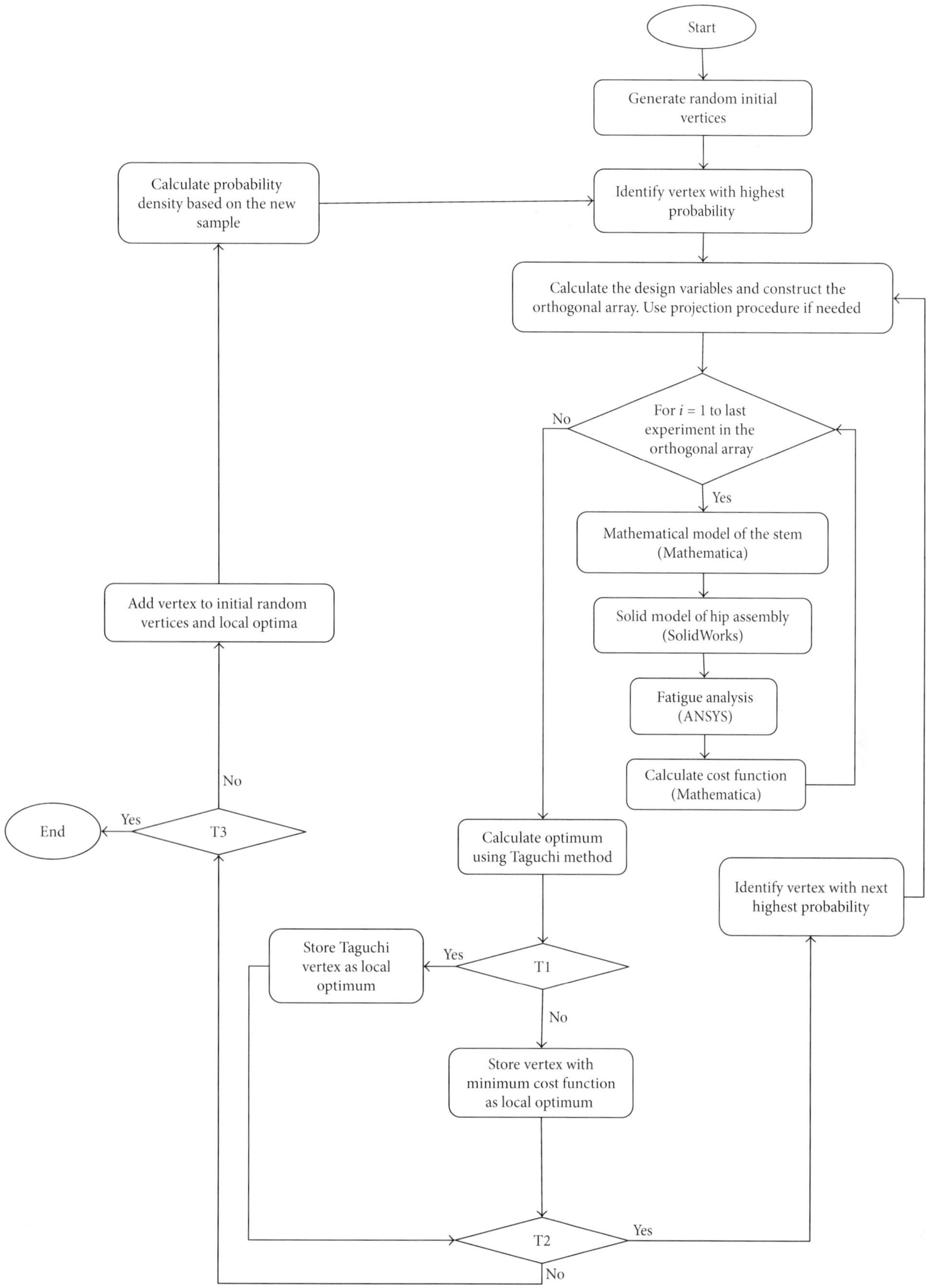

Figure 8: Global optimization. T1: Taguchi suggested optimum is best; T2: already known as an optimum; T3: maximum number of analyses is reached.

Table 1: Lower and upper bounds of the exponents over the cross sections in Figure 2.

	Cross section 1	Cross section 2	Cross section 3	Cross section 4	Cross section 5	Cross section 6
Lower bound	2	2	2	2	2	2
Upper bound	2	3	3	4	4	3

experiments and the process was repeated for the next optimum; the VVP ensures the globalization of the search since the next vertex selection is based on the largest distance among all vertices. There may be cases, however, when the new optimum is identical to one of the stored optima, that the suggested optimum is not better than one of the current vertices because of factor interactions, or that one or more of the vertex levels are not within the design space. In cases like these, we proceed as indicated in the diagram of Figure 8. The box projection procedure in (7) ensures that the levels are always selected within their search intervals.

$$x_i^k = x_i \mp 0.2\Delta x_i \quad k = 1,2,\ i = 1 \text{ to } 2 \tag{5}$$

$$p_i^k = p_i \mp 1 \quad k = 1,2,\ i = 1 \text{ to } 20 \tag{6}$$

$$x_i = \begin{cases} x_i^{\text{lower bound}} & \text{if } x < x_i^{\text{lower bound}} \\ x_i^{\text{upper bound}} & \text{if } x > x_i^{\text{upper bound}}. \end{cases} \tag{7}$$

3. Applications

In this section we shall represent the results of the application of the technique introduced in Section 2 to a cemented Titanium alloy and a functionally graded implant.

3.1. Optimization Setup. The radius of the circular cross section at the distal end was set to a fixed value of 6 mm, the total length of the implant was $L = 185$ mm, the upper and lower bounds of the exponent in (1) were set according to the first two rows in Table 1 for the cross sections in Figure 2, and a value of 2 corresponds to a circular or oval cross section, while values of 3 and 4 correspond to a trapezoid. The choice of these bounds was based on previous research [29], where it was demonstrated that circular and oval cross sections had maintained uniform stress distribution over the stem length while a change from an oval to a trapezoid produced more of a high to low stress distribution which is needed between the neck and prosthesis axes to minimize the stress concentration on the cement at these locations. The lowest and uppermost configurations corresponding, respectively, to the lowest and highest bounds of the search intervals are included in Figure 9. Ten random initial vertices were selected to start the optimization scheme described in Figure 8 and the maximum number of repetitive restarts was set to thirty. The results from each design of experiments along with the associated local optimum were stored for data analysis. Parallel computing with ten processor nodes was used in the FEA and in the calculation of the stress shielding coefficient and critical cement damage accumulation parameter.

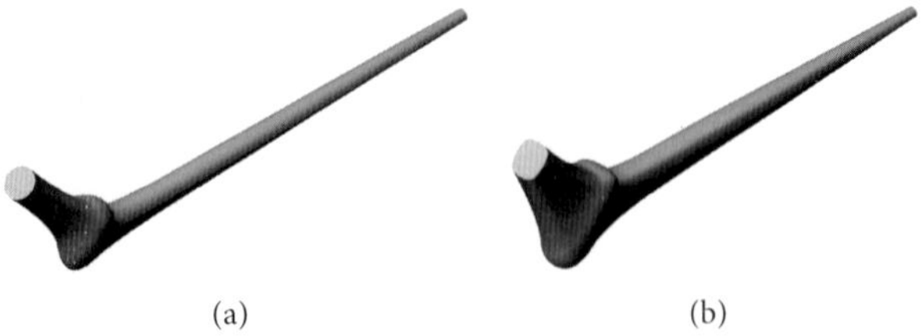

Figure 9: Lowest (a) and uppermost (b) implant configurations.

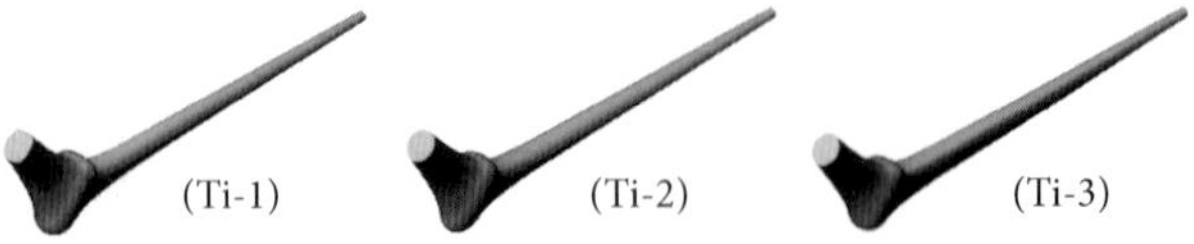

Figure 10: Optimal designs for the Titanium implant.

3.2. Application 1: Titanium Implant. In this application, Titanium alloy (Ti-6Al-4V) with uniform mechanical properties (modulus of elasticity of 110 GPa and a Poisson's ratio of 0.3 [39]) was used for the material of the implant.

Although several optimal configurations were identified upon the application of the methodology in Section 2, they did not contribute equally to the reduction in stress shielding and critical cement damage accumulation parameter. For brevity we discuss the most common results using three of the optimal configurations as depicted in Figure 10. The exponent (p) of the respective cross sections along with the critical cement damage accumulation parameter at 2.0×10^6 cycles is displayed in Table 2. All three designs had comparable critical cement damage accumulation parameters as indicated on the last column which can be attributed to the shape and size of the implant cross sections around the proximal cement. More explicitly, the size of the cross sections had increased and their profile broadened between the implant proximal end and the intersection of the neck and prosthesis axes (sections 6, 5, and 4) as depicted in Figure 11; the wider trapezoidal cross sections in contact with the proximal cement allowed for less stress concentration at these locations eventually delaying damage initiation.

In regard to the stress shielding coefficient, the Ti-1-bone assembly had the smallest value followed by the Ti-2 and Ti-3. The size and profile of the cross sections can also explain these differences as they affect the stiffness of the implant-bone assembly. In the scaled up cross-sectional view in Figure 11, Ti-1 had relatively smaller oval cross sections along the stem length (between cross sections 3 and 1); the relatively slender stem caused the implant-bone assembly to be relatively more flexible to bending. The reduced flexural strength resulted in

TABLE 2: Values of the exponents over the cross sections in Figure 2 along with the critical cement damage accumulation parameter at 2.0 × 10^6 cycles for three optimal configurations.

Optimal configurations	Exponents						Critical cement damage accumulation parameter (%)
	Cross section 1	Cross section 2	Cross section 3	Cross section 4	Cross section 5	Cross section 6	
Ti-1	2	2	2	4	3	3	2.1
Ti-2	2	2	2	3	3	2	2.9
Ti-3	2	3	3	4	2	2	2.6

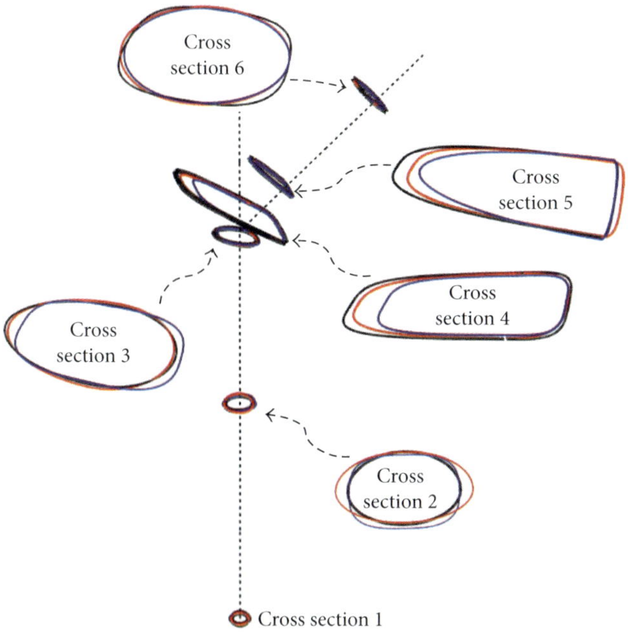

FIGURE 11: Change in the size and profile of the cross sections for all of Ti-1 (black), Ti-2 (red), and Ti-3 (blue) configurations.

an increase in the strain energy of the bone upon application of the body and adductor muscle forces which explains the relatively smaller stress shielding coefficient. By contrast, the wider trapezoidal cross sections along the stem length of the Ti-3 configuration caused the bending resistance of the assembly to increase which led to less strain energy in the bone and a relatively larger stress shielding coefficient. To justify these results we plotted the stress distribution (Von Mises stress) over the frontal and posterior external surfaces of the bone in Figures 12 and 13, respectively; there is a small increase in the stress over the proximal region of the bone, more noticeably over the posterior surface as the bending strain is relatively larger in these areas.

Overall, the reduced flexural strength of the implant-bone assembly owing to the slender medial to distal cross sections of the stem was responsible for reducing stress shielding as the strain energy of the bone had increased upon bending; it had also increased the stress over the proximal cement leading to more chances of early damage initiation. Balance was achieved during the global search by using wider trapezoidal cross sections that redistributed the stress and reduced stress concentration at these locations.

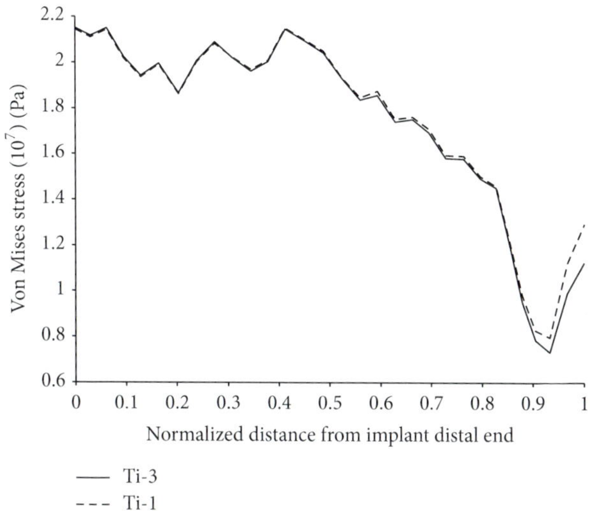

FIGURE 12: Von Mises stress over the external anterior surface of the bone.

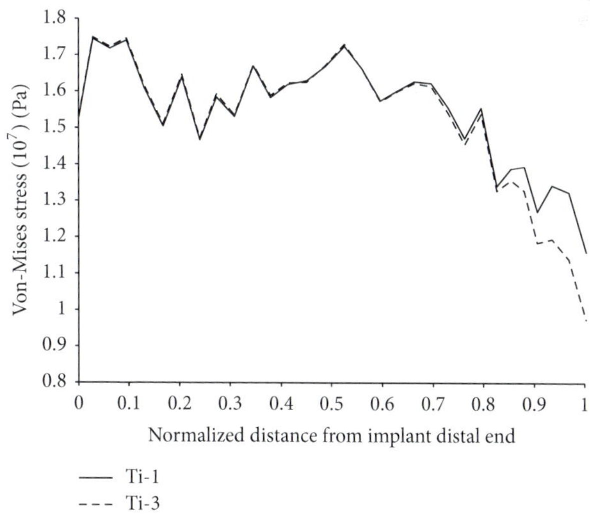

FIGURE 13: Von Mises stress over the external posterior surface of the bone.

3.3. Application 2: Functionally Graded Implant. Unlike materials with uniform composition, structural composites, in particular functionally graded materials (FGM), exhibit progressive change in composition, structure, and properties as a function of position within the material. Several

TABLE 3: Modulus of elasticity along the length of the functionally graded implant.

Layer #	1	2	3	4	5	6	7	8	9	10	11
Modulus of elasticity (GPa)	120	110	90	80	70	60	50	40	30	20	10

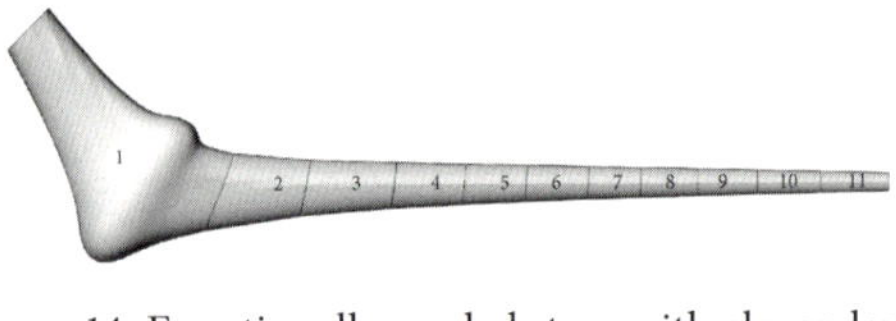

FIGURE 14: Functionally graded stem with eleven layers.

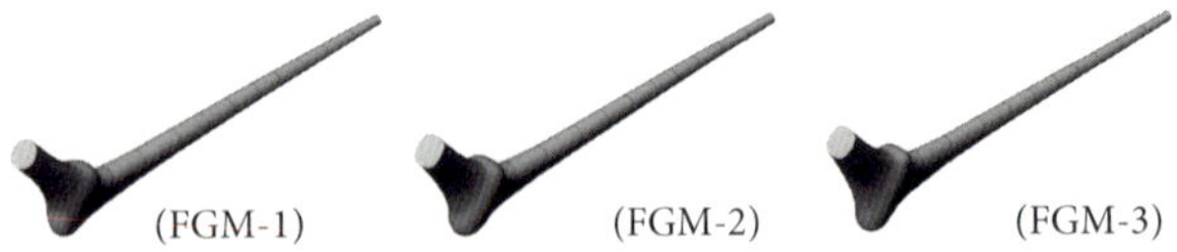

FIGURE 15: Optimal designs for the functionally graded implant.

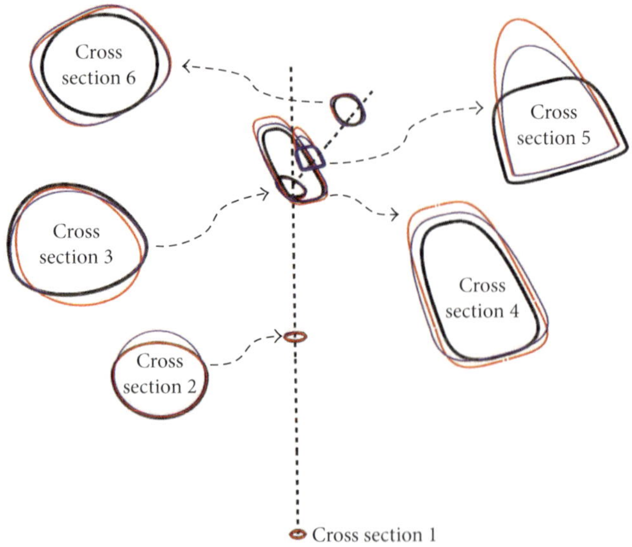

FIGURE 16: Change in the size and profile of the cross sections for all of FGM-1 (black), FGM-2 (red), and FGM-3 (blue) configurations.

processes have been reported to allow fabrication of such composites including plasma spraying, powder metallurgy, and physical vapor deposition [46–48]. A number of studies have demonstrated the suitability of these materials for use in various prostheses including hip, knee, and dental implants [49–52].

In the previous application, we attempted to increase the flexibility of the implant-bone assembly by modifying the profile and size of the stem cross sections. In the current application, a functionally graded material is used for the implant and the optimization technique introduced in Section 2 is applied to further balance stress shielding of the bone and cement damage.

The functionally graded implant was sliced into eleven lengthwise layers as indicated in Figure 14 and constant material properties were assigned to each layer. Layer #1 in particular had material properties identical to that of Titanium (Ti-6Al-4V) and extended over the proximal cement where the most likely sites of cement damage initiation occur. For the rest of the layers, material stiffness decreased according to the schedule described in Table 3. The length and number of layers were maintained throughout the analysis and Poisson's ratio was assumed constant overall and equal to 0.3. Insight into devising such a model stemmed from previous research [53] where it was demonstrated that stress shielding and interface shear stress were reduced upon decreasing implant material stiffness from the proximal to the distal end of the implant.

Several optimal configurations were identified upon the application of the methodology in Section 2; in the following we discuss the most common results using three of these designs as depicted in Figure 15. The critical cement damage accumulation parameters along with the exponents (p) for all six cross sections are displayed in Table 4. Like the Titanium configurations in Section 3.2, the designs in Figure 15 had oval cross sections over the stem length (cross sections 1 to 3) and trapezoidal cross sections around the intersection of the neck and prosthesis axes; additionally the sizes of the cross sections increased from the proximal end of the implant to the end of the neck axis and decreased afterward toward the distal end of the implant as illustrated in Figure 16.

FGM-1 had the smallest stress shielding coefficient followed by FGM-2 and FGM-3 and the size and profile of the cross sections can be used to explain these differences. FGM-1 had relatively smaller cross sections as can be demonstrated from the scaled up view in Figure 16; the smaller cross sections contributed to the implant enhanced flexibility to bending and to that of the assembly all together. As a result, the bone acquired more strain energy upon the application of the body and abductor muscle forces which lead to a relatively smaller stress shielding coefficient. Moreover, the gradual bending of the implant owing to the progressive softening of its material from the proximal to the distal end resulted in less stress over the proximal cement that was further redistributed using the broad trapezoidal cross sections leading to the smaller values in critical cement damage accumulation parameter. The cross sections in FGM-2 and FGM-3 were relatively larger overall resulting in an increase in the bending resistance of the assembly, eventually a relatively larger stress shielding coefficient. To justify these results we plotted in Figure 17 the stress distribution (Von Mises stress) over the external surface of the bone for two of the optimal configurations. There is a small increase in the stress when using FGM-1 implant which explains its relatively smaller stress shielding

TABLE 4: Values of the exponents over the cross sections in Figure 2 along with the critical cement damage accumulation parameter at 2.0 × 10^6 cycles for three optimal configurations.

Optimal configurations	Exponents						Critical cement damage accumulation parameter (%)
	Cross section 1	Cross section 2	Cross section 3	Cross section 4	Cross section 5	Cross section 6	
FGM-1	2	2	2	3	4	2	0.4
FGM-2	2	2	2	3	2	3	0.4
FGM-3	2	2	2	4	2	3	0.7

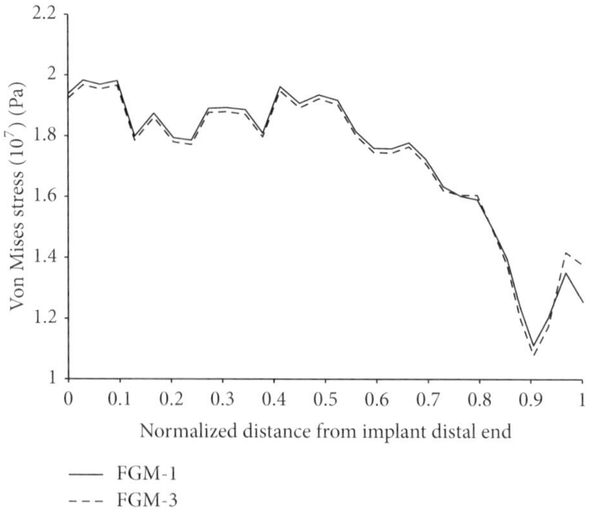

FIGURE 17: Von Mises stress over the external surface of the bone.

coefficient. Comparison with the optimal Titanium configurations revealed that FGMs induce less stress shielding and minimum cement damage (Tables 2 and 4).

4. Conclusion and Future Work

In this study, we introduced a novel methodology to realistically design cemented hip prostheses by controlling the size and profile of the implant cross sections. The self-regulated technique was used to assess the amount of stress shielding on the bone concurrently with the induced cement damage and then selects a local optimum that equally minimizes their individual effects. In a series of probabilistic restarts a fast global search is implemented and several optimal configurations are found. Stress shielding and cement damage are two conflicting effects nevertheless; a balance can be achieved through geometrical optimization of the implant cross sections. The degree of the balance depends on the material used since gradual softening of the material of the implant induces less stress shielding and minimum damage on the cement. The technique could be improved with a more realistic model of the femur and with accurate and evolutionary models of damage assessment; it can be modified to investigate additional effects such as the change in implant length and surface structure. The methodology can also be extended to other orthopedic joint implants, such as knee and shoulder implants.

Appendix

Variable Variance Probability Density (VVP)

The variable variance probability (VVP) density is based on the minimum distance to the points already sampled and is represented as

$$\Phi(x) = \frac{1}{\sqrt{2\pi}\sigma}\left(1 - e^{d_{\min}^2/2\sigma^2}\right)$$

$$d_{\min} = \underset{i=1,\ldots,m}{\min}\left\{d_i = \sqrt{\sum_{k=1}^{n}\left(\frac{x_{k,i} - x_k}{x_{k,u} - x_{k,l}}\right)^2}\right\}, \quad \text{(A.1)}$$

where $\Phi(x)$ is the sampling probability of a point x, n is the number of design variables, x_i is a point previously sampled, and m is the number of points already sampled. Length d_i is the nondimensional distance between point x and point x_i.

The variance of the normal probability density, which is updated in each restart, is given by

$$\sigma = \frac{1}{3\sqrt[n]{m}}. \quad \text{(A.2)}$$

The variance is gradually decreasing when the number of sampled points is increased.

Acknowledgments

The first author would like to express his gratitude to the Office of Research and Grants at the University of Central Oklahoma (UCO) for the financial support during this research.

References

[1] I. D. Learmonth, C. Young, and C. Rorabeck, "The operation of the century: total hip replacement," *Lancet*, vol. 370, no. 9597, pp. 1508–1519, 2007.

[2] S. Breusch and H. Malchau, *The Well-Cemented Total Hip Arthroplasty: Theory and Practice*, Springer, Dordrecht, The Netherlands, 1st edition, 2006.

[3] M. Jasty, W. J. Maloney, C. R. Bragdon, T. Haire, and W. H. Harris, "Histomorphological studies of the long-term skeletal responses to well fixed cemented femoral components," *Journal of Bone and Joint Surgery—Series A*, vol. 72, no. 8, pp. 1220–1229, 1990.

[4] M. Jasty, W. J. Maloney, C. R. Bragdon, D. O. O'Connor, T. Haire, and W. H. Harris, "The initiation of failure in cemented femoral components of hip arthroplasties," *Journal of Bone and Joint Surgery*, vol. 73, no. 4, pp. 551–558, 1991.

[5] R. L. Barrack, R. D. Jr. Mulroy, and W. H. Harris, "Improved cementing techniques and femoral component loosening in young patients with hip arthroplasty: a 12-year radiographic review," *Journal of Bone and Joint Surgery. Series B*, vol. 74, no. 3, pp. 385–389, 1992.

[6] T. Eisler, O. Svensson, V. Iyer et al., "Revision total hip arthroplasty using third-generation cementing technique," *Journal of Arthroplasty*, vol. 15, no. 8, pp. 974–981, 2000.

[7] J. G. Horne, W. Bruce, P. A. Devane, and H. H. Teoh, "The effect of different cement insertion techniques on the bone-cement interface," *Journal of Arthroplasty*, vol. 17, no. 5, pp. 579–583, 2002.

[8] A. D. Reading, A. W. McCaskie, M. R. Barnes, and P. J. Gregg, "A comparison of 2 modern femoral cementing techniques: analysis by cement-bone interface pressure measurements, computerized image analysis, and static mechanical testing," *Journal of Arthroplasty*, vol. 15, no. 4, pp. 479–487, 2000.

[9] Y. Wang, P. Han, W. Gu, Z. Shi, D. Li, and C. Wang, "Cement oscillation increases interlock strength at the cement-bone interface," *Orthopedics*, vol. 32, no. 5, article no. 325, 2009.

[10] C. J. Sychterz and C. A. Engh, "The influence of clinical factors on periprosthetic bone remodeling," *Clinical Orthopaedics and Related Research*, no. 322, pp. 285–292, 1996.

[11] C. J. Kershaw, R. M. Atkins, C. A. Dodd, and C. J. Bulstrode, "Revision THR for aseptic failure: a review of 276 cases," *The Journal of Bone & Joint Surgery—British Volume*, vol. 73, pp. 564–568, 1991.

[12] A. A. Hofmann, R. W. Wyatt, E. P. France, G. T. Bigler, A. U. Daniels, and W. E. Hess, "Endosteal bone loss after total hip arthroplasty," *Clinical Orthopaedics and Related Research*, no. 245, pp. 138–144, 1989.

[13] H. Kröger, P. Venesmaa, J. Jurvelin, H. Miettinen, O. Suomalainen, and E. Alhava, "Bone density at the proximal femur after total hip arthroplasty," *Clinical Orthopaedics and Related Research*, no. 352, pp. 66–74, 1998.

[14] C. A. Engh, T. F. McGovern, J. D. Bobyn, and W. H. Harris, "A quantitative evaluation of periprosthetic bone-remodeling after cementless total hip arthroplasty," *The Journal of Bone & Joint Surgery—American Volume*, vol. 74, no. 7, pp. 1009–1020, 1992.

[15] T. Karachalios, C. Tsatsaronis, G. Efraimis, P. Papadelis, G. Lyritis, and G. Diakoumopoulos, "The long-term clinical relevance of calcar atrophy caused by stress shielding in total hip arthroplasty: a 10-year, prospective, randomized study," *Journal of Arthroplasty*, vol. 19, no. 4, pp. 469–475, 2004.

[16] G. G. Polkowski, J. J. Callaghan, M. A. Mont, and J. C. Clohisy, "Total hip arthroplasty in the very young patient," *Journal of the American Academy of Orthopaedic Surgeons*, vol. 20, no. 8, pp. 487–497, 2012.

[17] F. Launay, J. Jouve, J. Guillaume, E. Viehweger, M. Jacquemier, and G. Bollini, "Total hip arthroplasty without cement in children and adolescents: 17 cases," *Revue de Chirurgie Orthopedique et Reparatrice de l'Appareil Moteur*, vol. 88, pp. 460–466, 2002.

[18] L. D. T. Topoleski, P. Ducheyne, and J. M. Cukler, "A fractographic analysis of in vivo poly(methyl methacrylate) bone cement failure mechanisms," *Journal of Biomedical Materials Research*, vol. 24, no. 2, pp. 135–154, 1990.

[19] T. P. Culleton, P. J. Prendergast, and D. Taylor, "Fatigue failure in the cement mantle of an artificial hip joint," *Clinical Materials*, vol. 12, no. 2, pp. 95–102, 1993.

[20] C. Li, C. Granger, H. D. Schutte Jr., S. B. Biggers Jr., J. M. Kennedy, and R. A. Latour Jr., "Progressive failure analysis of laminated composite femoral prostheses for total hip arthroplasty," *Biomaterials*, vol. 23, no. 21, pp. 4249–4262, 2002.

[21] J. A. Simões and A. T. Marques, "Design of a composite hip femoral prosthesis," *Materials and Design*, vol. 26, no. 5, pp. 391–401, 2005.

[22] S. Gross and E. W. Abel, "A finite element analysis of hollow stemmed hip prostheses as a means of reducing stress shielding of the femur," *Journal of Biomechanics*, vol. 34, no. 8, pp. 995–1003, 2001.

[23] W.-P. Chen, C.-L. Tai, M. S. Lee, P.-C. Lee, C.-P. Liu, and C.-H. Shih, "Comparison of stress shielding among different cement fixation modes of femoral stem in total hip arthroplasty—a three-dimensional finite element analysis," *Journal of Medical and Biological Engineering*, vol. 24, no. 4, pp. 183–187, 2004.

[24] R. M. Mahamood, E. T. Akinlabi, M. Shukla, and S. Pityana, "Functionally graded material: an overview," in *Proceedings of the World Congress on Engineering 2012 Vol III, WCE 2012, July 4–6, 2012, London, U.K.*, vol. 2199 of *Lecture Notes in Engineering and Computer Science*, pp. 1593–1597, International Association of Engineers, 2012.

[25] M. Hamadouche, A. Jahnke, C. Scemama et al., "Length of clinically proven cemented hip stems: state of the art or subject to improvement?" *International Orthopaedics*, vol. 39, no. 3, pp. 411–416, 2015.

[26] T. Ishida, I. Nishimura, H. Tanino, M. Higa, H. Ito, and Y. Mitamura, "Use of a genetic algorithm for multiobjective design optimization of the femoral stem of a cemented total hip arthroplasty," *Artificial Organs*, vol. 35, no. 4, pp. 404–410, 2011.

[27] H. Katoozian and D. T. Davy, "Effects of loading conditions and objective function on three-dimensional shape optimization of femoral components of hip endoprostheses," *Medical Engineering and Physics*, vol. 22, no. 4, pp. 243–251, 2000.

[28] H. Tanino, H. Ito, M. Higa et al., "Three-dimensional computer-aided design based design sensitivity analysis and shape optimization of the stem using adaptive p-method," *Journal of Biomechanics*, vol. 39, no. 10, pp. 1948–1953, 2006.

[29] A. L. Sabatini and T. Goswami, "Hip implants VII: finite element analysis and optimization of cross-sections," *Materials and Design*, vol. 29, no. 7, pp. 1438–1446, 2008.

[30] H. Katoozian and D. T. Davy, "Three-dimensional shape optimization of femoral components of total hip prostheses," in *Proceedings of the ASME Bioengineering Conference*, vol. 24, pp. 552–555, 1993.

[31] P. Kowalczyk, "Design optimization of cementless femoral hip prostheses using finite element analysis," *Journal of Biomechanical Engineering*, vol. 123, no. 5, pp. 396–402, 2001.

[32] P. B. Chang, B. J. Williams, K. S. B. Bhalla et al., "Design and analysis of robust total joint replacements: finite element model experiments with environmental variables," *Journal of Biomechanical Engineering*, vol. 123, no. 3, pp. 239–246, 2001.

[33] P. R. Fernandes, J. Folgado, and R. B. Ruben, "Shape optimization of a cementless hip stem for a minimum of interface

stress and displacement," *Computer Methods in Biomechanics and Biomedical Engineering*, vol. 7, no. 1, pp. 51–61, 2004.

[34] R. B. Ruben, J. Folgado, and P. R. Fernandes, "Three-dimensional shape optimization of hip prostheses using a multicriteria formulation," *Structural and Multidisciplinary Optimization*, vol. 34, no. 3, pp. 261–275, 2007.

[35] R. B. Ruben, P. R. Fernandes, and J. Folgado, "On the optimal shape of hip implants," *Journal of Biomechanics*, vol. 45, no. 2, pp. 239–246, 2012.

[36] H.-S. Park and X.-P. Dang, "Structural optimization based on CAD-CAE integration and metamodeling techniques," *CAD Computer Aided Design*, vol. 42, no. 10, pp. 889–902, 2010.

[37] J. R. T. Jeffers, M. Browne, A. B. Lennon, P. J. Prendergast, and M. Taylor, "Cement mantle fatigue failure in total hip replacement: experimental and computational testing," *Journal of Biomechanics*, vol. 40, no. 7, pp. 1525–1533, 2007.

[38] J. Stolk, N. Verdonschot, and R. Huiskes, "Hip-joint and abductor-muscle forces adequately represent in vivo loading of a cemented total hip reconstruction," *Journal of Biomechanics*, vol. 34, no. 7, pp. 917–926, 2001.

[39] K. A. Mann, D. L. Bartel, T. M. Wright, and A. H. Burstein, "Coulomb frictional interfaces in modeling cemented total hip replacements: a more realistic model," *Journal of Biomechanics*, vol. 28, no. 9, pp. 1067–1078, 1995.

[40] J. P. Davies, D. W. Burke, D. O. O'Connor, and W. H. Harris, "Comparison of the fatigue characteristics of centrifuged and uncentrifuged simplex P bone cement," *Journal of Orthopaedic Research*, vol. 5, no. 3, pp. 366–371, 1987.

[41] B. A. O. McCormack, P. J. Prendergast, and D. G. Gallagher, "An experimental study of damage accumulation in cemented hip prostheses," *Clinical Biomechanics*, vol. 11, no. 4, pp. 214–219, 1996.

[42] B. A. O. McCormack and P. J. Prendergast, "Microdamage accumulation in the cement layer of hip replacements under flexural loading," *Journal of Biomechanics*, vol. 32, no. 5, pp. 467–475, 1999.

[43] J.-P. Hung, J.-H. Chen, H.-L. Chiang, and J. Shih-Shyn Wu, "Computer simulation on fatigue behavior of cemented hip prostheses: a physiological model," *Computer Methods and Programs in Biomedicine*, vol. 76, no. 2, pp. 103–113, 2004.

[44] M. A. Hakulinen, H. Borg, A. Häkkinen, T. Parviainen, I. Kiviranta, and J. S. Jurvelin, "Quantification of bone density of the proximal femur after hip resurfacing arthroplasty-comparison of different DXA acquisition modes," *Journal of Clinical Densitometry*, vol. 13, no. 4, pp. 426–432, 2010.

[45] P. J. Ross, *Taguchi Techniques for Quality Engineering*, McGraw-Hill, New York, NY, USA, 1988.

[46] P. Shanmugavel, G. B. Bhaskar, M. Chandrasekaran, P. S. Mani, and S. P. Srinivasan, "An overview of fracture analysis in Functionally Graded Materials," *European Journal of Scientific Research*, vol. 68, no. 3, pp. 412–439, 2012.

[47] A. A. Atai, A. Nikranjbar, and R. Kasiri, "Buckling and post-buckling behaviour of semicircular functionally graded material arches: a theoretical study," *Proceedings of the Institution of Mechanical Engineers, Part C: Journal of Mechanical Engineering Science*, vol. 226, no. 3, pp. 607–614, 2012.

[48] C. Chenglin, Z. Jingchuan, Y. Zhongda, and W. Shidong, "Hydroxyapatite-ti functionally graded biomaterial fabricated by powder metallurgy," *Materials Science and Engineering A*, vol. 271, no. 1-2, pp. 95–100, 1999.

[49] D. Lin, Q. Li, W. Li, S. Zhou, and M. V. Swain, "Design optimization of functionally graded dental implant for bone remodeling," *Composites Part B: Engineering*, vol. 40, no. 7, pp. 668–675, 2009.

[50] H. Mishina, Y. Inumaru, and K. Kaitoku, "Fabrication of ZrO2/AISI316L functionally graded materials for joint prostheses," *Materials Science and Engineering A*, vol. 475, no. 1-2, pp. 141–147, 2008.

[51] J.-P. Zou, J.-M. Ruan, B.-Y. Huang, Z.-C. Zhou, and Y.-L. Liu, "Preparation and microstructure of HA-316L stainless steel fiber asymmetrical functionally gradient biomaterial," *Journal of Inorganic Materials*, vol. 20, no. 5, pp. 1181–1188, 2005.

[52] C. Chu, X. Xue, J. Zhu, and Z. Yin, "In vivo study on biocompatibility and bonding strength of Ti/Ti-20 vol.% HA/Ti-40 vol.% HA functionally graded biomaterial with bone tissues in the rabbit," *Materials Science and Engineering A*, vol. 429, no. 1-2, pp. 18–24, 2006.

[53] H. S. Hedia, M. A. N. Shabara, T. T. El-Midany, and N. Fouda, "A method of material optimization of cementless stem through functionally graded material," *International Journal of Mechanics and Materials in Design*, vol. 1, pp. 329–346, 2005.

26

Rasterstereographic Analysis of Lateral Shift in Patients with Lumbar Disc Herniation: A Case Control Study

Britta K. Krautwurst,[1] Jürgen R. Paletta,[2] Sylvia Mendoza,[3] Adrian Skwara,[2,4] and Melvin Mohokum[5]

[1] *Heidelberg University Clinics, Department for Orthopedics and Trauma Surgery, Schlierbacher Landstraße 200a, 66118 Heidelberg, Germany*
[2] *Department of Orthopedics and Rheumatology, University Hospital Marburg, Baldingerstrasse, 35043 Marburg, Germany*
[3] *Studiendekanat, Fachbereich Medizin, Dr. Reinfried Pohl-Zentrum für Medizinische Lehre (RPZ), University Hospital Marburg, Conradistraße 9, 35043 Marburg, Germany*
[4] *Orthopädische Gemeinschaftspraxis Ammenwerth / Skwara, Schildern 6, 33098 Paderborn, Germany*
[5] *SRH Hochschule für Gesundheit, University of Applied Health Science, Neue Str. 28–30, 07548 Gera, Germany*

Correspondence should be addressed to Melvin Mohokum; melvin.mohokum@srh.de

Guest Editor: Yasushi Oshima

Objective. Detection of a lateral shift (LS) in patients with diagnosed disc herniation compared to healthy controls. *Summary of Background Data.* A specific lateral shift (LS) pattern is observed in patients with disc herniation and low back pain, as shown in earlier studies. *Methods.* Rasterstereography (RS) was used to investigate the LS. Thirty-nine patients with lumbar disc herniation diagnosed by radiological assessment and low back pain and/or leg pain (mean age 48.2 years, mean BMI 28.5, 28 males and 11 females) and 36 healthy controls (mean age 47.4 years, mean BMI 25.7, 25 males and 11 females) were analysed. LS, pelvic tilt, pelvic inclination, lordotic angle, and trunk torsion were assessed. *Results.* The patient group showed a nonsignificant increase in LS, that is, 5.6 mm compared to the healthy controls with 5.0 mm ($p = 0.693$). However, significant differences were found between groups regarding pelvic tilt in degrees (patients 5.9°, healthy controls 2.0°; $p = 0.016$), trunk torsion (patients 7.5°, controls 4.5°; $p = 0.017$), and lordotic angle (patients 27.5°, healthy controls 32.7°; $p = 0.022$). The correlation between pain intensity and the FFbH-R amounted 0.804 ($p = < 0.01$), and that between pain intensity and the pain disability index was 0.785 ($p < 0.01$). *Discussion.* Although some studies have illustrated LS with disc herniation and low back pain, the present findings demonstrate no significant increase in LS in the patient group compared to healthy controls. *Conclusion.* The patients with lumbar disc herniation did not demonstrate an increased LS compared to healthy controls. Other parameters like pelvic tilt and inclination seemed to be more suitable to identify changes in posture measured by RS in patients with low back pain or disc herniation.

1. Introduction

Low back pain is currently a common problem with a considerable medical and therapeutic impact [1]. The lifetime prevalence amounts up to 80% and higher in the general population [2–4]. In approximately 85% of cases, the underlying cause is unknown, while in around 15%, the cause is known, for example, lumbar disc herniation [5]. Lumbar disc herniation has a high prevalence and affects the spine in younger and middle-aged patients [6–9]. For clinical decision making and to initiate a specific and appropriate therapy for the patient group, a systematic investigation of patients with lumbar disc herniation and low back pain is required. One parameter that can be assessed is the lateral shift (LS), which is an important clinical sign. It occurs ipsilaterally or contralaterally, with no relation to the side of pain [10]. There are different definitions available for the LS [11]. A LS is a deviation from the spinal midline. This is shown by the sagittal arrangement of the lumbar spinous processes. They are typically arranged asymmetrically. The upper body is clearly shifted to the side [11]. The LS can be determined with different methods, for example, visual investigation using a plumbline and palpation using the side-glide test sequence [12, 13]. The LS can be determined with an accuracy of 5 mm using the plumbline technique [14]. The prevalence of LS in patients with low back pain has been previously examined [10, 12]. In a collective of patients with an acute episode of low back pain, Gillan showed an abnormality in LS ranging from 5 to 50 mm and called it a "new phenomenon associated with the onset of back pain" [12]. Porter et al. examined 100 patients with back pain and LS; the majority (71 patients) reported pain distribution below the knee [10]. Healthy controls were not evaluated.

One measurement method that illustrates important spine parameters is rasterstereography [15]. RS is a contact-free, noninvasive technique to detect spinal deformities, for instance, scoliosis, on the basis of surface asymmetry. The validity and reliability of this method have been described elsewhere [16–22].

Khallaf examined 16 patients with lumbar disc herniation using rasterstereography [23]. The patients showed a significantly increased lateral pelvic tilt and an increased lordotic angle compared to healthy subjects. However, the lateral shift as an important clinical sign is not evaluated by Khallaf. Therefore, the primary aim of this study was to evaluate LS in patients with diagnosed lumbar disc herniation compared to healthy controls measured by RS. The secondary aim was to assess posture modifications in relation to spine, pelvic, and functional parameters. These parameters should be correlated to each other. According to the main aim of the study, the null hypothesis (H0) is that patients with lumbar disc herniation will have no LS compared to healthy controls. The alternative hypothesis (H1) is that patients with lumbar disc herniation will have a greater LS compared to healthy controls.

2. Methods

2.1. Patients and Recruitment Procedure. All participants were recruited in 2011. The individuals in the patient group were enrolled in a rehabilitation hospital with a special section for chronic spinal diseases at Montanus-Klinik Bad Schwalbach, Germany. The healthy individuals in the control group were recruited from the general population and were examined at a second hospital, that is, University Hospital in Marburg, Germany. Both hospitals used the same measurement system.

2.2. Patient Group. The inclusion criteria for the patient group were underwritten patient information and informed consent, the ability to speak the German language, the ability to stand free without any assistance, the ability to lay flat on their back, evidence of lumbar disc herniation or protrusion detected by magnetic resonance imaging (MRI), and low back pain and/or leg pain; all stadia of pain (acute, subacute, chronic) were included.

The exclusion criteria for the patient group were age younger than 18 years, cancer, previous spinal surgery, relevant bone degeneration, red flags, pension request, relevant tattoos or scars on the surface of the back, and no pain on a numeric rating scale (NRS = 0).

2.3. Control Group. The inclusion criteria for the healthy controls were the ability to speak the German language, no back or leg pain on a numeric rating scale (NRS = 0), the ability to stand free without any assistance, and the ability to lay flat on their back. The exclusion criteria were age younger than 18 years, cancer, previous spine surgery, relevant spinal degeneration, red flags, pension request, relevant tattoos or scars on the back, chronic low back pain, and lumbar low back pain and/or leg pain.

2.4. Ethical Aspects. The study received ethical approval from the independent ethics committee of University Hospital Marburg (reference number Az. 22/11). Information about the procedure and risks were included in the patient information. Participants in the patient and control groups had to provide written informed consent.

2.5. Methods of Measurement

2.5.1. Self-Assessment Questionnaire. All participants had to complete a general self-assessment questionnaire to provide individual data, for example, age, height, weight, comorbidities, pain anamneses, and a pain chart.

2.5.2. Numeric Rating Scale (NRS). The Numeric Rating Scale for Pain (NRS) was used to measure pain intensity. The numeric scale has 11 items with "0" representing no pain and "10" representing the worst pain imaginable [25].

2.5.3. Hannover Functional Ability Questionnaire (FFbH-R). The level of functional ability was measured by the Hannover Functional Ability Questionnaire (FFbH-R). This instrument was developed for patients with musculoskeletal disorders, comprising 12 short self-administered questionnaires on functional capacity in the activities of daily living [26].

2.5.4. Pain Disability Index (PDI). The PDI is a comprehensive self-administered questionnaire for assessing disability associated with pain. The respondents indicate the amount of perceived pain-related disability in seven different areas of daily living on an 11-point Likert scale with one end point of 0 (no disability) and the other end point set at 10 (maximum disability). The areas are home, social activities, recreational, occupational, sexual functioning, self-care, and life support activities. Higher scores indicate greater disability. The PDI has been shown to have a correlation of r = 0.7-0.9 with the Oswestry Disability Questionnaire in patients with low back pain [27].

2.5.5. Mainz Pain Staging System (MPSS). The MPSS is classified in three chronification levels. Four axes were considered: temporal aspects of pain, pain distribution, drug intake, and utilisation of health care. The final score described three chronification levels. On level I, the pain is intermittently, temporary, with changeable intensity, mostly in one

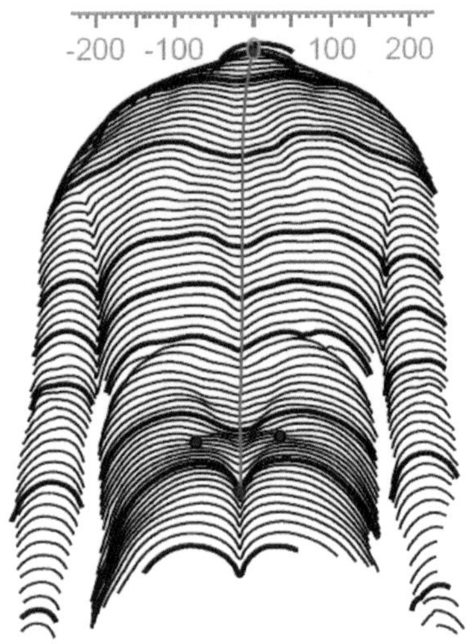

FIGURE 1: View of the raster lines on a patient's back. Blue dots: left and right lumbar dimples. Lower red dot: dimple mid-point (DM).

localization, adequate drug intake, visiting just one medical specialist, and not more than one stay in a hospital due to pain. Level II is characterized as follows: the pain during a longer time, more than one pain localization, drug abuse, changing medical consultations, and 2-3 clinical stays caused by pain. Continuous pain, pain on a large areal and changing localizations, long-time drug abuse, and more than three alterations of the medical specialist and clinical stays describe level III.

2.5.6. Straight Leg Raise (SLR). The SLR is widely used and is well suited for clinical investigations. The subject lies in a supine position with their head on the ground. The tester lifts the measured leg passively with an extended knee and ankle in the neutral position as high as possible. If the subject indicates pain or the investigator notices resistance, the investigator measures the hip flexion angle at the limit of the SLR using a plurimeter. A positive test result is associated with nerve root compression. The SLR is a reliable tool with a high intraclass reliability of 0.99 [28].

2.5.7. Rasterstereography (RS). RS is a noninvasive technique for analysing back and spinal deformities that uses the triangulation method [29]. Parallel white lines are projected onto the unclothed back of the subject (see Figure 1). This horizontal light raster is detected by a camera system. RS evaluates surface contours formed by the underlying tissue, for example, the spinous process. The system identifies anatomical fixed points with an accuracy of ±0.1 mm standard deviation [30, 31].

The lateral shift is a lateral deviation in the frontal plane. For the calculation the perpendicular from vertebrae prominence was dropped and the difference from this perpendicular to the DM was measured.

For this study, the following parameters were measured according to Degenhardt 2017 [32]:

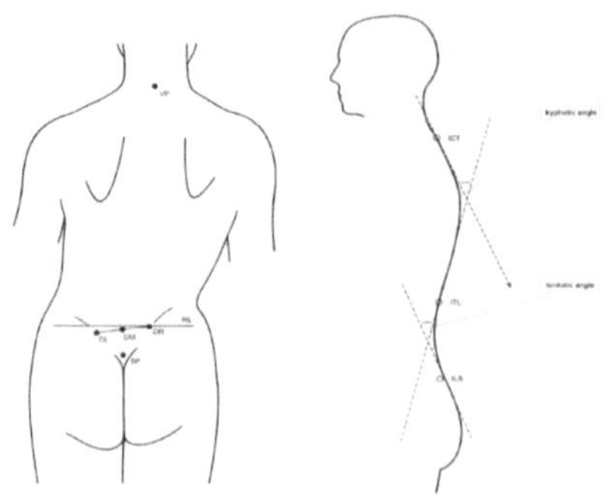

FIGURE 2: Rasterstereographic parameters: pelvic tilt (left) and lordotic angle (right) adapted by Lippold et al. [24].

(1) Pelvic tilt (PT): Difference in the height of the lumbar dimples is shown in Figure 2 [24]. A positive value indicates a higher right dimple than on the left and a negative value denotes the opposite. This value is quantified in millimetres (mm) and degrees (°).

(2) Pelvic inclination (PI dimples): A positive value indicates the vertical component of the left dimple and the right dimple is adjusted to the top; negative values denote the opposite. This value is provided in degrees.

(3) Pelvic inclination (PI symmetry line): This parameter is a symmetry line of the spinous processes. A positive value indicates an anterior pelvic inclination and a negative value indicates a posterior pelvic inclination. This value is provided in degrees.

(4) Lordotic angle (LA): There are two tangents estimated relating to the surface of the back. The angle between surface tangents of ITL (thoracic-lumbar transition) and ILS (lumbar-sacral transition) is shown in Figure 2 [24]. The higher the value is, the greater the degree of lumbar lordosis is. This value is provided in degrees.

(5) Trunk torsion (TT): This value is provided in degrees.

(6) Lateral shift (LS): This describes the difference in the translative shift (lateral shift) from L1 to DM. This value is provided in degrees. See Figure 3.

2.5.8. Measurement Setup. For this study, the Formetric® III 4 D system (Diers International GmbH, Schlangenbad, Germany) was applied for data collection. It can assess individual clinical parameters under static and dynamic conditions.

To avoid potential bias, the positioning of the subject was standardised. The subjects stood barefoot on a wooden platform with slightly extended knees. The upper extremities hung down lateral to the body, and the subject looked forward. One record took 6 seconds. Two pictures were taken per second. The mean of these 12 pictures of every record was used for the analysis.

2.5.9. Statistical Power Analysis and Statistics. The calculation of the power was based on the data of a pilot study. The difference of LS between healthy subjects and patients was 5.3 mm, the standard deviation 7.9 mm. The significance

TABLE 1: Characteristics of participants.

Parameter	Group	Mean	SD	p
Age (years)	Patient group	48.2	9.4	.721
	Healthy controls	47.4	9.5	
Height (cm)	Patient group	175.1	10.8	.898
	Healthy controls	175.4	10.1	
Weight (kg)	Patient group	87.4	15.0	.014*
	Healthy controls	79.3	12.6	
BMI (kg/m²)	Patient group	28.5	4.5	.002**
	Healthy controls	25.7	2.9	

Comparison between patient group and healthy controls: mean, standard deviation (SD), and p value were illustrated for age, height, weight, and BMI.
* Significance on the level of $p \leq .05$.
** Significance on the level of $p \leq .01$.

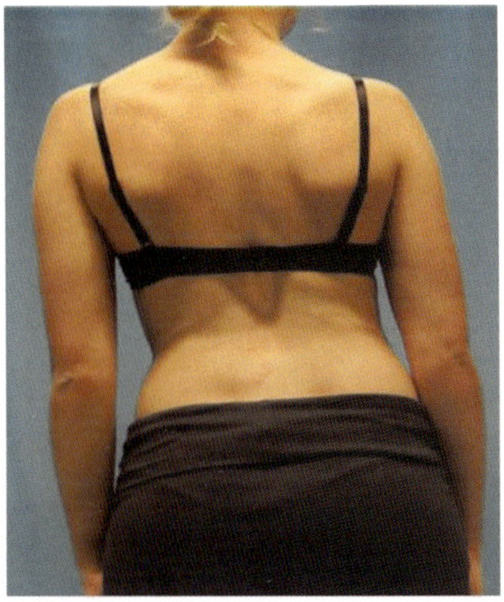

FIGURE 3: A person with a left LS from the posterior view.

level was 0.05 and power 0.8. The statistical power analysis suggested a minimal number of 35 subjects for each group (the patients and the healthy controls). A dropout rate of 10% for the sample size was estimated; therefore four additional volunteers were enrolled in each group as a safety margin.

Mean, minimum and maximum values, and standard deviations were calculated for all parameters. The Shapiro-Wilk-Test was used to estimate the normal distribution. The independent sample t-test was used to compare the patient and healthy controls. Correlations between the parameters were made using the Pearson correlation coefficient. Differences were accepted as significant when the probability was below 5% ($p < 0.05$). The comparisons of more than one parameter were performed by using one-way ANOVA, with the Bonferroni post hoc test. All statistical analyses were performed with SPSS Version 17 (SPSS Inc., Chicago, IL, USA).

3. Results

3.1. Characteristics of the Study Participants. In the patient group, 39 patients with a radiologically diagnosed herniated disc were enrolled. Out of the 36 healthy controls, three volunteers had to be excluded: one volunteer reported back pain, and two volunteers had scoliosis. Scoliosis is defined as a deviation of the spine greater than 10° in the coronal plane and an axial rotation [33]. The age range was 25–65 years with a mean age of 48.2 years in the patient group and 47.4 in the control group. 11 women were examined in each group, 28 male patients and 25 healthy men. The characteristics of the participants are shown in Table 1.

3.2. Lateral Shift. The lateral shift had a mean value of 5.6±6.0 mm in the patient group and 5.0±7.6 mm in the healthy controls. This difference was not significant (p = 0.693). The trunk of the participants with diagnosed disc herniation did not deviate laterally more than the healthy controls.

3.3. Lateral Shift in relation to SLR. The participants with a positive SLR demonstrated a slightly increased LS (5.5±5.0°) compared to the participants with negative SLR (5.2±8.1°). However, the difference was not significant ($p = 0.829$).

3.4. Trunk, Lumbar Spine, and Pelvis. The patients showed an increased pelvic tilt in [°] as well as [mm], a decreased anterior pelvic inclination (dimples [°] as well as symmetry [°]), an increased trunk torsion [°], and a decreased lordotic angle [°] compared to the healthy controls (Table 2).

3.5. Localization of Pain (Pain Chart). In relation to the localization of pain, there was a significant difference in pelvic tilt in degrees ($p = 0.036$) and pelvic inclination in degrees ($p = 0.017$). The localization of pain has a considerable influence on pelvic inclination (dimples). If pain is not present, the pelvis showed a more anterior tilt (17.8±6.9°) compared to pain up to the feet (11.4±6.6°) ($p = 0.022$).

3.6. Correlations between Rasterstereographic Parameters. There was a very high correlation between pelvic tilt [°] and pelvic tilt [mm] of 0.985 ($p \leq 0.001$) and between pelvic inclination (dimples) [°] and pelvic inclination (symmetry) [°] of 0.904 ($p \leq 0.001$). A lower correlation was found between trunk torsion [°] and pelvic tilt [°] of 0.390 ($p \leq 0.001$) and between trunk torsion [°] and pelvic tilt [mm] of 0.382 ($p \leq 0.001$).

TABLE 2: Parameters of trunk, lumbar spine, and pelvis.

Parameter	Group	Mean	SD	p
PT [°]	Patient group	5.9	9.2	.016*
	Healthy controls	2.0	2.4	
PT [mm]	Patient group	10.6	19.9	.033*
	Healthy controls	3.3	3.7	
PI (dimples) [°]	Patient group	12.5	7.5	.002**
	Healthy controls	17.8	6.9	
PI (symmetry) [°]	Patient group	15.0	10.2	.015*
	Healthy controls	20.4	8.5	
TT [°]	Patient group	7.5	6.2	.017*
	Healthy controls	4.5	4.1	
LA [°]	Patient group	27.5	9.6	.022*
	Healthy controls	32.7	9.5	

Comparison between patient group and healthy controls: mean, standard deviation (SD), and p value were illustrated for PT [°], PT [mm], PT (dimples), PI (symmetry) [°], TT [°], and LA [°].
PT = pelvic tilt; PI (dimples) = pelvic inclination (dimples); PI (symmetry) = pelvic inclination in relation to the symmetry line; TT = trunk torsion; LA = lordotic angle T12 – DM
* Significance on the level of $p \leq .05$.
** Significance on the level of $p \leq .01$.

TABLE 3: Correlations with the FFbH-R.

Parameter	Pearson r	p
BMI	0.310	.007**
MPSS	0.445	.005**
Pain chart	0.643	≤ .001**
NRS	0.804	≤ .001**
Drug intake	0.545	≤ .001**
PDI	0.793	≤ .001**

BMI, MPSS, pain chart, NRS, drug intake, and PDI were correlated with the FFbH-R.
* Significance on the level of $p \leq .05$.
** Significance on the level of $p \leq .01$.

3.7. Correlation to FFbH-R. The correlation between FFbH-R and pain intensity was 0.804 ($p < 0.001$), between FFbH-R and BMI 0.310 ($p = 0.007$), between FFbH-R and MPSS 0.445 ($p = 0.005$), between FFbH-R and drug intake 0.545 ($p < 0.001$), and between FFbH-R and PDI 0.793 ($p < 0.001$). A magnitude of 0.643 ($p < 0.001$) revealed the strength of the relationship between FFbH-R and pain chart. See Table 3.

3.8. Correlation with the PDI. The correlation between the PDI and weight was 0.246 ($p = 0.033$), between PDI and BMI 0.360 ($p = 0.002$), between PDI and MPSS 0.369 ($p = 0.021$), between PDI and pain chart 0.623 ($p \leq 0.001$), between PDI and drug intake 0.379 ($p \leq 0.001$), and between PDI and FFbH-R 0.793 ($p \leq 0.001$). As the pain intensity increased, then the disability in areas of living increased, too. The magnitude was r = 0.785 ($p \leq 0.001$). See Table 4.

4. Discussion

This study demonstrated that there is no significant LS in patients with diagnosed lumbar disc prolapse compared to healthy controls. Harrison et al. indicated a LS of the thoracic cage relative to the fixed pelvis with digitised anterior-posterior radiographs in a group of healthy volunteers [34]. The displacement was measured from T12 to S2 through a vertical line. The mean value in the left was 53.2±8.4 mm and in the right was 52.1±9.0 mm [34]. Although other studies have illustrated a LS with disc herniation and low back pain, this phenomenon could not be validated in this study. However, other studies did not compare their findings with a control group that included healthy individuals.

This is the first study to evaluate the lateral shift using the rasterstereography. The findings in the present study showed a mean LS in healthy controls of 5.0±7.6 mm and 5.6±6.0 mm in the patient group. This difference was not statistically significant ($p = 0.693$). Other studies did not define LS exactly. A threshold with a precise definition for the presence or absence of LS was also missing. However, in a study by Donahue et al., two therapists indicated a LS range of 1-7 mm in 26 out of 49 patients with low back pain [13]. Harrison and colleagues assessed a spinal rehabilitation program and the effect of LS in patients with chronic low back pain [35]. The control group demonstrated an average LS of 7.2±6.2 mm and an average LS of 15.0±5.9 mm in the treatment group. However, both studies

TABLE 4: Correlations with the PDI.

Parameter	Pearson r	p
Weight	0.246	.033*
BMI	0.360	.002**
MPSS	0.369	.021*
Pain chart	0.623	≤ .001**
NRS	0.785	≤ .001**
Drug intake	0.379	≤ .001**
FFbH-R	0.793	≤ .001**

Weight, BMI, MPSS, pain chart, NRS, drug intake, and FFbH-R were correlated with the PDI.
* Significance on the level of $p \leq .05$.
** Significance on the level of $p \leq .01$.

did not compare the results with healthy controls. Donahue et al. reported nonphysiological LS in their patient group [13]. If this phenomenon occurs in healthy subjects, it has not yet been reported. Therefore, in this case-control study, healthy volunteers were included. The LS in the healthy controls was not significant compared to that of the patient group. It is possible that the healthy volunteers had similar disc pathologies as there is a high prevalence of disc pathologies in asymptomatic patients [36, 37] which could explain the lateral shift also in healthy subjects in the current study. However, whether the healthy volunteers were suffering from disc herniation was not systematically investigated by MRI or CT. The healthy controls were only investigated clinically. This should be taken into account in further research.

There are different methods available to measure LS, for example, the plumbline method and the shadow method [13, 14, 38]. The plumbline technique investigated by McLean et al. indicates that it is possible to measure a trunk list within a reliability of 4 mm [14]. In the present study, RS was chosen as the method of measurement for LS. RS is a radiation-free, noninvasive technique that has demonstrated very good inter- and intratester reliability as well [18, 21].

Fritz and Georg analysed LS in patients with acute and chronic pain [39]. The present study included patients with acute or chronic back pain as well as healthy volunteers. The stage of chronification measured by the MPSS has no influence on the posture or the measured parameters.

The patients demonstrated a significant different posture compared to the healthy subjects which was shown also by Khallaf [23]. In both studies the pelvis is increased lateral tilted in patients. The lordotic angle was increased in the patient's group of Khallaf. In contrast to Khallaf, our patients demonstrated a decreased lordotic angle which fits to the decreased anterior inclined pelvis.

In our study, there was a significant difference with respect to the BMI in both groups. Liljenqvist and colleagues reported that the thickness of soft tissue may result in measurement inaccuracies [40]. In contrast, Mohokum et al. did not find any differences in accuracy between subgroups with respect to BMI in a collective of young, healthy volunteers. Therefore, we did not assume any coherence of our results in relation to BMI. The differences in body weight or BMI were not caused by gender effect. 11 women and 28/25 men were examined in both groups. One reason of an increased body weight in patients could be that the patients were not so sporty and agile compared to the healthy subjects due to their pain.

The force of gravity affects bone positions and trunk muscle activities. In the supine or standing position, these parameters are different. In patients with low back pain, the onset of symptoms typically decreases in the supine position and increases in the standing position. Therefore, an RS investigation is more functional than MRI or CT, which is often performed in the horizontal position. Some researchers have investigated LS by radiography [35, 41]. One limitation of the present study is that there was no reference standard used for detecting LS, for instance, radiography.

RS can be applied to monitor postural changes, but caution should be taken when comparing absolute values because RS uses reference contours only. Radiological methods can derive the position of the spinous process directly from the morphology of internal bone structures.

Further research on this topic needs to be done. An investigation should be performed into other spine pathologies to find a specific pattern and to define demarcations between different pathologies.

5. Conclusions

The rasterstereography can identify changes of the posture of the spine in all three dimensions. This is the first study which illustrated the lateral shift using RS. Patients with disc herniation and low back pain show no increase in LS compared to healthy controls. Maybe, a lateral shift is more common in healthy patients as supposed. Alternatively, patients with disc herniation demonstrate other distinctive, significant parameters: an increased pelvic tilt, a decreased anterior pelvic inclination, a lower lordotic angle, and a higher amplitude of trunk torsion. In a further study, patients should be grouped, for example, based on their pathology like radiculopathy and discogenic pain to evaluate differences in posture.

Acknowledgments

We thank the Montanus-Klinik Bad Schwalbach, Germany, that it was possible to examine patients in that clinic and for all support to recruit the patients. We are thankful for the reprint permission of Figure 2 [24].

References

[1] N. Patrick, E. Emanski, and M. A. Knaub, "Acute and chronic low back pain," *Medical Clinics of North America*, vol. 98, no. 4, pp. 777–789, 2014.

[2] J. Schumacher and E. Brähler, "The prevalence of pain in the German population: Results of population- based studies with the Giessen Subjective Complaints List (Giessener Beschwerdebogen GBB)," *Der Schmerz*, vol. 13, no. 6, pp. 375–384, 1999.

[3] C. O. Schmidt and T. Kohlmann, "What do we know about the symptoms of back pain? Epidemiological results on prevalence, incidence, progression and risk factors," *Zeitschrift für Orthopädie und ihre Grenzgebiete*, vol. 143, no. 3, pp. 292–298, 2005.

[4] C. O. Schmidt, H. Raspe, M. Pfingsten et al., "Back pain in the German adult population: Prevalence, severity, and sociodemographic correlates in a multiregional survey," *The Spine Journal*, vol. 32, no. 18, pp. 2005–2011, 2007.

[5] O. Airaksinen, J. I. Brox, C. Cedraschi et al., "Chapter 4: European guidelines for the management of chronic nonspecific low back pain," *European Spine Journal*, vol. 15, no. 2, pp. S192–S300, 2006.

[6] P. A. Anderson, P. C. McCormick, and P. D. Angevine, "Randomized controlled trials of the treatment of lumbar disk herniation: 1983-2007," *Journal of the American Academy of OrthopaedicSurgeons* , vol. 16, no. 10, pp. 566–573, 2008.

[7] M. Heliovaara, O. Impivaara, K. Sievers et al., "Lumbar disc syndrome in Finland," *Journal of Epidemiology and Community Health*, vol. 41, no. 3, pp. 251–258, 1987.

[8] G. Müller, "Problems of diagnostic assessment in low back patients," *Der Schmerz*, vol. 15, no. 6, pp. 435–441, 2001.

[9] M. N. Stienen, D. Cadosch, G. Hildebrandt, and O. P. Gautschi, "The lumbar disc herniation - Management, clinical aspects and current recommendations," *Praxis*, vol. 100, no. 24, pp. 1475–1485, 2011.

[10] R. W. Porter and C. G. Miller, "Back pain and trunk list," *The Spine Journal*, vol. 11, no. 6, pp. 596–600, 1986.

[11] R. A. McKenzie and S. May, *The Lumbar Spine. Mechanical Diagnosis and Therapy*, vol. 2, Spinal Publications New Zealand Limited, Wellington, New Zealand, Waikanae edition, 2003.

[12] M. G. C. Gillan, J. C. Ross, I. P. McLean, and R. W. Porter, "The natural history of trunk list, its associated disability and the influence of McKenzie management," *European Spine Journal*, vol. 7, no. 6, pp. 480–483, 1998.

[13] M. S. Donahue, D. L. Riddle, and M. S. Sullivan, "Intertester reliability of a modified version of McKenzie's lateral shift assessments obtained on patients with low back pain," *Physical Therapy in Sport*, vol. 76, no. 7, pp. 706–726, 1996.

[14] I. P. McLean, M. G. C. Gillan, J. C. Ross, R. M. Aspden, and R. W. Porter, "A comparison of methods for measuring trunk list: A simple plumbline is the best," *The Spine Journal*, vol. 21, no. 14, pp. 1667–1670, 1996.

[15] B. Drerup and E. Hierholzer, "Back shape measurement using video rasterstereography and three-dimensional reconstruction of spinal shape," *Clinical Biomechanics*, vol. 9, no. 1, pp. 28–36, 1994.

[16] L. Hackenberg, E. Hierholzer, W. Pötzl, C. Götze, and U. Liljenqvist, "Rasterstereographic back shape analysis in idiopathic scoliosis after posterior correction and fusion," *Clinical Biomechanics*, vol. 18, no. 10, pp. 883–889, 2003.

[17] L. Hackenberg, E. Hierholzer, W. Pötzl, C. Götze, and U. Liljenqvist, "Rasterstereographic back shape analysis in idiopathic scoliosis after anterior correction and fusion," *Clinical Biomechanics*, vol. 18, no. 1, pp. 1–8, 2003.

[18] M. Mohokum, S. Mendoza, W. Udo, H. Sitter, J. R. Paletta, and A. Skwara, "Reproducibility of rasterstereography for kyphotic and lordotic angles, trunk length, and trunk inclination: a reliability study," *Spine (Phila Pa 1976)*, vol. 35, no. 14, pp. 1353–1358, 2010.

[19] M. Mohokum, S. Schülein, and A. Skwara, "The validity of rasterstereography: A systematic review," *Orthopedic Reviews*, vol. 7, no. 3, pp. 68–73, 2015.

[20] R. J. Crawford, R. I. Price, and K. P. Singer, "The effect of interspinous implant surgery on back surface shape and radiographic lumbar curvature," *Clinical Biomechanics*, vol. 24, no. 6, pp. 467–472, 2009.

[21] S. Schülein, S. Mendoza, R. Malzkorn, J. Harms, and A. Skwara, "Rasterstereographic evaluation of interobserver and intraobserver reliability in postsurgical adolescent idiopathic scoliosis patients," *Journal of Spinal Disorders & Techniques*, vol. 26, no. 4, pp. E143–E149, 2013.

[22] A. Tabard-Fougère, A. Bonnefoy-Mazure, S. Hanquinet, P. Lascombes, S. Armand, and R. Dayer, "Validity and reliability of spine rasterstereography in patients with adolescent idiopathic scoliosis," *The Spine Journal*, vol. 42, no. 2, pp. 98–105, 2017.

[23] M. E. Khallaf, "Three dimensional analysis of spino-pelvic alignment in individuals with acutely herniated lumbar intervertebral disc," *Journal of Back and Musculoskeletal Rehabilitation*, vol. 30, no. 4, pp. 759–765, 2017.

[24] C. Lippold, T. Moiseenko, B. Drerup, M. Schilgen, A. Végh, and G. Danesh, "Spine deviations and orthodontic treatment of asymmetric malocclusions in children," *BMC Musculoskeletal Disorders*, vol. 13, 2012.

[25] G. A. Hawker, S. Mian, T. Kendzerska, and M. French, "Measures of adult pain: Visual Analog Scale for Pain (VAS Pain), Numeric Rating Scale for Pain (NRS Pain), McGill Pain Questionnaire (MPQ), Short-Form McGill Pain Questionnaire (SF-MPQ), Chronic Pain Grade Scale (CPGS), Short Form-36 Bodily Pain Scale (SF-36 BPS), and measure of Intermittent and Constant Osteoarthritis Pain (ICOAP)," *Arthritis Care & Research*, vol. 63, supplement 11, pp. S240–S252, 2011.

[26] T. Kohlmann and H. Raspe, "Hannover Functional Questionnaire in ambulatory diagnosis of functional disability caused by backache," *Rehabilitation (Stuttg)*, vol. 35, no. 1, pp. I–VIII, 1996.

[27] M. Gronblad, M. Hupli, P. Wennerstrand et al., "Intercorrelation and test-retest reliability of the Pain Disability Index (PDI) and the Oswestry Disability Questionnaire (ODQ) and their correlation with pain intensity in low back pain patients," *The Clinical Journal of Pain*, vol. 9, no. 3, pp. 189–195, 1993.

[28] T. Hall, A. Cacho, C. McNee, J. Riches, and J. Walsh, "Effects of the mulligan traction straight leg raise technique on range of movement," *Journal of Manual & Manipulative Therapy*, vol. 9, no. 3, pp. 128–133, 2001.

[29] B. Drerup, "Rasterstereographic measurement of scoliotic deformity," *Scoliosis*, vol. 9, no. 1, 2014.

[30] B. Drerup and E. Hierholzer, "Automatic localization of anatomical landmarks on the back surface and construction of a body-fixed coordinate system," *Journal of Biomechanics*, vol. 20, no. 10, pp. 961–970, 1987.

[31] B. Drerup and E. Hierholzer, "Objective determination of anatomical landmarks on the body surface: Measurement of

the vertebra prominens from surface curvature," *Journal of Biomechanics*, vol. 18, no. 6, pp. 467–474, 1985.

[32] B. Degenhardt, Z. Starks, S. Bhatia, and G.-A. Franklin, "Appraisal of the DIERS method for calculating postural measurements: An observational study," *Scoliosis and Spinal Disorders*, vol. 12, no. 1, 2017.

[33] S. Negrini, S. Donzelli, A. G. Aulisa et al., "2016 SOSORT guidelines: Orthopaedic and rehabilitation treatment of idiopathic scoliosis during growth," *Scoliosis and Spinal Disorders*, vol. 13, no. 1, 2018.

[34] D. E. Harrison, R. Cailliet, D. D. Harrison, T. J. Janik, S. J. Troyanovich, and R. R. Coleman, "Lumbar coupling during lateral translations of the thoracic cage relative to a fixed pelvis," *Clinical Biomechanics*, vol. 14, no. 10, pp. 704–709, 1999.

[35] D. E. Harrison, R. Cailliet, J. W. Betz et al., "A non-randomized clinical control trial of Harrison mirror image methods for correcting trunk list (lateral translations of the thoracic cage) in patients with chronic low back pain," *European Spine Journal*, vol. 14, no. 2, pp. 155–162, 2005.

[36] T. W. Stadnik, R. R. Lee, H. L. Coen, E. C. Neirynck, T. S. Buisseret, and M. J. C. Osteaux, "Annular tears and disk herniation: prevalence and contrast enhancement on MR images in the absence of low back pain or sciatica," *Radiology*, vol. 206, no. 1, pp. 49–55, 1998.

[37] C. W. Ernst, T. W. Stadnik, E. Peeters, C. Breucq, and M. J. C. Osteaux, "Prevalence of annular tears and disc herniations on MR images of the cervical spine in symptom free volunteers," *European Journal of Radiology*, vol. 55, no. 3, pp. 409–414, 2005.

[38] H. Razmjou, J. F. Kramer, and R. Yamada, "Intertester reliability of the McKenzie evaluation in assessing patients with mechanical low-back pain," *Journal of Orthopaedic & Sports Physical Therapy*, vol. 30, no. 7, pp. 368–389, 2000.

[39] J. M. Fritz and S. George, "The use of a classification approach to identify subgroups of patients with acute low back pain: Interrater reliability and short-term treatment outcomes," *The Spine Journal*, vol. 25, no. 1, pp. 106–114, 2000.

[40] U. Liljenqvist, H. Halm, E. Hierholzer, B. Drerup, and M. Weiland, "Three-dimensional surface measurement of spinal deformities using video rasterstereography," *Zeitschrift für Orthopädie und ihre Grenzgebiete*, vol. 136, no. 1, pp. 57–64, 1998.

[41] G. A. Arangio, S. M. Hartzell, and J. F. Reed, "Significance of lumbosacral list and low-back pain: A controlled radiographic study," *The Spine Journal*, vol. 15, no. 3, pp. 208–210, 1990.

27

Stability of the Subaxial Spine after Penetrating Trauma: Do Classification Systems Apply?

Jackson Rucker Staggers, Thomas Elliot Niemeier, William E. Neway III, and Steven Michael Theiss

Division of Orthopaedic Surgery, University of Alabama at Birmingham, Birmingham, Alabama, 35205, USA

Correspondence should be addressed to Jackson Rucker Staggers; rucker@uab.edu

Academic Editor: Hiroshi Hashizume

Objective. Blunt spinal trauma classification systems are well established and provide reliable treatment algorithms. To date, stability of the spine after civilian gunshot wounds (CGSWS) is poorly understood. Herein, we investigate the validity of trauma classification systems including the Thoracolumbar Injury Classification and Severity Score (TLICS), Subaxial Cervical Spine Injury Classification and Severity Score (SLIC), and Denis' three-column model when applied to spinal penetrating trauma from gunshots, while secondarily evaluating stability of these injuries. *Methods.* Gunshot injuries to the spine were identified from an institutional database from ICD-nine codes. Trauma scorings systems were applied using traditional criteria. Neurologic compromise and spinal stability were evaluated using follow-up clinic notes and radiographs. *Results.* Thirty-one patients with CSGSW were evaluated. There was an equal distribution of injuries amongst the spinal levels and spinal columns. Twenty patients had neurological deficits at presentation. Eight patient had a TLICS score >4. Three patients had a SLIC score >4. One patient had surgical treatment. Nonoperative treatment did not lead to spinal instability or adverse outcomes in any cases. The posterior column had a high correlation with neurologic compromise, though not statistically significant (p=.118). *Conclusions.* The TLICS, SLIC, and three-column classification systems cannot be applied to CSGSW to quantify injury severity, predict outcomes, or guide treatment decision-making. Despite significant neurologic injuries and disruption of multiple spinal columns, CSGSW do not appear to result in unstable injuries requiring operative intervention. Further research is needed to identify the rare spinal gunshot injury that would benefit from immediate surgical intervention.

1. Introduction

Civilian spinal gunshot wounds (CSGSW) are an increasingly common injury and carry significant morbidity and mortality [1–4]. Annually, CSGWS are the third most common cause of spinal injury and account for approximately 13-17% of all traumatic spinal injuries [1, 2, 5–9]. Despite the severity and frequency of CSGSW, there is little agreement on the universal classification and management of these injuries since surgeons continue to treat patients based on institutional, geographical, and surgeon preference [10–12]. As a result, numerous classification systems and stability concepts have been applied to these injuries in an attempt to improve care and optimize outcomes.

Three of the more popular spinal classification systems are the Thoracolumbar Injury Classification and Severity Score (TLICS), Subaxial Cervical Spine Injury Classification and Severity Score (SLIC), and Denis' three-column model. TLICS was introduced in 2005 and is a point-based system that utilizes the morphology of the injury, integrity of the posterior ligamentous complex (PLC) and neurologic status to evaluate an injury [10]. SLIC is another point-based system that was introduced in 2007 and is based on injury morphology, integrity of the disco-ligamentous complex, and neurologic status [13–15]. Both TLICS and SLIC give an injury score that correlates with injury severity, allowing the provider to quantify injury severity and guide treatment [13–15]. Denis' three-column model was introduced in 1983 and is based on radiographic findings [16, 17]. It divides the spine into three anatomic columns and defines instability as disruption of 2 or more columns [16, 17]. Although the three-column system provides an intuitive nomenclature for describing spinal injuries, it does not provide prognostic information or guide clinical decision-making [10].

These systems have been validated in many studies as reliable and reproducible for blunt force trauma; however, to date their use in penetrating trauma has not been validated [4, 10, 13–15]. Currently there are no spinal classification systems that were designed for penetrating trauma, and data in the literature is limited. This study seeks to assess the utility and legitimacy of the TLICS, SLIC, and three-column classification systems to quantify injury severity, predict outcomes, and guide treatment decision-making for CSGWS, while secondarily evaluating stability of these injuries.

2. Materials and Methods

After institutional review board (IRB) approval was obtained, we conducted a retrospective cohort review of patients who sustained low-velocity gunshot injuries to the spine from 2003-2016 using ICD-nine codes. Patients were treated by orthopedic and neurologic surgeons from a single level-one trauma center. All treatments were non-randomized and were at the discretions of the treating surgeon. Inclusion criteria included gunshot injuries that involved any aspect of the cervical, thoracic, lumbar, or sacral spine. Single and multiple gunshot injuries were included. Patients with non-spinal gunshot injuries were included as long as the injuries did not affect management of their spinal injuries. Patients who were unable to provide neurological exam due to clinical condition or with less than one month of follow up were excluded from the study. Also, patients without computed tomography (CT) imaging on the date of injury or radiographic or CT imaging at final follow up were excluded.

Standard patient demographic information was reviewed, including: age, date of injury, fracture morphology, fracture level, treatment, neurologic status, and final follow up data. Neurologic status was assessed using the American Spine Injury Association (ASIA) classification [18]. In some instances, a single ballistic injury resulted in multiple spinal level injuries due to an oblique sagittal tract. For these patients and for those with multiple spinal gunshot injuries, all spinal levels and columns involved were counted, but only the most severe injury was used for neurological and classification analysis. Initial CT evaluation was performed to assess fracture morphology, injury level, and coronal and sagittal alignment. The three-column system of spine stability was applied as classically described by Denis [16]. The Subaxial Cervical Spine Injury Classification and Severity Score (SLIC) and Thoracolumbar Injury Classification and Severity Score (TLICS) were calculated based off original papers by Vaccaro [10, 13]. In order to classify complex fracture patterns according to the pre-defined morphologic patterns of SLIC and TLICS systems, fractures that only affected the anterior column of the vertebral body were described as compression fractures and were assigned one point. Fractures that involved the anterior and middle columns were described as burst fractures and assigned two points. Injuries that involved the vertebral body and the posterior elements were assigned four points. Isolated posterior column injuries were given a morphologic score of zero. Patients with intact posterior elements were given no points whereas injuries that caused complete destruction of the posterior elements were classified as having a suspected PLC injury and given two points. On final follow-up, radiographs were evaluated for sagittal, coronal, and axial spinal alignment and final neurologic status was recorded.

Table 1: Demographic and injury data.

	Mean	SD
Age (yrs)	34.0	14.8
	Number	**% of Patients**
Sex		
Male	27	87.1
Female	4	12.9
Spinal Levels Involved		
Cervical	8	25.8
Thoracic	14	45.2
Lumbar	13	41.9
Sacral	1	3.2
Neurologic Grade		
ASIA A	9	28.0
ASIA B	2	6.0
ASIA C	3	9.0
ASIA D	6	19
ASIA E	11	34.0
Treatment		
Surgery	1	3.2
Nonoperative	30	96.8
Stability		
Stable	31	100.0
Unstable	0	0.0

Demographic information was evaluated using descriptive statistical analysis. Further statistical analysis was done using chi-squared tests. A $p < 0.05$ was considered statistically significant.

3. Results

Thirty-one patients (27 males, 4 females) with 33 spinal gunshot injuries met the inclusion criteria for the study. Mean age was 34.0+/- 14.8 years (range 17-63 years) with an average follow up of 2.0 +/- 2.6 years (range 1-99 months). Demographic, fracture, and neurologic information is shown in Table 1. ASIA neurological status was recorded in all patients with 20 of the 31 patients (64.5%) having neurologic deficits (ASIA A-D) and 11 patients without any neurologic deficits (ASIA E) immediately after presentation. Complete spinal cord injury (ASIA A) was the most commonly encountered deficit (9 patients). There was a nearly equal representation of CSGSW among cervical, thoracic, and lumbar regions, but

Table 2: TLICS Score.

	Thoracic Spine	Lumbar Spine	Total
TLICS Score 0-3	4	7	11
TLICS Score 4	3	1	4
TLICS Score >4	4	4	8

Table 3: SLIC Scores.

	Cervical Spine
SLIC Score 0-3	5
SLIC Score 4	0
SLIC Score >4	3

Table 4: Denis Classification.

	Number	%
Number of Columns Involved		
1 Column	12	38.7
2 Columns	9	29.0
3 Columns	10	32.2
Column Injuries		
Anterior	20	52.6
Middle	18	47.4
Posterior	20	52.6
Columns Involved		
Anterior only	3	7.9
Middle only	0	0.0
Posterior only	9	23.7
Anterior/Middle	11	28.9
Posterior/Middle	1	2.6
Anterior/Middle/Posterior	10	26.3

only one injury that involved the sacral spine. Twenty-one patients (67.7%) had injuries involving multiple vertebrae. Two patients (6.5%) had isolated intervertebral disk involvement. All but one patient were treated nonoperatively.

On follow up, no patients displayed significant change in spinal alignment or neurologic status. One patient with concomitant bowel injury developed spondylodiscitis and a progressive lumbar kyphosis secondary to near complete vertebral body collapse. This patient's CGSW injury was isolated to the posterior elements and their deformity was deemed unrelated to instability secondary to the initial trauma.

3.1. Thoracolumbar Injury Classification and Severity Score (TLICS). TLICS scores for each patient with thoracolumbar involvement are summarized in Table 2. Eleven patients of the 23 patients with thoracolumbar injuries (47.8%) had a TLICS score of 0-3 suggesting conservative therapy. Four patients (17.4%) scored a 4 suggesting that surgery is up to the surgeon's discretion. Eight patients (34.8%) had a TLICS score of greater than 4 suggesting surgical stabilization is appropriate. Despite the high number of patients for whom surgery is indicated according to TLICS, none had surgery.

3.2. The Subaxial Cervical Spine Injury Classification and Severity Score (SLIC). SLIC scores for each patient with cervical spine involvement are summarized in Table 3. Five of the 8 patients with cervical injuries (62.5%) had a SLIC score of 0-3, suggesting conservative therapy. Three patients (37.5%) scored greater than 4, suggesting surgical stabilization is appropriate. Only 1 patient (12.5%) with a SLIC score of 5 had surgical stabilization.

3.3. Denis' Three-Column Model. Table 4 summarizes the number of injuries per column as it pertains to Denis' three-column model. There was a near equal distribution of one-column (12), two-column (9), and three-column (10) injuries, as well as a near equal involvement of anterior (20), middle (18), and posterior columns (20). The association between column involvement and neurologic injury is described in Figures 1 and 2. One and two-column injuries involving the anterior and middle columns had a low correlation with neurological involvement. Though it was not statistically significant, there was a high correlation of the posterior column with neurologic involvement ($p = 0.118$). Of note, three-column injuries also had a high correlation with neurological involvement.

4. Discussion

Contemporary understanding of spinal injuries and their optimal management is continuously evolving. Classification systems have been used for decades for spinal trauma as a helpful resource, but there is little agreement on the universal classification across a broad spectrum of injuries. The TLICS, SLIC, and the three-column classifications have been validated in blunt trauma and provide useful information on the mechanical stability of the spine [4, 10, 13–15]. The current study investigated the utility of trauma classification systems in penetrating gunshot injuries, a topic that has yet to be discussed.

Ideally, a classification system should be able to provide prognostic information and help guide treatment. Application of TLICS and SLICS scores system were not able to predict injury severity or instability in our study. Eight patients (34.8%) with thoracolumbar injuries and 3 patients (37.5%) with cervical injuries had a TLICS or SLIC severity score that equated with recommendation for surgery. All but one of these patients were successfully managed conservatively with the one exception undergoing early surgical stabilization.

Fracture morphology was a major limiting factor for the general utility of TLICS and SLIC systems since penetrating

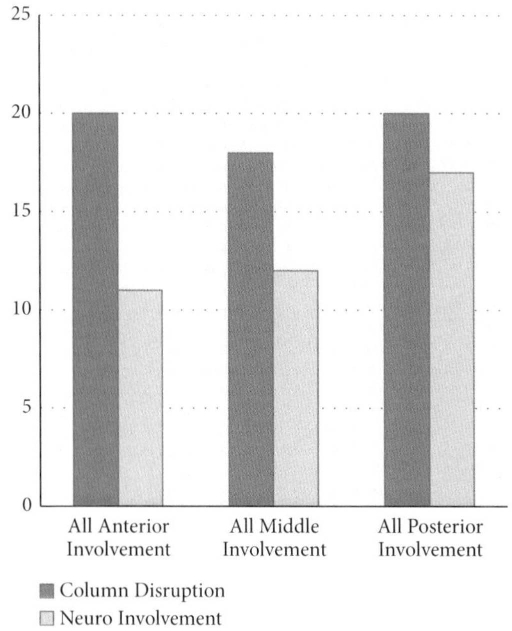

FIGURE 1: Correlation of neurologic injury and column disruption in Denis' three column stability system.

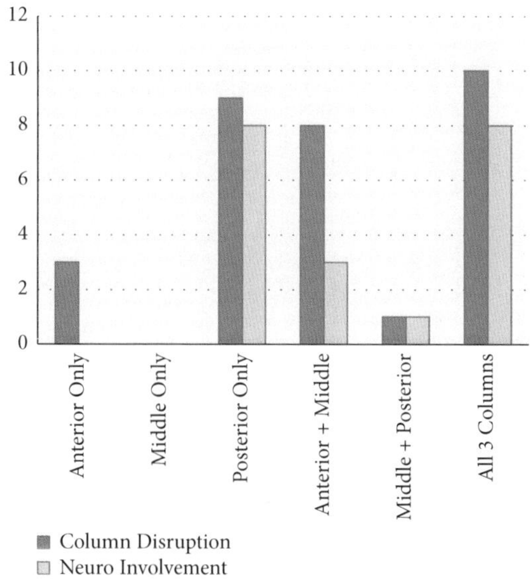

FIGURE 2: Correlation of neurologic injury and column disruption in Denis' three column stability system.

wounds do not usually result in classic fracture patterns. By definition, burst and compression fractures result in a loss of vertebral body height. In our cohort, nearly all of the CSGSW retained normal vertebral body alignment, intuitively making them more stable than their nomenclature suggested (Figure 3). This increased stability is thought to be the result of nearby supporting structures that are more likely to be maintained in penetrating trauma.

In TLICS and SLIC, neurologic status is used as a critical indicator of stability, but this may not have the same utility in CSGSW as it does in blunt force trauma. In our study, roughly

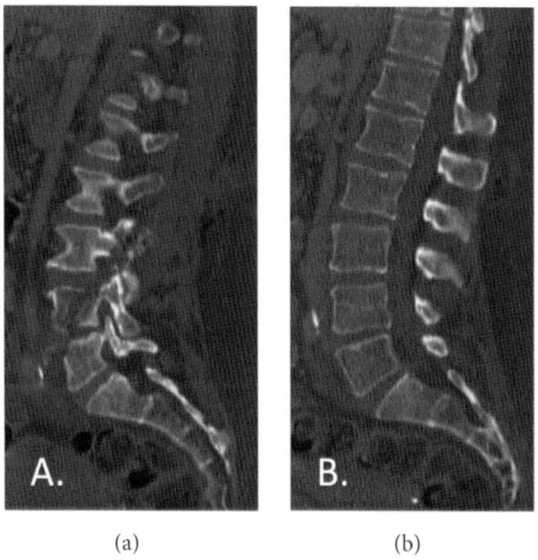

(a) (b)

FIGURE 3: (a) Parasagittal image demonstrating bullet tract involving multiple vertebral bodies and articulating facets joints. (b) Mid-sagittal image on the same patient seen in image 2A showing intact alignment despite CSGSW.

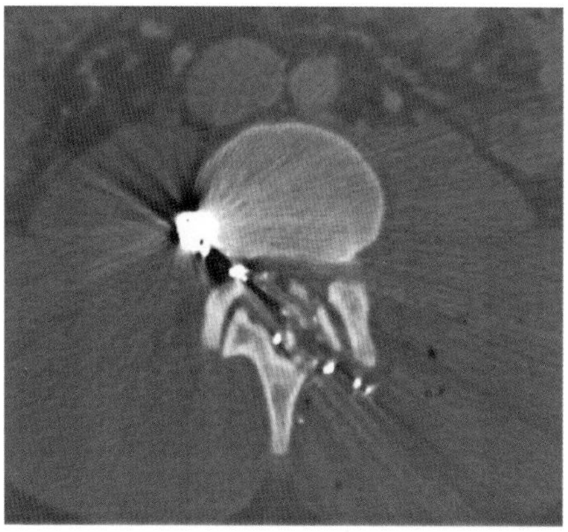

FIGURE 4: Bullet seen traversing spinal canal in a patient with complete neurologic injury (ASIA A).

two-thirds of patients had neurologic involvement without any patients showing spinal instability. This data is consistent with previous work by Bumpass et al. who showed a high rate of neurologic compromise despite low rates of biomechanical instability with CSGSW [19]. Prior studies suggest that in CSGSW, neural and spinal cord damage are generally due to direct impact, thermal energy, or blast effect (Figure 4) rather than compression or tension as seen in blunt force trauma [1, 20].

The Denis three-column spinal stability model provided no insight into instability or prognostic information for CSGSWS. Ten patients (32.2%) sustained three-column injuries as classified by Denis but all were successfully treated without surgical treatment. Though the posterior column had a high correlation with neurologic damage, this is believed to be related to classification system's basis on anatomy and the location of the spinal cord.

Our data is consistent with past studies supporting the inherit stability of the spine after CSGSW [2, 19, 21–23]. The authors of the current study find no value in classifying penetrating injuries with conventional spinal classification systems as they provide no appreciated information on mechanical stability. As previous studies have shown surgery frequently correlates with an increase in complications without improvement in outcome [19], the role of surgery should be limited to the rare patient with overt mechanical instability.

Our study is not without limitation, including its retrospective study design with a limited number of patients. Additionally, by design our study evaluates three spine trauma classification systems that were specifically designed for blunt force trauma in the setting of penetrating trauma. Though this provides little novel information, our study closes the literature gap on this topic and confirms current practices relating to penetrating trauma of the spine. A small number of patients were lost to follow-up and neurological exam required data extraction from numerous outpatient charts that were at times incomplete. Additionally, bullet fragments on CT scan serve a potential source of error as they proved to be a challenge in assess fracture morphology secondary to artifact.

5. Conclusion

We conclude that the TLICS, SLIC, and three-column classification systems cannot be applied to CSGSW to quantify injury severity, predict outcomes, or guide treatment decision-making. Despite significant neurologic injuries and disruption of multiple spinal columns, CSGSW do not appear to result in unstable injuries requiring immediate surgical stabilization. TLICS and SLIC grossly over-indicate surgery for many patients that actually did well when treated conservatively. Our data suggests that refraining from operative treatment does not result in worse outcomes; therefore, we propose that CSGSW warrant a trial of nonoperative management after injury. Further research is suggested to find the rare injury that would benefit from immediate surgical stabilization or debridement.

Disclosure

This research was presented at the Global Spine Congress 2015 in Buenos Aires, Argentina (podium presentation). Level of evidence is retrospective review, level 4.

References

[1] A. Jakoi, J. Iorio, R. Howell, and J. M. Zampini, "Gunshot injuries of the spine," *The Spine Journal*, vol. 15, no. 9, pp. 2077–2085, 2015.

[2] J. C. Farmer, A. R. Vaccaro, R. A. Balderston, T. J. Albert, and J. Cotler, "The changing nature of admissions to a spinal cord injury center: Violence on the rise," *Journal of Spinal Disorders & Techniques*, vol. 11, no. 5, pp. 400–403, 1998.

[3] C. S. Bartlett, "Clinical update: gunshot wound ballistics," *Clinical Orthopaedics and Related Research*, vol. 408, pp. 28–57, 2003.

[4] G. S. Sidhu, A. Ghag, V. Prokuski, A. R. Vaccaro, and K. E. Radcliff, "Civilian gunshot injuries of the spinal cord: a systematic review of the current literature," *Clinical Orthopaedics and Related Research*, vol. 471, no. 12, pp. 3945–3955, 2013.

[5] D. Gentleman and M. Harrington, "Penetrating injury of the spinal cord," *Injury*, vol. 16, no. 1, pp. 7-8, 1984.

[6] B. Aarabi, E. Alibaii, M. Taghipur, and A. Kamgarpur, "Comparative study of functional recovery for surgically explored and conservatively managed spinal cord missile injuries," *Neurosurgery*, vol. 39, no. 6, pp. 1133–1140, 1996.

[7] P. Chittiboina, A. D. Banerjee, S. Zhang, G. Caldito, A. Nanda, and B. K. Willis, "How bullet trajectory affects outcomes of civilian gunshot injury to the spine," *Journal of Clinical Neuroscience*, vol. 18, no. 12, pp. 1630–1633, 2011.

[8] S. S. Lin, A. R. Vaccaro, S. Reisch, M. Devine, and J. M. Cotler, "Low-velocity gunshot wounds to the spine with an associated transperitoneal injury," *Journal of Spinal Disorders & Techniques*, vol. 8, no. 2, pp. 136–144, 1995.

[9] D. P. Robertson and R. K. Simpson, "Penetrating injuries restricted to the cauda equina: a retrospective review," *Neurosurgery*, vol. 31, no. 2, pp. 265–270, 1992.

[10] A. A. Patel and A. R. Vaccaro, "Thoracolumbar spine trauma classification," *Journal of the American Academy of Orthopaedic Surgeons*, vol. 18, no. 2, pp. 63–71, 2010.

[11] N. Beaty, J. Slavin, C. Diaz, K. Zeleznick, D. Ibrahimi, and C. A. Sansur, "Cervical spine injury from gunshot wounds," *Journal of Neurosurgery: Spine*, vol. 21, no. 3, pp. 442–449, 2014.

[12] A. R. Vaccaro, C. Oner, C. K. Kepler et al., "AOSpine thoracolumbar spine injury classification system: fracture description, neurological status, and key modifiers," *The Spine Journal*, vol. 38, no. 23, pp. 2028–2037, 2013.

[13] A. R. Vaccaro, R. J. Hulbert, A. A. Patel et al., "The subaxial cervical spine injury classification system," *The Spine Journal*, vol. 32, no. 21, pp. 2365–2374, 2007.

[14] A. A. Patel, A. Dailey, D. S. Brodke et al., "Subaxial cervical spine trauma classification: The Subaxial injury classification system and case examples," *Neurosurgical Focus*, vol. 25, no. 5, article no. E8, 2008.

[15] A. A. Patel, R. J. Hurlbert, C. M. Bono, J. T. Bessey, N. Yang, and A. R. Vaccaro, "Classification and surgical decision making in acute subaxial cervical spine trauma," *The Spine Journal*, vol. 35, no. 21, pp. S228–S234, 2010.

[16] A. D. L. Baker, "The three column spine and its significance in the classification of acute thoracolumbar spinal injuries," *Class Pap Orthop*, vol. 8, pp. 289–292, 2014.

[17] F. Denis, "Spinal instability as defined by the three-column spine concept in acute spinal trauma," *Clinical Orthopaedics and Related Research*, no. 189, pp. 65–76, 1984.

[18] S. C. Kirshblum, S. P. Burns, F. Biering-Sorensen et al., "International standards for neurological classification of spinal cord injury (revised 2011)," *The Journal of Spinal Cord Medicine*, vol. 34, no. 6, pp. 535–546, 2011.

[19] D. B. Bumpass, J. M. Buchowski, A. Park et al., "An update on civilian spinal gunshot wounds," *The Spine Journal*, vol. 40, no. 7, pp. 450–461, 2015.

[20] J. D. Apfelbaum, S. V. Cantrill, and N. Waldman, "Unstable cervical spine without spinal cord injury in penetrating neck trauma," *The American Journal of Emergency Medicine*, vol. 18, no. 1, pp. 55–57, 2000.

[21] C. M. Bono and R. F. Heary, "Gunshot wounds to the spine," *The Spine Journal*, vol. 4, no. 2, pp. 230–240, 2004.

[22] T. Lustenberger, P. Talving, L. Lam et al., "Unstable cervical spine fracture after penetrating neck injury: A rare entity in an analysis of 1,069 patients," *Journal of Trauma - Injury Infection and Critical Care*, vol. 70, no. 4, pp. 870–872, 2011.

[23] J. C. Le Roux and R. N. Dunn, "Gunshot injuries of the spine - a review of 49 cases managed at the Groote Schuur Acute Spinal Cord Injury Unit," *South African Journal of Surgery*, vol. 43, no. 4, pp. 165–168, 2005.

28

3D Printing Aids Acetabular Reconstruction in Complex Revision Hip Arthroplasty

Andrew J. Hughes,[1] Cathal DeBuitleir,[1] Philip Soden,[1] Brian O'Donnchadha,[2] Anthony Tansey,[2] Ali Abdulkarim,[3] Colm McMahon,[4] and Conor J. Hurson[1,3]

[1] *Department of Orthopaedic Surgery, St. Vincent's University Hospital, Dublin 4, Ireland*
[2] *Department of Mechanical Engineering, Institute of Technology Tallaght, Dublin 24, Ireland*
[3] *Department of Orthopaedic Surgery, Cappagh National Orthopaedic Hospital, Dublin 11, Ireland*
[4] *Department of Radiology, St. Vincent's University Hospital, Dublin 4, Ireland*

Correspondence should be addressed to Andrew J. Hughes; hughesajk@gmail.com

Academic Editor: Allen L. Carl

Revision hip arthroplasty requires comprehensive appreciation of abnormal bony anatomy. Advances in radiology and manufacturing technology have made three-dimensional (3D) representation of osseous anatomy obtainable, which provide visual and tactile feedback. Such life-size 3D models were manufactured from computed tomography scans of three hip joints in two patients. The first patient had undergone multiple previous hip arthroplasties for bilateral hip infections, resulting in right-sided pelvic discontinuity and a severe left-sided posterosuperior acetabular deficiency. The second patient had a first-stage revision for infection and recurrent dislocations. Specific metal reduction protocols were used to reduce artefact. The images were imported into Materialise MIMICS 14.12®. The models were manufactured using selective laser sintering. Accurate templating was performed preoperatively. Acetabular cup, augment, buttress, and cage sizes were trialled using the models, before being adjusted, and resterilised, enhancing the preoperative decision-making process. Screw trajectory simulation was carried out, reducing the risk of neurovascular injury. With 3D printing technology, complex pelvic deformities were better evaluated and treated with improved precision. Life-size models allowed accurate surgical simulation, thus improving anatomical appreciation and preoperative planning. The accuracy and cost-effectiveness of the technique should prove invaluable as a tool to aid clinical practice.

1. Introduction

Total hip arthroplasty (THA) is one of the most successful and cost-effective interventions in medicine today, providing reliable pain relief and functional improvement to those with osteoarthritis or inflammatory arthritis of the hip [1, 2]. 90–95% of total hip replacement (THR) prostheses survive for at least 10 years, and there is an increasing demand within our population for such an intervention due to rising life expectancy among the ageing cohort with degenerative joint disease [3, 4]. Revision hip arthroplasty is indicated when a primary THR fails due to a variety of reasons, such as aseptic loosening (50%), instability (16%), infection (15%), debilitating pain, periprosthetic fractures, or component failure [5]. This complicated articular reconstructive procedure requires a comprehensive understanding of the abnormal bony anatomy. Surgeons must be able to appreciate areas of bony insufficiency, deficiency, and discontinuity, in order to conceptualise complex corrective reconstructions.

Conventional diagnostic imaging techniques provide only two-dimensional (2D) images of these deformities [6]. Orthopaedic surgeons develop experience in interpreting such 2D images when devising their operative strategies. More recently, advances in radiology combined with advances in computer and manufacturing technology have made the three-dimensional (3D) representation of anatomic structures relatively easily obtainable [7, 8]. Such images can be rotated and viewed from various angles, improving

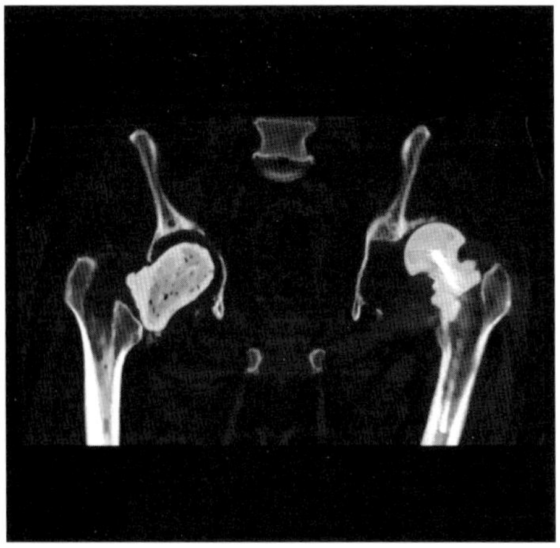

Figure 1: CT scan showing bilateral first-stage revision THR prostheses with right-sided pelvic discontinuity and a severe left-sided posterosuperior acetabular deficiency.

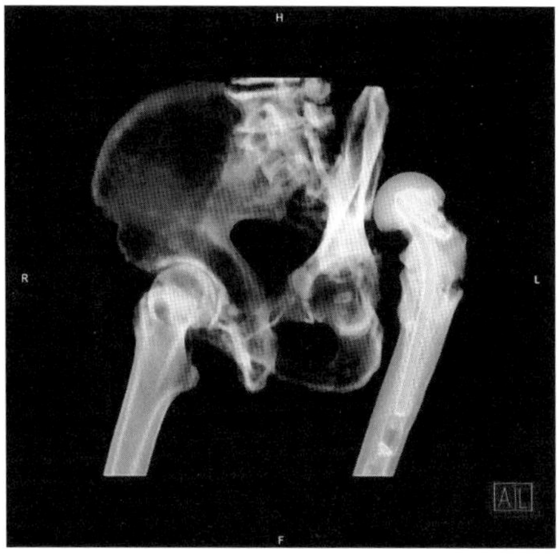

Figure 2: 3D CT reconstruction showing a dislocated left-sided THR secondary to a posterior acetabular wall deficiency.

anatomical appreciation, but they must still be viewed on a flat 2D computer screen. With the use of modern rapid prototyping techniques, 3D models of actual osseous anatomy can be manufactured from these 3D reconstructed images [9, 10].

Rapid prototyping, or 3D printing, is a term used to describe a group of techniques used to quickly fabricate a scale model of a physical part or assembly using three-dimensional computer aided design (CAD) data. The origins of this technique can be traced back to the 1960s when Professor Herbert Voelcker described theories and algorithms for 3D model fabrication. Carl Deckard developed a technique to bind metal powders to create a 3D model in the University of Texas in 1987, before Charles Hull patented the first 3D printer in 1988 in California [8, 11]. Rapid prototyping has been used in the medical industry since the early 2000s, initially in the production of dental implants and patient-specific prostheses [12]. Since then, the use of 3D printing in the field of medicine and surgery has been rapidly expanding to include the development of soft tissue, organs, blood vessels, implants, and anatomical models [13]. Also within orthopaedic surgery, 3D printed models have been shown to improve the preoperative understanding of complicated structures in neurosurgery, liver transplant surgery, and vascular aortic surgery [11, 12, 14].

Revision hip arthroplasty is one of the most complex orthopaedic disciplines. Each case provides the surgeon with a challenge specific to the patient's unique anatomy. Often, 3D images are studied closely, but, as mentioned above, appreciation of the abnormality in question may not always be obtained on a 2D screen. The individual variances of the human body make the use of 3D printed models a valuable asset to surgeons when preparing for a complex procedure [14]. A 3D printed model provides visual and tactile reproduction of the deficient pelvic bony anatomy. This enables an improved understanding of the anatomy prior to surgery and facilitates enhanced preoperative planning [15].

2. Methods and Results

Life-size 3D models were manufactured from the computed tomography (CT) scans of two patients with complex acetabular defects waiting for second-stage THRs.

2.1. Case 1. The first patient had a background of multiple bilateral hip arthroplasties for what was thought to have been aseptic loosening. Surgical intervention to date, however, had resulted in minimal symptomatic relief. Bilateral hip aspirations grew *Staphylococcus epidermidis* on enriched cultures. Bilateral first-stage hip revisions were subsequently performed, with bilateral antibiotic-coated spacers inserted. The postoperative CT scan of the pelvis showed right-sided pelvic discontinuity and a severe left-sided posterosuperior acetabular deficiency (see Figure 1). A six-week course of intravenous vancomycin and rifampicin was completed, as per the recommendation of the hospital's microbiology department.

2.2. Case 2. The second patient had undergone a first-stage hip revision, after preoperative aspiration confirmed an indolent *Staphylococcus epidermidis* periprosthetic joint infection, which had provoked multiple THR dislocations. Similar to the above, an antibiotic-coated spacer was inserted. A left-sided posterior acetabular wall deficiency was noted on the postoperative CT pelvis that was carried out (see Figure 2). Six weeks of intravenous daptomycin therapy was completed on consultation with the microbiology department. Both patients were listed for elective second-stage THRs as mentioned.

2.3. Rapid Prototyping. Specific metal reduction protocols were used to reduce artefact on the two mentioned CT scans, with the slice thickness set to 1 mm to improve the image quality. The CT scans obtained were converted to DIACOM images and were then imported into Materialise MIMICS 14.12, medical imaging processing software, in the Mechanical Engineering Department of the Institute of Technology Tallaght, in Dublin. Image thresholding was

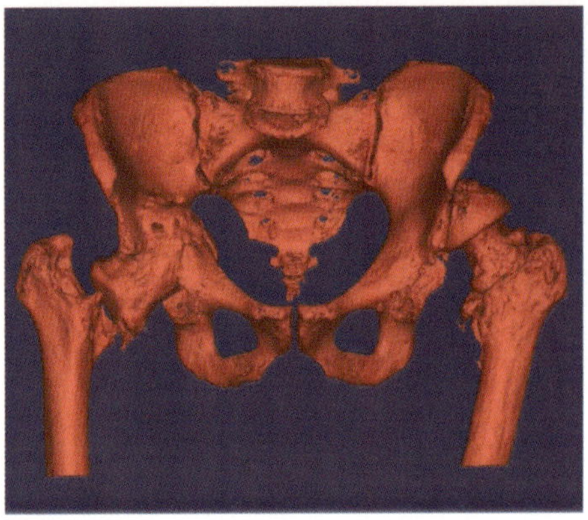

Figure 3: 3D pelvic image created from the CT scan using Materialise MIMICS 14.12.

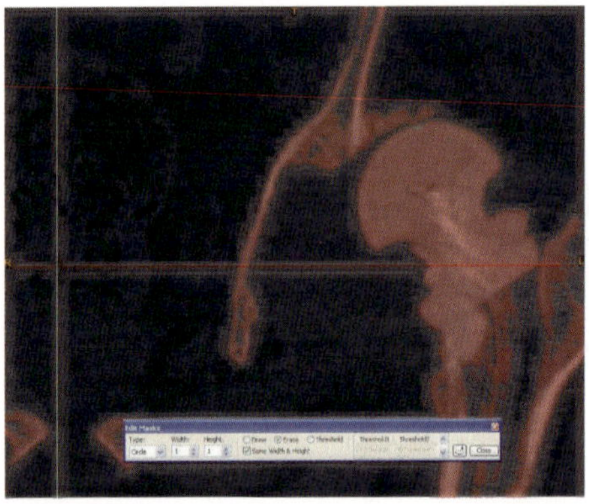

Figure 4: Segmenting the femur from the acetabulum using Materialise MIMICS 14.12.

performed, which allowed for bone to be differentiated from the surrounding soft tissue based on bone and soft tissue densities on the CT scan (see Figure 3). Using the region growing process, both femurs were digitally segmented from their corresponding pelvis by deleting the pixels that resulted in bony contact (see Figures 4, 5, and 6). The pelvis was isolated once both femurs were erased (see Figures 7 and 8). A 3D image of the isolated anatomy of interest was created on MIMICS. The imported file was saved in the .STL (stereolithographic) format which allows instructions related to the shape, thickness, and texture of the 3D image to be communicated to the 3D printer [8, 11]. The two models were manufactured using the rapid prototyping process, selective laser scintigraphy (SLS). SLS is one of many 3D printing methods, which builds the part in question via successive nylon powder layers as the substrate. The powder is selectively fused together in corresponding cross sections through the use of a programmed carbon dioxide laser beam. The use of fine nylon as the powder medium has been reported to enhance the accuracy of this technique. This allowed for two detailed models to be manufactured [16].

The first patient, with bilateral hip spacers in situ, required a full pelvic model to be constructed. The second patient needed only that of a hemipelvis. The larger pelvic model

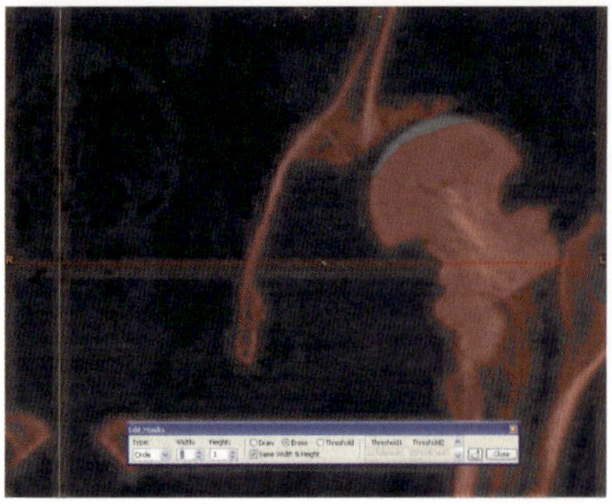

Figure 5: Segmenting the femur from the acetabulum using Materialise MIMICS 14.12.

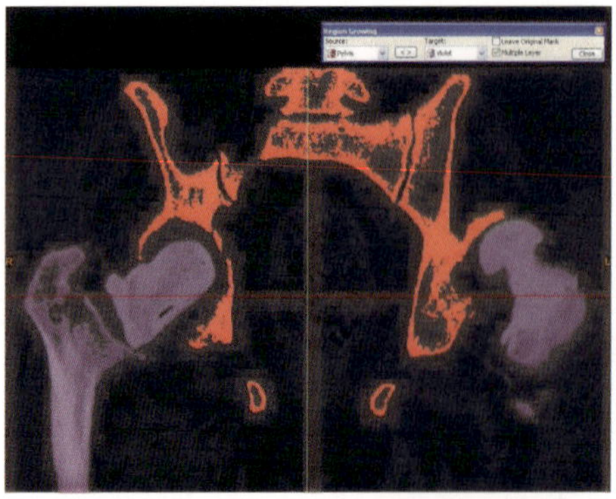

Figure 6: Thresholding of the pelvis and femoral bones.

contained minimal contact at a number of locations, in particular that of the pubic symphysis and both sacroiliac joints. Support bars were drawn across these articular surfaces, using MIMICS, so as to provide stabilisation and to prevent the model from collapsing once it was printed (see Figures 9 and 10).

2.4. 3D Models. The two 3D printed models provided the surgeon with visual and tactile appreciation of the three complex, irregular acetabula in question (see Figures 11 and 12). The two models cost $1450 ($400 and $1050) and were printed within twelve hours. Given the complexity of each case, these pelvic models allowed a life-size anatomical representation of the operative field to be closely examined. The operating surgeon described being able to identify and classify areas of bony deficiency. Following this, the team were able to plan and simulate a safe, successful surgical strategy. Templating was carried out by the surgeon in the weeks prior to surgery, and the implants were chosen accordingly. Acetabular cup, augment, and buttress sizes, as well as cage dimensions, were selected and trialled in advance. The malleable cage template was adjusted according to the contours of the model representing the patient's pelvic anatomy. This allowed prebending of the actual prosthesis prior to implantation before it was subsequently resterilised (see Figures 13, 14, and 15). The models were durable to

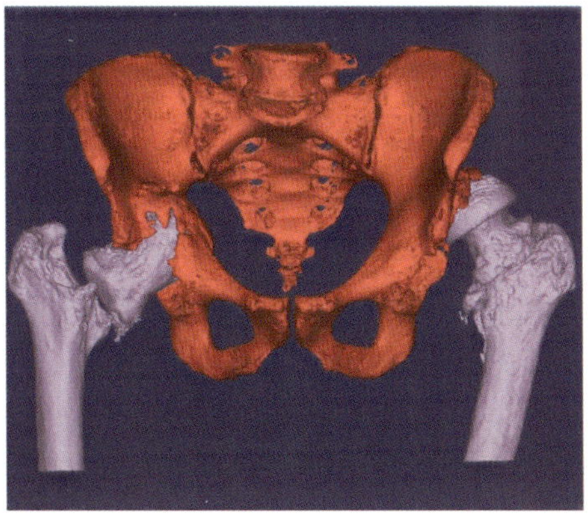

Figure 7: Thresholding and segmenting (deleting) the femoral bones from the pelvis.

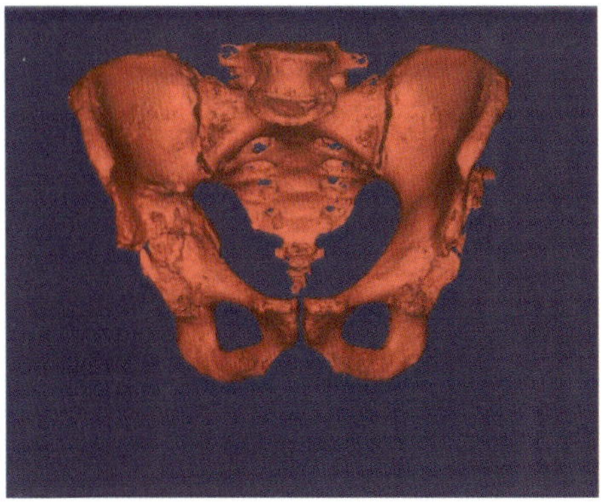

Figure 8: Thresholding and segmenting (deleting) the femoral bones from the pelvis.

a degree that allowed preoperative surgical simulation of drill trajectory and screw positioning in cortical bone.

The use of preoperative templating using these 3D models reduced operative time and blood loss and improved intraoperative surgical decision-making. Screw trajectory simulation was carried out on the models, allowing for improved accuracy and thus reducing the chance of intraoperative neurovascular injury. Screw position simulation allowed for the best use of available bone stock and helped ensure the best construct stability. Both patients underwent second-stage hip revision in Cappagh National Orthopaedic Hospital on an elective basis (see Figures 16 and 17). The outcome in both cases was satisfactory, with rehabilitation completed in a designated unit on discharge. Antibiotic therapy postoperatively was continued and completed as per the continued input of the microbiology department. Both patients are mobilising more than three years postoperatively with no signs of infection or loosening. The surgeon described overall satisfaction with the life-size pelvic models. Improved anatomical classification, preoperative surgical planning, and intraoperative accuracy resulted in a shorter, safer procedure with less perioperative morbidity and the efficient use of hospital resources.

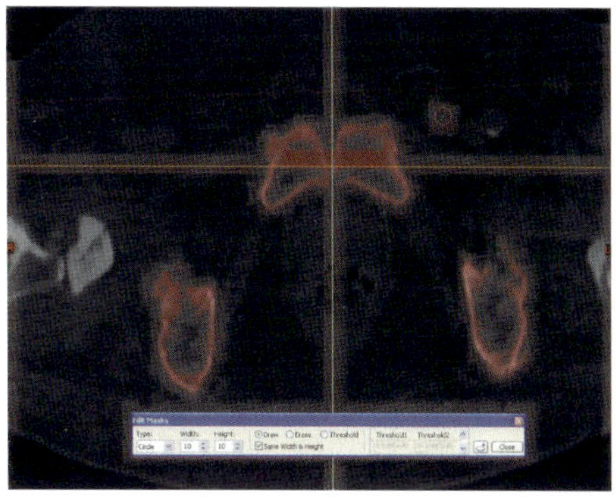

Figure 9: Support bars were drawn across the symphysis pubis and sacroiliac joints to avoid separation on printing the model.

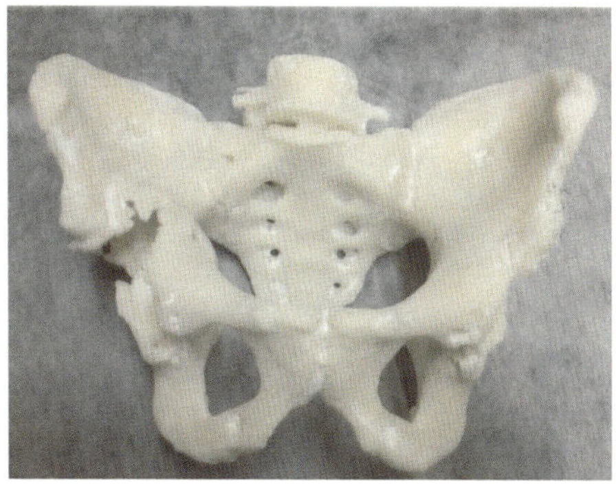

Figure 10: A life-size 3D printed model of the first patient's pelvis, providing the surgeon with visual and tactile appreciation of the defects in situ (note: these figures in print journal are two-dimensional, thus limiting the true demonstration of the value of 3D printed models in providing an accurate understanding and representation of the complex deformities and corrective reconstructive techniques).

3. Discussion

The complex anatomy of the pelvis and the acetabulum makes preoperative assessment of such abnormal bony deficiencies in revision hip arthroplasty notoriously difficult. With the use of 3D printing technology, pelvic deformities can be better evaluated by examining visual and tactile models of the patient's actual osseous anatomy. The internal structure is represented as a life-size 3D structure that can be held, rotated, and viewed by the operating team in advance of the procedure. As a result, complicated revision cases can be thoroughly evaluated and classified preoperatively, giving the surgeon an opportunity to treat the patient with improved surgical precision. Hurson et al. described the use of 3D models in assessing the acetabulum of 20 patients. In two of their cases, the initial surgical approach, having studied the patients' imaging, was altered based on further review of life-size anatomical 3D models [15].

The use of the models, combined with conventional imaging, has been shown to result in a greater understanding of abnormal bony anatomy, when compared to that of two- and three-dimensional imaging alone [11, 12]. 3D imaging

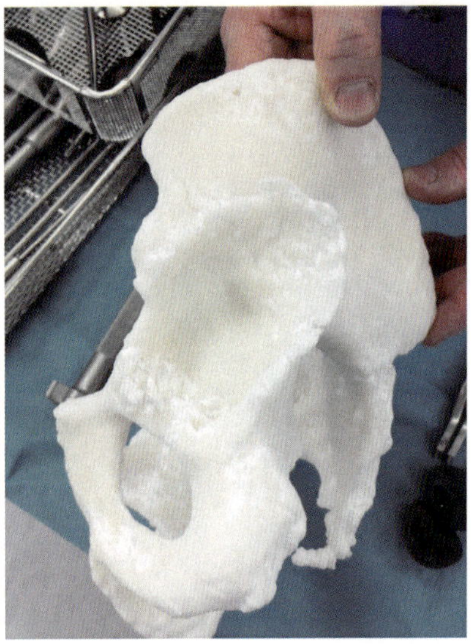

Figure 11: Examining the left acetabulum showing a posterosuperior deficiency. The right acetabulum shows significant central discontinuation due to bone loss (note: these figures in print journal are two-dimensional, thus limiting the true demonstration of the value of 3D printed models in providing an accurate understanding and representation of the complex deformities and corrective reconstructive techniques).

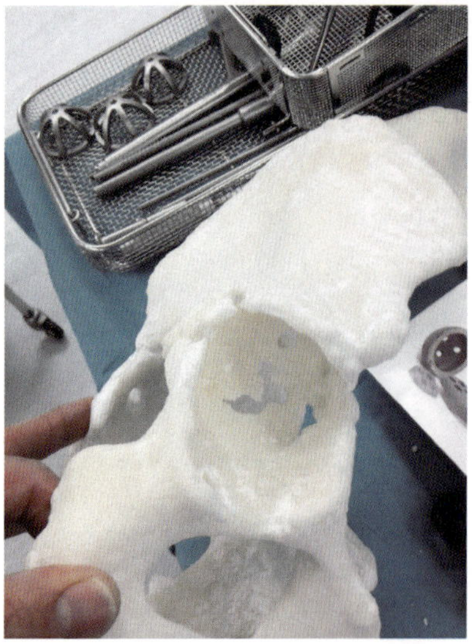

Figure 12: Examining the left acetabulum showing a posterosuperior deficiency. The right acetabulum shows significant central discontinuation due to bone loss (note: these figures in print journal are two-dimensional, thus limiting the true demonstration of the value of 3D printed models in providing an accurate understanding and representation of the complex deformities and corrective reconstructive techniques).

enhances the understanding of surgeons and radiologists when assessing bony deformities; however, they must be viewed on 2D screens. As a result, the true benefits of 3D imaging are often lost by this limitation. Tactile models have been shown to improve diagnostic accuracy and interobserver agreement when assessing abnormal acetabular anatomy. The combined use of conventional imaging modalities and anatomical models improved the accuracy further of trainees assessing acetabula and aided in their education by serving as demonstrative tools [15].

Life-size models allow accurate surgical simulation, enabling preoperative cup, augment, and buttress sizing, as well as cage templating and screw trajectory optimisation. Similar to our experience, Won et al. showed that this technique can reduce the intraoperative complications as described above [17]. 3D models have also been described to be of significant use in acetabular surgery preoperatively when implants require contouring in three planes. Performing this in advance of surgery, combined with trialling the implant's positioning, reduces operative and anaesthetic times [8].

In addition to their use in revision hip arthroplasty, 3D models use has also been described in spinal, dental, and maxillofacial surgery. Across the varying surgical specialties, 3D models have been used, similar to our experience, to gain preoperative insight into a patient's anatomy [12]. From a teaching perspective, the use of 3D models has been employed as a tool in subjects such as anatomy, obstetrics, dentistry, and embryology [8].

With regard to surgically applied anatomy, 3D models have been shown to be more cost-effective when compared to cadavers. 3D models allow the trainer to demonstrate the presence of pathology, which is not the case in cadaveric training. Having said this, the latter is recognised as being very beneficial when it comes to anatomical teaching, just less so when it comes to surgical simulation [11, 18].

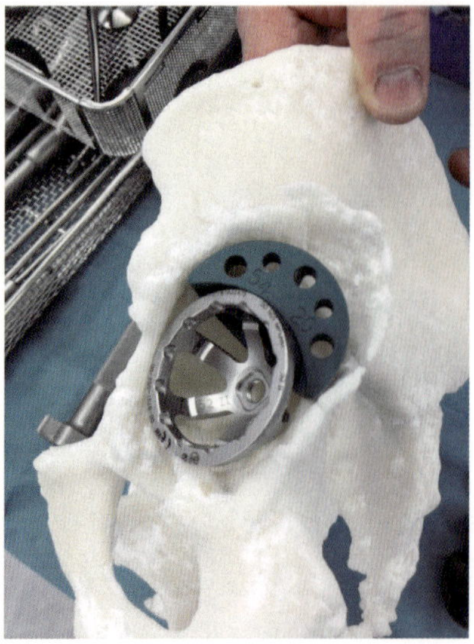

Figure 13: Preoperative templating, implant sizing, and surgical stimulation (note: these figures in print journal are two-dimensional, thus limiting the true demonstration of the value of 3D printed models in providing an accurate understanding and representation of the complex deformities and corrective reconstructive techniques).

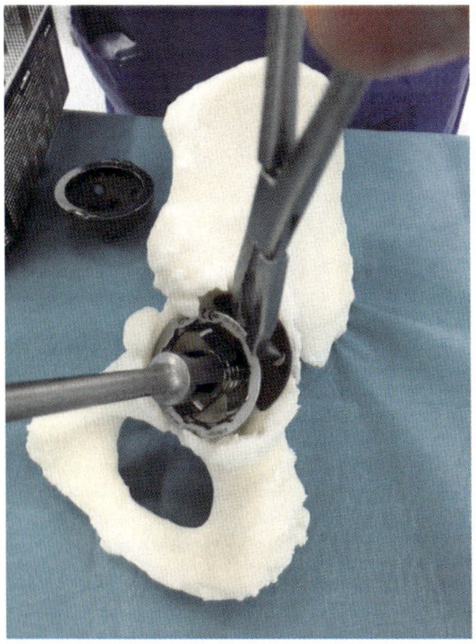

Figure 14: Preoperative templating, implant sizing, and surgical stimulation (note: these figures in print journal are two-dimensional, thus limiting the true demonstration of the value of 3D printed models in providing an accurate understanding and representation of the complex deformities and corrective reconstructive techniques).

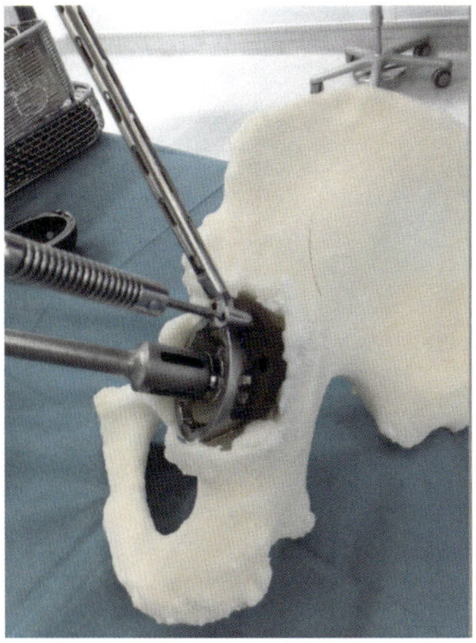

Figure 15: Preoperative templating, implant sizing, and surgical stimulation (note: these figures in print journal are two-dimensional, thus limiting the true demonstration of the value of 3D printed models in providing an accurate understanding and representation of the complex deformities and corrective reconstructive techniques).

Patient-specific implants and prostheses can now be manufactured worldwide within 24 hours. In complex cases, it can prove difficult to fit patients with a suitable prosthesis, in particular for those undergoing extensive limb salvaging oncological procedures. In other disciplines such as dental and maxillofacial surgery and neurosurgery, it is often not possible to use a standardised implant. As a result, availing of

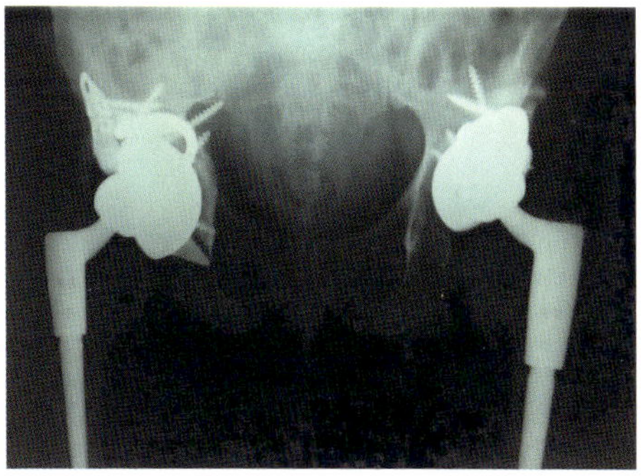

Figure 16: Postoperative anteroposterior pelvic plain film radiographs showing second-stage THR revisions in situ.

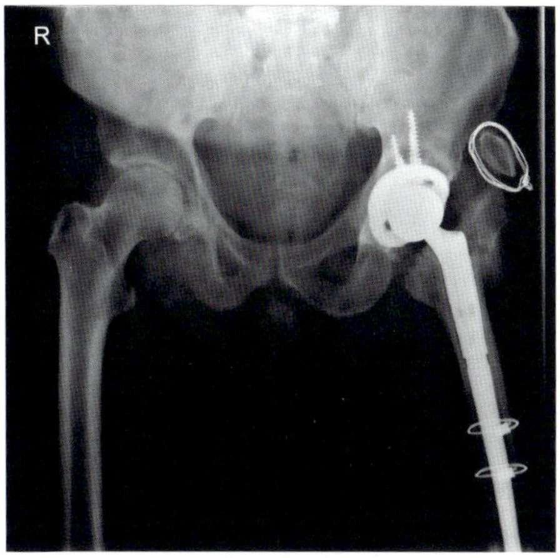

Figure 17: Postoperative anteroposterior pelvic plain film radiographs showing second-stage THR revisions in situ.

3D printing in unusual cases can produce a satisfactory result [12, 14, 18].

We described our experience of using rapid prototyping successfully in three complex revision hip arthroplasty cases in two patients. Whilst our results were encouraging, the number of documented cases in the literature remains relatively limited [19]. Our experience was one of satisfaction; however, there was no objective measurement of the benefit, and there was no comparison made with similar complex cases that did not use 3D printed models. The availability of 3D printing continues to improve and its cost continues to decline; however, barriers exist with regard to the regulation, safety, and security of the widespread use of 3D printing in surgery [19, 20].

4. Conclusion

Three complex second-stage hip revision cases were identified in two patients preoperatively. Rapid prototyping and 3D printing were used to produce life-size 3D models of three hips. Acetabular reconstruction was planned, trialled, and managed efficiently with improved surgical precision and reduced complications. The accuracy and cost-effectiveness of this technique in both cases as described were impressive and its increasing use should prove invaluable as a tool to aid clinical practice and education in the future.

References

[1] T. Eisler, O. Svensson, A. Tengström, and E. Elmstedt, "Patient expectation and satisfaction in revision total hip arthroplasty," *Journal of Arthroplasty*, vol. 17, no. 4, pp. 457–462, 2002.

[2] B. M. Wroblewski, "Current trends in revision of total hip arthroplasty," *International Orthopaedics*, vol. 8, no. 2, pp. 89–93, 1984.

[3] O. Furnes, S. A. Lie, B. Espehaug, S. E. Vollset, L. B. Engesaeter, and L. I. Havelin, "Hip disease and the prognosis of total hip replacements. A review of 53,698 primary total hip replacements reported to the Norwegian Arthroplasty Register 1987–99," *Journal of Bone and Joint Surgery B*, vol. 83, no. 4, pp. 579–586, 2001.

[4] J. Older, "Charnley low-friction arthroplasty: a worldwide retrospective review at 15 to 20 years," *The Journal of Arthroplasty*, vol. 17, no. 6, pp. 675–680, 2002.

[5] S. D. Ulrich, T. M. Seyler, D. Bennett et al., "Total hip arthroplasties: what are the reasons for revision?" *International Orthopaedics*, vol. 32, no. 5, pp. 597–604, 2008.

[6] J. M. Reagan and B. R. Moed, "Can computed tomography predict hip stability in posterior wall acetabular fractures?" *Clinical Orthopaedics and Related Research*, vol. 469, no. 7, pp. 2035–2041, 2011.

[7] E. McNamara, A. J. Hughes, C. J. Hurson, and D. Diamond, "3D Printing: potential in implants and surgery," *HPRA Medical Devices Newsletter*, vol. 1, no. 40, pp. 2–3, 2014.

[8] V. Bagaria, D. Rasalkar, S. J. Bagaria, and J. Ilyas, "Medical applications of rapid prototyping—a new horizon," in *Advanced Applications of Rapid Prototyping Technology in Modern Engineering*, INTECH, Rijeka, Croatia, 2016.

[9] R. Petzold, H.-F. Zeilhofer, and W. A. Kalender, "Rapid prototyping technology in medicine—basics and applications," *Computerized Medical Imaging and Graphics*, vol. 23, no. 5, pp. 277–284, 1999.

[10] G. A. Brown, K. Firoozbakhsh, T. A. DeCoster, J. R. Reyna Jr., and M. Moneim, "Rapid prototyping: the future of trauma surgery?" *Journal of Bone and Joint Surgery*, vol. 85, no. 4, pp. 49–55, 2003.

[11] C. L. Ventola, "Medical applications for 3D printing: current and projected uses," *P & T*, vol. 39, no. 10, pp. 704–711, 2014.

[12] B. C. Gross, J. L. Erkal, S. Y. Lockwood, C. Chen, and D. M. Spence, "Evaluation of 3D printing and its potential impact on biotechnology and the chemical sciences," *Analytical Chemistry*, vol. 86, no. 7, pp. 3240–3253, 2014.

[13] C. Schubert, M. C. Van Langeveld, and L. A. Donoso, "Innovations in 3D printing: a 3D overview from optics to organs," *British Journal of Ophthalmology*, vol. 98, no. 2, pp. 159–161, 2014.

[14] G. T. Klein, Y. Lu, and M. Y. Wang, "3D printing and neurosurgery—ready for prime time?" *World Neurosurgery*, vol. 80, no. 3-4, pp. 233–235, 2013.

[15] C. Hurson, A. Tansey, B. O'Donnchadha, P. Nicholson, J. Rice, and J. McElwain, "Rapid prototyping in the assessment, classification and preoperative planning of acetabular fractures," *Injury*, vol. 38, no. 10, pp. 1158–1162, 2007.

[16] M. B. Hoy, "3D printing: making things at the library," *Medical Reference Services Quarterly*, vol. 32, no. 1, pp. 94–99, 2013.

[17] S.-H. Won, Y.-K. Lee, Y.-C. Ha, Y.-S. Suh, and K.-H. Koo, "Improving pre-operative planning for complex total hip replacement with a Rapid Prototype model enabling surgical simulation," *The Bone & Joint Journal*, vol. 95, no. 11, pp. 1458–1463, 2013.

[18] J. Banks, "Adding value in additive manufacturing: researchers in the United Kingdom and Europe look to 3D printing for customization," *IEEE Pulse*, vol. 4, no. 6, pp. 22–26, 2013.

[19] H. H. Malik, A. R. J. Darwood, S. Shaunak et al., "Three-dimensional printing in surgery: a review of current surgical applications," *Journal of Surgical Research*, vol. 199, no. 2, pp. 512–522, 2015.

[20] A. E. M. Eltorai, E. Nguyen, and A. H. Daniels, "Three-dimensional printing in orthopedic surgery," *Orthopedics*, vol. 38, no. 11, pp. 684–687, 2015.

29

Traumatic Lumbosacral Dislocation: Current Concepts in Diagnosis and Management

Andrew S. Moon, Kivanc Atesok, Thomas E. Niemeier, Sakthivel R. Manoharan, Jason L. Pittman, and Steven M. Theiss

UAB Faculty Office Tower #960, 510 20th Street South, Birmingham, AL 35233, USA

Correspondence should be addressed to Andrew S. Moon; andy.s.moon@gmail.com

Academic Editor: Allen L. Carl

Traumatic lumbosacral dislocation is a rare, high-energy mechanism injury characterized by displacement of the fifth lumbar vertebra in relation to the sacrum. Due to the violent trauma typically associated with this lesion, there are often severe, coexisting injuries. High-quality radiographic studies, in addition to appropriate utilization of CT scan and MRI, are essential for proper evaluation and diagnosis. Although reports in the literature include nonoperative and operative management, most authors advocate for surgical treatment with open reduction and decompression with instrumentation and fusion. Despite advances in early diagnosis and management, this injury type is associated with significant morbidity and mortality, and long-term patient outcomes remain unclear.

1. Introduction

Traumatic lumbosacral dislocation is a rare clinical entity, characterized by unilateral or bilateral facet dislocations causing displacement at the level of the fifth lumbar vertebra in relation to the sacrum [1]. This injury pattern is caused by high-energy mechanisms such as motor vehicle collisions, falls from height, and crush injuries and is frequently associated with severe concomitant injuries [2].

There is some discrepancy in the literature with regard to the terminology describing injuries in this region; traumatic L5-S1 spondylolisthesis [3–7], lumbosacral/lumbopelvic dissociation [8–12], suicide jumper's fracture [13], spinopelvic dissociation [14–17], and spondylopelvic dissociation [18–20] have all been used to describe a spectrum of similar injuries. The terms spinopelvic and spondylopelvic dissociation are generally reserved for a more severe injury pattern with U-type, H-type, II-type, Y-type, or lambda type sacral fractures in conjunction with bilateral sacral fracture dislocations [17]. In this injury pattern, the spine and upper sacrum displace into the pelvis, separating from the remainder of the intact pelvic ring. However, to be a true lumbosacral dislocation, there must be dislocation of the facet joints between the fifth lumbar vertebrae and the sacrum.

Sacral fractures and lumbosacral dislocations are estimated to account for 1% of spinal fractures [21]. Current literature on lumbosacral dislocations is sparse, mainly consisting of case reports and small case series. The aim of this present study was to review the current literature on lumbosacral dislocation with regard to the relevant anatomy, biomechanics of injury, classification schemes, clinical evaluation, management, and prognosis.

2. Anatomy and Biomechanics of Injury

The lumbosacral junction consists of the L5 and S1 vertebra, as well as the corresponding intervertebral discs and apophyseal joints. It is a well-supported region stabilized by the local paraspinous musculature and iliolumbar ligamentous complex, which connects the transverse processes of L5 to the posterior iliac wing and crest. The ligamentous structures contributing to iliolumbosacral stability include the supraspinous ligament, ligamentum flavum, interspinous ligament, iliolumbar ligament, lateral lumbosacral ligament, and the facet joint capsule. The lumbosacral joint has an increased inclination in the sagittal plane and the facets at this junction have a more vertical, frontal plane orientation [22], resisting anterior translation and making dislocation a

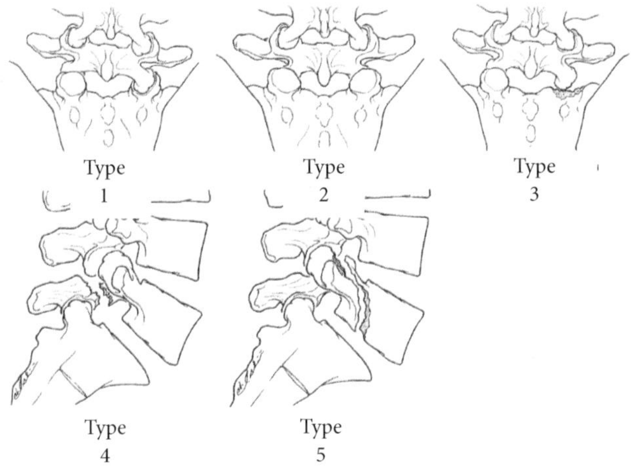

Figure 1: Classification of fracture-dislocation of the fifth lumbar vertebra according to Aihara et al. [1].

rare injury. Several authors have suggested that preexisting spondylolysis at the level of L5 may be a predisposing factor for the disruption of the lumbosacral junction with additional trauma [23–27].

This injury pattern is considered an unstable injury with disruption of virtually all stabilizing structures in that area, and may be suspected in cases where impact occurs cranial to or directly at the level of L5-S1. The direction of dislocation may vary depending on the traumatic force vector, and includes anterior, anterolateral, lateral, and posterior dislocations. Anterior dislocations, resulting in L5 anterior to S1, are most common [3, 23], while posterior dislocations are typically associated with more severe neurological injuries [3, 28–31].

Watson-Jones first described this injury pattern in 1940, and suggested forced hyperextension as the mechanism of injury [32]. However, Roaf et al. in 1960 demonstrated experimentally that the forces responsible for anterior dislocation were a combination of hyperflexion, axial rotation, and compression [33]. To date, the literature has shown hyperflexion to be the most common mechanism of injury [23]. However, isolated hyperflexion is unlikely to produce this type of injury in the lumbar spine [33]. Other contributing forces may include compression [6, 7, 34, 35], rotation [36–42], distraction [43, 44], translation [45–47], lateral translation [48–50], lateral bending [25, 36, 51], and direct traumatic vectors [44, 52].

Each variant of a lumbosacral dislocation is thought to occur through a slightly different combination of forces [7, 25, 28–32, 49, 53–56], and while multiple mechanisms have been postulated, no biomechanical study directly supporting a given mechanism of injury has been performed.

3. Classification

In 1998, Aihara et al. proposed a classification scheme specifically for fracture dislocations of the fifth lumbar vertebra based on the existing literature (Figure 1) [1]. Type 1 involved unilateral lumbosacral facet dislocation with or without facet fracture, with an intact contralateral facet. Type 2 involved bilateral lumbosacral facet dislocation with or without facet fracture. Type 3 involved unilateral lumbosacral facet dislocation and contralateral lumbosacral facet fracture. Type 4 involved dislocation of the body of L5 with bilateral fracture of the pars interarticularis (acute spondylolytic spondylolisthesis). Type 5 involved dislocation of the body of L5 with fracture of the body and/or pedicle with or without injury of the lamina and/or facet. This first attempt at a classification scheme did not distinguish between intact and unilateral/bilateral fractured facets, and other classification schemes based on varying anatomic factors exist in the literature [57, 58].

4. Clinical Evaluation

Given the substantial, high-energy trauma necessary for this injury, there are typically a variety of associated injuries involving bony, ligamentous, soft tissue and/or neurovascular elements [21], and the diagnosis may be easily overlooked on initial evaluation. Shen et al. reported that 10% of reported lumbosacral fracture dislocations were not initially recognized, though these were in patients where X-ray was the primary imaging modality [36]. Clinical presentation varies widely, [59–78] and may include severe lower back pain with exam findings such as flank hematomas, abrasions or palpable step-offs of the spinous processes.

Associated injuries are likely to occur locally, but may also involve other body cavities such as the abdomen, pelvis, thorax, and cranial cavity [21, 79]. Bony injuries may include vertebral fractures of the transverse processes, spinous processes, and sacral promontory, as well as distant fractures such as in the ribcage or femur [36]. Local soft tissue involvement includes the supraspinous ligaments, paraspinous musculature, facet joint capsules, dura and intervertebral disc [80, 81].

Typically associated neurological injuries include cauda equina syndrome and disruption of the lumbosacral plexus [36, 46, 82, 83]. Neurologic findings on exam may include hypoesthesia of the lower extremities, radiculopathy, bowel dysfunction, and urinary retention [84]. S1 is the most frequently affected nerve root [22, 39, 44, 49, 85], and more serious neurological injuries include paraplegia, although this is rare [81]. Neurologic compromise, as well as persistent neurologic deficits postoperatively, is more likely in bilateral dislocations or dislocations with fractures [25, 35, 58, 71, 72, 86].

There is a wide range of reported rates of neurological injury in the literature. Aihara et al. reported a 68.4% rate of neurologic deficit in 57 cases [1], while only 3 out of 11 patients (27.3%) in the series by Vialle et al. demonstrated neurological injury [58]. Grivas et al. reported a 58% rate of neurologic deficit for all lumbosacral fracture dislocations [2], while Arandi et al. found an 89% rate of neurological injury for complete lumbosacral dislocations [59].

5. Imaging

Initial work-up with high-quality standard radiographic studies will demonstrate an abnormal relationship between the lumbosacral facets. Clues to this pathology on the anteroposterior view include transverse process fractures (sentinel fractures), obliquity of L5 on sacrum, widening of the paravertebral soft tissue lines, widening of the interpedicular distance, and rotational deformity of the spinous processes [22, 27, 36, 85, 87]. On the lateral view, there may be an increased interspinous distance, kyphosis of L5 on S1, anterior or posterior subluxation of L5 on S1, anterior narrowing of height of disc space, disrupted spinolaminar lines, or amplification of lumbar lordosis [22, 27, 36, 87].

Advanced imaging modalities are now routinely used in virtually all high-energy trauma patients and will readily demonstrate the injury (Figure 2). A computed tomography (CT) study allows for visualization of injuries to the posterior elements and locked or fractured facet dislocations with displacement of L5 on S1 [22, 62, 88]. CT may show associated fractures, such as laminar or sacral fractures, as well as a "naked facet sign" on the axial plane, due to the L5 facets passing superiorly over the facets of S1 [22, 63, 87, 89, 90]. This gives the CT scan an image of empty or perched facets, and is indicative of facet dislocation. A magnetic resonance imaging (MRI) study will also demonstrate the dislocation, along with other local injuries including disc herniation, dural tears, torn discs, root compression, and degree of musculoligamentous injury. MRI can be instrumental in localizing sites of neural compression [22, 62, 87].

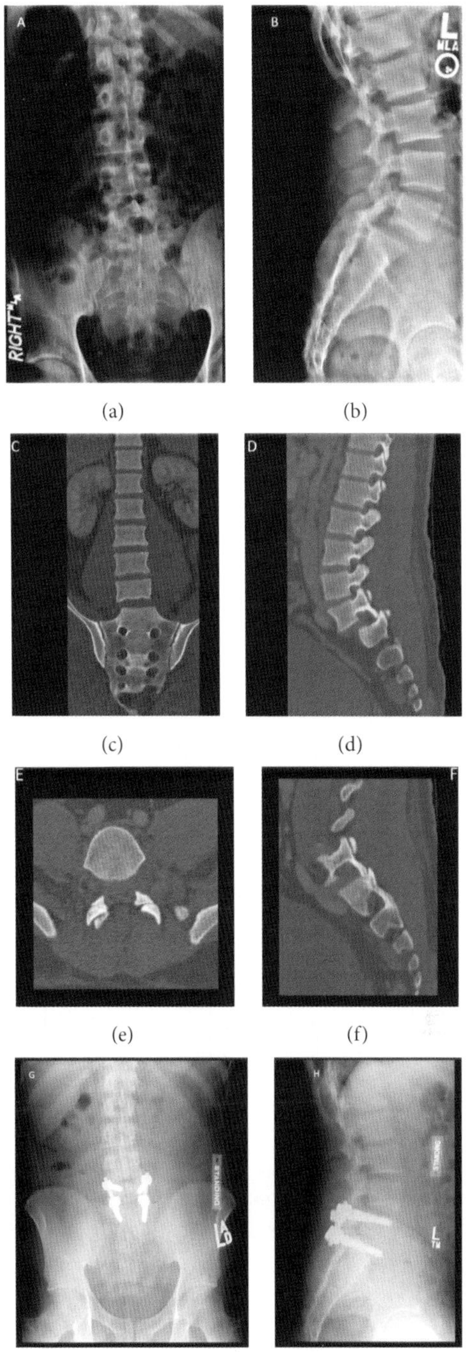

Figure 2: Imaging of a 25-year-old male patient who was involved in an all-terrain vehicle accident. He was ejected from the vehicle and presented with low back pain and intermittent bilateral lower extremity radicular pain with paresthesia. Figures (a) and (b) demonstrate anteroposterior and lateral radiographs, respectively. Coronal CT shows minimal lateralization of L5 over S1 (c). Sagittal view shows anterior dislocation of L5 over S1 with jumped facets (d). Axial (e) image cut through the same level as the sagittal image (f) shows bilateral jumped facets at L5-S1. The patient underwent posterior spinal instrumentation and fusion of the L5 and S1 vertebrae using pedicle screws and rods. Postoperative anteroposterior (g) and lateral (h) images demonstrate a reduced L5-S1 joint. (Courtesy of University of Alabama at Birmingham, Department of Orthopaedic Surgery, Spine Fellowship Program, Birmingham, Alabama, USA).

6. Management

Initial management includes appropriate evaluation, stabilization and resuscitation measures according to standard Advanced Trauma Life Support (ATLS) protocol, and emergent injuries should be treated first in order of priority [91]. There are a few published experiences with nonoperative management with techniques including closed reduction, traction and immobilization [26, 49, 56, 77, 92–95]. To the authors' knowledge, the last case report of an adult treated conservatively was published in 2000, with the authors opting for conservative treatment due to the patient's delayed presentation of three months [92].

In the pediatric population, nonsurgical treatment remains a consideration with any spinal condition due to concerns of disproportional growth of the anterior spine after isolated posterior fusion resulting in a progressive, iatrogenic deformity frequently referred to as the "crankshaft phenomenon." [96] However, with closed reduction and immobilization, studies have documented risk of secondary neurological injury during external reduction maneuvers [46, 56, 58, 93]. In addition, prior reports have documented an increased risk of progressive back pain, deformity, and neurologic deterioration with conservative treatment [4, 26, 31].

Acute lumbosacral dislocations are unstable, and a growing body of literature recommends early surgical reduction with instrumentation [1, 59, 71, 81, 92, 97, 98]. Historic techniques for instrumentation have included a wide range of constructs including interspinous screws, posterior articular screws, sublaminar wiring, Harrington hooks and rods, and osteosynthesis with posterior plates or with

Cotrel-Dubousset-type instrumentation [23, 25, 27, 30, 40, 54, 64, 84, 99–104].

Currently, treatment should consist of pedicle screws in L5 and S1, assuming the pedicles at these levels are intact. While this short segment construct may be sufficient in patients with good facet apposition following reduction, fixation may need to be extended proximally to L4 or distally to the pelvis when bony support is poor after reduction. The lumbosacral canal should be examined intraoperatively for any bone or disc fragments, if MRI indicates neurocompression [3, 54, 58]. Spinal cord monitoring can be used to confirm intact peripheral nerve function during reduction maneuvers and significant distraction should be avoided during reduction.

All dislocation injuries should also be treated with fusion. While there is little literature describing the superiority of one fusion method over another, options include posterior arthrodesis [1, 59], circumferential arthrodesis [27, 70, 72], and interbody fusion, which is often used in cases of significant disc disruption [24, 64, 99]. Partial facetectomy may be performed in patients with traumatic lumbosacral dislocation to facilitate reduction [34, 46, 70, 85, 99], although intact apophyseal joints are preferred to prevent redislocation [34].

Numerous case reports support decompression in patients with evidence of neurologic compromise [1, 59, 71, 81, 92, 97, 98]. The authors of the current study suggest surgical decompression is patient-dependent, and recommend selective decompression based on the patient's clinical exam and sites of neurologic compression as evidenced on MRI. In cases of cauda equina syndrome or delayed reduction, decompressive laminectomy may be performed [40, 43, 70, 83]. However, this may lead to increased instability and is not indicated in the absence of neurologic compromise [68, 77, 85].

7. Prognosis and Complications

Although there have been a few reports of satisfactory outcomes after nonoperative management [56, 92, 93], many patients initially treated conservatively eventually required fusion due to progression of listhesis and/or neurological deficit [5–7, 22, 40, 51, 54]. However, even with surgical intervention there may be residual disability and permanent neurological dysfunction [1, 98, 100–103]. The degree of residual translational displacement and kyphosis postoperatively may be associated with clinical outcomes following surgery. Perioperative surgical complications include infection and wound dehiscence, not unlike other surgeries in this region. Additional complications include mechanical issues such as instrumentation failure that can occur late, requiring reoperation years after the initial surgery [68, 92, 102]. Adelved et al. published long-term results in a small series of patients with traumatic lumbosacral dissociation, showing that functional impairments, pain, and poor patient-reported health were common, along with high rates of neurologic, urinary, and sexual dysfunction [8]. Conversely, De lure et al. demonstrated successful long-term clinical outcomes in a small cohort of patients who underwent lumboiliac fixation for lumbosacral dislocation injuries [92]. Long-term prognosis is unclear due to the small number of reported cases with limited follow-up and heterogeneous results.

8. Summary

Traumatic lumbosacral dislocation is a rare injury pattern resulting from high-energy trauma. It often presents with multiple concomitant injuries, and may be easily overlooked on initial evaluation. Acute complete dislocations are highly unstable, three-column injury patterns, requiring surgical intervention with open reduction and internal fixation. Early diagnosis and treatment are likely to improve clinical outcomes. Despite advances in diagnosis and management, these injuries are associated with significant morbidity and mortality.

References

[1] T. Aihara, K. Takahashi, M. Yamagata, and H. Moriya, "Fracture-dislocation of the fifth lumbar vertebra," *The Journal of Bone & Joint Surgery (British Volume)*, vol. 80, no. 5, pp. 840–845, 1998.

[2] T. B. Grivas, "Unilateral Lumbosacral Dislocation: Case Report and a Comprehensive Review," *The Open Orthopaedics Journal*, vol. 6, no. 1, pp. 473–477, 2012.

[3] M. Robbins, Z. Mallon, R. Roberto, R. Patel, M. Gupta, and E. Klineberg, "Traumatic spondylopelvic dissociation: A report of two cases of spondylolisthesis at l5-s1 and review of literature," *Global Spine Journal*, vol. 5, no. 3, pp. 225–230, 2015.

[4] M. Reinhold, C. Knop, and M. Blauth, "Acute traumatic L5-S1 spondylolisthesis: A case report," *Archives of Orthopaedic and Trauma Surgery*, vol. 126, no. 9, pp. 624–630, 2006.

[5] S. J. Reddy, W. N. Al-Holou, J.-C. Leveque, F. La Marca, and P. Park, "Traumatic lateral spondylolisthesis of the lumbar spine with a unilateral locked facet: Description of an unusual injury, probable mechanism, and management: Report of two cases," *Journal of Neurosurgery: Spine*, vol. 9, no. 6, pp. 576–580, 2008.

[6] M. Lamm, S.-E. H. Henriksen, and S. Eiskjœr, "Acute Traumatic L5-S1 Spondylolisthesis," *Journal of Spinal Disorders & Techniques*, vol. 16, no. 6, pp. 524–527, 2003.

[7] D. Fabris, S. Costantini, U. Nena, and V. Lo Scalzo, "Traumatic L5-S1 spondylolisthesis: Report of three cases and a review of the literature," *European Spine Journal*, vol. 8, no. 4, pp. 290–295, 1999.

[8] A. Adelved, A. Tötterman, T. Glott, J. C. Hellund, J. E. Madsen, and O. Røise, "Long-term functional outcome after traumatic lumbosacral dissociation. A retrospective case series of 13 patients," *Injury*, vol. 47, no. 7, pp. 1562–1568, 2016.

[9] M. D. Helgeson, R. A. Lehman Jr., P. Cooper, M. Frisch, R. C. Andersen, and C. Bellabarba, "Retrospective review of lumbosacral dissociations in blast injuries," *The Spine Journal*, vol. 36, no. 7, pp. E469–E475, 2011.

[10] P. M. Formby, S. C. Wagner, D. G. Kang, G. S. Van Blarcum, and R. A. Lehman, "Operative management of complex lumbosacral dissociations in combat injuries," *The spine journal : official journal of the North American Spine Society*, vol. 16, no. 10, pp. 1200–1207, 2016.

[11] D. G. Kang, J. P. Cody, and R. A. Lehman Jr., "Combat-related lumbopelvic dissociation treated with L4 to ilium posterior fusion," *The Spine Journal*, vol. 12, no. 9, pp. 860-861, 2012.

[12] J. P. Cody, D. G. Kang, and R. A. Lehman Jr., "Combat-related lumbopelvic dissociation treated with percutaneous sacroiliac screw placement," *The Spine Journal*, vol. 12, no. 9, pp. 858-859, 2012.

[13] R. Roy-Camille, G. Saillant, G. Gagna, and C. Mazel, "Transverse fracture of the upper sacrum: Suicidal jumper's fracture," *The Spine Journal*, vol. 10, no. 9, pp. 838–845, 1985.

[14] S. K. Williams and S. M. Quinnan, "Percutaneous lumbopelvic fixation for reduction and stabilization of sacral fractures with spinopelvic dissociation patterns," *Journal of Orthopaedic Trauma*, vol. 30, no. 9, pp. e318–e324, 2016.

[15] J. Lindahl, T. J. Mäkinen, S. K. Koskinen, and T. Söderlund, "Factors associated with outcome of spinopelvic dissociation treated with lumbopelvic fixation," *Injury*, vol. 45, no. 12, pp. 1914–1920, 2014.

[16] M. A. Ayoub, "Displaced spinopelvic dissociation with sacral cauda equina syndrome: Outcome of surgical decompression with a preliminary management algorithm," *European Spine Journal*, vol. 21, no. 9, pp. 1815–1825, 2012.

[17] C. Yi and D. J. Hak, "Traumatic spinopelvic dissociation or U-shaped sacral fracture: A review of the literature," *Injury*, vol. 43, no. 4, pp. 402–408, 2012.

[18] M. P. Sullivan, H. E. Smith, J. M. Schuster, D. Donegan, S. Mehta, and J. Ahn, "Spondylopelvic dissociation," *Orthopedic Clinics of North America*, vol. 45, no. 1, pp. 65–75, 2014.

[19] E. J. Vresilovic, S. Mehta, R. Placide, and R. A. Milam IV, "Traumatic spondylopelvic dissociation: A report of two cases," *The Journal of Bone & Joint Surgery*, vol. 87, no. 5, pp. 1098–1103, 2005.

[20] R. T. Bents, J. C. France, J. M. Glover, and K. L. Kaylor, "Traumatic spondylopelvic dissociation: A case report and literature review," *The Spine Journal*, vol. 21, no. 15, pp. 1814–1819, 1996.

[21] M. R. Leventhal, "Fractures, Dislocations, and Fracture-Dislocations of Spine," in *Campbell's Operative Orthopaedics*, S. T. Canale, Ed., vol. 2, pp. 1597–1690, 10th edition, 2003.

[22] C. Tohme-Noun, L. Rillardon, A. Krainik, P. Guigui, Y. Menu, and A. Feydy, "Imaging features of traumatic disclocation of the lumbosacral joint associated with disc herniation," *Skeletal Radiology*, vol. 32, no. 6, pp. 360–363, 2003.

[23] K. Saiki, S. Hirabayashi, H. Sakai, and K. Inokuchi, "Traumatic anterior lumbosacral dislocation caused by hyperextension mechanism in preexisting L5 spondylolysis: A case report and a review of literature," *Journal of Spinal Disorders & Techniques*, vol. 19, no. 6, pp. 455–462, 2006.

[24] P. A. Robertson, M. J. Sherwood, and A. T. Hadlow, "Lumbosacral dislocation injuries: Management and outcomes," *Journal of Spinal Disorders & Techniques*, vol. 18, no. 3, pp. 232–237, 2005.

[25] R. Vialle, S. Wolff, F. Pauthier et al., "Traumatic Lumbosacral Dislocation: Four Cases and Review of Literature," *Clinical Orthopaedics and Related Research*, no. 419, pp. 91–97, 2004.

[26] A. S. Hilibrand, A. G. Urquhart, G. P. Graziano, and R. N. Hensinger, "Acute spondylolytic spondylolisthesis. Risk of progression and neurological complications," *The Journal of Bone & Joint Surgery*, vol. 77, no. 2, pp. 190–196, 1995.

[27] P. J. Connolly, S. I. Esses, M. H. Heggeness, and S. S. Cook, "Unilateral facet dislocation of the lumbosacral junction," *The Spine Journal*, vol. 17, no. 10, pp. 1244–1248, 1992.

[28] J. A. Finkelstein, R. W. Hu, and T. Al-Harby, "Open posterior dislocation of the lumbosacral junction: A case report," *The Spine Journal*, vol. 21, no. 3, pp. 378–380, 1996.

[29] S. D. Gertzbein, "Posterior dislocation of the lumbosacral joint: A case report," *Journal of Spinal Disorders & Techniques*, vol. 3, no. 2, pp. 174–178, 1990.

[30] S. L. Cohn, L. Keppler, and B. A. Akbarnia, "Traumatic retrolisthesis of the lumbosacral junction: A case report," *The Spine Journal*, vol. 14, no. 1, pp. 132–134, 1989.

[31] J. B. Griffin and G. H. Sutherland, "Traumatic posterior fracture-dislocation of the lumbosacral joint," *Journal of Trauma - Injury Infection and Critical Care*, vol. 20, no. 5, pp. 426–428, 1980.

[32] R. Watson-Jones, *Fractures and Joint Injuries*, Williams & Wilkins, Baltimore, Maryland, USA, 1940.

[33] R. Roaf, "A study of the mechanics of spinal injuries," *The Journal of Bone & Joint Surgery*, vol. 42-B, no. 4, pp. 810–823, 1960.

[34] S. Das De and S. W. McCreath, "Lumbosacral fracture-dislocations. A report of four cases," *The Journal of Bone & Joint Surgery (British Volume)*, vol. 63, no. 1, pp. 58–60, 1981.

[35] G. S. Miz and G. L. Engler, "Unilateral dislocation of a lumbosacral facet," *The Spine Journal*, vol. 13, no. 8, pp. 956-957, 1988.

[36] F. H. Shen, A. Crowl, T. E. Shuler, J. A. Feldenzer, and S. W. Leivy, "Delayed Recognition of Lumbosacral Fracture Dislocations in the Multitrauma Patient: The Triad of Transverse Process Fractures, Unilateral Renal Contusion and Lumbosacral Fracture Dislocation," *Journal of Trauma - Injury Infection and Critical Care*, vol. 56, no. 3, pp. 700–705, 2004.

[37] JP. Atanasiu, I. Brechet, and E. Renault, "Fracture dislocation of L5-S1: a case report with review of the literature," *Ann Orthop Ouest*, vol. 25, pp. 121–123, 1993.

[38] H. Halm, U. Liljenqvist, J. Steinbeck, and D. Jeszenszky, "Lumbosacral fracture dislocation in a lumberjack," *European Spine Journal*, vol. 4, no. 6, pp. 354–356, 1995.

[39] M. E. Wilchinsky, "Traumatic lumbosacral dislocation. A case report and review of the literature," *Orthopedics*, vol. 10, no. 9, pp. 1271–1274, 1987.

[40] L. D. Herron and R. C. Williams, "Fracture-Dislocation of the Lumbosacral Spine," *Clinical Orthopaedics and Related Research*, vol. 186, pp. 205–211, 1984.

[41] B. D. A. Morris, "Unilateral dislocation of a lumbosacral facet. A case report," *The Journal of Bone & Joint Surgery*, vol. 63, no. 1, pp. 164-165, 1981.

[42] R. Roy-Camille, P. Gagnon, Y. Catonne, and J. P. Benazet, "Antero-lateral dislocation of the lumbo-sacral spine: A rare lesion," *Revue de Chirurgie Orthopédique et Traumatologique*, vol. 66, no. 2, pp. 105–109, 1980.

[43] J. J. Verlaan, F. C. Oner, W. J. A. Dhert, and A. J. Verbout, "Traumatic lumbosacral dislocation: Case report," *The Spine Journal*, vol. 26, no. 17, pp. 1942–1944, 2001.

[44] P.-H. Roche, H. Dufour, N. Graziani, J. Jolivert, and F. Grisoli, "Anterior lumbosacral dislocation: Case report and review of the literature," *World Neurosurgery*, vol. 50, no. 1, pp. 11–16, 1998.

[45] H. Miyamoto, M. Sumi, O. Kataoka, M. Doita, M. Kurosaka, and S. Yoshiya, "Traumatic spondylolisthesis of the lumbosacral spine with multiple fractures fo the posterior elements," *The Journal of Bone & Joint Surgery (British Volume)*, vol. 86, no. 1, pp. 115–118, 2004.

[46] P. Dewey and P. S. Browne, "Fracture-dislocation of the lumbosacral spine with cauda equina lesion," *The Journal of Bone & Joint Surgery (British Volume)*, vol. 50, no. 3, pp. 635–638, 1968.

[47] R. G. Lambert and E. L. Billings, "Traumatic spondylolisthesis," *Journal of Bone and Joint Surgery*, vol. 43, p. 310, 1961.

[48] R. Vialle and C. Court, "Traumatic lateral lumbosacral dislocation: One cose and review of literature," *Journal of Spinal Disorders & Techniques*, vol. 18, no. 3, pp. 286–289, 2005.

[49] J. Beguiristain, D. Schweitzer, G. Mora, and V. Pombo, "Traumatic lumbosacral dislocation in a 5-year-old boy with eight years follow-up," *The Spine Journal*, vol. 20, no. 3, pp. 362–366, 1995.

[50] A. Barquet, J. Menendez, A. Dubra, R. Masliah, and D. Pereyra, "Anterolateral dislocation of the lumbosacral junction," *Canadian Association of Radiologists Journal*, vol. 44, no. 2, pp. 129–132, 1993.

[51] J. R. Carlson, J. G. Heller, F. L. Mansfield, and F. X. Pedlow Jr., "Traumatic open anterior lumbosacral fracture dislocation: A report of two cases," *The Spine Journal*, vol. 24, no. 2, pp. 184–188, 1999.

[52] W. I. El Assuity, M. A. El Masry, and D. Chan, "Acute traumatic spondylolisthesis at the lumbosacral junction," *Journal of Trauma - Injury Infection and Critical Care*, vol. 62, no. 6, pp. 1514–1516, 2007.

[53] F. Magerl, M. Aebi, S. D. Gertzbein, J. Harms, and S. Nazarian, "A comprehensive classification of thoracic and lumbar injuries," *European Spine Journal*, vol. 3, no. 4, pp. 184–201, 1994.

[54] R. Schmid, M. Reinhold, and M. Blauth, "Lumbosacral dislocation: A review of the literature and current aspects of management," *Injury*, vol. 41, no. 4, pp. 321–328, 2010.

[55] J. K. Burkus and F. Denis, "Shear fracture-dislocations of the thoracic and lumbar spine associated with forceful hyperextension (Lumberjack paraplegia)," *The Spine Journal*, vol. 17, no. 2, pp. 156–161, 1992.

[56] R. L. M. Newell, "Lumbosacral fracture-dislocation: a case managed conservatively, with return to heavy work," *Injury*, vol. 9, no. 2, pp. 131–134, 1977.

[57] L. L. Wiltse, P. H. Newman, and I. Macnab, "Classification of spondylolisis and spondylolisthesis," *Clinical Orthopaedics and Related Research*, no. 117, pp. 23–29, 1976.

[58] R. Vialle, S. Charosky, L. Rillardon, N. Levassor, and C. Court, "Traumatic dislocation of the lumbosacral junction diagnosis, anatomical classification and surgical strategy," *Injury*, vol. 38, no. 2, pp. 169–181, 2007.

[59] N. R. Arandi, G. M. Mundis, N. Kabirian, D. Zhang, and S. Schroerlucke, "Traumatic complete lateral dislocation at the lumbosacral junction: A case report," *Journal of Spinal Disorders & Techniques*, vol. 28, no. 1, pp. E56–E60, 2015.

[60] L. Rizzi and C. Castelli, "Open pelvic fracture associated with lumbosacral dislocation and extensive perineal injury," *Injury*, vol. 46, pp. S44–S47, 2015.

[61] A. Safaie Yazdi, F. Omidi-Kashani, and A. Baradaran, "Intrapelvic Lumbosacral Fracture Dislocation in a Neurologically Intact Patient: A Case Report," *Archives of Trauma Research*, vol. 4, no. 3, 2015.

[62] K. Shinohara, S. Soshi, Y. Kida, A. Shinohara, and K. Marumo, "A rare case of spinal injury: Bilateral facet dislocation without fracture at the lumbosacral joint," *Journal of Orthopaedic Science*, vol. 17, no. 2, pp. 189–193, 2012.

[63] R. Blecher, A. Geftler, Y. Anekstein, and Y. Mirovsky, "Isolated unilateral facet dislocation of the lumbosacral junction," *The Journal of Bone & Joint Surgery (British Volume)*, vol. 92, no. 10, pp. 1456–1459, 2010.

[64] X. Lu, C. Hou, W. Yuan, Z. Zhang, and A. Chen, "Complete traumatic anterior dislocation of the lumbosacral joint: A case report," *The Spine Journal*, vol. 34, no. 14, pp. E488–E492, 2009.

[65] M. D. Vilela, M. Gelfenbeyn, and C. Bellabarba, "U-shaped sacral fracture and lumbosacral dislocation as a result of a shotgun injury: Case report," *Neurosurgery*, vol. 64, no. 1, pp. E193–E194, 2009.

[66] A. M. Hidalgo-Ovejero, S. Garcia-Mata, T. Izco-Cabezon, J. Martinez de Morentin, P. Lasanta, and M. Martinez-Grande, "Posttraumatic lumbosacral dislocation.," *American journal of orthopedics (Belle Mead, N.J.)*, vol. 34, no. 1, pp. 38–42, 2005.

[67] S. D. Hodges, J. Shuster, M. A. Asher, and S. J. Mcclarty, "Traumatic L5-S1 spondylolisthesis," *Southern Medical Journal*, vol. 92, no. 3, pp. 316–320, 1999.

[68] A. A. Davis and E. J. Carragee, "Bilateral facet dislocation at the lumbosacral joint: A report of a case and review of literature," *The Spine Journal*, vol. 18, no. 16, pp. 2540–2544, 1993.

[69] F. Pellise, J. Bago, and C. Villanueva, "Double-level spinal injury resulting in "en bloc" dislocation of the lumbar spine. A case report," *Acta Orthopœdica Belgica*, vol. 58, no. 3, pp. 349–352, 1992.

[70] A. Carl and B. Blair, "Unilateral lumbosacral facet fracture-dislocation," *The Spine Journal*, vol. 16, no. 2, pp. 218–220, 1991.

[71] J. G. Van Savage, L. E. Dahners, J. B. Renner, and C. C. Baker, "Fracture-Dislocation of the lumbosacral spine: Case report and review of the literature," *Journal of Trauma - Injury Infection and Critical Care*, vol. 33, no. 5, pp. 779–784, 1992.

[72] K. M. Kramer and A. M. Levine, "Unilateral facet dislocation of the lumbosacral junction. A case report and review of the literature," *The Journal of Bone & Joint Surgery*, vol. 71, no. 8, pp. 1258–1261, 1989.

[73] CS. Resnik, CE. Scheer, and RS. Adelaar, "Lumbosacral dislocation," *Canadian Association of Radiologists Journal*, vol. 36, pp. 259–261, 1985.

[74] D. C. Boger, R. W. Chandler, J. G. Pearce, and A. Balciunas, "Unilateral facet dislocation at the lumbosacral junction. Case report and literature review," *The Journal of Bone & Joint Surgery*, vol. 65, no. 8, pp. 1174–1178, 1983.

[75] R. A. Nicholson, "Lateral lumbosacral fracture dislocation: a case report," *Injury*, vol. 15, no. 1, pp. 41–43, 1983.

[76] R. H. Jackson, R. G. Quisling, and A. L. Day, "Fracture and complete dislocation of the thoracic or lumbosacral spine: Report of three cases," *Neurosurgery*, vol. 5, no. 2, pp. 250–253, 1979.

[77] L. C. Samberg, "Fracture dislocation of the lumbosacral spine. A case report," *The Journal of Bone & Joint Surgery*, vol. 57, no. 7, pp. 1007-1008, 1975.

[78] R. K. White, "Complete lumbosacral dislocation. Report of a case," *The American Journal of Surgery*, vol. 102, no. 1, pp. 103-104, 1961.

[79] S. Anderson, M. H. Biros, and R. F. Reardon, "Delayed diagnosis of thoracolumbar fractures in multiple-trauma patients," *Academic Emergency Medicine*, vol. 3, no. 9, pp. 832–839, 1996.

[80] M. Krbec and P. Hraběta, "Unilateral isolated dislocation at the lumbosacral junction: Lateral flexion-distraction as a major vector in the mechanism of injury: Case report and trauma mechanism analysis," *European Spine Journal*, vol. 20, no. 2, pp. S166–S171, 2011.

[81] R. Cruz-Conde, A. Rayo, R. Rodriguez de Oya, P. Berjano, and E. Gárate, "Acute traumatic lumbosacral dislocation treated by open reduction internal fixation and fusion," *The Spine Journal*, vol. 28, no. 3, pp. E51–E53, 2003.

[82] S. K. Cho, L. G. Lenke, and D. Hanson, "Traumatic noncontiguous double fracture-dislocation of the lumbosacral spine," *The Spine Journal*, vol. 6, no. 5, pp. 534–538, 2006.

[83] D. F. Fardon, "Displaced fracture of the lumbosacral spine with delayed cauda equina deficit. Report of a case and review of literature," *Clinical Orthopaedics and Related Research*, vol. 120, pp. 155–158, 1976.

[84] C. Angthong, S. Wunnasinthop, and S. Sanpakit, "Complex lumbosacral fracture-dislocation with pelvic ring disruption and vertical shear sacral fracture: A case report of late presentation and review of the literature," *Ulusal Travma ve Acil Cerrahi Dergisi*, vol. 16, no. 6, pp. 561–566, 2010.

[85] A. I. Tsirikos, A. Saifuddin, M. H. Noordeen, and S. K. Tucker, "Traumatic lumbosacral dislocation: report of two cases.," *The Spine Journal*, vol. 29, no. 8, pp. E164–168, 2004.

[86] H. T. Hee, J. Thambiah, A. Nather et al., "A case report of neurologically unstable fracture of the lumbosacral spine in a patient with ankylosing spondylitis," *Annals Academy Of Medicine Singapore*, vol. 31, pp. 115–118, 2002.

[87] R. M. Stuart and S. J. Song, "Unilateral lumbosacral facet joint dislocation without associated fracture," *Journal of Medical Imaging and Radiation Oncology*, vol. 48, no. 2, pp. 224–229, 2004.

[88] N. A. Ebraheim, E. R. Savolaine, P. Shapiro, T. Houston, and W. T. Jackson, "Unilateral lumbosacral facet joint dislocation associated with vertical shear sacral fracture," *Journal of Orthopaedic Trauma*, vol. 5, no. 4, pp. 498–503, 1991.

[89] V. B. Graves, J. S. Keene, and C. M. Strother, "CT of bilateral lumbosacral facet dislocation," *American Journal of Neuroradiology (AJNR)*, vol. 9, pp. 809-810, 1988.

[90] D. K. Steinitz, D. I. Alexander, R. K. Leighton, and J. J. O'Sullivan, "Late displacement of a fracture dislocation at the lumbosacral junction: A case study," *The Spine Journal*, vol. 22, no. 9, pp. 1024–1027, 1997.

[91] ATLS Subcommittee, American College of Surgeons' Committee on Trauma, and International ATLS working group, "Advanced trauma life support (ATLS): The ninth edition," *Journal of Trauma and Acute Care Surgery*, vol. 74, no. 5, pp. 1363–1366, 2013.

[92] L. M. Veras Del Monte and J. Bagó, "Traumatic lumbosacral dislocation," *The Spine Journal*, vol. 25, no. 6, pp. 756–759, 2000.

[93] J. D. Zoltan, L. A. Gilula, and W. A. Murphy, "Unilateral facet dislocation between the fifth lumbar and first sacral vertebrae. Case report," *The Journal of Bone & Joint Surgery*, vol. 61, no. 5, pp. 767–769, 1979.

[94] M. C. Boyd and W. Y. Yu, "Closed reduction of lumbosacral fracture dislocations," *World Neurosurgery*, vol. 23, no. 3, pp. 295–298, 1985.

[95] D. C. Boger, R. W. Chandler, P. G. Pearce, and A. Balciunas, "Unilateral facet dislocation at the lumbosacral junction. Case report and literature review," *The Journal of Bone & Joint Surgery*, vol. 65, no. 8, pp. 1174–1178, 1983.

[96] R. F. Murphy and J. F. Mooney, "The Crankshaft Phenomenon," *Journal of the American Academy of Orthopaedic Surgeons*, vol. 25, no. 9, pp. e185–e193, 2017.

[97] S. S. Kaplan, N. M. Wright, K. D. Yundt, and C. Lauryssen, "Adjacent fracture-dislocations of the lumbosacral spine: Case report," *Neurosurgery*, vol. 44, no. 5, pp. 1134–1137, 1999.

[98] F. Holdsworth, "Fractures, dislocations, and fracture-dislocations of the spine.," *The Journal of Bone & Joint Surgery*, vol. 52, no. 8, pp. 1534–1551, 1970.

[99] R. Xu, C. Solakoglu, R. M. Kretzer, M. J. McGirt, T. F. Witham, and A. Bydon, "Bilateral traumatic dislocation without fracture of the lumbosacral junction: Case report and review of the literature," *The Spine Journal*, vol. 36, no. 10, pp. E662–E668, 2011.

[100] H. Pascal-Moussellard, C. Hirsch, and R. Bonaccorsi, "Osteosynthesis in sacral fracture and lumbosacral dislocation," *Orthopaedics & Traumatology: Surgery & Research*, vol. 102, 1, pp. S45–S57, 2016.

[101] H.-C. Liu, Y.-Z. Chen, X.-G. Sang, and L. Qi, "Management of lumbosacropelvic fracture-dislocation using lumbo-iliac internal fixation," *Injury*, vol. 43, no. 4, pp. 452–457, 2012.

[102] K. Soultanis, G. I. Karaliotas, D. Mastrokalos, V. I. Sakellariou, K. A. Starantzis, and P. N. Soucacos, "Lumbopelvic fracture-dislocation combined with unstable pelvic ring injury: One stage stabilisation with spinal instrumentation," *Injury*, vol. 42, no. 10, pp. 1179–1183, 2011.

[103] M. R. Sobhan, S. M. J. Abrisham, M. Vakili, and S. Shirdel, "Spinopelvic fixation of sacroiliac joint fractures and fracture-dislocations: A clinical 8 years follow-up study," *Archives of Bone and Joint Surgery*, vol. 4, no. 4, pp. 381–386, 2016.

[104] F. De Iure, M. Cappuccio, M. Palmisani, R. Pascarella, and M. Commessatti, "Lumboiliac fixation in lumbosacral dislocation and associated injuries of the pelvis and lumbosacral junction: a long-term radiological and clinical follow-up," *Injury*, vol. 47, pp. S44–S48, 2016.

Allograft Reconstruction of the Extensor Mechanism after Resection of Soft Tissue Sarcoma

Daniel A. Müller,[1] Giovanni Beltrami,[2] Guido Scoccianti,[2] Pierluigi Cuomo,[2] Francesca Totti,[2] and Rodolfo Capanna[3]

[1]*Department of Orthopedic Surgery, Balgrist University Hospital, Forchstrasse 340, 8008 Zürich, Switzerland*
[2]*Department of Orthopedic Oncology, Azienda Ospedaliero-Universitaria Careggi, Largo Brambilla 3, 50134 Firenze, Italy*
[3]*Department of Orthopedic Surgery, Azienda Ospedaliero-Universitaria Pisana, Via Paradisa 2, Cisanello, 56125 Pisa, Italy*

Correspondence should be addressed to Daniel A. Müller; daniel.a.mueller@me.com

Academic Editor: Panagiotis Korovessis

Introduction. Soft tissue tumors around the knee joint still pose problems for the excision and subsequent reconstruction. *Methods.* In the 6 included patients the soft tissue sarcoma has its base on the anterior surface of the extensor mechanism and expands towards the skin. The entire extensor apparatus (quadriceps tendon, patella, and patellar tendon) was resected and replaced by a fresh-frozen allograft. *Results.* The mean follow-up was 6.7 years (range: 2–12.4 years). In two patients a local recurrence occurred, resulting in a 5-year local recurrence-free rate of 66.7% (95% CI: 19.5%–90.4%). Distant metastases were found in 4 patients resulting in a 5-year metastasis-free rate of 33.3% (95% CI: 4.6%–67.5%). Two patients underwent at least one revision surgery, including one patient in whom the allograft had to be removed. According to the ISOLS function score 24.7 points (range: 19–28 points) were achieved at the last follow-up. The mean active flexion of the knee joint was 82.5° (range: 25–120°) and a mean extension lag of 10° (range: 0–30°) was observed. *Conclusions.* The replacement of the extensor mechanism by an allograft is a reasonable option, allowing wide margins and restoration of active extension in most patients. *Trial Registration.* The presented study is listed on the ISRCTN registry with trial number ISRCTN63060594.

1. Introduction

Soft tissue sarcomas represent a heterogeneous group of lesions that are often subtle in presentation and have a wide variation in extent of malignant behavior. Because of the rarity and vast histological varieties, they frequently pose diagnostic problems. The knee joint and the adjacent structures are quite uncommon locations for soft tissue sarcoma [1]. The most common entities are liposarcoma (25%) and synovial sarcoma (25%), followed by fibrosarcoma (9%) and undifferentiated pleomorphic sarcoma (8%) [1].

Over the recent decades, limb-sparing surgery has become an accepted method of treatment for most patients with soft tissue sarcomas. Advances in surgical techniques, prosthetic design, and bone allograft banking have opened the avenue for reconstruction procedures after wide excision of bone and soft tissues. This allows the surgeon to achieve adequate margins while salvaging the limb and its function. Yet, soft tissue tumors around the knee joint still pose problems for the excision and subsequent reconstruction. Extension of the tumor in the joint or in the extensor mechanism is a challenging situation to achieve adequate margins and a good functional limb. There is no current consensus as to the best method of reconstruction of the extensor mechanism of the knee [2]. Few reconstructive options are available to avoid knee arthrodesis including tendon transfers or local grafts [3], synthetic materials [4], and allograft tissues [5]. Regardless of the used reconstruction technique, the principal technical difficulty remains to be restoration of the extensor function and the provision of soft tissue coverage. In the current literature, no data is available considering specifically the demanding situation of soft tissue sarcomas involving the extensor mechanism of the knee. This study aims to highlight the surgical difficulties as well as the oncological and functional results after a resection of the extensor apparatus due to a soft tissue sarcoma.

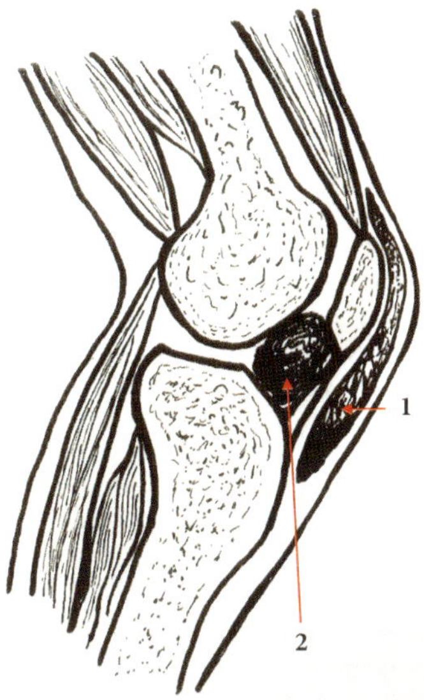

FIGURE 1: *Inclusion criteria of the patients according to the tumor localization.* Schematic illustration of a knee joint (lateral view). The patients were divided into 2 groups according the tumor localization. Patients with a superficially spreading lesion and no joint involvement were included in this study (indicated as number 1). If the tumor site is deep and involves the joint space (indicated as number 2) an extra-articular resection of the knee was performed.

2. Materials and Methods

2.1. Patients. Between 2002 and 2012 17 patients were treated for a soft tissue sarcoma involving the knee extensor apparatus in one institution. We observed mainly two different extension and growth patterns of the tumor (see Figure 1): 11 patients showed an intra-articular expansion of the tumor mass with contamination of the joint cavity, whereas in 6 patients the soft tissue sarcoma has its base on the anterior surface of the extensor mechanism and expands towards the skin. The 11 patients with involvement of the joint space needed an extra-articular knee resection and an allograft prosthetic composite reconstruction as formerly described [6] and were therefore excluded from this study.

All patients ($n = 6$), who have undergone a surgical resection of a soft tissue sarcoma affecting the quadriceps tendon, the patella, and/or the patellar tendon without apparent joint involvement were included in this study. The tumors were adherent and fixed to the underlying extensor mechanism.

These cases were often misdiagnosed as a chronic inflammation process of the prepatellar bursa prior to the referral to our institution. Therefore, all the included patients underwent an inadequate and intralesionally previous surgery before our treatment. The presence of either microscopic (R1) or macroscopic (R2) residual tumor was classified as inadequate resection. The histological diagnosis was based on the primary excision of the tumor. All the external histology samples were ordered and reviewed by the institutional pathology. The detailed characteristics of the included patients are indicated in Table 1.

2.2. Surgical Technique. It must be assumed that tumor cells were implanted in the surrounding tissue after the first inadequate surgery outside. During the reexcision the whole area which is theoretically contaminated should be removed. In all the included cases the previous surgeries were small with short incisions. The presented surgical technique was only performed, if the whole previous surgical area could be removed completely. If this was not possible, an extra-articular resection or an above-knee amputation was considered.

Only in the patient who underwent an arthroscopy the area of the possible iatrogenic spread of tumor cells was difficult to define. As the tumor was outside the joint capsule and not touched by the arthroscopy portals, we considered a limb salvage procedure feasible. However, it is important to bear in mind that a compartmental resection was not achieved in this case with the presented technique. The only remaining alternative surgical option would be an above-knee amputation, which the patient refused categorically.

The crucial criterion for the surgical indication in the presented patients was the absence of tumor involvement of the joint cavity. All the presented patients had an MRI before the initial surgery in the referral hospital. The MRI before and after the initial inadequate surgery were both available and evaluated in our institution. If no effusion was found in the clinical examination and all available MRI revealed no tumor mass deep to the extensor mechanism, we resigned an extra-articular knee resection. Instead, the whole extensor apparatus was resected in its entire length including distal part of quadriceps tendon, patella, and patellar ligament through a midline anterior approach (Figure 2). The quadriceps tendon was spared as much as the tumor expansion allowed. In all patients, a size-matched fresh-frozen nonirradiated allograft harvested from donors younger than 40 years was used to restore the extensor mechanism. The allograft consists of the quadriceps tendon, the patella, the patellar tendon, and the tibia tuberosity. First the allograft bone block of the tuberosity was fixed to the host tibia by screws. Then the allograft quadriceps tendon was sutured to the remaining host tendon and to the medial and lateral edges of the quadriceps muscle in full extension of the knee joint. This important tendon to tendon suture was done by modified Mason Allen stitches [7] with nonabsorbable fibers.

In 5 out of 6 patients, a free or rotational flap was necessary for sufficient soft tissue coverage: a rotational medial gastrocnemius flap was performed in one and a free fasciocutaneous flap (anterolateral thigh flap from the contralateral limb) in 4 patients.

2.3. Surgical Aftercare and Follow-Up. The affected knee was maintained in a plaster splint for 5 weeks. After removal of the splint, patients began active and passive mobilization assisted by a physiotherapist. For the first 5 weeks, an ambulation with 2 crutches and non-weight bearing was allowed. The weight bearing was increased stepwise until full weight bearing was usually achieved 3 months after the surgery. The patients were followed with serial clinical and radiographic examinations of the limb, combined with CT imaging of the chest. For the first 3 months, clinical and radiographic follow-ups were obtained

Table 1: Characteristics of included patients.

Patient number	Diagnosis	Localization	Previous surgery	Margins at previous surgery	Chemotherapy	Radiotherapy	Flap
1	Myxofibrosarcoma	Patella	Inadequate excision	R1	None	Postoperative	Anterolateral thigh, free flap
2	Myxofibrosarcoma (recurrent)	Patellar tendon	Inadequate excision	R1	None	Postoperative	Anterolateral thigh, free flap
3	Pleomorphic sarcoma (recurrent)	Patellar tendon	2 inadequate excisions	R2	Postoperative	Preoperative	Medial gastrocnemius
4	Synovial sarcoma (recurrent)	Patellar tendon	Arthroscopy; 2 inadequate excisions	R2	Pre- and postoperative	None	None
5	Synovial sarcoma	Patella	Inadequate excision	R2	Preoperative	None	Anterolateral thigh, free flap
6	Pleomorphic sarcoma	Patella	Inadequate excision	R1	None	None	Anterolateral thigh, free flap

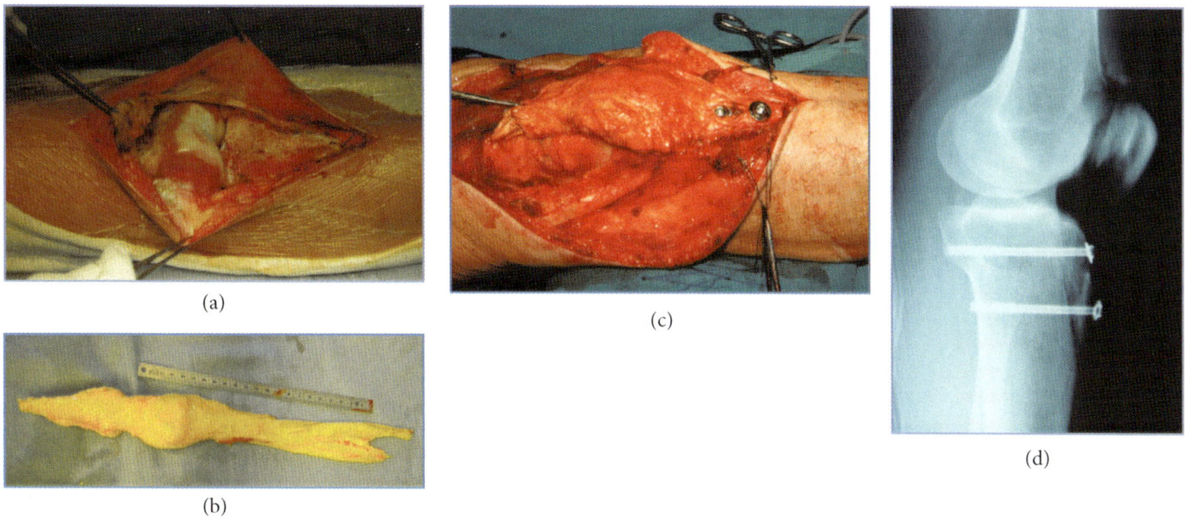

FIGURE 2: *Surgical technique.* Clinical case (patient number 4) as example for the surgical technique used in the described study population. (a) Complete resection of lesion and extensor apparatus; (b) preparation of the osteotendinous allograft; (c) fixation of the allograft with screws distally and direct end-to-end suture proximally; (d) postoperative radiography.

monthly. Afterwards the intervals were extended to 3 months in the first 2 years, 4 months in the 3rd year, 6 months in the 4th, 5th, and 6th years, and finally once a year until the 10th year after the surgery.

2.4. Oncological Treatment. The indication and the sequence of adjuvant therapies such as chemotherapy or irradiation were discussed in a multidisciplinary sarcoma board. Compared to other soft tissue sarcomas, synovial sarcomas are relatively chemosensitive [8]. For this reason, both patients diagnosed with synovial sarcoma received a systemic treatment with doxorubicin and ifosfamide. Patient number 3 had a high grade pleomorphic sarcoma with a high probability of developing metastatic disease. The interdisciplinary board decided to apply a preoperative "prophylactic" chemotherapy and radiation therapy. In patient numbers 1 and 2 the surgical margins were either marginal or tumor-free but "close." These two patients received a postoperative radiation therapy to improve local control.

2.5. Measurements and Statistical Analysis. As indicators for the knee function the active range of motion, active flexion, and extension lag were measured and the International Society of Limb Salvage (ISOLS) score was calculated [4] at the last follow-up.

Survival curves were generated using the Kaplan-Meier method. Statistical analyses were done by the help of the software Stata version 12.1 (Statacorp, College Station TX, USA). P values < 0.05 were considered significant.

3. Results and Discussion

3.1. Results. The mean follow-up was 6.7 years (range: 2–12.4 years). An overview considering the complications of the treatment and oncological outcome is highlighted in Table 2.

3.1.1. Complications. In 2 patients, at least one revision surgery was necessary including 1 patient in whom the allograft had to be removed: Patient number 1 fell on the operated knee 12 years after the surgery and suffered consecutively from an extension deficit. A rupture of the quadriceps tendon was identified at the musculotendinous transition zone. The ruptured tendon was replaced by a new allograft of the extensor apparatus and reinforced by an artificial ligament. The second case who needed a surgical revision (patient number 6) showed a partial necrosis of the primary flap during the first two weeks postoperatively. A secondary coverage was achieved by skin transplantation harvested from the inguinal region.

In one case (patient number 2) a traumatic fracture of the allograft happened 6 years after the surgery, affecting the tibia tuberosity. As the fracture showed no displacement and the integrity of the extensor mechanism was not disturbed, conservative treatment achieved complete healing of the bone.

3.1.2. Functional Results. The different functional outcomes for every patient are indicated in Table 3. On average 24.7 points (range: 19–28 points) were achieved using the ISOLS score. The mean active flexion of the knee joint was 82.5° (range: 25–120°). Patients were suffering from a mean extension lag of 10° (0–30°). Due to this lag, the range of motion averaged with 72.5° (range: 25–100°) lower than the flexion alone. No obvious correlation between the preoperative (all the patients had a ROM of at least 90° and more before the surgery in our institution) and the postoperative function was found. The poor ROM of patient number 6 was due to the difficult soft tissue situation. The primary flap was necrotic and a revision surgery was performed. A complete closure of the surgical field was achieved, but the flexion was restricted because of scar tissue and adhesions.

Table 2: Oncological results and complications.

Patient number	Follow-up (months)	Oncological result	Local recurrence (months)	Metastasis (months)	Complications
1	149	CDF	None	None	Rupture of quadriceps tendon
2	145	NED	27	None	Fracture of tibia tuberosity
3	62	DOD	None	15	None
4	22	DOD	16	17	None
5	76	AWD	None	6	None
6	28	AWD	None	6	Partial necrosis of flap

CDF: continuously disease-free; DOD: dead of disease; AWD: alive with disease; NED: no evidence of disease.

Table 3: Functional results.

Patient number	Follow-up (months)	ISOLS score (points)	Active ROM (degree °)	Active Flexion (degree °)	Extension Lag (degree °)
1	149	28	60	90	30
2	145	19	90	100	10
3	62	28	100	120	20
4	22	23	60	60	0
5	76	24	100	100	0
6	28	26	25	25	0

ROM: range of motion.

3.1.3. Oncological Results. At the last follow-up one patient was disease-free, 2 patients were alive with disease and 2 patients died because of the disease. In one patient no evidence of disease was found after treating a local recurrence. The disease specific 5-year survival of the patients was 62.5% (95% CI: 21.3–89.3%).

The histological examination of the resected tumor revealed 5 wide surgical margins and one case with marginal margins. In all patients, residual tumor cells were found in the reexcision samples. Especially in the deep surface against the extensor mechanism the margins were all inadequate, probably because the previous surgeons were afraid to injure the patellar ligament.

The patient with marginal margins had a local recurrence after 16 months. Furthermore, one local recurrence occurred after an adequate surgery with wide margins. As shown in Figure 3 the 5-year local recurrence-free rate is 66.7% (95% CI: 19.5%–90.4%). Distant metastases were found in 4 patients resulting in a 5-year metastasis-free rate of 33.3% (95% CI: 4.6%–67.5%).

The effect of the applied radiotherapy for local control and the chemotherapy for systemic disease was not measurable as the numbers are too small and the histologic types of the sarcomas are too heterogeneous. The radiation therapy was applied as planned with the favored dose in all 3 patients concerned. As the tumors were all superficial, skin reactions were common. But no complication due to the radiation therapy was observed.

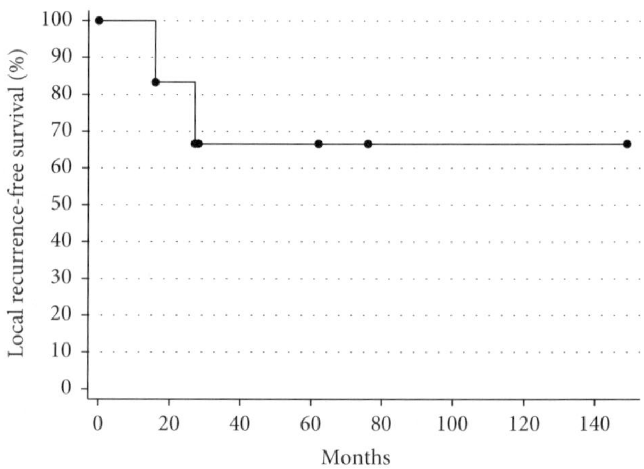

Figure 3: *Local recurrence-free survival curve.* Kaplan-Meier curve for local recurrence-free survival.

3.2. Discussion. A soft tissue sarcoma of the extensor mechanism poses a particularly demanding surgical situation. The oncologic surgeon does handle the difficulties not only to achieve adequate margins in a surgical field of sparse soft tissue coverage, but also to reconstruct the extensor mechanism providing good functional results.

The aim of the study was to evaluate the (1) complications, (2) functional outcome, and (3) oncological results in patients suffering from a soft tissue sarcoma of the knee extensor mechanism with absence of joint invasion.

3.2.1. Limitations. Our presented case series has some limitations. First, as with other series dealing with reconstruction of the knee extensor mechanism, the number of included patients is small, although relatively large compared to the available studies in the literature. Second, our series of tumors was heterogeneous for type, stage, and adjuvant treatment.

These variables certainly affect rates of survival but not whether adequate margins or restored function was achieved. Third, different procedures for soft tissue coverage were performed, according to the case-specific situation.

3.2.2. Reconstruction Technique. The use of an allograft extensor mechanism proved to be a valid strategy for the reconstruction. The presented technique is mainly for primary tumors without any previous surgery. These are the preferred conditions for an oncological correct resection providing the best local control. Experience in using an allograft extensor mechanism in the tumor setting is lacking completely in literature. Although in a nononcological setting (major revision in total knee arthroplasties), previous reports confirm the safety and functionality of the reconstructive procedure [2, 9–12]. Our functional results regarding active range of motion, active flexion, and extension lag are consistent with these series [2, 9, 10, 12]. There is only one existing case study which can be compared to our results. Imanishi et al. described 4 cases [5] in whom the patellar tendon was resected due to a soft tissue sarcoma. The patellar tendon was reconstructed with a bone-tendon-bone allograft and fixed by wires and screws to the residual patella and tibia tuberosity. This technique presupposes the preservation of the quadriceps tendon together with some residual patella. In all our patients this would have led to inadequate excision of the tumor. The functional results were excellent in the series of Imanishi et al. [5] as all patients achieved virtually full range of motion and 28–30 points in the MSTS score. The difference to our results probably lies in the extent of the resection. All of our patients had to undergo a complete resection of the previous surgical area. In addition to the defect of the extensor mechanism, large soft tissue defects resulted. The need of extensive resections certainly has a negative influence on the functional outcome.

Different alternative reconstructions were previously described in the oncologic setting. As substitute for the patellar tendon a fascia lata graft [3, 13], autologous achilles tendon [14], or hamstring tendon grafts [15, 16], as well as a latissimus dorsi flap [17], were proposed. In contrast to all these case reports Muramatsu et al. [18] described a complete resection of the extensor apparatus including quadriceps tendon, patella, and patellar tendon. After treating the resected specimen with liquid nitrogen intraoperatively, the extensor mechanism was reimplanted as recycled autograft. We have some reservations concerning this recycled autograft technique, as in our opinion the oncologic safety is questionable.

3.2.3. Complication Rate. In our presented reconstruction technique, the short- and long-term morbidity rates were acceptable for tumors, which widely involved the knee. No deep infection was observed. Possible explanation is the use of an aggressive perioperative antibiotic prophylaxis. Two of the three complications were attributed to the allograft: one allograft fracture and one rupture of the quadriceps tendon. The fracture was treated conservatively, meaning that a total of one allograft (16.7%) needed to be surgically revised. This is slightly higher than previous reported case in revision surgeries of failed extensor mechanism due to total knee arthroplasties [19]. Fracture and rupture of the allograft both occurred late in clinical course and had clear traumatic reason. Assuming the healing was complete after this time, the complications are hardly attributable to the reconstruction technique. Nevertheless, Imanishi et al. [5] observed a fracture of the allograft, too. So, the structural weakness of the allograft substitute seems to be the major reason for failure.

3.2.4. Oncologic Outcome. The residual tumor and the whole area of the previous surgery were removed in one piece allowing a reliable histological work-up. In all the included patients an above-knee amputation was a valid option. In general, the safety of tumor removal must always be weighed against the remaining limb function. In all the presented patients we decided against an amputation after a comprehensive discussion.

However, it is not clear whether amputation would have improved the oncological result. The metastatic rate cannot be influenced by local measures and depends mainly on size and histologic grading of the tumor [20]. Regarding the local recurrence current studies showed that the outcome is worse if an unplanned excision in a nononcological setting was done prior to the referral in a tertiary sarcoma center, independent of the anatomical location [21–23].

The oncological outcome is difficult to compare with other series in the literature as no specific results for the extensor mechanism are available and the prognostic among soft tissue sarcomas varies widely according to histologic type, grade size, and location [24–27]. Local recurrence rates after radiation and resection have been reported as high as 20% [28]; however most recent series report number at 10% or less [24, 25, 29]. In overall, our local recurrence rate seems to be much higher compared to other localizations. All patients have undergone an inadequate previous surgery before the referral to our tertiary care center. Because of the superficial location of the lesions and the proximity to the prepatellar bursa, they were all misdiagnosed as benign tumors or chronic bursitis. An unplanned excision of soft tissue sarcomas or an inadequate biopsy is associated with a poor local control [21–23]. At least in our series, unplanned resections of soft tissue sarcomas before a correct diagnosis seem to pose a serious problem around the knee joint. One patient had even undergone an arthroscopy before the sarcoma diagnosis. Although the arthroscopic procedure was independent of the tumor excision, there is still the risk of wide spreading of tumor cells through the used liquid. At the time of the reexcision in our institution no evidence for joint involvement was found but the decision for a joint-preserving resection remains debatable in this situation. Unfortunately, a local recurrence occurred indeed, and the patient died from the disease due to systemic metastasis.

A recent published case study reported similar oncologic problems: 3 out 4 patients included in their series had an unplanned excision of a sarcoma affecting the patellar tendon [5]. But, the present case series is inhomogeneous with respect to former surgery and the potential contamination status before the index operation in our institution. This may additionally cause the bias of high local recurrence rates.

4. Conclusions

In summary, the treatment of soft tissue sarcoma involving the extensor apparatus of the knee is associated with a high rate of previous inadequate surgeries and high local recurrence and metastatic rates. The replacement of the extensor mechanism by an allograft is a reasonable option, allowing wide margins and restoration of active extension in most patients.

References

[1] P. M. Picci, N. Fabbri, M. Gambarotti, and D. Vanel, *Atlas of Musculoskeletal Tumors and Tumorlike Lesions*, Springer International Publishing, 1st edition, 2014.

[2] N. Maffulli, F. Spiezia, L. La Verde, M. A. Rosa, and F. Franceschi, "The management of extensor mechanism disruption after total Knee Arthroplasty: A systematic review," *Sports Medicine and Arthroscopy Review*, vol. 25, no. 1, pp. 41–50, 2017.

[3] J. Chahla, N. N. DePhillipo, M. E. Cinque et al., "Open Repair of Quadriceps Tendon With Suture Anchors and Semitendinosus Tendon Allograft Augmentation," *Arthroscopy Techniques*, 2017.

[4] G. M. Hobusch, P. T. Funovics, C. Hourscht et al., "Erratum to "LARS® band and tube for extensor mechanism reconstructions in proximal tibial modular endoprostheses after bone tumors" (The Knee (2016) 23(5) (905–910) (S0968016016300060) (10.1016/j.knee.2016.04.002))," *The Knee*, vol. 23, no. 6, p. 1173, 2016.

[5] J. Imanishi, D. Grinsell, and P. F. M. Choong, "Bone-patellar tendon-bone allograft reconstruction for peri-patellar tendon sarcomas: case series," *SpringerPlus*, vol. 4, no. 1, article no. 740, pp. 1–7, 2015.

[6] R. Capanna, G. Scoccianti, D. A. Campanacci, G. Beltrami, and P. De Biase, "Surgical technique: Extraarticular knee resection with prosthesis-proximal tibia-extensor apparatus allograft for tumors invading the knee," *Clinical Orthopaedics and Related Research*, vol. 469, no. 10, pp. 2905–2914, 2011.

[7] C. Gerber, A. G. Schneeberger, M. Beck, and U. Schlegel, "Mechanical strength of repairs of the rotator cuff," *The Journal of Bone & Joint Surgery—British Volume*, vol. 76, no. 3, pp. 371–380, 1994.

[8] I. M. Desar, E. D. Fleuren, and W. T. van der Graaf, "Systemic Treatment for Adults with Synovial Sarcoma," *Current Treatment Options in Oncology*, vol. 19, no. 2, 2018.

[9] R. S. J. Burnett, R. A. Berger, W. G. Paprosky, C. J. D. Valle, J. J. Jacobs, and A. G. Rosenberg, "Extensor mechanism allograft reconstruction after total knee arthroplasty: a comparison of two techniques," *The Journal of Bone & Joint Surgery*, vol. 86, no. 12, pp. 2694–2699, 2004.

[10] D. G. Nazarian and R. E. Booth, "Extensor Mechanism Allografts in Total Knee Arthroplasty," *Clinical Orthopaedics and Related Research*, vol. 367, pp. 123–129, 1999.

[11] B. D. Springer and C. J. Della Valle, "Extensor Mechanism Allograft Reconstruction After Total Knee Arthroplasty," *The Journal of Arthroplasty*, vol. 23, no. 7, pp. 35–38, 2008.

[12] C. T. Lim, D. F. Amanatullah, J. I. Huddleston et al., "Reconstruction of Disrupted Extensor Mechanism After Total Knee Arthroplasty," *The Journal of Arthroplasty*, vol. 32, no. 10, pp. 3134–3140, 2017.

[13] H. Nakashima, M. Yoshida, and K. Miyamoto, "Anatomical reconstruction of the patellar tendon using the fascia lata attached to the iliac bone following resection for soft tissue sarcoma: A case report," *Upsala Journal of Medical Sciences*, vol. 117, no. 4, pp. 460–464, 2012.

[14] T. Osanai, T. Tsuchiya, and T. Ogino, "Gastrocnemius muscle flap including Achilles tendon after extensive patellectomy for soft tissue sarcoma," *Journal of Plastic Surgery and Hand Surgery*, vol. 42, no. 3, pp. 161–163, 2008.

[15] N. Fukui, N. Cho C., T. Tashiro, and K. Nakamura, "Anatomical reconstruction of the patellar tendon: A new technique with hamstring tendons and iliotibial tract," *Journal of Orthopaedic Trauma*, vol. 13, no. 5, pp. 375–379, 1999.

[16] A. B. Peyser and J. T. Makley, "Patellar tendon reconstruction augmented by a free autograft of the biceps tendon attached to the fibular head," *Orthopedics*, vol. 19, no. 6, pp. 545–549, 1996.

[17] H.-G. Machens, F. Siemers, M. Kaun et al., "Patellar tendon reconstruction using a free latissimus dorsi flap following resection of a prepatellar myxofibrosarcoma: Case report," *Journal of Reconstructive Microsurgery*, vol. 21, no. 4, pp. 235–238, 2005.

[18] K. Muramatsu, K. Yoshida, K. Fujii, T. Okazaki, A. Moriya, and T. Toshihiko, "Anatomical reconstruction of the knee extensor apparatus for prepatellar myxofibrosarcoma," *Orthopedics*, vol. 33, no. 10, 2010.

[19] N. M. Brown, T. Murray, S. M. Sporer, N. Wetters, R. A. Berger, and C. J. Della Valle, "Extensor mechanism allograft reconstruction for extensor mechanism failure following total knee arthroplasty," *Journal of Bone and Joint Surgery - American Volume*, vol. 97, no. 4, pp. 279–283, 2015.

[20] M. W. Kattan, D. H. Y. Leung, and M. F. Brennan, "Postoperative nomogram for 12-year sarcoma-specific death," *Journal of Clinical Oncology*, vol. 20, no. 3, pp. 791–796, 2002.

[21] M. A. Smolle, P.-U. Tunn, E. Goldenitsch et al., "The Prognostic Impact of Unplanned Excisions in a Cohort of 728 Soft Tissue Sarcoma Patients: A Multicentre Study," *Annals of Surgical Oncology*, vol. 24, no. 6, pp. 1596–1605, 2017.

[22] G. Bianchi, A. Sambri, S. Cammelli et al., "Impact of residual disease after "unplanned excision" of primary localized adult soft tissue sarcoma of the extremities: evaluation of 452 cases at a single Institution," *Musculoskeletal Surgery*, vol. 101, no. 3, pp. 243–248, 2017.

[23] J. Pretell-Mazzini, M. D. Barton, S. A. Conway, and H. T. Temple, "Current concepts review—unplanned excision of soft-tissue sarcomas: current concepts for management and prognosis," *The Journal of Bone & Joint Surgery—American Volume*, vol. 97, no. 7, pp. 597–603, 2015.

[24] K. R. Gundle, L. Kafchinski, S. Gupta et al., "Analysis of Margin Classification Systems for Assessing the Risk of Local Recurrence After Soft Tissue Sarcoma Resection," *Journal of Clinical Oncology*, vol. 36, no. 7, pp. 704–709, 2018.

[25] W. M. Guerrero and J. L. Deneve, "Local Recurrence of Extremity Soft Tissue Sarcoma," *Surgical Clinics of North America*, vol. 96, no. 5, pp. 1157–1174, 2016.

[26] K. Maretty-Nielsen, N. Aggerholm-Pedersen, A. Safwat et al., "Prognostic factors for local recurrence and mortality in adult soft tissue sarcoma of the extremities and trunk wall," *Acta Orthopaedica*, vol. 85, no. 3, pp. 323–332, 2014.

[27] L. Cai, R.-O. Mirimanoff, E. Mouhsine et al., "Prognostic factors in adult soft tissue sarcoma treated with surgery combined

with radiotherapy: A retrospective single-center study on 164 patients," *Rare Tumors*, vol. 5, no. 4, article no. e55, pp. 178–182, 2013.

[28] G. K. Zagars, M. T. Ballo, P. W. T. Pisters et al., "Prognostic factors for patients with localized soft-tissue sarcoma treated with conservation surgery and radiation therapy: an analysis of 1225 patients," *Cancer*, vol. 97, no. 10, pp. 2530–2543, 2003.

[29] D. A. Müller, G. Beltrami, G. Scoccianti, F. Frenos, and R. Capanna, "Combining limb-sparing surgery with radiation therapy in high-grade soft tissue sarcoma of extremities – Is it effective?" *European Journal of Surgical Oncology*, vol. 42, no. 7, pp. 1057–1063, 2016.

Clinical and Radiological Outcomes of Extracorporeal Shock Wave Therapy in Early-Stage Femoral Head Osteonecrosis

Abdulrahman D. Algarni[1] **and Hassan M. Al Moallem**[2]

[1]*Department of Orthopedic Surgery, King Saud University, Riyadh, Saudi Arabia*
[2]*Department of Surgery, Prince Mohammed Bin Abdulaziz Hospital, Riyadh, Saudi Arabia*

Correspondence should be addressed to Abdulrahman D. Algarni; abdulrahmanga@gmail.com

Academic Editor: Panagiotis Korovessis

Objective. Femoral head osteonecrosis is a progressive clinical condition with significant morbidity and long-term disability. Several treatment modalities including both surgical and nonsurgical options have been used with variable levels of success. High-energy extracorporeal shock wave therapy is a nonoperative treatment option that has been described for early-stage disease. We aimed to assess the functional and radiological outcomes of extracorporeal shockwave therapy (ESWT) in the treatment of osteonecrosis of the femoral head (ONFH). *Methods.* Thirty-three hips of 21 patients were included in this study. Adult patients with ONFH of any etiology and in the precollapse stage were included. Clinical (visual analogue scale [VAS] and Harris hip score [HHS]) and radiological (plain radiographs and magnetic resonance imaging [MRI]) evaluations were performed before and after intervention. We used 3000–4500 pulses in a single session performed under general anesthesia. *Results.* At an average of 8 months after ESWT, pain scores and HHS were significantly improved compared with the preintervention scores ($p<0.001$). The overall clinical outcomes were improved in 21 hips (63.3%), unchanged in 5 hips (15.15%), and worsened in 7 hips (21.2%). A trend toward a decrease in the size of the ONFH was observed although not of clinical significance ($p=0.235$). MRI revealed significant resolution of bone marrow edema ($p<0.003$). Regression was observed in 9 lesions (42.9%) and progression in 1 lesion (4.7%); no change was observed in the remaining 23 lesions (52.4%). *Conclusion.* ESWT is a viable noninvasive treatment option for early-stage ONFH. It significantly improves clinical outcomes and may halt or delay the radiographic progression of the disease in the precollapse stage.

1. Introduction

Osteonecrosis of the femoral head (ONFH) was originally described in 1925 as an ischemic necrosis of the hip area [1]. ONFH can affect any joint but most commonly occurs in the hip joint. Its pathology is poorly understood; however, it is known to decrease blood flow to the femoral head leading to cellular death, fractures, and collapse of the articular surface [2, 3].

ONFH is a multifactorial disease with different etiologies ranging from genetic to idiopathic to certain risk factors such as trauma, hematological disorders, and steroid intake [4]. Such pathology is frequently observed in relatively young adults, and most of the untreated patients with ONFH progress to total hip arthroplasty (THA) with a collapse rate of 67% and 85% in asymptomatic and symptomatic patients, respectively [5].

Although the optimal management protocol for patients in the precollapse stage remains unestablished, early intervention before collapse is critical for a successful outcome [1, 5]. High-energy extracorporeal shock wave therapy (ESWT) is a noninvasive procedure that has been successfully used for the last 20 years to manage various orthopedic conditions [6]. ESWT is a sound wave with high pressure and velocity that forms precipitation on the interface between soft tissue and bone [3]. The positive effect of ESWT has been attributed to the reflection and precipitation of shock waves. Multiple studies have demonstrated the therapeutic potential of ESWT in ONFH [7, 8].

Table 1: Patient demographic characteristics.

Variable	Values
Patients/hips (no.)	21 (33)
Age∗ (years)	37.5 ± 4.8 (21-54)
Male/female (no. of patients)	9/12
Right/left (no. of hips)	14/19
Bilateral disease (no. of patients)	12
Duration of symptoms∗ (months)	6 ± 3 (3-9)
ARCO grade (no. of patients/hips)	
Grade-I	4/5
Grade-II	17/28
Medical history (no. of patients/hips)	
Sickle cell disease	11/18
Systemic lupus erythematosus	2/3
Steroid intake	3/3
History of trauma	3/5
Idiopathic	2/4
Length of follow-up∗ (years)	5 ± 3.5 (2-9)

∗The values are given as the mean and standard deviation with the range in parentheses. ARCO: the Association Research Circulation Osseous.

In this study, we aimed to assess the short-term clinical and radiological outcomes of ESWT in patients with early-stage ONFH.

2. Patients and Methods

The institutional review board of our hospital approved this study. Between September 2006 and September 2011, all patients who presented to our institution and met the inclusion criteria were enrolled in this study. Each patient provided informed consent before participating in the study. Adult patients with ONFH due to any etiology in the precollapse stage, grades I or II according to the Association Research Circulation Osseous (ARCO) classification system, were included in this study. Immunocompromised patients and patients with a history of infection were excluded. The patient demographics are summarized in Table 1.

The evaluation parameters before and after intervention included clinical assessment of pain with a visual analog scale (VAS), where 0 indicated no pain and 10 indicated severe pain, and assessment of function, activity, and motion of the hip using Harris hip score (HHS). Anteroposterior and lateral plain radiographs were obtained before ESWT; at 3, 6, and 12 months after ESWT; and once a year subsequently. Plain radiographs of the hip were used to assess the size of the lesion, the extent of subchondral bone collapse, and the presence of degenerative changes in the hip joint. Magnetic resonance imaging (MRI) was performed before ESWT, at 6 and 12 months after ESWT, and then once a year. These images were used to evaluate bone marrow edema, the size of the lesion, femoral head congruency, the presence of a crescent sign, and degenerative changes in the hip joint. Plain radiographs and MRI images were evaluated by a senior musculoskeletal radiologist who was blinded to the nature of the treatment.

The clinical outcome was defined as "improved" if the patient had ≥50% improvement in VAS and HHS scores, "unchanged" if the patient had <50% improvement in VAS and HHS scores, and "worse" if the patient experienced more severe hip pain and had further restricted hip function than that before intervention [9].

2.1. Treatment Protocol. We used the shock wave device OssaTron (HMT High Medical Technologies AG, Switzerland) with a therapy head capable of 350° rotation. After preparing the therapy apparatus and fixing the limb of the affected hip in adduction and internal rotation, ONFH was marked using fluoroscopy in 2–3 points depending on the size of the lesion. We used 3000–4500 pulses (1500 pulses of shock waves for each point); frequency was set at 4/s at 26 kV in a single session, performed with the patient under general anesthesia. The femoral artery was palpated before and after treatment, and lidocaine gel was applied to the skin to maximize shock wave penetration. Local complications such as formation of hematoma, petechial hemorrhage, swelling, deep vein thrombosis, and superficial infection were all recorded.

After the shock wave treatment, the patients were instructed to walk on crutches with non-weight-bearing on the affected extremity for 6 weeks. Follow-up at the outpatient department was performed at 6 weeks, once every 3 months, and then once a year for a minimum of 2 years.

Statistical analysis was performed with SPSS statistical software version 22 (IBM Corp., Armonk, NY, USA). The Student's t-test was used to compare the pre- and postintervention values of VAS and HHS scores. The outcome end points were clinical improvement and conversion to THA. Statistical significance was based on 2-sided p values <0.05.

3. Results

Twenty-three patients met our inclusion criteria; of those, 1 patient was excluded owing to inadequate documentation, and 1 patient was lost to follow-up. A total of 21 patients comprising 33 hips with ONFH were included. The average follow-up was 5 years (range, 2–9 years).

At an average of 8 months after ESWT, pain scores and HHS were significantly improved compared with the preintervention scores ($p<0.001$). The values of VAS and HHS before and after ESWT are summarized in Table 2. The overall clinical outcomes after ESWT are summarized in Table 3. Improvement was seen in 21 hips (63.3%), whereas no change was seen in 5 hips (15.15%) and 7 hips (21.2%) worsened. At the most recent follow-up, 4 hips were converted to THA as their symptoms had deteriorated at an average of 3.7 years after ESWT (range, 2–8 years).

The changes on plain radiographs and MRIs before and after ESWT are summarized in Table 4. Although a trend toward a decrease in the size of the ONFH after ESWT compared with the preintervention size was seen, it was not clinically significant ($p=0.23$). On plain radiographs, 2 lesions (6.06%) showed improvement and 5 lesions (15.1%) showed progression. No change was seen in the remaining 26 lesions (78.78%). MRI showed regression of 9 lesions (42.9%; 7 of

Table 2: The VAS and Harris hip scores before and after ESWT.

Variable	Before ESWT	After ESWT (months) 3	6	12	24
VAS*	6.7 ± 2.1 (3-9)	2.4 ± 2.2 (0-5)	1.3 ± 1.2 (0-4)	0.5 ± 0.4 (0-2)	0.8 ± 1.1 (0-3)
P-value		<0.001	<0.001	<0.001	<0.001
HSS*	73.2 ± 9.8 (53-89)	88.7 ± 7.1 (62-100)	91.7 ± 7.8 (65-100)	97.2 ± 2.2 (72-100)	96.7 ± 3.1 (73-100)
P-value		<0.001	<0.001	<0.001	<0.001

* The values are given as the mean and standard deviation with the range in parentheses. VAS: visual analog scale; ESWT: extracorporeal shock wave therapy; and HSS = Harris hip score.

Table 3: The overall clinical outcomes after ESWT.

Clinical outcome	ARCO grade-I ($n = 5$ hips) no. (%)	ARCO grade-II ($n = 28$ hips) no. (%)	Total series ($n = 33$ hips) no. (%)
Improved	4 (80%)	17 (60.7%)	21 (63.3%)
Unchanged	1 (20%)	4 (14.3%)	5 (15.15%)
Worse	0 (0%)	7 (25%)	7 (21.2%)
Total hip arthroplasty	0 (0%)	4 (14.3%)	4 (12.1%)

ESWT: extracorporeal shock wave therapy; ARCO: the Association Research Circulation Osseous.

Table 4: Changes on plain radiographs and MRI images before and after ESWT.

Variable	Before ESWT	After ESWT	P-value
Size of ONFH* (%)	59 ± 32 (5-76)	28 ± 16 (0-63)	0.235
Bone marrow edema			
Grade 0	3	20	
Grade 1	9	9	
Grade 2	16	4	0.003
Grade 3	3	0	
Grade 4	2	0	

*The values, given as the mean and standard deviation with the range in parentheses, represent the percentage of the involved area of the femoral head. ESWT: extracorporeal shockwave therapy; ONFH = osteonecrosis of the femoral head.

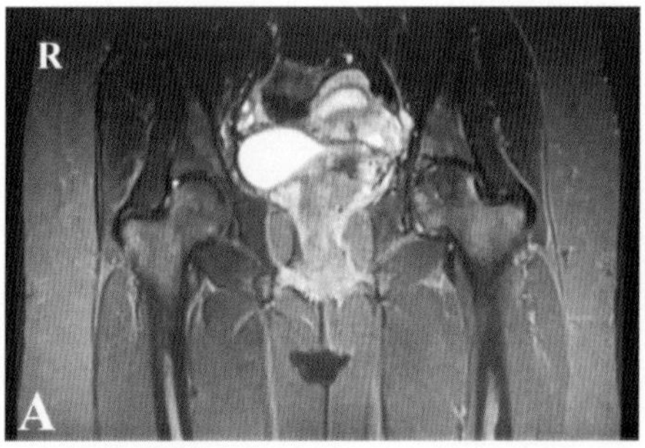

(a)

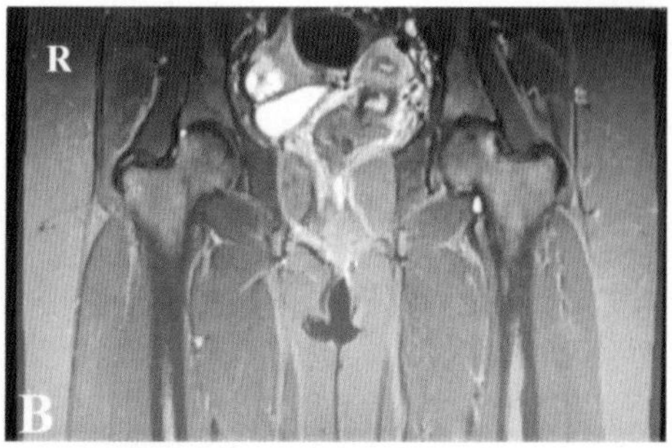

(b)

Figure 1: T1-weighted MRI image showing grade II ONFH of the left hip before ESWT (a). The lesion regressed to grade I at 2-year follow-up after ESWT (b).

grade II and 2 of grade I) and progression of 1 lesion (4.7%; of grade II to III). The remaining 23 lesions (52.4%) showed no change (Figure 1). MRI revealed a significant overall improvement of bone marrow edema (p<0.003) after ESWT compared with the preintervention images. Bone marrow edema decreased among patients from grades 3–4 to 2–1 after ESWT (grade 0 stands for no bone marrow edema, 1 for perinecrotic bone marrow edema, 2 for bone marrow edema extended into the femoral head, 3 for bone marrow edema extended into the neck of the femur, and 4 for bone marrow edema extended into the inter-trochanteric region) [10].

There was no difference in clinical or radiological outcomes according to the etiology of the ONFH. No major complications were seen. Nine hips (27.3%) developed device-related petechial hemorrhage in the groin at the site of ESWT application that spontaneously resolved in few days.

4. Discussion

Management of ONFH depends on the stage of the disease. For an early-stage disease (grade I and II), before subchondral collapse, both conservative and surgical treatment options have been described. Among the different femoral head preservation procedures (core decompression, muscle-pedicle grafting, and derotational osteotomy), core decompression with bone grafting is considered the gold standard surgical option [11]. Similarly, various conservative treatment modalities have been proposed in the literature as a standalone treatment or in combination with each other [12] These include restriction of weight-bearing, pharmacologic agents (bisphosphonates, low-molecular-weight heparin, statins, and prostaglandins), and biophysical modalities (hyperbaric oxygen, ESWT, and pulsed electromagnetic field therapy) [13]. Lack of sufficient evidence precludes strongly recommending a certain type of conservative treatment in early-stage ONFH; however, the existing evidence favors ESWT [1, 12]. Weight-bearing restriction alone is insufficient; evidence recommending pharmacologic agents is limited, and they have potential side effects. Remaining biophysical modalities (hyperbaric oxygen and pulsed electromagnetic field therapy) have both limited availability and high cost [11–13]. Conservative treatment may be a major focus for orthopedic studies in the future to determine which modality carries the best cost-benefit ratio to establish a standard of care for the treatment of ONFH. Regardless of the selected treatment method, the aim is to improve quality of life, prevent femoral head collapse, improve the speed and quality of repair at the molecular level, and avoid surgical intervention, if possible. The results of this study show that ESWT could help and improve the clinical outcome and possibly cease or retard the progression of the disease eventually.

ESWT is an effective therapeutic option for ONFH, particularly for early-stage disease [7, 8, 14–19]. At grade III and beyond, it is a less viable treatment option [12]. Only few studies with an objective similar to our study exist in the literature [14–17]. Most existing studies highlight the improvement in pain and function, while radiological results varied among these studies. The clinical improvement seen in our study is similar to that reported in previous studies [14, 15]. Although the findings of this study are in agreement with those of other studies with regard to lesion regression after ESWT as seen on MRI, conflicting evidence also exists, mandating further research in this regard [18, 19]. In fact, most studies, including our study, included a small patient population and had limitations such as being uncontrolled and not blinded, which precludes drawing a definitive conclusion. However, evidence indicates that ESWT can resolve bone marrow edema and at least halt disease progression. In the present study, patients had similar clinical and radiographic outcomes regardless of the etiology of ONFH. This finding is consistent with reports by other authors [14, 20].

The exact mechanism of action of ESWT remains unknown. Experimental animal studies demonstrated a significant increase in the ingrowth of neovascularization associated with increased expressions of angiogenic growth indicators in tendon, bone, and tendon-bone interface, which might play a role in the improvement of blood supply and healing, which in turn can improve subchondral bone remodeling and prevent femoral head collapse [21–23]. A close relationship between the decrease of substance P release and consecutive pain reduction after shock wave treatment has also been reported [24–26]. Based on these findings, we can argue that the enhanced angiogenic and osteogenic mechanisms together with hyperstimulation analgesia might play a role in the improvement of blood supply to the femoral head and promotion of bone regeneration.

Reports suggest that although ESWT is an effective standalone treatment modality, combining it with other conservative modalities does not improve its curative benefit [18, 27]. Wang et al. [28] compared the outcomes of ESWT alone and in combination with alendronate in 2 randomly distributed groups. The authors found that clinical outcomes were improved in 83% and 77% of the patients in the ESWT alone group and the combined group, respectively. They concluded that ESWT is an effective treatment with or without the concurrent use of alendronate. Similarly, Hsu et al. [29] have compared the outcomes of ESWT alone and as part of a cocktail treatment consisting of ESWT, hyperbaric oxygen, and alendronate. The authors reported improvement in 79.2% of the patients in the ESWT group, without a significant difference between both groups. In the current study, the therapeutic effect of ESWT, as a conservative treatment, is comparable to that reported following femoral head core decompression for early-stage ONFH. Sen et al. [30] reported a success rate of 63.5% in their series of femoral head core decompression for ONFH. Furthermore, Wang et al. [16] reported even better long-term outcomes with ESWT than with core decompression and bone grafting for early-stage ONFH.

This study has limitations inherent to a retrospective cohort study. Other limitations include the small sample size and the lack of a control group for comparison.

5. Conclusion

ESWT is a safe, noninvasive treatment method for ONFH. It helped to improve clinical outcomes in our patients and may delay the radiographic progression in early-stage disease and therefore mitigate the need for surgery. It is a suitable treatment option to be considered, particularly in the precollapse stage of the disease. Further studies are required to validate the long-term and sustained effects of ESWT in ONFH.

Disclosure

The study was self-funded by the authors.

Authors' Contributions

All authors have made substantial contributions to the study and the manuscript.

References

[1] J. Moya-Angeler, A. L. Gianakos, J. C. Villa, A. Ni, and J. M. Lane, "Current concepts on osteonecrosis of the femoral head," *World Journal of Orthopedics*, vol. 6, no. 8, pp. 590–601, 2015.

[2] F. Mwale, H. Wang, A. J. Johnson, M. A. Mont, and J. Antoniou, "Abnormal vascular endothelial growth factor expression in mesenchymal stem cells from both osteonecrotic and osteoarthritic hips," *Bulletin of the NYU Hospital for Joint Diseases*, vol. 69, no. 1, pp. S56–S61, 2011.

[3] K. Ohzono, K. Takaoka, S. Saito, M. Saito, M. Matsui, and K. Ono, "Intraosseous arterial architecture in nontraumatic avascular necrosis of the femoral head: microangiographic and histologic study," *Clinical Orthopaedics and Related Research*, vol. 277, pp. 79–88, 1992.

[4] A. J. Johnson, M. A. Mont, A. K. Tsao, and L. C. Jones, "Treatment of femoral head osteonecrosis in the United States: 16-year analysis of the nationwide inpatient sample," *Clinical Orthopaedics and Related Research*, vol. 472, no. 2, pp. 617–623, 2014.

[5] C. Wang, J. Peng, and S. Lu, "Summary of the various treatments for osteonecrosis of the femoral head by mechanism: A review," *Experimental and Therapeutic Medicine*, vol. 8, no. 3, pp. 700–706, 2014.

[6] C. Schmitz, N. B. M. Császár, S. Milz et al., "Efficacy and safety of extracorporeal shock wave therapy for orthopedic conditions: a systematic review on studies listed in the PEDro database," *British Medical Bulletin*, vol. 116, no. 1, pp. 115–138, 2015.

[7] J. Ludwig, S. Lauber, H.-J. Lauber, U. Dreisilker, R. Raedel, and H. Hotzinger, "High-energy shock wave treatment of femoral head necrosis in adults," *Clinical Orthopaedics and Related Research*, no. 387, pp. 119–126, 2001.

[8] C.-J. Wang, J.-H. Cheng, C.-C. Huang, H.-K. Yip, and S. Russo, "Extracorporeal shockwave therapy for avascular necrosis of femoral head," *International Journal of Surgery*, vol. 24, pp. 184–187, 2015.

[9] J. M. van der Waal, C. B. Terwee, D. A. W. M. van der Windt, L. M. Bouter, and J. Dekker, "The impact of non-traumatic hip and knee disorders on health-related quality of life as measured with the SF-36 or SF-12. A systematic review," *Quality of Life Research*, vol. 14, no. 4, pp. 1141–1155, 2005.

[10] S. Russo, F. Sadile, R. Esposito et al., "Italian experience on use of E.S.W. therapy for avascular necrosis of femoral head," *International Journal of Surgery*, vol. 24, pp. 188–190, 2015.

[11] R. Klumpp and C. Trevisan, "Aseptic osteonecrosis of the hip in the adult: Current evidence on conservative treatment," *Clinical Cases in Mineral and Bone Metabolism*, vol. 12, pp. 39–42, 2015.

[12] F. Osmani, S. Thakkar, and J. Vigdorchik, "The utility of conservative treatment modalities in the management of osteonecrosis: A systematic review," *Bulletin of the Hospital for Joint Diseases*, vol. 75, no. 3, pp. 186–192, 2017.

[13] D. Kusz, A. Franek, R. Wilk et al., "The effects of treatment the avascular necrosis of the femoral head with extracorporeal focused shockwave therapy. preliminary report," *Ortopedia Traumatologia Rehabilitacja*, vol. 14, no. 5, pp. 435–442, 2012.

[14] F. Gao, W. Sun, Z. Li et al., "High-Energy Extracorporeal Shock Wave for Early Stage Osteonecrosis of the Femoral Head: A Single-Center Case Series," *Evidence-Based Complementary and Alternative Medicine*, vol. 2015, 2015.

[15] C.-J. Wang, F.-S. Wang, C.-C. Huang, K. D. Yang, L.-H. Weng, and H.-Y. Huang, "Treatment for osteonecrosis of the femoral head: comparison of extracorporeal shock waves with core decompression and bone-grafting," *The Journal of Bone and Joint Surgery—American Volume*, vol. 87, no. 11, pp. 2380–2387, 2005.

[16] C.-J. Wang, C.-C. Huang, J.-W. Wang, T. Wong, and Y.-J. Yang, "Long-term results of extracorporeal shockwave therapy and core decompression in osteonecrosis of the femoral head with eight- to nine-year follow-up," *Biomedical Journal*, vol. 35, no. 6, pp. 481–485, 2012.

[17] J. Y. Lee, J. W. Kwon, J. S. Park et al., "Osteonecrosis of Femoral Head Treated with Extracorporeal Shock Wave Therapy: Analysis of Short-term Clinical Outcomes of Treatment with Radiologic Staging," in *Hip & pelvis*, pp. 250–257, 2015.

[18] M. C. Vulpiani, M. Vetrano, D. Trischitta et al., "Extracorporeal shock wave therapy in early osteonecrosis of the femoral head: prospective clinical study with long-term follow-up," *Archives of Orthopaedic and Trauma Surgery*, vol. 132, no. 4, pp. 499–508, 2012.

[19] Q. Zhang, L. Liu, W. Sun, F. Gao, L. Cheng, and Z. Li, "Extracorporeal shockwave therapy in osteonecrosis of femoral head a systematic review of now available clinical evidences," *Medicine (United States)*, vol. 96, no. 4, 2017.

[20] J.-M. Chen, S.-L. Hsu, T. Wong, W.-Y. Chou, C.-J. Wang, and F.-S. Wang, "Functional outcomes of bilateral hip necrosis: total hip arthroplasty versus extracorporeal shockwave," *Archives of Orthopaedic and Trauma Surgery*, vol. 129, no. 6, pp. 837–841, 2009.

[21] A. Notarnicola and B. Moretti, "The biological effects of extracorporeal shock wave therapy (eswt) on tendon tissue," *Muscle, Ligaments and Tendons Journal*, vol. 2, no. 1, pp. 33–37, 2012.

[22] C.-J. Wang, F.-S. Wang, J.-Y. Ko et al., "Extracorporeal shockwave therapy shows regeneration in hip necrosis," *Rheumatology*, vol. 47, no. 4, pp. 542–546, 2008.

[23] V. Visco, M. C. Vulpiani, M. R. Torrisi, A. Ferretti, A. Pavan, and M. Vetrano, "Experimental studies on the biological effects of extracorporeal shock wave therapy on tendon models. A review of the literature," *Muscle, Ligaments and Tendons Journal*, vol. 4, no. 3, pp. 357–361, 2014.

[24] C. Ertürk, M. A. Altay, I. Özardali, N. Altay, H. Çeçe, and U. E. Işikan, "The effect of extracorporeal shockwaves on cartilage end-plates in rabbits: A preliminary MRI and histopathological study," *Acta Orthopaedica et Traumatologica Turcica*, vol. 46, no. 6, pp. 449–454, 2012.

[25] E. M. Alves, A. T. Angrisani, and M. B. Santiago, "The use of extracorporeal shock waves in the treatment of osteonecrosis of the femoral head: A systematic review," *Clinical Rheumatology*, vol. 28, no. 11, pp. 1247–1251, 2009.

[26] F. Gao, W. Sun, Z. Li, W. Guo, N. Kush, and K. Ozaki, "Intractable bone marrow edema syndrome of the hip," *Orthopedics*, vol. 38, no. 4, pp. e263–e270, 2015.

[27] Y.-C. Hong, R.-B. Luo, T. Lin, H.-M. Zhong, and J.-B. Shi, "Efficacy of alendronate for preventing collapse of femoral head in adult patients with nontraumatic osteonecrosis," *BioMed Research International*, vol. 2014, 2014.

[28] C.-J. Wang, F.-S. Wang, K. D. Yang et al., "Treatment of osteonecrosis of the hip: comparison of extracorporeal shockwave with shockwave and alendronate," *Archives of Orthopaedic and Trauma Surgery*, vol. 128, no. 9, pp. 901–908, 2008.

[29] S.-L. Hsu, C.-J. Wang, M. S.-S. Lee, Y.-S. Chan, C.-C. Huang, and K. D. Yang, "Cocktail therapy for femoral head necrosis of the hip," *Archives of Orthopaedic and Trauma Surgery*, vol. 130, no. 1, pp. 23–29, 2010.

[30] R. K. Sen, "Management of avascular necrosis of femoral head at pre-collapse stage," *Indian Journal of Orthopaedics*, vol. 43, no. 1, pp. 6–16, 2009.

Percutaneous Injection of Strontium Containing Hydroxyapatite versus Polymethacrylate Plus Short-Segment Pedicle Screw Fixation for Traumatic A2- and A3/AO-Type Fractures in Adults

Panagiotis Korovessis, Eva Mpountogianni, Vasileios Syrimpeis, Andreas Baikousis, and Vasileios Tsekouras

Orthopaedics Department, General Hospital of Patras, Tsertidou Str. 1, 26224 Rio, Greece

Correspondence should be addressed to Vasileios Syrimpeis; siva@upatras.gr

Academic Editor: Kivanc Atesok

Introduction. Polymethacrylate (PMMA) is commonly used in vertebroplasty and balloon kyphoplasty, but its use has been associated with complications. This study tests three hypotheses: (1) whether strontium hydroxyapatite (Sr-HA) is equivalent to PMMA for restoring thoracolumbar vertebral body fractures, (2) whether the incidence of PMMA leakage is similar to that of Sr-HA leakage, and (3) whether Sr-HAis is resorbed and substituted by new vertebral bone. *Materials and Methods*. Two age- and sex-matched groups received short percutaneous pedicle screw fixation plus PEEK implant (Kiva, VCF Treatment System, Benvenue Medical, Santa Clara, CA, USA) filled with either Sr-HA (Group A) or PMMA (Group B) after A2- and A3/AO-type thoracolumbar vertebral body fractures. The Visual Analog Scale (VAS) score and imaging parameters, which included segmental kyphosis angle (SKA), vertebral body height ratios (VBHr), spinal canal encroachment (SCE), bone cement leakage, and Sr-HA resorption, were compared between the two groups. *Results*. The average follow-up was 28 months. No differences in VAS scores between Groups A and B were observed at baseline. Baseline back pain in both groups improved significantly three months postoperatively. Anterior, middle, and posterior VBHr did not differ between the two groups at any time point. SKA was improved insignificantly in both groups. SCE decreased insignificantly in both groups on 12-month follow-up using computed tomography (CT). PMMA leakage was observed in one patient, while no Sr-HA paste leakages occurred. Sr-HA resorption and replacement with vertebral bone were observed, and no new fractures were observed. *Conclusions*. As all hypotheses were confirmed, the authors recommend the use of Sr-HA instead of PMMA in traumatic spine fractures, although more patients and longer follow-up will be needed to strengthen these results. This trial is registered with NCT03431519.

1. Introduction

Polymethacrylate (PMMA) is commonly used in vertebroplasty (VP) and balloon kyphoplasty (BK) for osteoporotic and fresh thoracolumbar fractures. VP and BK can be used either alone or in combination with pedicle screw constructs. However, PMMA has been reported to be associated with undesirable properties such as high setting temperature, leakage (7–10%), lung and distal emboli, lack of osseointegration, and significant stiffness mismatch with bone leading to subsequent adjacent fractures or even refracture of the augmented vertebra [1]. In consideration of these potential complications, biological and bioactive bone substitutes (calcium phosphate, Sr-HA, etc.) have been used in an attempt to reduce the undesirable events associated with PMMA, while enhancing the mechanical stability of osteoporotic vertebral compression fractures. Compared with PMMA, significantly lower leakage rates have been reported with biologic and bioactive bone cements [1–7].

Strontium (Sr) is an antiosteoporosis agent, which has dual effects on bone metabolism [8]. Sr restores the bone turnover balance, especially when the treatment of bone fractures caused by osteoporosis is challenging [9, 10]. *In vitro* studies have shown that Sr acts through the calcium-sensing receptor to increase the mRNA level of osteoprotegerin and decrease the mRNA levels of the receptor activator of nuclear factor-kappaB ligand [11]. Furthermore, Sr promotes bone formation by stimulating the differentiation of osteoblasts, as well as by blocking bone resorption through inhibition of osteoclast differentiation [11]. A 10-year clinical trial reported that Sr reduces the risk of vertebral and nonvertebral fractures and increases bone mineral density [11].

Sr-HA exhibits radiopacity three times greater than that of cortical bone and thus has enhanced visibility compared to bone. This is an advantage from the perspective of clinical imaging when it is used to assess implant placement and osseointegration at the bone-implant interface [12, 13].

Previous investigations have not identified any adverse reactions associated with Sr-HA use (such as foreign body reaction, inflammation, or bone necrosis). This is likely because of the nontoxicity of bisphenol-A bis(2-hydroxypropyl)methacrylate (BISGMA) and the lower setting temperature of Sr-HA [6, 12, 14].

Clinical studies reporting the use of Sr-HA in VP and BK for vertebral compression fractures are lacking [5]. An experimental study showed that Sr-HA facilitated reconstruction and maintenance of vertebral body height. It was also reported that Sr-HA is incorporated in the fractured vertebral body during bone remodeling by 3 to 6 months after the VP [5]. In an animal study, new lamellar bone grew onto the Sr-HA, soon after surgery [15].

Since biologic and bioactive cements do not provide immediate stability like PMMA can, several authors are currently performing BK and VP procedures for A2- and A3/AO-type thoracolumbar fractures using titanium stents and PEEK devices, supplemented with short-segment pedicle screws, to increase immediate stability [16–18].

Taking into consideration the biological properties of Sr-HA bioactive bone cement, the authors of this study have been using Sr-HA with PEEK implants together with percutaneous pedicle screw fixation in selected young adult patients with fresh, severely compressed, A2- and A3/AO-type thoracolumbar fractures. The aim of this preliminary comparative study was to examine the short- to medium-term efficacy of percutaneous vertebral body reconstruction by vertebral body augmentation with Sr-HA paste plus short-segment pedicle screw fixation in fresh fractures, as well as evaluate Sr-HA resorption/substitution. The hypotheses tested in this prospective comparative controlled study were as follows: (1) whether Sr-HA is equivalent to PMMA for restoring the fractured thoracolumbar vertebral body, (2) whether leakage of Sr-HA is less than that of PMMA, and (3) whether Sr-HA is completely resorbed and replaced by cancellous bone.

2. Methods

2.1. Patients. This study was approved by the institutional ethical committee and all patients gave written informed consent. From April to December 2013, thirty-eight (38) consecutive adult female patients were selected and divided into two groups, each consisting of 19 age-matched individuals. Each of the subjects had a single, severely (>40%) compressed A2- and A3/AO-type thoracolumbar (T10-L3) fracture, without any serious concomitant injuries. For treatment of the fractures, the subjects received VP with PEEK and either Sr-HA (Group A) or PMMA (Group B). A total of 8 patients (4 in each group) were excluded from the final evaluation for the following reasons: one patient was excluded because her intraoperative biopsy revealed metastatic disease; six patients were excluded because they were not available for further evaluation after the 3-month follow-up; and one patient was excluded because of a deep-tissue infection. Finally, each of the two groups included 15 age-matched ($P = 0.52$) adult female patients. Group A included 15 women aged 45.7 ± 8 years (range: 38–53 years), and Group B included 15 women aged 46 ± 6 years (range: 40–52 years) at the time of the index surgery. The body mass index (BMI) of the subjects in Group A averaged 28 ± 5 (range: 19–39) and in Group B averaged 26 ± 3 (range: 22–30) ($P = 0.32$). All patients from both groups were attended by the same senior spine surgeon and underwent percutaneous short pedicle screw fixation plus vertebroplasty with PEEK implants (Kiva, VCF Treatment System, Benvenue Medical, Santa Clara, CA, USA) filled with either Sr-HA paste (Neogel, Teknimed, Vic-en-Bigorre, France) (Group A) or low-viscosity PMMA (Group B).

Patients were excluded from the study in cases of polytrauma, neurologic impairment, spinal deformity, known malignancy, and previous fracture or surgery in the same or adjacent vertebrae. Back pain intensity was recorded using the VAS scoring system (10-point scale).

Patients were randomly assigned to receive either Sr-HA or PMMA, and the process was blinded by the following method: the second author randomized the patients to receive either PMMA or Sr-HA without knowledge of the patients' names. The surgeons were unaware of which patients would receive Sr-HA or PMMA.

The operation was performed in the prone position. Two multiaxial, cannulated pedicle screws with diameters of 6-7 mm were inserted into the vertebrae immediately superior and inferior to the fractured vertebra via stab incisions using an image intensifier. One PEEK implant was introduced unilaterally through the pedicle to reduce the likelihood of vertebral body collapse, and subsequently the filling material, PMMA or Sr-HA, was injected. A column of either PMMA or Sr-HA was constructed inside the PEEK implant. Next, two longitudinal, appropriately contoured rods were percutaneously inserted and assembled with the pedicle screws in each side. Supine, anteroposterior, and lateral digital roentgenograms of the thoracolumbar spine were taken on admission. Standing digital roentgenograms of the whole spine were taken on the second postoperative day, 6 months postoperatively, and at the final observation (average follow-up of 28 months). CT scans were performed preoperatively and at 12 months postoperatively to evaluate the spinal canal remodeling, the Sr-HA resorption, and the bone healing state in the fractured vertebral body.

The following roentgenographic parameters were measured at the time of admission and postoperatively: (a) segmental kyphotic deformity (SKD) (defined by the angle formed from the lines drawn on the lower endplate of the

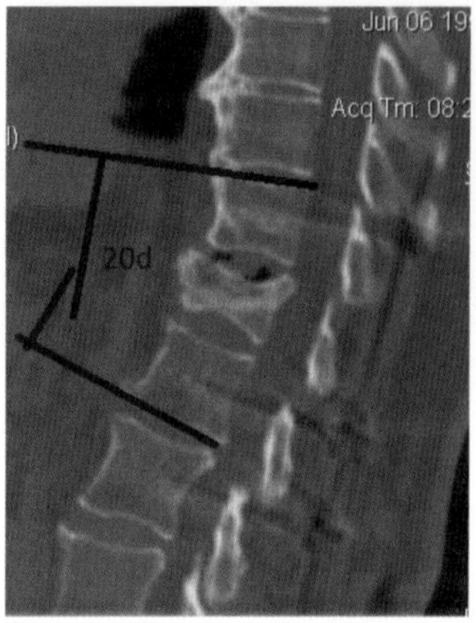

(a) Preoperative CT scan of a 61-year-old woman with an L1 fracture and posttraumatic L1 vertebral body wedging of 20°

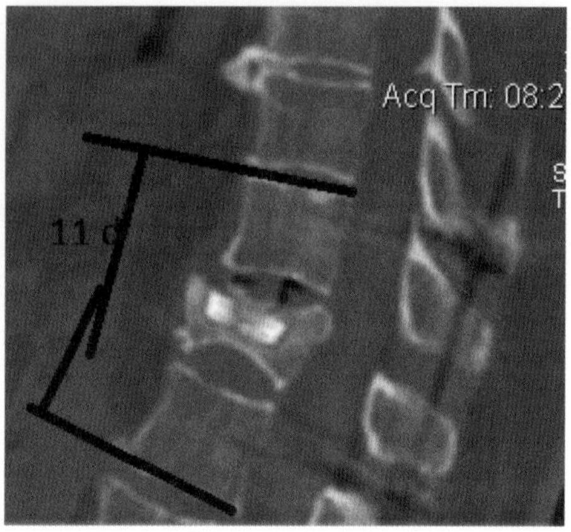

(b) Postoperative CT scan of the patient in (a) obtained 27 months postoperatively showing the PEEK implant with Sr-HA in the correct position and a reduction of segmental kyphosis to 11°; Note the resorption of the paste inside the PEEK loops

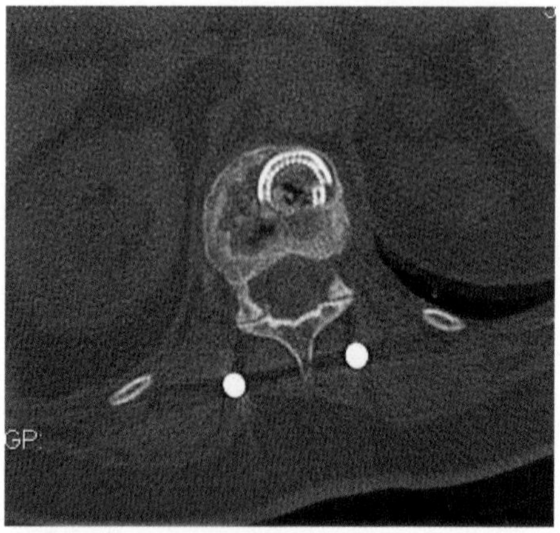

(c) Postoperative CT scan 12 months after surgery in a 67-year-old woman showing complete resorption of Sr-HA and bone healing around the PEEK implant; no Sr-HA traces are shown inside the PEEK loops

FIGURE 1

intact vertebra inferior to the fractured vertebra and the upper endplate of the adjacent vertebra superior to the fractured vertebra), (b) anterior vertebral body height ratio (AVBHr), (c) middle vertebral body height ratio (MVBHr), (d) posterior vertebral body height ratio (PVBHr) (vertebral body height ratios are equal to the fractured vertebral body height divided by the average of the vertebral body heights of the adjacent intact vertebrae superior and inferior to the fractured vertebra), (e) refractures, and (f) adjacent or remote vertebral fractures.

On axial CT scans, the percentages (%) of spinal canal encroachment (SCE) and spinal canal clearance (SCC) (the narrowest anteroposterior spinal canal diameter divided by the average anteroposterior diameter of the two adjacent noninjured vertebrae) were evaluated.

One senior orthopedic spine surgeon and one senior orthopedic radiologist were asked to evaluate the following parameters on axial CT scan slices: cement (Sr-HA or PMMA) leakage and Sr-HA resorption and bone substitution within the cylinder formed by the implanted PEEK loops. Since there is no available method for quantitative or qualitative evaluation of bone cement resorption, the evaluation of Sr-HA resorption and cancellous bone formation (Group A) inside the column constructed by the PEEK loops was rated as present (+) or absent (−) based on different axial CT scan slices taken 12 months postoperatively (Figures 1(a)–1(c)). Patients were encouraged to walk wearing a 3-point fixation brace from the first day following surgery and for a period of 6 weeks.

2.2. Statistical Analysis. Statistical analysis was performed with paired (change of variables in the same group) and unpaired (change of a variable in different groups) t-tests for changes in every radiographic parameter. The kappa value for agreement was used for the radiological evaluation of Sr-HA resorption only, since the digital roentgenograms and

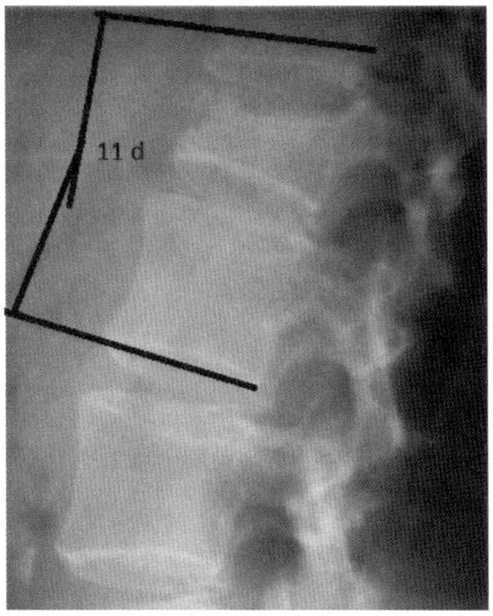

(a) Lateral roentgenogram of a 54-year-old woman who sustained a traumatic L3 A3/AO-type fracture

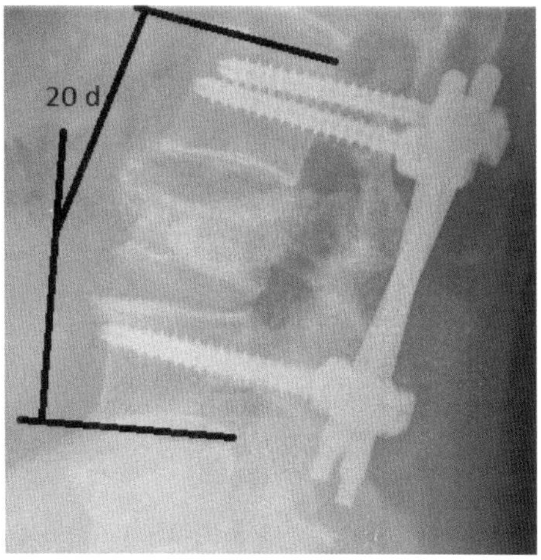

(b) Lateral roentgenogram of the patient in (a) obtained 27 months postoperatively following Sr-HA injection and short-segment pedicle screw fixation; there is a correction of the preoperative 11° kyphosis to a 20° lordosis and reduction of the L2 endplates

Figure 2

CT scans are highly reliable. The interobserver reliability was measured by the kappa values. Kappa values between 0.61 and 0.80 were considered to indicate "substantial agreement."

2.3. Implant Characteristics. Sr-HA paste is a radiopaque, osteoconductive, and osteocompatible bone substitute that was used in this study, together with the PEEK implant, for vertebral body augmentation in all 15 patients of Group A. Sr-HA consists of highly pure synthetic, fully resorbable, nanocrystalline hydroxyapatite (HA) with strontium (Sr) and water. Sr-HA is gradually resorbed and replaced by bone during the remodeling process, and the strontium-developed drug acts as an effective antiosteoporotic therapy in postmenopausal women with osteoporosis [19, 20].

Previous studies have reported the occurrence of osteogenesis early after the implantation, while the histological integration of Sr-HA in sheep's vertebrae revealed excellent osteogenic and osteoconductive properties. No adverse events (cytotoxicity or hemolysis), rejections, or osteolyses have been recorded [6, 21, 22]. The reported compressive strength of Sr-HA is 40.9 MPa, which is 2 to 9.9 times lower than that of PMMAs (80–396 MPa) and 2–8 times higher than that of cancellous bone (6–24 MPa) [14]. Its bending strength is 31.3 MPa, which is 50% lower than that of PMMAs (67–72 MPa) and 10 times stronger than that of cancellous bone (3 MPa) [12, 14].

3. Results

All patients in both groups were followed up for an average of 28 months (range: 24–33 months).

The *operative time* in both groups averaged 65 minutes (range: 55–80 minutes). The *fluoroscopy exposure time* ranged from 1.05 to 4.2 minutes, with an average time of 1.3 ± 1.14 min, and this was similar in both groups ($P = 0.72$). The *volume of injected liquid* of Sr-HA (Group A) per vertebra averaged 1.5 ml (range: 1-2 ml) and did not differ from PMMA with average volumes of 2 ml (range: 1–2.5 ml) (Group B) ($P = 0.64$).

No significant amount of perioperative *blood loss* was observed in either group. No significant decrease in hemoglobin was observed postoperatively, and no blood transfusion was given to any patient in both groups. The *hospital stay* in both groups averaged 2 days (range: 1–3 days).

Baseline *VAS back pain* scores in both groups improved significantly by 3 months postoperatively ($P < 0.000$). Improvements of VAS scores in Group A averaged 2 ± 3, and the average in Group B was 1.6 ± 2. There was no difference in VAS changes between the two groups ($P = 0.7$). No further significant changes in VAS score were seen in the patients of either group.

The *kappa values* among the two observers after evaluating the roentgenographic and CT parameters ranged from 0.96 to 0.98. The baseline and follow-up radiographic and CT scan parameters values did not differ significantly between the two groups (Table 1, Figures 2(a) and 2(b)).

PMMA leakage without sequelae was observed in one patient in Group B, while no Sr-HA paste leakage was observed in Group A. No loss of correction of SKA, AVBHr, and PVBHr and no change of SCC were measured at the latest observation point (average follow-up of 28 months) in both groups (Table 1). Sr-HA resorption and replacement with vertebral bone were observed by 12 months postoperatively in all the spines of Group A (Figures 1(a), 1(b), and 1(c)). No adjacent or remote new fractures were observed in the latest follow-up (average follow-up of 28 months).

4. Discussion

This preliminary comparative study examined the short- and medium-term efficacy of percutaneous VP with PEEK

TABLE 1: Comparative presentation of radiological changes observed in Group A and Group B preoperatively till the last follow-up.

Parameters	PREOP		GrA/GrB	Postop		GrA/GrB	3 months		GrA/GrB	6 months		GrA/GrB	Last follow-up		GrA/GrB
	GrA	GrB	*P* value	GrA	GrB	*P* value	GrA	GrB	*P* value	GrA	GrB	*P* value	GrA	GrB	*P* value
AVBHr	0.59 ± 0.11	0.63 ± 0.14	0.48	0.79 ± 0.12	0.87 ± 0.15	0.22	0.75 ± 0.12	0.86 ± 0.17	0.1	0.7 ± 0.15	0.9 ± 0.20	0.089	0.71 ± 0.16	0.91 ± 0.19	0.09
MVBHr	0.53 ± 0.12	0.68 ± 0.16	**0.054**	0.66 ± 0.08	0.86 ± 0.13	**0.06**	0.73 ± 0.15	0.8 ± 0.20	0.24	0.63 ± 0.2	0.8 ± 0.12	0.21	0.6 ± 0.18	0.82 ± 0.13	0.23
PVBHr	0.95 ± 0.15	0.97 ± 0.18	0.77	0.97 ± 0.07	1 ± 0.09	0.069	1 ± 0.12	1 ± 0.11	0.13	0.98 ± 0.13	1 ± 0.18	0.4	1 ± 12	1.1 ± 0.17	0.45
⁺SKA	14.7 ± 8.7	13.9 ± 8	0.81	8.6 ± 7	9 ± 4	0.88	13 ± 8	10 ± 6	0.40	10 ± 6	12 ± 8	0.65	12 ± 5	14 ± 9.8	0.66
SCE (%)	22 ± 17	26 ± 19	0.46							15 ± 13*	10 ± 15*	0.49			

*SCE values on CT scan 12 months following surgery. GrA: Group A; GrB: Group B; AVBHr: anterior vertebral body height ratio; MVBHr: middle vertebral body height ratio; PVBHr: posterior vertebral body height ratio; SCE: spinal canal encroachment. ⁺SKA in Cobb degrees.

and Sr-HA or PMMA plus short-segment pedicle screw fixation for single fresh A2- and A3/AO-type thoracolumbar fractures. We also evaluated the amount of Sr-HA resorption and substitution with cancellous bone. All three hypotheses in this study were confirmed: (1) Sr-HA and PMMA equally restored the fractured thoracolumbar vertebral body angulation and heights, (2) bone cement leakage in VP with Sr-HA was less than that with PMMA, and (3) Sr-HA paste was resorbed and replaced by cancellous bone.

Previous clinical studies showed that percutaneous VP with PEEK and low-viscosity PMMA for osteoporotic vertebral body fractures in elderly patients exhibited PMMA containment [13, 16]. However, because of the exothermic reaction and heat released during the PMMA hardening process, an active membrane is created around the PMMA cement, which is considered to be a potential disadvantage of PMMA osseointegration [3, 23, 24]. It seems that osseointegration provides a critical advantage of Sr-HA over PMMA. This advantage of Sr-HA may result in better long-term outcomes and fewer potential adverse reactions than those reported with PMMA, in cemented hip and knee arthroplasties. Previous studies reported no adverse reactions associated with Sr-HA use, probably because of the nontoxic nature of bisphenol-A bis(2-hydroxypropyl)methacrylate (BISGMA) and the lower setting temperature of Sr-HA [6, 12, 14].

HA is a biocompatible and osteoconductive material. The mechanism of formation and strengthening of the bone-HA interface has been studied using high-resolution transmission electron microscopy and energy-dispersive X-ray analysis [25]. It was suggested that the transition of crystalline to amorphous HA is the first critical step in bone-to-implant bonding. The osseointegration of an implant as a function of the biological response to HA can be significantly enhanced by pharmaceutical agents [26, 27]. It was found that apatites obtained by partial substitution of Ca^{++} by Sr yield higher solubility compared to pure HA [28]. Both Sr and Ca^{++} have common chemical properties, while Sr is characterized as "a bone seeking element" having a similar charge/size ratio to Ca^{++}.

A previous study showed an increase in bone mass following oral intake of Sr-HA for osteoporosis [9]. Sr is beneficial for bone health in postmenopausal osteoporotic women, because it assists in the replication of preosteoblastic cells promoting bone formation [29] and, to a lesser extent, decreases bone resorption *in vivo* [30].

Oral administration of Sr salts results in adsorption of Sr ions on the apatite surface or in the substitution of Ca^{++} ions in the apatite crystal lattice at low ion exchange rates. Only about 10% of the Ca^{++} ions are substituted by Sr ions [31]. The procedure of ion exchange is more profoundly realized in new bone during remodeling. There is some controversy regarding the beneficial effects of Sr on bone because it is dose-dependent, and although low doses stimulate bone formation, high doses have deleterious effects on bone mineralization [9, 32–34]. Increased attention has been paid to the repair of osteoporotic fractures by Sr-modified bioceramics with improved osseointegration capabilities. Moreover, biocompatible Sr-doped HAs enhance the peri-implant bone formation more efficiently than the administered strontium [35].

Recently, Li et al. [36] published a thought-provoking study of doped hydroxyapatite (Sr-HA) in ovariectomized rats, comparing HA and Sr-HA. In this study, Li et al. [36] clearly showed that Sr-HA is a promising material for bone tissue engineering, because it promotes osteogenesis and improves the trabecular microarchitecture under osteoporotic conditions. The osteoconductive properties of different Sr-doped biocomposites have been investigated in numerous bone defects [37, 38]. It has been reported that the implantation of Sr-containing HA materials promotes bone repair and healing in both normal [39] and ovariectomized [36, 40] animals.

A previous study regarding the use of VP for osteoporotic single spine fractures revealed that Sr-HA is incorporated during the bone remodeling as early as 3 to 6 months after implantation [5]. In an animal research study, newly formed bone grew onto the Sr-HA by 4 months following surgery [15]. Complete Sr-HA resorption was documented on CT scans 12 months postoperatively in all 15 patients of Group A, justifying the previously mentioned study. This means that the Sr-HA ingredients (hydroxyapatite and strontium) are resorbed without interference during the vertebral bone healing process and probably induce osteogenesis.

Another advantage of the use of bioactive cements is their lower leakage rate [5, 13]. A leakage rate of 22% was reported with the use of PMMA in fresh thoracolumbar vertebral body fractures, whereas the leakage rate with calcium phosphate was 15% [13]. A clinical study reporting on the use of Sr-HA in VP for the augmentation of single osteoporotic thoracolumbar fractures revealed maintenance of the vertebral body height with only 3 (13%) cases of slight Sr-HA leakage into the spinal canal, but none of the patients developed any neurologic sequela [5]. In the present study, the leakage rate with PEEK was 7.5% when using PMMA and 0% when using Sr-HA.

The addition of pedicle screws together with the PEEK implant secured the vertebral body stiffness against compression and rotational forces acting across the thoracolumbar spine immediately following surgery and thus, at least theoretically, enhanced the process of bone healing and new bone formation. There were no reactions, either local or systemic, to Sr-HA injections in any of the patients.

In contrast to Sr-HA, which is a resorbable bioactive bone cement, PMMA is not resorbable. Taking into consideration the extensive experience gained in clinical practice with PMMA and its low cost, efforts have been made recently to improve the bioactivity of PMMA [41]. Researchers have attempted to improve PMMA bioactivity and osseointegration by incorporating Sr-containing borate bioactive glass (SrBG) as a reinforcement phase and bioactive filler for the PMMA cement [41]. The prepared SrBG/PMMA composite cements showed evidence of significantly decreased polymerization temperatures, when compared with PMMA alone. The composite also retained the properties of appropriate setting times and great mechanical strength. The bioactivity of the SrBG/PMMA composite cements was confirmed *in vitro*, as evidenced by ion release (Ca^{+2} P, B, and Sr) from

SrBG particles. It has been demonstrated *in vitro* that SrBG incorporation may promote adhesion, migration, proliferation, and collagen secretion by cells. Consequently, the SrBG/PMMA composite cement may be a better alternative to cement made from PMMA alone, in clinical applications, and it has promising applications in minimally invasive orthopedic surgery.

A limitation of this study is that it is a pilot study, with a small (n = 30) number of patients. Further, it has limited power, since the results may be subject to a Type II error.

5. Conclusions

Based on the results of the present preliminary study and taking into consideration the small number of individuals included, the authors recommend using Sr-HA bioactive bone cement instead of PMMA, supplemented by short pedicle screw construction, in adults with osteoporotic and fresh traumatic thoracolumbar fractures. However, further studies, with a greater number of patients and longer follow-up, are needed.

Ethical Approval

All the authors certified that the study was performed in accordance with the ethical standards in the 1964 Declaration of Helsinki; therefore, the ethical committee approved the study.

Disclosure

An earlier version of this work was presented as a poster at the Global Spine Congress (GSC), 6th Annual Meeting for AOSpine 2017 [42].

Acknowledgments

The authors would like to thank Editage (https://www.editage.com) for English language editing.

References

[1] J. C. Eck, D. Nachtigall, S. C. Humphreys, and S. D. Hodges, "Comparison of vertebroplasty and balloon kyphoplasty for treatment of vertebral compression fractures: a meta-analysis of the literature," *The Spine Journal*, vol. 8, no. 3, pp. 488–497, 2008.

[2] P. Korovessis, A. Hadjipavlou, and T. Repantis, "Minimal invasive short posterior instrumentation plus balloon kyphoplasty with calcium phosphate for burst and severe compression lumbar fractures," *The Spine Journal*, vol. 33, no. 6, pp. 658–667, 2008.

[3] W. F. Mousa, M. Kobayashi, S. Shinzato et al., "Biological and mechanical properties of PMMA-based bioactive bone cements," *Biomaterials*, vol. 21, no. 21, pp. 2137–2146, 2000.

[4] G. Lewis, "Injectable bone cements for use in vertebroplasty and kyphoplasty: state-of-the-art review," *Journal of Biomedical Materials Research Part B: Applied Biomaterials*, vol. 76, no. 2, pp. 456–468, 2006.

[5] K. M. C. Cheung, W. W. Lu, K. D. K. Luk et al., "Vertebroplasty by use of a strontium-containing bioactive bone cement," *The Spine Journal*, vol. 30, no. 17, pp. S84–S91, 2005.

[6] W. W. Lu, K. M. C. Cheung, Y. W. Li et al., "Bioactive bone cement as a principal fixture for spinal burst fracture: An in vitro biomechanical and morphologic study," *The Spine Journal*, vol. 26, no. 24, pp. 2684–2690, 2001.

[7] Y. W. Li, J. C. Y. Leong, W. W. Lu et al., "A novel injectable bioactive bone cement for spinal surgery: A developmental and preclinical study," *Journal of Biomedical Materials Research Part B: Applied Biomaterials*, vol. 52, no. 1, pp. 164–170, 2000.

[8] E. Bonnelye, A. Chabadel, F. Saltel, and P. Jurdic, "Dual effect of strontium ranelate: Stimulation of osteoblast differentiation and inhibition of osteoclast formation and resorption in vitro," *Bone*, vol. 42, no. 1, pp. 129–138, 2008.

[9] S. G. Dahl, P. Allain, P. J. Marie et al., "Incorporation and distribution of strontium in bone," *Bone*, vol. 28, no. 4, pp. 446–453, 2001.

[10] P. J. Marie, P. Ammann, G. Boivin, and C. Rey, "Mechanisms of action and therapeutic potential of strontium in bone," *Calcified Tissue International*, vol. 69, no. 3, pp. 121–129, 2001.

[11] A. P. Trouvin and V. Goeb, "Receptor activator of nuclear factor-kappaB ligand and osteoprotegerin: maintaining the balance to prevent bone loss," *Clinical Interventions in Aging*, vol. 5, pp. 345–354, 2010.

[12] K. Kühn, *Determination of The Setting Temperature/Time According to ISO 5833: Bone Cements*, Springer, Berlin, Germany, 2000.

[13] P. Korovessis, K. Vardakastanis, T. Repantis, and V. Vitsas, "Transpedicular vertebral body augmentation reinforced with pedicle screw fixation in fresh traumatic A2 and A3 lumbar fractures: comparison between two devices and two bone cements," *European Journal of Orthopaedic Surgery and Traumatology*, vol. 24, supplement 1, pp. 183–191, 2014.

[14] M. M. Panjabi and A. A. White, *Biomechanics in The Musculoskeletal System*, Churchill Livingstone, Philadelphia, Penn, USA, 2001.

[15] C. T. Wong, W. W. Lu, W. K. Chan et al., "In vivo cancellous bone remodeling on a strontium-containing hydroxyapatite (sr-HA) bioactive cement," *Journal of Biomedical Materials Research Part B: Applied Biomaterials*, vol. 68A, no. 3, pp. 513–521, 2004.

[16] P. Korovessis, T. Repantis, L. E. Miller, and J. E. Block, "Initial clinical experience with a novel vertebral augmentation system for treatment of symptomatic vertebral compression fractures: A case series of 26 consecutive patients," *BMC Musculoskeletal Disorders*, vol. 12, article 206, 2011.

[17] R. F. McLain, E. Sparling, and D. R. Benson, "Early failure of short-segment pedicle instrumentation for thoracolumbar fractures. A preliminary report," *Journal of Bone and Joint Surgery - Series A*, vol. 75, no. 2, pp. 162–167, 1993.

[18] T. McCormack, E. Karaikovic, and R. W. Gaines, "The load sharing classification of spine fractures," *The Spine Journal*, vol. 19, no. 15, pp. 1741–1744, 1994.

[19] I. F. Vasconcelos, M. A. Pimenta, and A. S. B. Sombra, "Optical properties of $Bi_{12}SiO_{20}$ (BSO) and $Bi_{12}TiO_{20}$ (BTO) obtained by mechanical alloying," *Journal of Materials Science*, vol. 36, no. 3, pp. 587–592, 2001.

[20] O. A. Adebanjo, H. K. Anandatheerthavarada, A. P. Koval et al., "A new function for CD38/ADP-ribosyl cyclase in nuclear Ca2+ homeostasis," *Nature Cell Biology*, vol. 1, no. 7, pp. 409–414, 1999.

[21] G. Romieu, X. Garric, S. Munier, M. Vert, and P. Boudeville, "Calcium-strontium mixed phosphate as novel injectable and radio-opaque hydraulic cement," *Acta Biomaterialia*, vol. 6, no. 8, pp. 3208–3215, 2010.

[22] E. Gentleman, Y. C. Fredholm, G. Jell et al., "The effects of strontium-substituted bioactive glasses on osteoblasts and osteoclasts in vitro," *Biomaterials*, vol. 31, no. 14, pp. 3949–3956, 2010.

[23] Y. Okada, K. Kawanabe, H. Fujita, K. Nishio, and T. Nakamura, "Repair of segmental bone defects using bioactive bone cement: Comparison with PMMA bone cement," *Journal of Biomedical Materials Research Part B: Applied Biomaterials*, vol. 47, no. 3, pp. 353–359, 1999.

[24] Y. Senaha, T. Nakamura, J. Tamura, K. Kawanabe, H. Iida, and T. Yamamuro, "Intercalary replacement of canine femora using a new bioactive bone cement," *The Journal of Bone & Joint Surgery*, vol. 78, no. 1, pp. 26–31, 1996.

[25] Q. Z. Chen, C. T. Wong, W. W. Lu, K. M. C. Cheung, J. C. Y. Leong, and K. D. K. Luk, "Strengthening mechanisms of bone bonding to crystalline hydroxyapatite in vivo," *Biomaterials*, vol. 25, no. 18, pp. 4243–4254, 2004.

[26] Z. Evis and T. J. Webster, "Nanosize hydroxyapatite: Doping with various ions," *Advances in Applied Ceramics*, vol. 110, no. 5, pp. 311–320, 2011.

[27] J. Terra, E. R. Dourado, J. Eon, D. E. Ellis, G. Gonzalez, and A. M. Rossi, "The structure of strontium-doped hydroxyapatite: an experimental and theoretical study," *Physical Chemistry Chemical Physics*, vol. 11, no. 3, pp. 568–577, 2009.

[28] W. Zhang, Y. Shen, H. Pan et al., "Effects of strontium in modified biomaterials," *Acta Biomaterialia*, vol. 7, no. 2, pp. 800–808, 2011.

[29] E. Canalis, M. Hott, P. Deloffre, Y. Tsouderos, and P. J. Marie, "The divalent strontium salt S12911 enhances bone cell replication and bone formation in vitro," *Bone*, vol. 18, no. 6, pp. 517–523, 1996.

[30] J. Buehler, P. Chappuis, J. L. Saffar, Y. Tsouderos, and A. Vignery, "Strontium ranelate inhibits bone resorption while maintaining bone formation in alveolar bone in monkeys (Macaca fascicularis)," *Bone*, vol. 29, no. 2, pp. 176–179, 2001.

[31] S. Pors Nielsen, "The biological role of strontium," *Bone*, vol. 35, no. 3, pp. 583–588, 2004.

[32] M. D. Grynpas, E. Hamilton, R. Cheung et al., "Strontium increases vertebral bone volume in rats at a low dose that does not induce detectable mineralization defect," *Bone*, vol. 18, no. 3, pp. 253–259, 1996.

[33] L. Cianferotti, F. D'Asta, and M. L. Brandi, "A review on strontium ranelate long-term antifracture efficacy in the treatment of postmenopausal osteoporosis," *Therapeutic Advances in Musculoskeletal Disease*, vol. 5, no. 3, pp. 127–139, 2013.

[34] I. Pernicova, E. T. Middleton, and M. Aye, "Rash, strontium ranelate and DRESS syndrome put into perspective. European Medicine Agency on the alert," *Osteoporosis International*, vol. 19, no. 12, pp. 1811-1812, 2008.

[35] E. Landi, A. Tampieri, G. Celotti, S. Sprio, M. Sandri, and G. Logroscino, "Sr-substituted hydroxyapatites for osteoporotic bone replacement," *Acta Biomaterialia*, vol. 3, no. 6, pp. 961–969, 2007.

[36] Y. Li, E. Luo, S. Zhu, J. Li, L. Zhang, and J. Hu, "Cancellous bone response to strontium-doped hydroxyapatite in osteoporotic rats," *Journal of Applied Biomaterials & Functional Materials*, vol. 13, no. 1, pp. 28–34, 2015.

[37] U. Thormann, S. Ray, U. Sommer et al., "Bone formation induced by strontium modified calcium phosphate cement in critical-size metaphyseal fracture defects in ovariectomized rats," *Biomaterials*, vol. 34, no. 34, pp. 8589–8598, 2013.

[38] S. Chandran, S. Suresh Babu, V. S. Hari Krishnan, H. K. Varma, and A. John, "Osteogenic efficacy of strontium hydroxyapatite micro-granules in osteoporotic rat model," *Journal of Biomaterials Applications*, vol. 31, no. 4, pp. 499–509, 2016.

[39] I. Elgali, A. Turri, W. Xia et al., "Guided bone regeneration using resorbable membrane and different bone substitutes: Early histological and molecular events," *Acta Biomaterialia*, vol. 29, pp. 409–423, 2016.

[40] K. Lin, L. Xia, H. Li et al., "Enhanced osteoporotic bone regeneration by strontium-substituted calcium silicate bioactive ceramics," *Biomaterials*, vol. 34, no. 38, pp. 10028–10042, 2013.

[41] X. Cui, C. Huang, M. Zhang et al., "Enhanced osteointegration of poly(methylmethacrylate) bone cements by incorporating strontium-containing borate bioactive glass," *Journal of the Royal Society Interface*, vol. 14, no. 131, Article ID 20161057, 2017.

[42] P. Korovessis, E. Mpoutogianni, V. Syrimpeis, A. Baikousis, and V. Tsekouras, "P355 - percutaneous injection of strontium containing hydroxyapatite (Sr-HA) versus polymethacrylate (PMMA) plus short segment pedicle screw fixation for traumatic A2 and A3 AO-type fractures in adults: a preliminary prospective case control study," *Global Spine Journal*, vol. 7, no. 2S, pp. 190S–373S, 2017.

33

Use of Common Inflammatory Markers in the Long-Term Screening of Total Hip Arthroprosthesis Infections: Our Experience

Gabriele Falzarano,[1] Antonio Piscopo,[2] Predrag Grubor,[3] Giuseppe Rollo,[4] Antonio Medici,[1] Valerio Pipola,[5] Michele Bisaccia,[6] Auro Caraffa,[6] Elizabeth Mary Barron,[7] Francesco Nobile,[8] Raffaele Cioffi,[1] and Luigi Meccariello[6]

[1]*Department of Orthopedics and Traumatology, Azienda Ospedaliera "Gaetano Rummo", Benevento, Italy*
[2]*Department of Orthopedics and Traumatology, Sacro Cuore di Gesù Fatebenefratelli Hospital, Benevento, Italy*
[3]*Clinic of Traumatology, University Hospital Clinical Center Banja Luka, Banja Luka, Bosnia and Herzegovina*
[4]*Department of Orthopedics and Traumatology, Vito Fazzi Hospital, Lecce, Italy*
[5]*Rizzoli Orthopedic Institute, University of Bologna, Bologna, Italy*
[6]*Division of Orthopedics and Trauma Surgery, University of Perugia, S. Maria della Misericordia Hospital, Perugia, Italy*
[7]*School of Medicine, Central Michigan University, Mount Pleasant, MI, USA*
[8]*Department of Orthopedics and Traumatology, Hospital "Santa Maria alla Gruccia", Montevarchi, Arezzo, Italy*

Correspondence should be addressed to Luigi Meccariello; drlordmec@gmail.com

Academic Editor: Elizaveta Kon

Orthopedic implants have become essential components of modern medicine. The risk of infection of total hip arthroplasty (THA) is 1.5%–2%. Are the C-reactive protein (CRP), the erythrocyte sedimentation rate (ESR), and procalcitonin (PCT) good markers for THA infection screenings? From February 2009 to December 2012 at our Department of Orthopedics and Traumatology, 1248 patients were treated with THA. No prosthesis was cemented. All patients received antibiotic prophylaxis. All patients were discharged approximately 7.4 days after surgery with this clinical and radiographic follow-up program at 15 days and 1, 3, 6, 12, 24, and 36 months after surgery. Blood samples to determine ESR, CRP, and PCT values were taken at 1 hour before surgery and 15 days and 1, 3, 6, 12, 24, and 36 months after surgery. During follow-ups there were 22 cases of THA infections; according the Widmer classification, infections are hematogenous ones in 16 cases, late chronic ones in 5 cases, and early postoperative ones in 1 case. In all cases the three markers were considered positive; in 6 cases there were no radiological signs of septic loosening. ESR, CRP, and PCT proved to have a greater diagnostic accuracy than X-rays in predicting late chronic and early postoperative infections. These markers are valuable support for the surgeon in monitoring the prosthetic implant lifespan.

1. Introduction

The number of primary total hip arthroplasties (THAs) performed in the United States each year continues to increase, as does the incidence of septic complications. The changing profile of antibiotic resistant bacteria has made the prevention and the treatment of primary THA infections increasingly complex [1]. The incidence of PJI (prosthetic joint infections) varies depending on the joint involved; the rate of arthroplasties becoming infected is as follows: 1.7% of primary and 3.2% of nonprimary hip arthroplasties [2]. A correct and early diagnosis is essential in order to provide the most appropriate therapy. If a correct and timely microbiological diagnosis of infections is done within 4 weeks, it could be possible to follow a conservative approach on the prosthesis, since microorganisms are not yet organized in biofilms. A delayed diagnosis (>4 weeks) of early and late infections involves the necessity of prosthesis removal [3] due to the production of a structurated and mature microbial biofilm. Biofilm is an aggregate of microcolony of microbial cells adherent to a living or nonliving surface embedded in an extracellular polymeric matrix. Biofilm renders bacteria highly tolerant to antibiotics and host defenses [4].

The definition of PJI was recently revised by the International Consensus Group on Periprosthetic Joint Infection. According to PJI Consensus Group, patients should be considered to have a PJI if they meet one of the major criteria or at least three of the minor criteria. Major criteria are as follows: two positive periprosthetic cultures with phenotypically identical organisms; a sinus tract communicating with the joint. Minor criteria are as follows: elevated serum C-reactive protein and erythrocyte sedimentation rate; elevated synovial fluid white blood cell (WBC) count or ++ change on leukocyte esterase test strip; elevated synovial fluid polymorphonuclear neutrophil percentage; positive histological analysis of periprosthetic tissue; a single positive culture [5].

The aim of our study is to investigate the rationale and the utility of a long-term screening of prosthetic hip infections by use of common inflammatory markers [3]: erythrocyte sedimentation rate (ESR), C-reactive protein (CRP), and procalcitonin (PCT).

2. Material and Methods

From January 2009 to December 2012 a cohort of 1248 patients, who had undergone single hip arthroplasty at Department of Orthopedics and Traumatology of the "G. Rummo" Hospital of Benevento, the Sacred Heart Hospital Fatebenefratelli (Benevento, Italy), and the Clinical Center of Banja Luka (BIH), had been prospectively followed to detect the onset of prosthesis infection.

The population of our group at the time of the implant (THA) had an average age of 73.4 years (range 21–85); the relationship between sexes (M : F) was of 1.15 (658 : 570). The relationship between osteoarthritis and femoral fractures was 2.59 (900 : 348). The ASA physical status classification system was used to assess the anesthesiological risk of the patients (ASA I: 338 (27.08%); ASA II: 792 (63.46%); and ASA III: 118 (9.46%)) and the number of patients transferred to the intensive care unit after surgery, 59 (4.73%), with an average stay of 2.8 days (range 1–6 days). The average days of hospital stay were 6.7 days (range 4–15 days). 40 patients (3.2%) were operated on with anterior surgical access, 926 (74.2%) with direct lateral surgical approach, and 282 (22.6%) with posterior-lateral approach. On average, the surgical wound was 11.6 cm long (range of 10.3–16.5 cm). The average time for the THA surgery was 56.3 minutes (range 48.3–90.8 minutes). 523 patients (41.19%) received general anesthesia and 725 patients (58.81%) spinal anesthesia (Table 1).

No THA was cemented. All patients received short term cefazolin for antibiotic prophylaxis (2 gr before the surgery and 1 gr every 8 hours for five times after the surgery). The THA surfaces were the following: ceramic on polyethylene in 53.7% (n = 670 patients), ceramic on ceramic in 38.6% (n = 482 patients), and metal on metal in 7.7% (n = 96 patients).

Patients were treated according to the ethical standards of the Helsinki Declaration and were invited to read, understand, and sign the informed consent form.

The number of comorbidities was 1561 (Table 2). Cardiovascular diseases which affected 356 patients (28.53%) were the most frequent comorbidities (Table 2).

Follow-ups were performed with clinical and radiographic evaluations with pelvic and hip projections (AP, LL, and axial femur) at 15 days, 1 month, 3 months, 6 months, 12 months, 24 months, and 36 months after surgery. Blood tests were conducted to determine ESR, CRP, and PCT values: one hour before surgery, 15 days, 1 month, 3 months, 6 months, 12 months, 24 months, and 36 months after surgery. During this period, complications were evaluated and the possible infections were listed according to the Widmer classification.

The evaluation endpoint was set at 36 months. The exclusion criteria were the voluntary withdrawal from the scheduled follow-up program.

Furthermore, to confirm suspected infections, the surgeon examines the joint fluid (cytochemical and microbiological), the histological and microbiological periprosthetic tissue, and the prosthetic components.

No PJI Consensus Group criteria were followed in the suspicion of PJI because the study started before their publication and the study protocol was set as explained above.

All parameters were recorded into a spreadsheet for further processing and statistical analysis.

Descriptive statistics were used to summarize the characteristics of the study group and subgroups, including means and standard deviations of all continuous variables. The t-test was used to compare continuous outcomes. The Chi-square test or Fisher (in subgroups smaller than 10 patients) exact test was used to compare categorical variables.

The statistical significance was defined as $p < 0.05$.

3. Results

There were 387 complications not related to the THA system (Table 3). The most common complication during the 36-month period was the infection of the urinary tract in 168 patients (13.46%). 4 of them died during follow-up (Table 3). The ESR, CRP, and procalcitonin trends, shown in Figures 1, 2, and 3, are on average not dissimilar to the limits of the work. 1.76% of the patients (n = 22) had a PTA infection.

According to the Widmer classification (Table 4), there were one case of implant infection in the first four weeks after surgery (with WBCs: 24,000; ESR: 36; CRP: 35; PCT: 2.3), 5 cases of prosthetic infection between 5 weeks and the 23 months after surgery (average values: white blood cells: 18,356; ESR: 52.6; CRP: 42.3; PCT: 2.8), and 16 cases of prosthetic infection after 24 months after surgery (average values: white blood cells: 16,300; ESR: 56; CRP: 22.9; 14.2 PCT).

We had 20 patients with false positive values of CRP: 4 during the first month; 14 between the first month and 2 years; 2 patients after two years.

Before the prosthetic implant revision, aspiration under fluoroscopy of the intra-articular hip fluid was performed

Table 1: Description of population.

Description	
Numbers of patients	1248
Average age of patients	73,40 years
Range of age	21–85 years
Gender ratio (M : F)	1,15 (658 : 570)
Diseases ratio (arthritis/fractures)	2,59 (900 : 348)
ASA physical status classification system	ASA I: 338 (27,08%) ASA II: 792 (63,46%) ASA III: 118 (9,46%)
Number of patients who needed intensive care after surgery	59 (4,73%)
Average days in intensive care	2,8
Range of days in intensive care	1–6
Average days of hospitalization	6,7
Range of days of hospitalization	4–15
Surgical approach	Anterior approach: 40 (3,20%) Laterolateral approach: 926 (74,20%) Posterolateral approach: 282 (22,6%)
Average length of surgical wound	11.6 cm
Range of length of surgical wound	10.3–16.5 cm
Average length of surgery	56.3 minutes
Range of length of surgery	48.3–90.8 minutes
General anesthesia	523 (41,19%)
Spinal anesthesia	725 (58,81%)

Table 2: Number of comorbidities (%).

Respiratory disease	256 (20,51%)
Renal disease	108 (8,65%)
Diabetes mellitus	72 (5,77%)
Rheumatoid disease	243 (19,47%)
Parkinson disease	16 (1,28%)
Severe mental deterioration in old age	3 (0,24%)
Paget disease	12 (0,96%)
Current smokers	160 (12,82%)
Enteral steroids	281 (22,51%)
Number of comorbidities in patient	
1	476
2	894
≥3	191

to determine the number of white blood cells and the presence of pathogens. The pathogens were classified as follows: coagulase-negative staphylococci in 12 cases (54.54%), Gram-negative bacilli in 7 cases (31.82%), and enterococci in 3 patients (13.64%). After 5 days from the intra-articular aspiration, an implant revision was performed in two stages for late chronic and hematogenous infections and 1 stage for the early infection. There were no new cases of reinfection after revision. We did not perform intra-articular aspiration to all patients but only in those whose value of white blood cell was over 10.000 or those with elevated value of CRP and ESR. In some patients we performed an intra-articular aspiration without finding a joint infection because of false positive values of ESR and CRP due to other conditions that could rise their value [6].

4. Discussion

The total hip arthroplasty infections represent a serious problem given the increasing number of implants performed each year for both arthritis and hip fractures. Early detection of infection is the main objective orthopedists need in order to adopt an appropriate treatment procedure.

The incidence of primary hip arthroplasty infections of this study is 1.76%. This value is in line with the incidence of hip prosthetic infections present in the literature which is

TABLE 3: Number of perioperative complications.

	Number (%)
Chest infection	24 (1,92%)
Cardiac failure	60 (4,80%)
DVT/PE	27 (2,16%)
Urinary tract infection	168 (13,46%)
Gastrointestinal haemorrhage	27 (2,16%)
Myocardial infarction	54 (4,33%)
Stroke	27 (2,16%)
Number of complications	
1	170
2	89
≥3	128
Total of complications	387
Died before the second year of follow-up	4

TABLE 4: Description of THA infection.

Infection category	Typical onset after surgery	Type	Signs and symptoms	Representative microorganism
Early postoperative	≤2–4 weeks	Acute (type I)	Persistent pain after surgery, fever, redness, swelling after surgery	*Staphylococcus aureus*, coagulase-negative staphylococci
Late chronic	≥1 month	Chronic (type II)	Insidious onset, persisting pain after surgery	Coagulase-negative staphylococci, *Propionibacterium* species, anaerobes, *S. aureus*
Hematogenous	>2 years	Acute (type III)	Fever, pain, redness, swelling after a long period of wellness	Streptococci, *S. aureus*, gram-negative bacilli

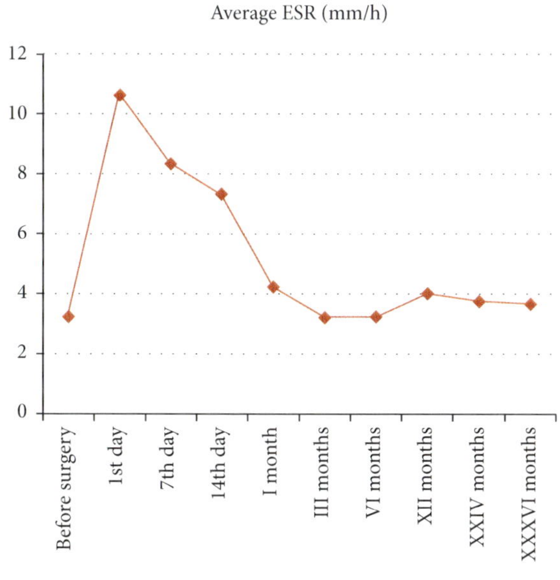

FIGURE 1: Trend of ESR during 36 months of follow-up.

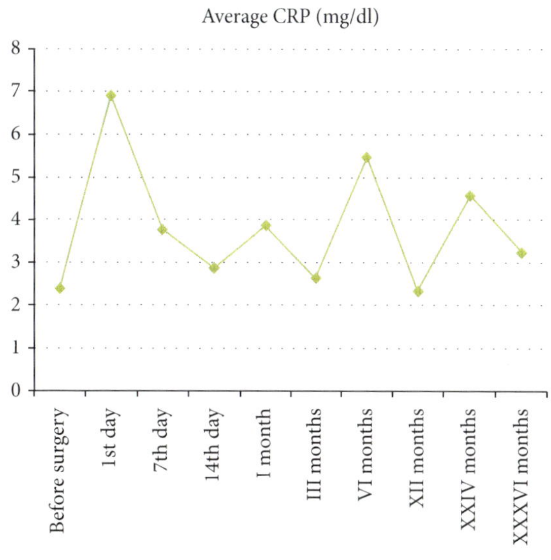

FIGURE 2: Trend of CRP during 36 months of follow-up.

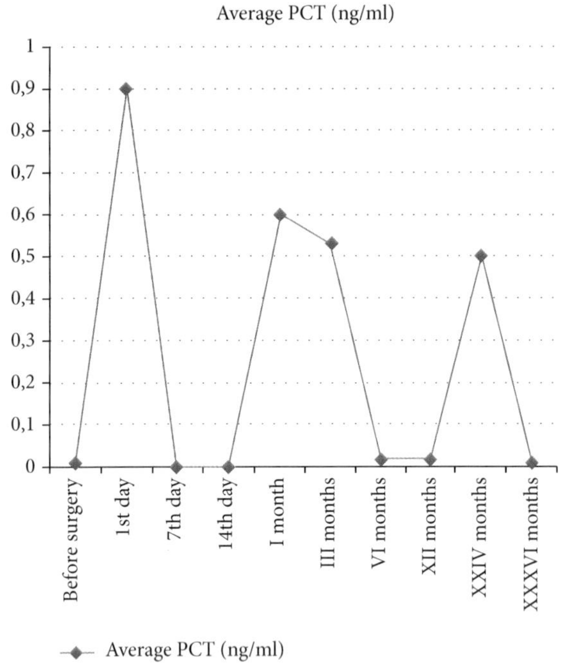

FIGURE 3: Trend of PCT during 36 months of follow-up.

comprised between 0.3% and 1.7% of primary implants [3, 7]. Patients developing an infection at follow-up had a history of more than three comorbidities [8–12].

Prosthetic infections are usually listed according to the Widmer classification: early postoperative if they occur during the first 2–4 weeks after surgery; late chronic after the first month; hematogenous after two years [1].

The purpose of the study is to evaluate the hematological parameters showing an early diagnosis of primary implant suspected infection. The following indexes are used: CRP, ESR, and PCT. CRP and PCT show a statistically significant peak during the first week after primary hip arthroplasty and then return to similar preintervention values in the first 14 days [3]. CRP has no sensitivity of 100%, so some cases of infection may go unrecognized because of low-grade infections or due to encapsulated bacteria associated with a less intense systemic response with a more modest rise of inflammatory markers. The PCT also increases the sensitivity of CRP and permits avoiding false positive results, as it is a more specific marker for bacterial infections [5], although the trauma and surgery show a transient increase. The assessment of the time of the laboratory indexes permits pointing out, in cases of infection, that the average CRP, ESR, and PCT values show a statistically significant peak compared to the average of uninfected patients' values at the same time. The early postoperative infections resulted in an increase of CRP, ESR, and PCT greater than that associated with trauma and surgery [13] which occurs in the first 2 weeks after surgery. This is an extremely important fact because it emphasizes the importance of CRP, ESR, and PCT for the diagnosis of early infections by showing suspicious markers which enable the orthopedic surgeon to implement the best diagnostic-therapeutic protocol.

In a study conducted at Isfahan's educational treatment centers from 2009 to 2011, 80 patients, candidates for THA and TKA, were examined. 35 patients were candidates for TKA and 45 others for THA. ESR and CRP were analyzed on the day before surgery, the day of operation, and after 1, 2, 5, and 15 days and 1, 3, 6, and 12 months after total joint replacement. The mean ESR had an upward trend during the first 5 days and then decreased gradually, lasting up to 3 months. After 1 year it increased to a level higher than that before operation but its value was not statistically significant. The same happened for CRP. Patients with high ESR and CRP that do not follow the normalization process have to be studied to evaluate the presence of prosthetic infection [14].

In a study done in an academic center in Spain on patients who had undergone THA and TKA operations, the level of CRP was measured before operation and 1, 2, 3, 15, 42, and 150 days after operation, in which the maximum level was related to 2 days after surgery. CRP returned to preoperative level in 150 days. Patients who showed an increase of CRP after 3 days with a persisting level after the 42nd day were worthy of study to evaluate the presence of prosthetic infection [15].

The use of these markers in the screening of THA infections is associated with a percentage of false positive and false negative results. False positives are linked to the increasing of these markers both in inflammatory and in infection processes. Instead, false negatives depend on the fact that in same patients they rise only in a clinical infection. False positive and false negative results depend on the sensibility and specificity of ESR, CRP, and PCT. ESR has a sensitivity of 0.93 and a specificity of 0.86; CRP has a sensitivity of 0.91 and a specificity of 0.86 [16].

In our retrospective cohort study, discrepancies between C-reactive protein and erythrocyte sedimentation rate have been reported in 12.5% of patients. Patients with raised C-reactive protein and a normal erythrocyte sedimentation rate usually have infection but some have other tissue damage (e.g., myocardial infarction or venous thromboembolism). These discrepancies may be due to timing, with the rise in C-reactive protein manifesting itself before the sedimentation rate elevates, or simply because the sedimentation rate does not change with minor inflammation. Patients with a high erythrocyte sedimentation rate and normal C-reactive protein mostly have conditions without demonstrable systemic inflammation such as malignancy [17].

However, there are two circumstances when the sedimentation rate can be a better marker of an inflammatory process: some low-grade bone and joint infections (e.g., in joint prosthesis infections due to low-level pathogens such as coagulase-negative staphylococci); autoimmune disease, in particular some people with systemic lupus erythematosus [6].

Seriate controls of such markers in the first 4 weeks after surgery fairly indicate a primary implant suspected infection as the study of the temporal trend may help in discriminating between infection and postoperative inflammatory phase [14]. In addition, the use of these markers makes it possible to avoid the indiscriminate use of imaging tests such XR controls, scintigraphy [15], and PET/CT and resort to them only when there is reasonable suspect of infection [7].

Intra-articular aspiration can give false positive results. In fact, Meermans and Haddad performed a prospective study of 120 patients who underwent aspiration and biopsy for suspected joint infection (64 with THAs and 56 with TKAs). The sensitivity reported was 83% for aspiration, 79% for biopsy, and 90% for the combination of both techniques [18].

In a prospective study conducted at the ENDO Klinik, Bonanzinga et al. enrolled 156 patients with chronically (>90 days) painful total joint arthroplasties (65 TKAs, 91 THAs). Diagnosis of PJI was made according to the PJI Consensus Group criteria. Patients diagnosed as having PJI underwent a single-stage direct exchange following the ENDO Klinik protocol if the microorganisms were known in advance or two-stage surgery if the bacteriology was not known after preoperative diagnostics. Intraoperative aspiration was performed after surgical incision, preparation of soft tissues, and exposure of capsule without opening the joint and sending to laboratory for the alpha-defensin immunoassay test. In 29 patients with PJI confirmed intraoperatively, alpha-defensin assay was positive in 28 patients and negative in 1 patient. On the other hand, in 127 confirmed aseptic painful total joint arthroplasties alpha-defensin test was positive in four cases (2 with metallosis, 1 with severe polyethylene wear with osteolysis, and 1 with unknown origin). Statistical analysis reveals that alpha-defensin immune assay sensibility was 97%, specificity was 97%, positive predictive value was 88%, and the negative predictive value was 99% [19].

In a retrospective study including data from 106 hip and knee arthroplasties with PJI diagnosed more than 90 days after primary surgery, alpha-defensin assay showed higher sensitivity in diagnosing PJI among patients given antibiotics when compared with ESR, CRP, fluid PMN%, and fluid culture [20].

Unlike the cases of late chronic and hematogenous infections that occur from the first month after surgery in which the use of laboratory indexes, object of study, is definitely of help in confirming the suspected diagnosis, in these cases, given the striking clinical manifestations, it would be more beneficial to use imaging tests such as X-rays, scans, and eventually PET/CT showing signs of implant infection rather than resorting to seriated CRP, ESR, and PCT [7, 16, 17] controls. The analysis of such markers therefore has a favorable impact on cost management for patients with early infections, rather than using imaging methods such X-rays, scans, and PET/CT. For patients with late chronic and hematogenous infections undergoing a long follow-up through regular CRP, ESR, and PCT evaluations and for those undergoing primary hip arthroplasty, the diagnostic suspect may be helpful but it represents an unnecessary expense if compared to the costs of diagnostic imaging methods [7, 21]. Synovial fluid biomarkers, such as alpha-defensin, represent a breakthrough in the scenario of late chronic and hematogenous PJI and may represent in the next future a valid tool in the diagnosis of PJI.

In our experience, only in the cases of late chronic infections we had X-ray findings of septic loosening. In the other cases, X-rays were normal.

In conclusion, according to our experience, we suggest the use of seriated CRP, ESR, and PCT controls for patients undergoing total hip arthroplasty in the first 4 weeks after surgery; their evaluation during this period allows discriminating between early postoperative infection and reactive inflammatory phenomena and implementing, after an initial assessment of these indexes, appropriate investigations with diagnostic imaging if there is a suspect of late chronic and hematogenous infection.

Ethical Approval

For this type of study no statement related to studies on humans and animals is required. All procedures involving human participants were in accordance with the 1964 Helsinki declaration and its later amendments.

References

[1] A. F. Widmer, "New developments in diagnosis and treatment of infection in orthopedic implants," *Clinical Infectious Diseases*, vol. 33, Suppl 2, no. 5, pp. S94–S106, 2001.

[2] S. Leone, S. Borrè, A. D. Monforte et al., "Consensus document on controversial issues in the diagnosis and treatment of prosthetic joint infections," *International Journal of Infectious Diseases*, vol. 14, no. 4, pp. S67–S77, 2010.

[3] S. Battistelli, M. Fortina, S. Carta, R. Guerranti, F. Nobile, and P. Ferrata, "Serum C-reactive protein and procalcitonin kinetics in patients undergoing elective total hip arthroplasty," *BioMed Research International*, vol. 2014, Article ID 565080, 2014.

[4] T. M. Myckatyn, J. Cohen, and R. A. Chole, "Clarification of the definition of a "Biofilm"," *Plastic and Reconstructive Surgery*, vol. 137, no. 1, pp. 237-238, 2016.

[5] W. Cats-Baril, T. Gehrke, K. Huff, D. Kendoff, M. Maltenfort, and J. Parvizi, "International consensus on periprosthetic joint infection: Description of the consensus process," *Clinical Orthopaedics and Related Research*, vol. 471, no. 12, pp. 4065–4075, 2013.

[6] M. Harrison, "Erythrocite sedimentation rate and C-reactive protein," *Australian Prescriber*, vol. 38, no. 3, pp. 93-94, 2015.

[7] A. J. Tande and R. Patel, "Prosthetic joint infection," *Clinical Microbiology Reviews*, vol. 27, no. 2, pp. 302–345, 2014.

[8] L. Fisichella, D. Fenga, and M. A. T. Rosa, "Surgical Site Infection In Orthopaedic Surgery: Correlation Between Age, Diabetes, Smoke And Surgical Risk," *Folia medica*, vol. 56, no. 4, pp. 259–263, 2014.

[9] P. F. M. Choong, M. M. Dowsey, D. Carr, J. Daffy, and P. Stanley, "Risk factors associated with acute hip prosthetic joint infections and outcome of treatment with a rifampinbased regimen," *Acta Orthopaedica*, vol. 78, no. 6, pp. 755–765, 2007.

[10] B. H. Kapadia, R. A. Berg, J. A. Daley, J. Fritz, A. Bhave, and M. A. Mont, "Periprosthetic joint infection," *The Lancet*, vol. 387, no. 10016, pp. 386–394, 2016.

[11] S. Marmor and Y. Kerroumi, "Patient-specific risk factors for infection in arthroplasty procedure," *Orthopaedics & Traumatology: Surgery & Research*, vol. 102, 1, no. 1, pp. S113–S119, 2016.

[12] M. D. Wimmer, T. M. Randau, M. J. Friedrich et al., "Outcome predictors in prosthetic joint infections - Validation of a risk stratification score for prosthetic joint infections in 120 cases," *Acta Orthopaedica Belgica*, vol. 82, no. 1, pp. 143–148, 2016.

[13] M. K. Wasko, K. Bobecka-Wesołowska, R. Tomasiuk, and J. Kowalczewski, "Measurement of the inflammatory response in the early postoperative period after hip and knee arthroplasty," *Clinical Chemistry and Laboratory Medicine*, vol. 53, no. 11, pp. 1785–1792, 2015.

[14] M. Rothenburger, A. Markewitz, T. Lenz et al., "Detection of acute phase response and infection. The role of procalcitonin and C-Reactive protein," *Clinical Chemistry and Laboratory Medicine*, vol. 37, no. 3, pp. 275–279, 1999.

[15] Z. Ouyang, H. Li, X. Liu, Z. Zhai, and X. Li, "Prosthesis infection: diagnosis after total joint arthroplasty with three-phase bone scintigraphy," *Annals of Nuclear Medicine*, vol. 28, no. 10, pp. 994–1003, 2014.

[16] L. Brammen, C. Palestro, and H. Sinzinger, "Radionuclide imaging: Past, present and future outlook in the diagnosis of infected prosthetic joints," *Hellenic Journal of Nuclear Medicine*, vol. 18, pp. 95–102, 2015.

[17] A. d. Arco and M. L. Bertrand, "The diagnosis of periprosthetic infection," *The Open Orthopaedics Journal*, vol. 7, no. 1, pp. 178–183, 2013.

[18] G. Meermans and F. S. Haddad, "Is there a role for tissue biopsy in the diagnosis of periprosthetic infection?" *Clinical Orthopaedics and Related Research®*, vol. 468, no. 5, pp. 1410–1417, 2010.

[19] T. Bonanzinga, A. Zahar, M. Dütsch, C. Lausmann, D. Kendoff, and T. Gehrke, "How Reliable Is the Alpha-defensin Immunoassay Test for Diagnosing Periprosthetic Joint Infection? A Prospective Study," *Clinical Orthopaedics and Related Research*, vol. 475, no. 2, pp. 408–415, 2017.

[20] A. Shahi, J. Parvizi, G. S. Kazarian et al., "The Alpha-defensin Test for Periprosthetic Joint Infections Is Not Affected by Prior Antibiotic Administration," *Clinical Orthopaedics and Related Research*, vol. 474, no. 7, pp. 1610–1615, 2016.

[21] B. H. Kapadia, S. Banerjee, J. J. Cherian, K. J. Bozic, and M. A. Mont, "The Economic Impact of Periprosthetic Infections After Total Hip Arthroplasty at a Specialized Tertiary-Care Center," *Journal of Arthroplasty*, vol. 31, no. 7, pp. 1422–1426, 2016.

Permissions

All chapters in this book were first published in AO, by Hindawi Publishing Corporation; hereby published with permission under the Creative Commons Attribution License or equivalent. Every chapter published in this book has been scrutinized by our experts. Their significance has been extensively debated. The topics covered herein carry significant findings which will fuel the growth of the discipline. They may even be implemented as practical applications or may be referred to as a beginning point for another development.

The contributors of this book come from diverse backgrounds, making this book a truly international effort. This book will bring forth new frontiers with its revolutionizing research information and detailed analysis of the nascent developments around the world.

We would like to thank all the contributing authors for lending their expertise to make the book truly unique. They have played a crucial role in the development of this book. Without their invaluable contributions this book wouldn't have been possible. They have made vital efforts to compile up to date information on the varied aspects of this subject to make this book a valuable addition to the collection of many professionals and students.

This book was conceptualized with the vision of imparting up-to-date information and advanced data in this field. To ensure the same, a matchless editorial board was set up. Every individual on the board went through rigorous rounds of assessment to prove their worth. After which they invested a large part of their time researching and compiling the most relevant data for our readers.

The editorial board has been involved in producing this book since its inception. They have spent rigorous hours researching and exploring the diverse topics which have resulted in the successful publishing of this book. They have passed on their knowledge of decades through this book. To expedite this challenging task, the publisher supported the team at every step. A small team of assistant editors was also appointed to further simplify the editing procedure and attain best results for the readers.

Apart from the editorial board, the designing team has also invested a significant amount of their time in understanding the subject and creating the most relevant covers. They scrutinized every image to scout for the most suitable representation of the subject and create an appropriate cover for the book.

The publishing team has been an ardent support to the editorial, designing and production team. Their endless efforts to recruit the best for this project, has resulted in the accomplishment of this book. They are a veteran in the field of academics and their pool of knowledge is as vast as their experience in printing. Their expertise and guidance has proved useful at every step. Their uncompromising quality standards have made this book an exceptional effort. Their encouragement from time to time has been an inspiration for everyone.

The publisher and the editorial board hope that this book will prove to be a valuable piece of knowledge for researchers, students, practitioners and scholars across the globe.

List of Contributors

Takanori Miura, Toshihito Ebina, Takayuki Tani and Shuichi Chida
Department of Orthopedic Surgery, Kakunodate General Hospital, 3-Iwase Kakunodatemachi, Semboku, Akita 014-0394, Japan

Hiroaki Kijima, Naohisa Miyakoshi and Yoichi Shimada
Department of Orthopedic Surgery, Akita University Graduate School of Medicine, 1-1-1 Hondo, Akita 010-8543, Japan

Noriyuki Ishikawa, Tetsuya Suzuki, Satoshi Yumto and Hiroshi Tazawa
Department of Orthopedic Surgery, Akita Red Cross Hospital, Kamikitate Saruta, Aza-Naeshirosawa 222-1, Akita 010-1406, Japan

Michael Schlegelmilch
Faculty of Medicine and Dentistry, University of Alberta, Edmonton, AB, Canada

Michael Schlegelmilch, Saifee Rashiq and Barbara Moreau
Canadian Association of Medical Teams Abroad, Edmonton, AB, Canada

Saifee Rashiq and Anderson Chuck
Department of Anesthesiology and Pain Medicine, University of Alberta, Edmonton, AB, Canada

Patricia Jarrín
Fundación Tierra Nueva, Quito, Ecuador

Bach Tran and Anderson Chuck
Institute of Health Economics, Edmonton, AB, Canada

Ramazan Erden Erturer, Bahadir Gokcen, Sinan Erdogan, Kursat Kara and Cagatay Ozturk
Department of Orthopedics, Istinye University, Istanbul, Turkey

Bekir Eray Kilinc
Orthopedics Clinic, Golhisar State Hospital, Burdur, Turkey

Nobuhiro Tanaka, Kazuyoshi Nakanishi, Naosuke Kamei, Toshio Nakamae, Shinji Kotaka and Nobuo Adachi
Department of Orthopaedic Surgery, Institute of Biomedical and Health Sciences, Hiroshima University, Hiroshima, Japan

Kivanc Atesok
Department of Orthopaedic Surgery, University of Alabama at Birmingham, Birmingham, AL, USA

Jeffrey M. Pearson, Thomas E. Niemeier and Sakthivel Rajaram Manoharan
Department of Orthopedic Surgery, University of Alabama at Birmingham, Birmingham, AL, USA

Gerald McGwin
Department of Epidemiology, University of Alabama at Birmingham, Birmingham, AL, USA

Juan M. Giugale, Mitchell S. Fourman and John R. Fowler
Department of Orthopaedic Surgery, University of Pittsburgh Medical Center, Pittsburgh, PA, USA

Deidre L. Bielicka
Department of Orthopaedic Surgery, Rutgers-RobertWood Johnson Medical Center, New Brunswick, NJ, USA

Eric Robinson, Dani Gaillard-Campbell and Thomas P. Gross
Midlands Orthopaedics and Neurosurgery, 1910 Blanding Street, Columbia, SC 29201, USA

Thomas S. Moores, Benjamin D. Chatterton, Matthew J. Walker and Phillip J. Roberts
Department of Trauma and Orthopaedics, Royal Stoke University Hospital, Stoke-on-Trent, Staffordshire, UK

Timothy A. Damron and Kenneth A. Mann
SUNY Upstate Medical University, Syracuse, New York, USA

Freyja Hálfdanardóttir and Kristín Briem
Faculty of Medicine, School of Health Sciences, University of Iceland, Saemundargata 2, 101 Reykjavík, Iceland

Dan K. Ramsey
Department of Health Professions Education, D'Youville College, 220 Koessler Administration Building (KAB), 320 Porter Ave, Buffalo, NY 14201, USA

Christopher Jackson, Mina Tanios and Nabil Ebraheim
Department of Orthopedic Surgery, University of ToledoMedical Center, Toledo, OH 43614-5807, USA

Riccardo Luigi Alberio, Matteo Del Re and Federico Alberto Grassi
Department of Orthopedics and Traumatology, University of East Piedmont, Hospital "Maggiore della Carità", Via Mazzini 18, Novara, Italy

Brian T. Grisez, Andrew E. Hanselman, Karim W. Boukhemis, Trapper A. J. Lalli and Brock A. Lindsey
Department of Orthopaedics, West Virginia University, Morgantown, WV 26506-9196, USA

Panagiotis Korovessis, Vasileios Syrimpeis, Vasileios Tsekouras and Konstantinos Vardakastanis
Orthopaedics Department, General Hospital of Patras, Tsertidou Str 1, 26224, Greece

Peter Fennema
AMR AdvancedMedical Research GmbH, Hofenstrasse 89b, CH-8708 Männedorf, Switzerland

P. Koenen, M. M. Schneider, T. R. Pfeiffer, B. Bouillon and H. Bäthis
Department of Orthopaedics, Trauma Surgery and Sports Medicine, Cologne-Merheim Medical Center, University ofWitten/Herdecke, Cologne, Germany

Frank W. M. Faber and Paulien M. van Kampen
Department of Orthopaedic Surgery, Bergman Clinics, Rijswijk, Netherlands

Monique J. L. Mastboom and Sabine T. van Vliet-Koppert
Department of Orthopaedic Surgery, LUMC, Leiden, Netherlands

Ilse C. E. Bouman
Department of Orthopaedic Surgery, HAGA Hospital, The Hague, Netherlands

J.M.Wilson, C. A. Staley, A. R. Boissonneault, A.M. Schwartz and M. L. Schenker
Department of Orthopaedic Surgery, Emory University School of Medicine, Atlanta, Georgia, USA

A. L. Boden
Emory University School of Medicine, Atlanta, Georgia, USA

Eric W. Edmonds, Joanna H. Roocroft, John Munch and Tracey P. Bastrom
Rady Children's Hospital, San Diego, CA, USA

Eric W. Edmonds
University of California, San Diego, CA, USA

John W. Kemppainen
Helen DeVos Children's Hospital, Grand Rapids, MI, USA

Anna-Lena Robinson
Stockholm Spine Center, Upplands Väsby, Sweden

Anna-Lena Robinson, Claes Olerud and Yohan Robinson
Department of Surgical Sciences, Uppsala University Hospital, Uppsala, Sweden

Hiroaki Kijima, Naohisa Miyakoshi, Yuji Kasukawa, Yoshinori Ishikawa, Hayato Kinoshita, Masazumi Suzuki, Nozomi Kaga, Shuichi Chida and Yoichi Shimada
Department of Orthopedic Surgery, Akita University Graduate School of Medicine, 1-1-1 Hondo, Akita 010-8543, Japan

Hiroaki Kijima, Kentaro Ohuchi, Chie Sato and Yoichi Shimada
Akita Sports, Arthroscopy, and Knee Group (ASAKG), 1-1-1 Hondo, Akita 010-8543, Japan

Vincenzo De Luna, Federico Mancini, Fernando De Maio, Gabriele Bernardi, Ernesto Ippolito and Roberto Caterini
Department of Orthopaedic Surgery, University of Rome Tor Vergata, Viale Oxford 81, 00133 Rome, Italy

Hideto Irifune and Suguru Hirayama
Department of Emergency Medicine Advanced Critical Care and Emergency Center, Sapporo Medical University School of Medicine, Sapporo, Japan

Hideto Irifune, Nobuyuki Takahashi, Mitsumasa Chiba and Toshihiko Yamashita
Department of Orthopedic Surgery, Sapporo Medical University School of Medicine, Sapporo, Japan

Jennifer J. Beck
Orthopedic Institute for Children/UCLA, Los Angeles, CA, USA

Dai Sugimoto and Lyle Micheli
The Micheli Center for Sports Injury Prevention, Waltham, MA, USA
Boston Children's Hospital Orthopaedics and Sports Medicine, Boston, MA, USA
Department of Orthopaedic Surgery, Harvard Medical School, Boston, MA, USA

Kivanc Atesok, Donald Deinlein, Sakthivel Rajaram Manoharan, Jason Pittman and Steven Theiss
Department of Orthopaedic Surgery, University of Alabama at Birmingham, Birmingham, AL, USA

Nobuhiro Tanaka
Department of Orthopaedic Surgery, Hiroshima University, Hiroshima, Japan

Andrew O'Brien
Royal Victoria Hospital and Royal Belfast Hospital for Sick Children, Belfast, UK

Yohan Robinson
Department of Surgical Sciences, Uppsala University Hospital, Uppsala, Sweden

Dachling Pang
Department of Pediatric Neurosurgery, University of California, Davis, CA, USA
Regional Centre for Paediatric Neurosurgery, Kaiser Permanente Hospitals, Oakland, CA, USA
Great Ormond Street Hospital For Children, NHS Trust, London, UK

Abdellah Ait Moussa, Justin Fischer, Rohan Yadav and Morshed Khandaker
Department of Engineering and Physics, University of Central Oklahoma, Edmond, OK, USA

Britta K. Krautwurst
Heidelberg University Clinics, Department for Orthopedics and Trauma Surgery, Schlierbacher Landstraße 200a, 66118 Heidelberg, Germany

Jürgen R. Paletta and Adrian Skwara
Department of Orthopedics and Rheumatology, University Hospital Marburg, Baldingerstrasse, 35043 Marburg, Germany

Sylvia Mendoza
Studiendekanat, Fachbereich Medizin, Dr. Reinfried Pohl-Zentrum für Medizinische Lehre (RPZ), University Hospital Marburg, Conradistraße 9, 35043 Marburg, Germany

Adrian Skwara
Orthopädische Gemeinschaftspraxis Ammenwerth / Skwara, Schildern 6, 33098 Paderborn, Germany

Melvin Mohokum
SRH Hochschule für Gesundheit, University of Applied Health Science, Neue Str. 28–30, 07548 Gera, Germany

Jackson Rucker Staggers, Thomas Elliot Niemeier, William E. Neway III and Steven Michael Theiss
Division of Orthopaedic Surgery, University of Alabama at Birmingham, Birmingham, Alabama, 35205, USA

Andrew J. Hughes, Cathal DeBuitleir, Philip Soden and Conor J. Hurson
Department of Orthopaedic Surgery, St. Vincent's University Hospital, Dublin 4, Ireland

Brian O'Donnchadha and Anthony Tansey
Department of Mechanical Engineering, Institute of Technology Tallaght, Dublin 24, Ireland

Ali Abdulkarim and Conor J. Hurson
Department of Orthopaedic Surgery, Cappagh National Orthopaedic Hospital, Dublin 11, Ireland

Colm McMahon
Department of Radiology, St. Vincent's University Hospital, Dublin 4, Ireland

Andrew S. Moon, Kivanc Atesok, Thomas E. Niemeier, Sakthivel R. Manoharan, Jason L. Pittman and Steven M. Theiss
UAB Faculty Office Tower #960, 510 20th Street South, Birmingham, AL 35233, USA

Daniel A. Müller
Department of Orthopedic Surgery, Balgrist University Hospital, Forchstrasse 340, 8008 Zürich, Switzerland

Giovanni Beltrami, Guido Scoccianti, Pierluigi Cuomo and Francesca Totti
Department of Orthopedic Oncology, Azienda Ospedaliero-Universitaria Careggi, Largo Brambilla 3, 50134 Firenze, Italy

Rodolfo Capanna
Department of Orthopedic Surgery, Azienda Ospedaliero-Universitaria Pisana, Via Paradisa 2, Cisanello, 56125 Pisa, Italy

Abdulrahman D. Algarni
Department of Orthopedic Surgery, King Saud University, Riyadh, Saudi Arabia

Hassan M. Al Moallem
Department of Surgery, Prince Mohammed Bin Abdulaziz Hospital, Riyadh, Saudi Arabia

Panagiotis Korovessis, Eva Mpountogianni, Vasileios Syrimpeis, Andreas Baikousis and Vasileios Tsekouras
Orthopaedics Department, General Hospital of Patras, Tsertidou Str. 1, 26224 Rio, Greece

Gabriele Falzarano, Antonio Medici and Raffaele Cioffi
Department of Orthopedics and Traumatology, Azienda Ospedaliera "Gaetano Rummo", Benevento, Italy

Antonio Piscopo
Department of Orthopedics and Traumatology, Sacro Cuore di Gesù Fatebenefratelli Hospital, Benevento, Italy

Predrag Grubor
Clinic of Traumatology, University Hospital Clinical Center Banja Luka, Banja Luka, Bosnia and Herzegovina

Giuseppe Rollo
Department of Orthopedics and Traumatology, Vito Fazzi Hospital, Lecce, Italy

Valerio Pipola
Rizzoli Orthopedic Institute, University of Bologna, Bologna, Italy

Michele Bisaccia, Auro Caraffa and Luigi Meccariello
Division of Orthopedics and Trauma Surgery, University of Perugia, S. Maria della Misericordia Hospital, Perugia, Italy

Elizabeth Mary Barron
School of Medicine, Central Michigan University, Mount Pleasant, MI, USA

Francesco Nobile
Department of Orthopedics and Traumatology, Hospital "Santa Maria alla Gruccia", Montevarchi, Arezzo, Italy

Index